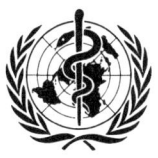

WORLD HEALTH ORGANIZATION

INTERNATIONAL AGENCY FOR RESEARCH ON CANCER

IARC Handbooks of Cancer Prevention

Retinoids

Volume 4

This publication represents the views and expert opinions
of an IARC Working Group on the
Evaluation of Cancer-preventive Agents,
which met in Lyon,

24–30 March 1999

Published by the International Agency for Research on Cancer,
150 cours Albert Thomas, F-69372 Lyon cedex 08, France

Distributed by Oxford University Press, Walton Street, Oxford, OX2 6DP, UK (Fax: +44 1865 267782) and in
the USA by Oxford University Press, 2001 Evans Road, Carey, NC 27513, USA (Fax: +1 919 677 1303).
All IARC publications can also be ordered directly from IARC*Press*
(Fax: +33 4 72 73 83 02; E-mail: press@iarc.fr).

IARC Library Cataloguing in Publication Data

Retinoids/
    IARC Working Group on the Evaluation of
    Cancer Preventive Agents (1999 : Lyon, France)

(IARC handbooks of cancer prevention ; 4)

1. Retinoids – congresses. I. IARC Working Group on the Evaluation of Cancer
    Preventive Agents II Series

ISBN 92 832 3004 3   (NLM Classification: W1)
ISSN 1027-5622

Printed in France

International Agency For Research On Cancer

The International Agency for Research on Cancer (IARC) was established in 1965 by the World Health Assembly, as an independently financed organization within the framework of the World Health Organization. The headquarters of the Agency are in Lyon, France.

The Agency conducts a programme of research concentrating particularly on the epidemiology of cancer and the study of potential carcinogens in the human environment. Its field studies are supplemented by biological and chemical research carried out in the Agency's laboratories in Lyon and, through collaborative research agreements, in national research institutions in many countries. The Agency also conducts a programme for the education and training of personnel for cancer research.

The publications of the Agency contribute to the dissemination of authoritative information on different aspects of cancer research. A complete list is printed at the back of this book. Information about IARC publications, and how to order them, is also available via the Internet at: **http://www.iarc.fr/**

Note to the Reader

Anyone who is aware of published data that may influence any consideration in these *Handbooks* is encouraged to make the information available to the Unit of Chemoprevention, International Agency for Research on Cancer, 150 Cours Albert Thomas, 69372 Lyon Cedex 08, France

Although all efforts are made to prepare the *Handbooks* as accurately as possible, mistakes may occur. Readers are requested to communicate any errors to the Unit of Chemoprevention, so that corrections can be reported in future volumes.

Acknowledgements

The Foundation for Promotion of Cancer Research, Japan, is gratefully acknowledged for its generous support to the meeting of the Working Group and the production of this volume of the *IARC Handbooks of Cancer Prevention*.

Contents

List of participants
Volume 4. Retinoids

Lyon, 24–30 March 1999

Members[1]

J.S. Bertram
Cancer Research Center of Hawaii
University of Hawaii
1236 Lauhala Street
Honolulu, HI 96813
USA

W.S. Blaner
Hammer Health Sciences Building
Room 502, Department of Medicine
Columbia University
701 West 168th Street
New York, NY 10032
USA

R.A. Chandraratna
Vice-President, Retinoid Research
Allergan
2525 Dupont Drive
PO Box 19534
Irvine, CA 92623–9534
USA

C. Chomienne
Laboratoire de Biologie Cellulaire Hématopoïétique
Hôpital Saint Louis
1 avenue Claude Vellefaux
75010 Paris
France

J.A. Crowell
Chemoprevention Branch
Division of Cancer Prevention and Control
National Institutes of Health
National Cancer Institute
Bethesda, MD 20892
USA

M.I. Dawson
Molecular Medicine Research Institute
325 East Middlefield Road
Mountain View, CA 94043
USA

F. Formelli
Istituto Nazionale per lo Studio e la Cura dei Tumori
Via Venezian 1
20133 Milan
Italy

E.R. Greenberg *(Vice-Chairman)*
Norris Cotton Cancer Center
Dartmouth-Hitchcock Medical Center
One Medical Center Drive
Lebanon, NH 03756
USA

H. Gronemeyer
Institut de Génétique et de Biologie Moléculaire et
Cellulaire
BP 163
67404 Illkirch Cedex
France

D.L. Hill
Chemoprevention Center
University of Alabama at Birmingham
1675 University Boulevard
Webb Building #310
Birmingham, AL 35294–3361
USA

R.J. Kavlock
Reproductive Toxicology Division
Environmental Protection Agency
Research Triangle Park, NC27711
USA

R. Lotan
Department of Thoracic/Head and Neck Medical
Oncology
University of Texas
M.D. Anderson Cancer Center
1515 Holcombe Boulevard
Houston, TX 77030
USA

---

[1] **Unable to attend:** F.R. Khuri, Associate Professor of Medicine, University of Texas, M.D. Anderson Cancer Center, 1515 Holcombe Boulevard, Box 80, Houston, TX 77030, USA

M. Maden
Division of Biomedical Sciences
King's College
26–29 Drury Lane
London WC2B 5RL
United Kingdom

R.G. Mehta
University of Illinois at Chicago
Department of Surgical Oncology and Pharmacology
840 South Wood Street
Chicago, IL 60912–7322
USA

T.E. Moon
Clinical Research Department
Ligand Pharmaceuticals Inc.
10275 Science Center Drive
San Diego, CA 92121
USA

H. Nau
Department of Food Toxicology
Centre of Food Sciences
School of Veterinary Medicine Hannover
Bischofsholer Damm 15
30173 Hannover
Germany

P. Nettesheim
National Institute of Environmental Health Sciences
Research Triangle Park, NC 27709
USA

J.A. Olson
Iowa State University
Biochemistry, Biophysics and Molecular Biology
  Department
Ames, IA 50011
USA

M.P. Rosin
British Columbia Cancer Agency
Cancer Control Research Program
600 West 10th Avenue
Vancouver, British Columbia
Canada V5Z 1E6

B.W. Stewart *(Chairman)*
Cancer Control Program
South Eastern Sydney Area Health Service
PO Box 88
Randwick, NSW 2031
Australia

C.C. Willhite
State of California
Department of Toxic Substances Control
700 Heinz Street, Suite 200
Berkeley, CA 94710–2737
USA

R.A. Woutersen
Department of General Toxicology
TNO-Nutrition and Food Research Institute
Toxicology Division
PO Box 360
3700 AJ Zeist
The Netherlands

Secretariat
R. Baan
E. Heseltine *(Editor)*
C. Malaveille
A.B. Miller (*Responsible Officer*)
C. Partensky
R. Sankaranarayanan
A.L. Van Kappel-Dufour
J. Wilbourn

Technical assistance
A. Meneghel
D. Mietton
J. Mitchell
E. Perez
S. Reynaud
S. Ruiz
J. Thévenoux

Preamble to the *IARC Handbooks of Cancer Prevention*

The prevention of cancer is one of the key objectives of the International Agency for Research on Cancer (IARC). This may be achieved by avoiding exposures to known cancer-causing agents, by increasing host defences through immunization or chemoprevention or by modifying lifestyle. The aim of the *IARC Monographs* programme is to evaluate carcinogenic risks of human exposure to chemical, physical and biological agents, providing a scientific basis for national or international decisions on avoidance of exposures. The aim of the series of *IARC Handbooks of Cancer Prevention* is to evaluate scientific information on agents and interventions that may reduce the incidence of or mortality from cancer. This preamble is divided into two parts. The first addresses the general scope, objectives and structure of the *Handbooks*. The second describes the procedures for evaluating cancer-preventive agents.

Part One

Scope

Cancer-preventive strategies embrace chemical, immunological, dietary and behavioural interventions that may retard, block or reverse carcinogenic processes or reduce underlying risk factors. The term 'chemoprevention' is used to refer to interventions with pharmaceuticals, vitamins, minerals and other chemicals to reduce cancer incidence. The *IARC Handbooks* address the efficacy, safety and mechanisms of cancer-preventive strategies and the adequacy of the available data, including those on timing, dose, duration and indications for use.

Preventive strategies can be applied across a continuum of: (1) the general population; (2) subgroups with particular predisposing host or environmental risk factors, including genetic susceptibility to cancer; (3) persons with precancerous lesions; and (4) cancer patients at risk for second primary tumours. Use of the same strategies or agents in the treatment of cancer patients to control the growth, metastasis and recurrence of tumours is considered to be patient management, not prevention, although data from clinical trials may be relevant when making a *Handbooks* evaluation.

Objective

The objective of the *Handbooks* programme is the preparation of critical reviews and evaluations of evidence for cancer-prevention and other relevant properties of a wide range of potential cancer-preventive agents and strategies by international working groups of experts. The resulting *Handbooks* may also indicate when additional research is needed.

The *Handbooks* may assist national and international authorities in devising programmes of health promotion and cancer prevention and in making benefit–risk assessments. The evaluations of IARC working groups are scientific judgements about the available evidence for cancer-preventive efficacy and safety. No recommendation is given with regard to national and international regulation or legislation, which are the responsibility of individual governments and/or other international authorities. No recommendations for specific research trials are made.

IARC Working Groups

Reviews and evaluations are formulated by international working groups of experts convened by the IARC. The tasks of each group are: (1) to ascertain that all appropriate data have been collected; (2) to select the data relevant for the evaluation on the basis of scientific merit; (3) to prepare accurate summaries of the data to enable the reader to follow the reasoning of the Working Group; (4) to evaluate the significance of the available data from human studies and experimental models on cancer-preventive activity, carcinogenicity and other beneficial and adverse effects; and (5) to evaluate data relevant to the understanding of mechanisms of action.

Working Group participants who contributed to the considerations and evaluations within a particular *Handbook* are listed, with their addresses, at the beginning of each publication. Each participant serves as an individual scientist and not as a representative of any organization, government or industry. In addition, scientists nominated by national and international agencies, industrial associations and consumer and/or environmental organizations may be invited as observers. IARC staff involved in the preparation of the *Handbooks* are listed.

Working procedures

Approximately 13 months before a working group meets, the topics of the *Handbook* are announced, and participants are selected by IARC staff in consultation with other experts. Subsequently, relevant clinical, experimental and human data are collected by the IARC from all available sources of published information. Representatives of producer or consumer associations may assist in the preparation of sections on production and use, as appropriate.

About eight months before the meeting, the material collected is sent to meeting participants to prepare sections for the first drafts of the *Handbooks*. These are then compiled by IARC staff and sent, before the meeting, to all participants of the Working Group for review. There is an opportunity to return the compiled specialized sections of the draft to the experts, inviting preliminary comments, before the complete first-draft document is distributed to all members of the Working Group.

Data for *Handbooks*

The *Handbooks* do not necessarily cite all of the literature on the agent or strategy being evaluated. Only those data considered by the Working Group to be relevant to making the evaluation are included. In principle, meeting abstracts and other reports that do not provide sufficient detail upon which to base an assessment of their quality are not considered.

With regard to data from toxicological, epidemiological and experimental studies and from clinical trials, only reports that have been published or

accepted for publication in the openly available scientific literature are reviewed by the Working Group. In certain instances, government agency reports that have undergone peer review and are widely available are considered. Exceptions may be made on an ad-hoc basis to include unpublished reports that are in their final form and publicly available, if their inclusion is considered pertinent to making a final evaluation. In the sections on chemical and physical properties, on production, on use, on analysis and on human exposure, unpublished sources of information may be used.

The available studies are summarized by the Working Group, with particular regard to the qualitative aspects discussed below. In general, numerical findings are indicated as they appear in the original report; units are converted when necessary for easier comparison. The Working Goup may conduct additional analyses of the published data and use them in their assesment of the evidence; the results of such supplementary analyses are given in square brackets. When an important aspect of a study, directly impinging on its interpretation, should be brought to the attention of the reader, a comment is given in square brackets.

Criteria for selection of topics for evaluation

Agents, classes of agents and interventions to be evaluated in the *Handbooks* are selected on the basis of one or more of the following criteria.

- The available evidence suggests potential for significantly reducing the incidence of cancers.
- There is a substantial body of human, experimental, clinical and/or mechanistic data suitable for evaluation.
- The agent is in widespread use and of putative protective value, but of uncertain efficacy and safety.
- The agent shows exceptional promise in experimental studies but has not been used in humans.
- The agent is available for further studies of human use.

Outline of data presentation scheme for evaluating cancer-preventive agents

1. **Chemical and physical characteristics**

2. **Occurrence, production, use, analysis and human exposure**

    2.1 Occurrence
    2.2 Production
    2.3 Use
    2.4 Human exposure
    2.5 Analysis

3. **Metabolism, kinetics and genetic variation**

    3.1 Humans
    3.2 Experimental models

4. **Cancer-preventive effects**

    4.1 Humans
        4.1.1 Epidemiological studies
        4.1.2 Intervention trials
        4.1.3 Intermediate end-points
    4.2 Experimental models
        4.2.1 Cancer and preneoplastic lesions
        4.2.2 Intermediate biomarkers
        4.2.3 *In-vitro* models
    4.3 Mechanisms of cancer-prevention

5. **Other beneficial effects**

6. **Carcinogenicity**

    6.1 Humans
    6.2 Experimental models

7. **Other toxic effects**

    7.1 Adverse effects
        7.1.1 Humans
        7.1.2 Experimental models

    7.2 Reproductive and developmental effects
        7.2.1 Humans
        7.2.2 Experimental models
    7.3 Genetic and related effects
        7.3.1 Humans
        7.3.2 Experimental models

8. **Summary of data**

    8.1 Chemistry, occurrence and human exposure
    8.2 Metabolism and kinetics
    8.3 Cancer-preventive effects
        8.3.1 Humans
        8.3.2 Experimental models
        8.3.3 Mechanisms of cancer prevention
    8.4 Other beneficial effects
    8.5 Carcinogenicity
        8.5.1 Humans
        8.5.2 Experimental models
    8.6 Other toxic effects
        8.6.1 Humans
        8.6.2 Experimental models

9. **Recommendations for research**

10. **Evaluation**

    10.1 Cancer-preventive activity
        10.1.1 Humans
        10.1.2 Experimental animals
    10.2 Overall evaluation

11. **References**

Part Two

Evaluation of cancer-preventive agents

A wide range of findings must be taken into account before a particular agent can be recognized as preventing cancer. On the basis of experience from the *IARC Monographs* programme, a systematized approach to data presentation is adopted for *Handbooks* evaluations.

1. Chemical and physical characteristics of the agent

The Chemical Abstracts Services Registry Number, the latest Chemical Abstracts Primary Name, the IUPAC Systematic Name and other definitive information (such as genus and species of plants) are given as appropriate. Information on chemical and physical properties and, in particular, data relevant to identification, occurrence and biological activity are included. A description of technical products of chemicals includes trade names, relevant specifications and available information on composition and impurities. Some of the trade names given may be those of mixtures in which the agent being evaluated is only one of the ingredients.

2. Occurrence, production, use, analysis and human exposure

2.1 Occurrence

Information on the occurrence of an agent or mixture in the environment is obtained from data derived from the monitoring and surveillance of levels in occupational environments, air, water, soil, foods and animal and human tissues. When available, data on the generation, persistence and bioaccumulation of the agent are included. For mixtures, information is given about all agents present.

2.2 Production

The dates of first synthesis and of first commercial production of a chemical or mixture are provided; for agents that do not occur naturally, this information may allow a reasonable estimate to be made of the date before which no human use of, or exposure to, the agent could have occurred. The dates of first reported occurrence of an exposure are also provided. In addition, methods of synthesis used in past and present commercial production and methods of production that may give rise to different impurities are described.

2.3 Use

Data on production, international trade and uses and applications are obtained for representative regions. Some identified uses may not be current or major applications, and the coverage is not necessarily comprehensive. In the case of drugs, mention of their therapeutic applications does not necessarily represent current practice, nor does it imply judgement as to their therapeutic efficacy.

2.4 Analysis

An overview of current methods of analysis or detection is presented. Methods for monitoring human exposure are also given, when available.

2.5 Human exposure

Human uses of, or exposure to, the agent are described. If an agent is used as a prescribed or over-the-counter pharmaceutical product, then the type of person receiving the product in terms of health status, age, sex and medical condition being treated are described. For nonpharmaceutical agents, particularly those taken because of cultural traditions, the characteristics of use or exposure and the relevant populations are described. In all cases, quantitative data, such as dose–response relationships, are considered to be of special importance.

3. Metabolism, kinetics and genetic variation

In evaluating the potential utility of a suspected cancer-preventive agent or strategy, a number of different properties, in addition to direct effects upon cancer incidence, are described and weighed. Furthermore, as many of the data leading to an evaluation are expected to come from studies in experimental animals, information that facilitates interspecies extrapolation is particularly important; this includes metabolic, kinetic and genetic data. Whenever possible, quantitative data, including information on dose, duration and potency, are considered.

Information is given on absorption, distribution (including placental transfer), metabolism and excretion in humans and experimental animals. Kinetic properties within the target species may affect the interpretation and extrapolation of dose–response relationships, such as blood concentrations, protein binding, tissue concentrations, plasma half-lives and elimination rates. Comparative information on the relationship between use or exposure and the dose that reaches the target site may be of particular importance for extrapolation between species. Studies that indicate the metabolic pathways and fate of the agent in humans and experimental animals are summarized, and data on humans and experimental animals are compared when possible. Observations are made on inter-individual variations and relevant metabolic polymorphisms. Data indicating long-term accumulation in human tissues are included. Physiologically based pharmacokinetic models and their parameter values are relevant and are included whenever they are available. Information on the fate of the compound within tissues and cells (transport, role of cellular receptors, compartmentalization, binding to macromolecules) is given.

Genotyping will be used increasingly, not only to identify subpopulations at increased or decreased risk for cancers but also to characterize variation in the biotransformation of, and responses to, cancer-preventive agents.

This subsection can include effects of the compound on gene expression, enzyme induction or inhibition, or pro-oxidant status, when such data are not described elsewhere. It covers data obtained in humans and experimental animals, with particular attention to effects of long-term use and exposure.

4. Cancer-preventive effects

4.1 Human studies

Types of study considered. Human data are derived from experimental and non-experimental study designs and are focused on cancer, precancer or intermediate biological end-points. The experimental designs include randomized controlled trials and short-term experimental studies; non-experimental designs include cohort, case–control and cross-sectional studies.

Cohort and case–control studies relate individual use of, or exposure to, the agents under study to the occurrence of cancer in individuals and provide an estimate of relative risk (ratio of incidence or mortality in those exposed to incidence or mortality in those not exposed) as the main measure of association. Cohort and case–control studies follow an observational approach, in which the use of, or exposure to, the agent is not controlled by the investigator.

Intervention studies are experimental in design — that is, the use of, or exposure to, the agent is assigned by the investigator. The intervention study or clinical trial is the design that can provide the strongest and most direct evidence of a protective or preventive effect; however, for practical and ethical reasons, such studies are limited to observation of the effects among specifically defined study subjects of interventions of 10 years or fewer, which is relatively short when compared with the overall lifespan.

Intervention studies may be undertaken in individuals or communities and may or may not involve randomization to use or exposure. The differences between these designs is important in relation to analytical methods and interpretation of findings.

In addition, information can be obtained from reports of correlation (ecological) studies and case series; however, limitations inherent in these approaches usually mean that such studies carry limited weight in the evaluation of a preventive effect.

Quality of studies considered. The *Handbooks* are not intended to summarize all published studies. It is important that the Working Group consider the following aspects: (1) the relevance of the study; (2) the appropriateness of the design and analysis to the question being asked; (3) the adequacy and completeness of the presentation of the data; and (4) the degree to which chance, bias and confounding may have affected the results.

Studies that are judged to be inadequate or irrelevant to the evaluation are generally omitted. They may be mentioned briefly, particularly when the information is considered to be a useful supplement to that in other reports or when it provides the only data available. Their inclusion does not imply acceptance of the adequacy of the study design, nor of the analysis and interpretation of the results, and their limitations are outlined.

cancer-preventive activity; and (4) the number and structural diversity of carcinogens whose activity can be reduced by the agent being evaluated.

An important variable in the evaluation of the cancer-preventive response is the time and the duration of administration of the agent in relation to any carcinogenic treatment, or in transgenic or other experimental models in which no carcinogen is administered. Furthermore, concurrent administration of a cancer-preventive agent may result in a decreased incidence of tumours in a given organ and an increase in another organ of the same animal. Thus, in these experiments it is important that multiple organs be examined.

For all these studies, the nature and extent of impurities or contaminants present in the cancer-preventive agent or agents being evaluated are given when available. For experimental studies of mixtures, consideration is given to the possibility of changes in the physicochemical properties of the test substance during collection, storage, extraction, concentration and delivery. Chemical and toxicological interactions of the components of mixtures may result in nonlinear dose–response relationships.

As certain components of commonly used diets of experimental animals are themselves known to have cancer-preventive activity, particular consideration should be given to the interaction between the diet and the apparent effect of the agent being studied. Likewise, restriction of diet may be important. The appropriateness of the diet given relative to the composition of human diets may be commented on by the Working Group.

Qualitative aspects. An assessment of the experimental prevention of cancer involves several considerations of qualitative importance, including: (1) the experimental conditions under which the test was performed (route and schedule of exposure, species, strain, sex and age of animals studied, duration of the exposure, and duration of the study); (2) the consistency of the results, for example across species and target organ(s); (3) the stage or stages of the neoplastic process, from preneoplastic lesions and benign tumours to

malignant neoplasms, studied and (4) the possible role of modifying factors.

Considerations of importance to the Working Group in the interpretation and evaluation of a particular study include: (1) how clearly the agent was defined and, in the case of mixtures, how adequately the sample composition was reported; (2) the composition of the diet and the stability of the agent in the diet; (3) whether the source, strain and quality of the animals was reported; (4) whether the dose and schedule of treatment with the known carcinogen were appropriate in assays of combined treatment; (5) whether the doses of the cancer-preventive agent were adequately monitored; (6) whether the agent(s) was absorbed, as shown by blood concentrations; (7) whether the survival of treated animals was similar to that of controls; (8) whether the body and organ weights of treated animals were similar to those of controls; (9) whether there were adequate numbers of animals, of appropriate age, per group; (10) whether animals of each sex were used, if appropriate; (11) whether animals were allocated randomly to groups; (12) whether appropriate respective controls were used; (13) whether the duration of the experiment was adequate; (14) whether there was adequate statistical analysis; and (15) whether the data were adequately reported. If available, recent data on the incidence of specific tumours in historical controls, as well as in concurrent controls, are taken into account in the evaluation of tumour response.

Quantitative aspects. The probability that tumours will occur may depend on the species, sex, strain and age of the animals, the dose of carcinogen (if any), the dose of the agent and the route and duration of exposure. A decreased incidence and/or decreased multiplicity of neoplasms in adequately designed studies provides evidence of a cancer-preventive effect. A dose-related decrease in incidence and/or multiplicity further strengthens this association.

Statistical analysis. Major factors considered in the statistical analysis by the Working Group include the adequacy of the data for each treatment group: (1) the initial and final effective numbers of animals studied and the survival rate; (2) body weights; and (3) tumour incidence and multiplicity. The statistical methods used should be clearly stated and should be the generally accepted techniques refined for this purpose. In particular, the statistical methods should be appropriate for the characteristics of the expected data distribution and should account for interactions in multifactorial studies. Consideration is given as to whether the appropriate adjustment was made for differences in survival.

4.2.2   Intermediate biomarkers

Other types of study include experiments in which the end-point is not cancer but a defined preneoplastic lesion or tumour-related, intermediate biomarker.

The observation of effects on the occurrence of lesions presumed to be preneoplastic or the emergence of benign or malignant tumours may aid in assessing the mode of action of the presumed cancer-preventive agent. Particular attention is given to assessing the reversibility of these lesions and their predictive value in relation to cancer development.

4.2.3   In-vitro models

Cell systems *in vitro* contribute to the early identification of potential cancer-preventive agents and to elucidation of mechanisms of cancer prevention. A number of assays in prokaryotic and eukaryotic systems are used for this purpose. Evaluation of the results of such assays includes consideration of: (1) the nature of the cell type used; (2) whether primary cell cultures or cell lines (tumorigenic or nontumorigenic) were studied; (3) the appropriateness of controls; (4) whether toxic effects were considered in the outcome; (5) whether the data were appropriately summated and analysed; (6) whether appropriate quality controls were used; (7) whether appropriate concentration ranges were used; (8) whether adequate

numbers of independent measurements were made per group; and (9) the relevance of the end-points, including inhibition of mutagenesis, morphological transformation, anchorage-independent growth, cell–cell communication, calcium tolerance and differentiation.

4.3   Mechanisms of cancer prevention

Data on mechanisms can be derived from both human studies and experimental models. For a rational implementation of cancer-preventive measures, it is essential not only to assess protective end-points but also to understand the mechanisms by which the agents exert their anticarcinogenic action. Information on the mechanisms of cancer-preventive activity can be inferred from relationships between chemical structure and biological activity, from analysis of interactions between agents and specific molecular targets, from studies of specific end-points *in vitro*, from studies of the inhibition of tumorigenesis *in vivo*, from the effects of modulating intermediate biomarkers, and from human studies. Therefore, the Working Group takes account of data on mechanisms in making the final evaluation of cancer prevention.

Several classifications of mechanisms have been proposed, as have several systems for evaluating them. Cancer-preventive agents may act at several distinct levels. Their action may be: (1) extracellular, for example, inhibiting the uptake or endogenous formation of carcinogens, or forming complexes with, diluting and/or deactivating carcinogens; (2) intracellular, for example, trapping carcinogens in non-target cells, modifying transmembrane transport, modulating metabolism, blocking reactive molecules, inhibiting cell replication or modulating gene expression or DNA metabolism; or (3) at the level of the cell, tissue or organism, for example, affecting cell differentiation, intercellular communication, proteases, signal transduction, growth factors, cell adhesion molecules, angiogenesis, interactions with the extracellular matrix, hormonal status and the immune system.

Many cancer-preventive agents are known or suspected to act by several mechanisms, which may operate in a coordinated manner and allow them a broader spectrum of anticarcinogenic activity. Therefore, multiple mechanisms of action are taken into account in the evaluation of cancer-prevention.

Beneficial interactions, generally resulting from exposure to inhibitors that work through complementary mechanisms, are exploited in combined cancer-prevention. Because organisms are naturally exposed not only to mixtures of carcinogenic agents but also to mixtures of protective agents, it is also important to understand the mechanisms of interactions between inhibitors.

5.   Other beneficial effects

This section contains mainly background information on preventive activity; use is described in Section 2.3. An expanded description is given, when appropriate, of the efficacy of the agent in the maintenance of a normal healthy state and the treatment of particular diseases. Information on the mechanisms involved in these activities is described. Reviews, rather than individual studies, may be cited as references.

The physiological functions of agents such as vitamins and micronutrients can be described briefly, with reference to reviews. Data on the therapeutic effects of drugs approved for clinical use are summarized.

6.   Carcinogenicity

Some agents may have both carcinogenic and anticarcinogenic activities. If the agent has been evaluated within the *IARC Monographs on the Evaluation of Carcinogenic Risks to Humans*, that evaluation is accepted, unless significant new data have appeared that may lead the Working Group to reconsider the evidence. When a re-evaluation is necessary or when no carcinogenic evaluation has been made, the procedures described in the Preamble to the *IARC Monographs on the Evaluation of Carcinogenic Risks to Humans* are adopted as guidelines.

7.   Other toxic effects

Toxic effects are of particular importance in the case of agents that may be used widely over long periods in healthy populations. Data are given on acute and chronic toxic effects, such as organ toxicity, increased cell proliferation, immunotoxicity and adverse endocrine effects. If the agent occurs naturally or has been in clinical use previously, the doses and durations used in cancer-prevention trials are compared with intakes from the diet, in the case of vitamins, and previous clinical exposure, in the case of drugs already approved for human use. When extensive data are available, only summaries are presented; if adequate reviews are available, reference may be made to these. If there are no relevant reviews, the evaluation is made on the basis of the same criteria as are applied to epidemiological studies of cancer. Differences in response as a consequence of species, sex, age and genetic variability are presented when the information is available.

Data demonstrating the presence or absence of adverse effects in humans are included; equally, lack of data on specific adverse effects is stated clearly.

Findings in human and experimental studies are presented sequentially under the headings 'Adverse effects', 'Reproductive and developmental effects' and 'Genetic and related effects'.

The section 'Adverse effects' includes information on immunotoxicity, neurotoxicity, cardiotoxicity, haematological effects and toxicity to other target organs. Specific case reports in humans and any previous clinical data are noted. Other biochemical effects thought to be relevant to adverse effects are mentioned.

The section on 'Reproductive and developmental effects' includes effects on fertility, teratogenicity, foetotoxicity and embryotoxicity. Information from nonmammalian systems and *in vitro* are presented only if they have clear mechanistic significance.

The section 'Genetic and related effects' includes results from studies in mammalian and nonmammalian systems *in vivo* and *in vitro*. Information on whether DNA damage occurs via direct interaction with the agent or via indirect mechanisms (e.g. generation of free radicals) is included, as is information on other genetic effects such as mutation, recombination, chromosomal damage, aneuploidy, cell immortalization and transformation, and effects on cell–cell communication. The presence and toxicological significance of cellular receptors for the cancer-preventive agent are described.

The adequacy of epidemiological studies of toxic effects, including reproductive outcomes and genetic and related effects in humans, is evaluated by the same criteria as are applied to epidemiological studies of cancer. For each of these studies, the adequacy of the reporting of sample characterization is considered and, where necessary, commented upon. The available data are interpreted critically according to the end-points used. The doses and concentrations used are given, and, for experiments *in vitro*, mention is made of whether the presence of an exogenous metabolic system affected the observations. For studies *in vivo*, the route of administration and the formulation in which the agent was administered are included. The dosing regimens, including the duration of treatment, are also given. Genetic data are given as listings of test systems, data and references; bar graphs (activity profiles) and corresponding summary tables with detailed information on the preparation of genetic activity profiles are given in appendices. Genetic and other activity in humans and experimental mammals is regarded as being of greater relevance than that in other organisms. The *in-vitro* experiments providing these data must be carefully evaluated, since there are many trivial reasons why a response to one agent may be modified by the addition of another.

Structure–activity relationships that may be relevant to the evaluation of the toxicity of an agent are described.

Studies on the interaction of the suspected cancer-preventive agent with toxic and subtoxic doses of other substances are described, the objective being to determine whether there is inhibition or enhancement, additivity, synergism or potentiation of toxic effects over an extended dose range.

Biochemical investigations that may have a bearing on the mechanisms of toxicity and cancer-prevention are described. These are carefully evaluated for their relevance and the appropriateness of the results.

8. Summary of data

In this section, the relevant human and experimental data are summarized. Inadequate studies are generally not summarized; such studies, if cited, are identified in the preceding text.

8.1 Chemistry, occurrence and human exposure

Human exposure to an agent is summarized on the basis of elements that may include production, use, occurrence in the environment and determinations in human tissues and body fluids. Quantitative data are summarized when available.

8.2 Metabolism and kinetic properties

Data on metabolism and kinetic properties in humans and in experimental animals are given when these are considered relevant to the possible mechanisms of cancer-preventive, carcinogenic and toxic activity.

8.3 Cancer-preventive effects

8.3.1 Human studies

The results of relevant studies are summarized, including case reports and correlation studies when considered important.

8.3.2 Experimental models

Data relevant to an evaluation of cancer-preventive activity in experimental models are summarized. For each animal species and route of administration, it is stated whether a change in the incidence of neoplasms or preneoplastic lesions was observed, and the tumour sites are indicated. Negative findings are also summarized. Dose– response relationships and other quantitative data may be given when available.

8.3.3 *Mechanism of cancer-prevention*

Data relevant to the mechanisms of cancer-preventive activity are summarized.

8.4 Other beneficial effects

When beneficial effects other than cancer prevention have been identified, the relevant data are summarized.

8.5 Carcinogenic effects

The agent will has reviewed and evaluated within the *IARC Monographs* programme, that summary is used with the inclusion of more recent data, if appropriate.

8.5.1 *Human studies*

The results of epidemiological studies that are considered to be pertinent to an assessment of human carcinogenicity are summarized.

8.5.2 *Experimental models*

Data relevant to an evaluation of carcinogenic effects in animal models are summarized. For each animal species and route of administration, it is stated whether a change in the incidence of neoplasms or preneoplastic lesions was observed, and the tumour sites are indicated. Negative findings are also summarized. Dose–response relationships and other quantitative data may be mentioned when available.

8.6 Other toxic effects

Adverse effects in humans are summarized, together with data on general toxicological effects and cytotoxicity, receptor binding and hormonal and immunological effects. The results of investigations on the reproductive, genetic and related effects are summarized. Toxic effects are summarized for whole animals, cultured mammalian cells and non-mammalian systems. When available, data for humans and for animals are compared.

Structure–activity relationships are mentioned when relevant to toxicity.

9. Recommendations for research

During the evaluation process, it is likely that opportunities for further research will be identified. These are clearly stated, with the understanding that the areas are recommended for future investigation. It is made clear that these research opportunities are identified in general terms on the basis of the data currently available.

10. Evaluation

Evaluations of the strength of the evidence for cancer-preventive activity and carcinogenic effects from studies in humans and experimental models are made, using standard terms. These terms may also be applied to other beneficial and adverse effects, when indicated. When appropriate, reference is made to specific organs and populations.

It is recognized that the criteria for these evaluation categories, described below, cannot encompass all factors that may be relevant to an evaluation of cancer-preventive activity. In considering all the relevant scientific data, the Working Group may assign the agent or other intervention to a higher or lower category than a strict interpretation of these criteria would indicate.

10.1 Cancer-preventive activity

The evaluation categories refer to the strength of the evidence that an agent prevents cancer. The evaluations may change as new information becomes available.

Evaluations are inevitably limited to the cancer sites, conditions and levels of exposure and length of observation covered by the available studies. An evaluation of degree of evidence, whether for a single agent or a mixture, is limited to the materials tested, as defined physically, chemically or biologically. When the agents evaluated are considered by the Working Group to be sufficiently closely related, they may be grouped for the purpose of a single evaluation of degree of evidence.

Information on mechanisms of action is taken into account when evaluating the strength of evidence in humans and in experimental animals, as well as in assessing the consistency of results between studies in humans and experimental models.

10.1.1 Cancer-preventive activity in humans

The evidence relevant to cancer prevention in humans is classified into one of the following categories.

- *Sufficient evidence of cancer-preventive activity*
  The Working Group considers that a causal relationship has been established between use of the agent and the prevention of human cancer in studies in which chance, bias and confounding could be ruled out with reasonable confidence.
- *Limited evidence of cancer-preventive activity*
  The data suggest a reduced risk for cancer with use of the agent but are limited for making a definitive evaluation either because chance, bias or confounding could not be ruled out with reasonable confidence or because the data are restricted to intermediary biomarkers of uncertain validity in the putative pathway to cancer.
- *Inadequate evidence of cancer-preventive activity*
  The available studies are of insufficient quality, consistency or statistical power to permit a conclusion regarding a cancer-preventive effect of the agent, or no data on the prevention of cancer in humans are available.
- *Evidence suggesting lack of cancer-preventive activity*
  Several adequate studies of use or exposure are mutually consistent in not showing a preventive effect.

The strength of the evidence for any carcinogenic effect is assessed in parallel.

Both cancer-preventive activity and carcinogenic effects are identified and, when appropriate, tabulated by organ site. The evaluation also cites the population subgroups concerned, specifying age, sex, genetic or environmental predisposing risk factors and the relevance of precancerous lesions.

10.1.2 Cancer-preventive activity in experimental animals

Evidence for cancer prevention in experimental animals is classified into one of the following categories.

- *Sufficient evidence of cancer-preventive activity*
  The Working Group considers that a causal relationship has been established between the agent and a decreased incidence and/or multiplicity of neoplasms.
- *Limited evidence of cancer-preventive activity*
  The data suggest a cancer-preventive effect but are limited for making a definitive evaluation because, for example, the evidence of cancer prevention is restricted to a single experiment, the agent decreases the incidence and/or multiplicity only of benign neoplasms or lesions of uncertain neoplastic potential or there is conflicting evidence.
- *Inadequate evidence of cancer-preventive activity*
  The studies cannot be interpreted as showing either the presence or absence of a preventive effect because of major qualitative or quantitative limitations (unresolved questions regarding the adequacy of the design, conduct or interpretation of the study), or no data on cancer prevention in experimental animals are available.
- *Evidence suggesting lack of cancer-preventive activity*
  Adequate evidence from conclusive studies in several models shows that, within the limits of the tests used, the agent does not prevent cancer.

10.2 Overall evaluation

Finally, the body of evidence is considered as a whole, and summary statements are made that encompass the effects of the agents in humans with regard to cancer-preventive activity, carcinogenic effects and other beneficial and adverse effects, as appropriate.

General Remarks

1. Introduction and definitions

This is the fourth handbook in the series of *Handbooks of Cancer Prevention*. Previous volumes represented the views and expert opinions of working groups that met in 1997 and 1998 which considered non-steroidal anti-inflammatory drugs (IARC, 1997), carotenoids (IARC, 1998a) and vitamin A (IARC, 1998b). The present volume completes the consideration of vitamin A-related compounds — so-called retinoids — some of which, like all-*trans*-retinoic acid, the prototypic family member, exert potential cancer preventive effects.

Although it is not the intention that the *IARC Handbooks of Cancer Prevention* be restricted to chemoprevention, the drugs and micronutrients that have been considered until now are potential chemopreventive agents. All of the retinoids discussed in the present volume are the result of a deliberate attempt to identify or synthesize compounds that prevent cancer and simultaneously reduce toxicity and teratogenicity, thus increasing the therapeutic ratio.

Chemoprevention can be defined as the inhibition or reversal of any stage of carcinogenesis by intervention with chemical agents before an overt malignancy is detectable. Chemoprevention can theoretically act at any of the multiple stages of carcinogenesis, although most of the agents evaluated in this handbook do so at relatively early stages of cancer development.

As the efficacy of a chemopreventive agent that is not in use in the general population cannot be evaluated by conventional, observational, analytical epidemiology studies (case–control and cohort studies), the evidence considered in this volume is derived almost exclusively from randomized clinical trials which have either development of cancer as the end-point or some intermediate biomarker of carcinogenesis, usually precancerous lesions. Thus, almost all of the data considered to date in this series (with the exception of that for sulindac in Volume 1) are derived from experimental situations or from trials involving small groups of individuals. In considering the trials that had cancer as the end-point, the Working Group had to satisfy themselves that the end-point considered was a second primary tumour rather than a recurrence of the original tumour, because agents that are effective in preventing recurrence of a cancer are therapeutic and therefore outside the purview of this series. The distinction between chemoprevention and therapy was sometimes difficult to make, especially for organs that show multiple primary tumours. For example, in this handbook, of the studies that relate to the potential prevention of recurrences of superficial tumours of the urinary bladder, only those in which the patients no longer had any evidence of overt neoplasia at the time of initiation of the trial were retained.

The availability of data from clinical trials was of considerable value to the Working Group, since in such studies bias and confounding have largely been eliminated; however, the conclusions are necessarily restricted to the population studied. Since many of the clinical trials cited here relate to patients known to be at substantial risk of a second primary tumour, at the same or a different site but with similar etiology, extrapolation to other groups, whether at high risk for the relevant cancer or more like members of the general population, would be tenuous at best and potentially in serious error.

Other considerations arise when markers of intermediate steps in the carcinogenesis process are considered, either as a means of selecting patients for study or, more problematically, as an end-point of the investigation. Studies that involve precancerous lesions as an end-point allow more rapid identification of putative chemopreventive agents than studies in which cancer is the end-point, but they cannot be given as much weight since the proportion of lesions that progress to cancer is usually small. It is anticipated that biomarkers that can be used in studies in both animals and humans will be the subject of a more detailed evaluation by a special group convened by IARC in the near future.

1.1 Use of biomarkers in studies of chemoprevention

Many malignancies develop over a period of one to two decades, during which time the multistep process of carcinogenesis evolves, culminating in the appearance of invasive and metastatic cancer. While this 'latent period' of cancer development offers a chance to interrupt the process at various stages by chemical or physical means, it poses a challenge to trials of cancer chemopreventive agents, because the outcome may not be known for many years. Therefore, investigators are searching for intermediate or surrogate biomarkers of cancer, in order to identify individuals at increased (or high) risk of developing cancer and to have an early indication of the effectiveness of intervention strategies.

Biomarkers can be used to detect exposure to carcinogenic influences, to identify individuals susceptible to cancer and as indicators of prognosis or diagnosis. Much of the initial work on the identification and validation of biomarkers that characterize the neoplastic process was carried out in cellular or whole-animal models, and the results may not reflect the usefulness of a marker in humans. Biomarkers that are useful in chemoprevention have measurable biological or chemical properties that are highly correlated to cancer incidence in humans and can therefore serve as indicators of the incidence or progression of cancer.

Several types of biomarkers are being considered:
- gene mutations, activated oncogenes and inactivated tumour suppressor genes;
- markers indicative of exposure of molecular targets, such as DNA adducts;
- biochemical changes, such as high plasma concentrations of insulin-like growth factor in breast cancers; and
- cytological and tissue lesions considered to be precancerous.

Although numerous oncogenes and tumour suppressor genes are being identified that help to define early events in the process of carcinogenesis, subsequent events are critical in the actual occurrence of cancer, and interventions at all stages of carcinogenesis may lead to cancer prevention.

Precancerous lesions (dysplasia and carcinoma *in situ*) have been used as the starting point for intervention in a number of studies of the efficacy of chemical agents in inhibiting progression of lesions to frank malignancy. Because not all such lesions progress to carcinoma, identifying the critical events in progression may permit identification of strategies to reverse the process that would otherwise lead to the occurrence of invasive cancer, even at relatively late stages of carcinogenesis.

An alternative approach is to use precancerous lesions as the end-point of an intervention, i.e. to determine the extent to which the earlier stages of carcinogenesis that eventually result in the development of a precancerous lesion can be terminated. Unfortunately, this approach has two practical drawbacks. The first is that the earliest stages of carcinogenesis may begin early in life, when the subjects who would be studied would not be regarded as being at substantial risk for cancer. The more critical problem is that precancerous lesions almost invariably occur in a much higher proportion of the population than does frank malignancy. Thus, prevention of the development of some of these lesions may not guarantee that those that eventually progress and result in the occurrence of cancer have been ablated.

Recent advances in our understanding of the molecular and tissue lesions that occur during the development of hereditary and sporadic colon cancer indicate that a combination of molecular and morphological end-points could be useful predictive measures of neoplastic development in other organ systems as well.

The genetic markers of precancerous lesions that are currently undergoing phase II trials include cytogenetic manifestations such as chromosomal aberrations and micronuclei, abnormal DNA content, DNA and protein adducts and genetic alteration in oncogenes, as well as markers of abnormal cell proliferation, growth regulation and differentiation. These biomarkers have not yet been validated in relation to subsequent cancer occurrence, and they are not yet being tested as the definitive end-points in phase III trials.

1.2   Data from animal models

Data from studies of chemoprevention in animal models are useful for evaluating the potential role of chemopreventive agents in humans but are not sufficient of themselves. A number of studies designed to evaluate whether retinoids inhibit the development of malignant tumours have been conducted on transplanted tumours, often of human origin, as xenografts in nude mice. Studies with this model were not considered in this handbook because it is considered to be a model of the treatment of established cancer rather than of chemoprevention of cancer.

Collectively, the results of the studies reviewed in this handbook suggest that the chemopreventive effects of retinoids are species- and tissue-dependent because of differences in variables such as tissue distribution, retinoid metabolism and cognate receptor levels and activity.

1.3   Agents considered in this handbook

The retinoids are a class of compounds structurally related to vitamin A. Synthesis of retinoids by chemical modification of the vitamin A molecule was begun in 1968, with the objective of identifying retinoids with a better risk–benefit ratio than vitamin A (Bollag & Holdener, 1992). More than 2500 retinoids have since been synthesized and tested biologically. all-*trans*-Retinoic acid and 13-*cis*-retinoic acid were synthesized and then recognized as occurring naturally. The second generation of retinoids included the aromatic compounds etretinate and acitretin, which had an enhanced therapeutic ratio, and the third generation included the polyaromatic retinoids with or without polar end groups.

The retinoids selected for evaluation in this handbook are those for which there were sufficient data in humans and/or animals to permit evaluation. Thus, a number of retinoids at various stages of development or being considered for use in humans were left out, were some that have been studied but are no longer under consideration for use.

In studies of retinoids, care must be taken over their handling in various media to ensure that what is being measured clearly reflects the compound of interest. When blood is collected for assay of retinoids, it should be heparinized or clotted in the dark, centrifuged to obtain plasma or serum and then protected from light and oxygen. Other anticoagulants such as oxalate, citrate and ethylene diamine tetra-acetic acid should be avoided because they reduce the recovery of retinoid (Nierenberg, 1984). Serum or plasma samples for analysis should be stored at – 20 °C or less. An internal standard is usually used to correct for incomplete extraction. To minimize oxidation of retinoids during their extraction, an antioxidant such as butylated hydroxytoluene is added to all the solvents at a final concentration of approximately 100 mg/ml.

The relationship between the toxicity of an agent and its beneficial effects (the therapeutic index) is critical in chemoprevention because the people subjected to this form of cancer prevention are healthy and the probability that they will not develop cancer is usually substantially greater than the probability that they will develop cancer, except for carriers of the rare dominant cancer susceptibility genes. These considerations are less germane for patients at risk for second primary tumours, as they may be prepared to tolerate side-effects of chemoprevention as an extension of their therapy. Toxicity is also likely to be less of a problem when the agent is used as therapy for a malignancy, such as all-*trans*-retinoic acid in the treatment of acute promyelocytic leukaemia. Section 7 of each handbook therefore addresses the toxicity of these compounds. A disappointing outcome of the review is that the therapeutic index of the retinoids considered in this volume appears to be too strongly balanced to the risk side, suggesting that any role of these agents in chemoprevention should be restricted to people at high risk for cancer, who are willing to suffer the almost inevitable side-effects.

1.4   Nomenclature of the retinoids

The natural retinoids consist of four isoprenoid units joined in a head-to-tail manner (IUPAC–IUB Joint Commission on Biochemical Nomenclature, 1983). The term 'vitamin A' is a generic descriptor of retinoids that qualitatively

Table 1. Abbreviations and standardized expressions

all-*trans*-*N*-Ethylretinamide (NER)

Etretinate, acitretin, *N*-(4-hydroxyphenyl)retinamide, *N*-ethyl retinamide, and LGD1550 are assumed to have the all-*trans* configuration unless denoted otherwise.

all-*trans*-*N*-(4-Hydroxyphenyl)retinamide (4-HPR)

all-*trans*-4-Hydroxyretinoic acid (all-*trans*-4-hydroxy-RA)

all-*trans*-4-Oxoretinoic acid (all-*trans*-4-oxo-RA)

all-*trans*-Retinoic acid (all-*trans*-RA; ATRA)

13-*cis*-Retinoic acid (13-*cis*-RA)

9-*cis*-Retinoic acid (9-*cis*-RA)

9,13-Di-*cis*-retinoic acid

Retinoic acid, if an isomeric designation is not given, is a generic indicator or is assumed to be a mixture of isomers.

all-*trans*-Retinol

have the biological activity of retinol. Retinoic acid contains a carboxyl group in place of the primary alcohol group of retinol.

The initial numbering system of the IUPAC (International Union of Pure and Applied Chemistry) for the 20 carbon atoms in retinol and retinoic acid, in keeping with the systematic convention of organic chemistry, started with 1 at the carboxyl group. This terminology proved to be awkward, however, inasmuch as the IUPAC-approved number of the corresponding carbon atom in the biological precursor of retinol and retinoic acid, all-*trans*-β-carotene, was 15 (IUPAC Commission on the Nomenclature of Biological Chemistry, 1960). A nomenclature in which the trimethylcyclohexane ring of vitamin A was considered as the parent compound (IUPAC–IUB Commission on Biochemical Nomenclature, 1966) suffered from the same drawback. Thus, in more recent recommendations of the IUPAC–IUB (International Union of Biochemistry) Joint Commission on Biochemical Nomenclature, the oxygen-bearing carbon in retinol and retinoic acid was labelled C-15 and the *gem*-dimethyl carbon atom in the β-ionone ring was called C-1 (IUPAC–IUB Joint Commission

on Biochemical Nomenclature, 1983), in keeping with carotenoid numbering. That nomenclature has been retained to the present (e.g. Anon., 1990).

The IUPAC–IUBMB (International Union of Biochemistry and Molecular Biology) Joint Commission on Biochemical Nomenclature (1998) has suggested in its newsletter that aromatic acidic compounds that control epithelial differentiation and prevent metaplasia without having the full range of activities of vitamin A be termed 'retinoate analogues' rather than 'retinoids'. This suggestion is pending. Although a reasonable argument was presented in favour of this change, the term 'retinoids' is used to refer to the compounds considered in this handbook, as there is no single universally accepted definition of retinoids. Usage and abbreviations of retinoids are shown in Table 1.

2. Endogenous metabolism of retinoids

Since retinoic acid is both a naturally occuring retinoid and a pharmacological agent that may be effective in preventing and/or treating cancer, both its endogenous or physiological metabolism and its metabolism after administration as a pharmacological agent must be considered. The endogenous metabolism of all-*trans*-, 13-*cis*- and 9-*cis*-retinoic acid is considered mainly in this section, whereas the metabolism of each isomer that is relevant to its pharmacological use is considered in the individual handbooks.

Most of the information on the synthesis and oxidation of retinoic acid is derived from studies carried out in animal models. The studies in humans consist mainly of metabolic studies of the uptake, plasma turnover and/or metabolism of physiological or pharmacological doses or biochemical studies of the enzymes or processes responsible for the formation or oxidation of retinoic acid in human tissues or cultured cells. Comparisons of the results of metabolic studies in humans and in animal models show marked differences in metabolite profiles, but biochemical investigations of enzymes and enzymatic processes that are important for retinoic acid formation and/or metabolism suggest that they do not differ widely in humans and other higher animals. Thus, although humans and species such as the rat and mouse probably have similar enzymatic pathways for retinoic acid synthesis and oxidation, there are probably important differences in how the pathways are regulated and how balances between them are maintained.

2.1 Studies in humans
2.1.1 Metabolism
It is generally accepted that all-*trans*-retinoic acid facilitates most of the gene-modulating actions of vitamin A in humans. Other natural forms of retinoic acid, including all-*trans*-3,4-didehydroretinoic acid and all-*trans*-4-oxo-retinoic acid, can also induce retinoic acid receptor (RAR) *trans*-activation *in vitro*, and these forms of retinoic acid are probably important for facilitating the effects of retinoids in birds and amphibians *in vivo* (Hofmann & Eichele, 1994; Mangelsdorf *et al.*, 1994). Moreover, 9-*cis*-retinoic acid is the putative physiological ligand for the retinoid X receptor (RXR) nuclear receptors. 13-*cis*-Retinoic acid, which only weakly activates transcription (Mangelsdorf *et al.*, 1994), is found in human and animal tissues and blood (Blaner & Olson, 1994). All of these forms of retinoic acid are in large part derived from all-*trans*-retinol (vitamin A or vitamin A alcohol). A hypothetical metabolic scheme for the formation of these active retinoic acid forms from all-*trans*-retinol is shown in Figure 1, which provides a framework for the metabolism and transport of all-*trans*-, 13-*cis*- and 9-*cis*-retinoic acid.

It is generally believed that the synthesis of retinoic acid initially involves the oxidation of retinol to retinal, catalysed by a number of alcohol dehydrogenases which, because they can use retinol as a substrate, are referred to subsequently as 'retinol dehydrogenases'. The retinal formed through the action of a retinol dehydrogenase undergoes subsequent oxidation to retinoic acid with one of several aldehyde dehydrogenases, which are also referred to as retinal dehydrogenase because of their substrate preference. The oxidative metabolism of retinoic acid is not solely deactivating since

both the 4-hydroxy and 4-oxo derivatives of retinoic acid show activity in *trans*-activation assays. The metabolism is, however, catabolic, since many of the oxidized metabolites of all-*trans*-retinoic acid are excreted.

Numerous enzymes have been proposed to be involved in the synthesis and oxidative metabolism of retinoic acid (Table 2).

2.1.1.1 Biosynthesis of all-trans-*retinoic acid* — Oxidation of retinol
The identity of the enzymes in humans that catalyse the formation of all-*trans*-retinal from all-*trans*-retinol, the first of the two oxidative steps in the formation of retinoic acid, has not yet been established unequivocally, and it is unknown whether only some or all of the enzymes described in the literature as important are indeed physiologically essential in humans. *In vitro*, all-*trans*-retinol is oxidized to all-*trans*-retinoic acid by multiple enzymes present in the cytosol or in microsomes (Duester, 1996; Napoli, 1996). The cytosolic enzymes that catalyse retinol oxidation have been identified as alcohol dehydrogenases (ADHs) with 40-kDa subunits (Boleda *et al.*, 1993). These medium-chain ADHs are encoded in humans by nine genes. The ADH isoenzymes have been grouped into six classes on the basis of their catalytic properties and primary structures. All the members of this enzyme family are dimeric zinc metalloenzymes that require NAD$^+$ to catalyse the oxidation of a variety of primary, secondary and cyclic alcohols (Jörnvall & Höög, 1995). Several human and rat ADH isozymes (classes I, II and IV) oxidize retinol to retinal *in vitro* (Duester, 1996; Napoli, 1996). The class IV ADH human isozyme (ADH4) is the most efficient catalyser of retinol oxidation (Yang *et al.*, 1994) and consequently has been proposed to contribute importantly to retinoic acid biosynthesis *in vivo*.

all-*trans*-Retinol and 9-*cis*-retinol, but not 13-*cis*-retinol, are good substrates for human ADH4, and the apparent K_m values for the reverse (reduction) reactions were very similar to those determined for the two retinol isomers (Allali-Hassani *et al.*, 1998). Kedishvili *et al.* (1998) used purified recombinant human ADH4 and purified recombinant rat cellular

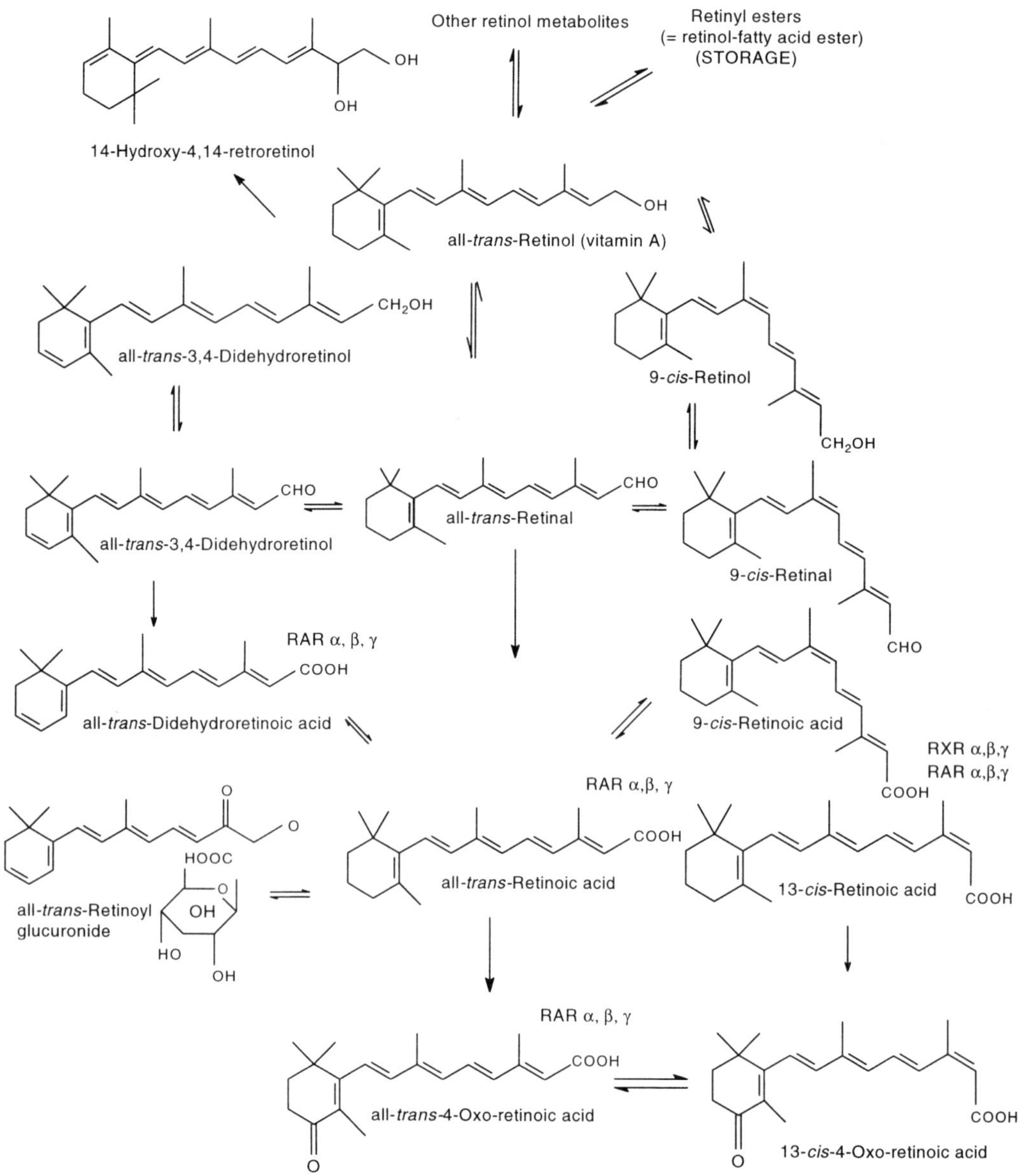

Figure 1. Hypothetical scheme for the metabolism of all-*trans*-retinol

Although all of the metabolic interconversions of vitamin A species indicated in this scheme have not been unequivocally demonstrated experimentally, they have been postulated to take place in some living organism. The reader should focus on the metabolic transformations described in the text, which are those most extensively studied and involve oxidative metabolism of retinol to retinoic acid and oxidative and conjugative transformation of retinoic acid to more polar metabolites. The *cis*–*trans* isomerizations proposed in the figure are less well understood.

Table 2. Nomenclature and abbreviations of enzymes proposed to be involved in the metabolism of retinoic acid

Enzyme	Abbreviation	Reference
Oxidation of retinol		
Short-chain dehydrogenase/reductase	SCDR	Jörnvall & Höög (1995)
Medium-chain alcohol dehydrogenases	ADH	Jörnvall *et al.* (1995)
Retinol dehydrogenase, type I	RoDH(I)	Boerman & Napoli (1995)
Retinol dehydrogenase, type II	RoDH(II)	Chai *et al.* (1995)
Retinol dehydrogenase, type III	RoDH(III)	Chai *et al.* (1996)
Retinol dehydrogenase, type IV	RoDH-4	Gough *et al.* (1998)
Retinol short-chain dehydrogenase/reductase	RetSDR1	Haeseleer *et al.* (1998)
9-*cis*-Retinol dehydrogenase	9cRDH	Mertz *et al.* (1997)
11-*cis*-Retinol dehydrogenase	11cRDH	Saari (1994)
cis-Retinol/3α-hydroxysteroid dehydrogenase, I	CRADI	Chai *et al.* (1997)
cis-Retinol/3α-hydroxysteroid II dehydrogenase, II	CRADII	Su *et al.* (1998)
Alcohol dehydrogenase, class I	ADH1	Jörnvall & Höög (1995)
Alcohol dehydrogenase, class III	ADH3	Jörnvall & Höög (1995)
Alcohol dehydrogenase, class IV	ADH4	Jörnvall & Höög (1995)
Oxidation of retinal		
Liver aldehyde dehydrogenase	ALDH1	Bhat & Samaha (1999)
Retinal dehydrogenase, type I	Ra1DH(I)	El Akawi & Napoli (1994)
Retinal dehydrogenase, type II	Ra1DH(II)	Wang *et al.* (1996a); Niederreither *et al.* (1997)
Oxidative metabolism		
Cytochrome P450 26	CYP26	Ray *et al.* (1997); White *et al.* (1997a); Fujii *et al.* (1997)

This list is not comprehensive. The abbreviations given here and used in the text are those coined in the original citation.

retinol-binding protein, type I (CRBP I), to demonstrate that retinol bound to CRBP I cannot be channelled to the active site of ADH4. They concluded that the contribution of ADH isozymes to retinoic acid biosynthesis depends on the amount of free retinol present in a cell. Since most retinol within a cell is thought to be bound to CRBP I and since human ADH4 catalyses the oxidation of free retinol and not retinol bound to CRBP I, the physiological relevance of ADH4 in the formation of retinoic acid is questionable (Duester, 1996; Napoli, 1996).

Other reports indicate that the oxidation of all-*trans*-retinol to all-*trans*-retinal is catalysed by microsomal enzymes that can use all-*trans*-retinol bound to CRBP I as a substrate. These enzymes are members of the short-chain dehy-drogenase/reductase (SCDR) family, over 60 members of which have been identified. They consist of peptides of 28–32 kDa and do not require zinc for activity. Many of the members of this family are reported to catalyse oxidation or reduction of hydroxysteroids and prosta-glandins (Baker, 1994; Jörnvall *et al.*, 1995; Baker, 1998). Several of the SCDRs that oxidize retinol prefer retinol bound to CRBP I or cellular retinaldehyde-binding protein as a substrate rather than unbound retinol (Saari, 1994; Duester, 1996; Napoli, 1996).

A human liver SCDR with all-*trans*-retinol dehydrogenase activity has been cloned by Gough *et al.* (1998). This NAD⁺-dependent enzyme comprises 317 amino acids and has strong primary sequence similarity to rat retinol dehydrogenase (RoDH)(I), RoDH(II) and RoDH(III). This microsomal protein, designated RoDH-4, is expressed strongly in adult liver and weakly in the lung and not in heart, brain, placenta, skeletal muscle or pancreas. RoDH-4 has also been found to be expressed in human fetal liver and lung but not in fetal brain or kidney. The apparent K_m values of RoDH-4 for 5α-androstene-3α,17β-diol, androsterone and dihydrotestosterone were reported to be well under 1 mmol/L, similar to those of RoDH(I) for these hydroxysteroids (Biswas & Russell, 1997). Gough et al. (1998) further reported that all-trans-retinol is a much better substrate for RoDH-4 than 13-cis-retinol. all-trans-Retinol and 13-cis-retinol bound to CRBP I were relatively potent inhibitors of RoDH-4-catalysed androsterone oxidation, whereas apo-CRBP I had no effect. Thus, Gough et al. (1998) suggested that one enzyme may be involved in the metabolism of both steroids and retinoids.

Links between the metabolism of retinoids and steroids were first suggested by Biswas and Russell (1997), who studied 17β- and 3-hydroxy-steroid dehydrogenases cloned from rat and human prostate and found that the human prostate hydroxysteroid dehydrogenase shares a high degree of primary sequence homology with rat RoDH(I). This observation led the investigators to hypothesize that the microsomal retinol dehydrogenases might also use hydroxysteroids as substrates. Both rat and human recombinant RoDH(I) catalyse the oxidation of 5α-androstan-3,17-diol to dihydro-testosterone, with apparent K_m values of 0.1 mmol/L, as compared with approximately 2 mmol/L for rat RoDH(I) for retinol-CRBP I (Boerman & Napoli, 1995).

Chai et al. (1997) and Su et al. (1998) identified two previously unknown members of the SCDR enzyme family that can use both sterols and retinols as substrates. These rat enzymes, cis-retinol/3α-hydroxysteroid dehydrogenases (CRADs), catalyse the oxidation of cis-retinols. The existence of the CRADs adds further weight to the suggestion that steroid and retinoid metabolism intersects at key multifunctional enzymes.

Haeseleer et al. (1998) cloned a human SCDR that can catalyse oxidation of all-trans-retinol and reduction of all-trans-retinal. This enzyme, called 'retinol short-chain dehydrogenase/reductase' (retSDR1), was cloned from human, bovine and mouse retinal tissue cDNA libraries, and the human, bovine and murine enzymes show approximately 35% amino acid similarity to rat RoDH(I), RoDH(II) and RoDH(III). Human retSDR1 was found by northern blot analysis to be expressed in heart, liver, kidney, pancreas and retina. Recombinant retSDR1 catalyses the reduction of all-trans-retinal but not 11-cis-retinal, indicating that it is specific for all-trans-retinoids. The authors proposed that one physiological action of retSDR1 is to reduce the bleached visual pigment, all-trans-retinal, to all-trans-retinol.

2.1.1.2 Biosynthesis of all-trans-retinoic acid — Oxidation of retinal

Several distinct cytosolic aldehyde dehydrogenases have been identified that catalyse the oxidation of retinal to retinoic acid. These enzymes show strong preference for NAD+ as a substrate. The irreversible nature of the reaction catalysed by these enzymes indicates why retinoic acid cannot restore vision in retinol-deficient animals. Only a few studies of retinal oxidation by human aldehyde dehydrogenases have been reported.

The kinetics of a human liver cytosolic aldehyde dehydrogenase (ALDH1) for retinal isomers has been explored (Bhat & Samaha, 1999). Human ALDH1 shares 87% amino acid identity with a rat kidney retinal dehydrogenase described previously (Bhat et al., 1995). The human isozyme catalyses the oxidation of all-trans-, 9-cis- and 13-cis-retinal, and all-trans-retinol was found to be a potent, noncompetitive inhibitor of retinal oxidation. Unlike human ALDH1, all-trans-retinol also inhibits the rat kidney retinal dehydrogenase homologue, but competitively (Bhat et al., 1995). It was therefore suggested that human ALDH1 and rat kidney aldehyde dehydrogenases have different actions in retinal metabolism (Bhat & Samaha, 1999).

*2.1.1.3   Oxidative metabolism of all-*trans*-retinoic acid*

Duell *et al.* (1996) demonstrated that application of all-*trans*-retinoic acid onto human skin markedly increases the activity of retinoic acid 4-hydroxylase. The inducible 4-hydroxylase activity was present in microsomes and could catalyse 4-hydroxylation of all-*trans*-retinoic acid but not of 9-*cis*- or 13-*cis*-retinoic acid *in vitro*. Neither all-*trans*-retinol nor all-*trans*-retinal could compete with all-*trans*-retinoic acid as a substrate for 4-hydroxylase. The inducible 4-hydroxylase activity was inhibited by addition of the cytochrome P450 (CYP) inhibitor ketoconazole to skin microsomes.

Han and Choi (1996) reported that treatment of human breast cancer T47-D cells with all-*trans*-retinoic acid induced the activity of all-*trans*-retinoic acid 4- and 18-hydroxylases. The induction was time- and dose-dependent and appeared to be regulated at the transcriptional level. The retinoic acid-inducible 4- and 18-hydroxylase activities present in microsomes from T47-D cells showed high specificity for all-*trans*-retinoic acid and could be inhibited by treatment with the CYP inhibitor liarazole. On the basis of these and other data, the authors suggested that these enzymes are new CYP isozymes.

The metabolism and isomerization of all-*trans*- and 9-*cis*-retinoic acid were studied in primary cultures of human umbilical cord endothelial cells and in primary human and HepG2 hepatocytes by Lansink *et al.* (1997), who observed that all-*trans*-retinoic acid was quickly metabolized by both cell types. all-*trans*-Retinoic acid induced its own metabolism in endothelial cells but not hepatocytes. Liarazole and ketoconazole at 10 mmol/L inhibited oxidation of all-*trans*-retinoic acid in both endothelial cells and hepatocytes. Interestingly, 9-*cis*-retinoic acid was degraded slowly by endothelial cells, whereas hepatocytes metabolized this isomer very quickly.

White *et al.* (1997a) cloned a specific human CYP isoform that is very rapidly induced within cells and tissues after exposure to all-*trans*-retinoic acid. This novel isoform, called CYP26, catalyses the oxidative metabolism of the retinoic acid. Like the zebrafish enzyme (White

et al., 1996), with which human CYP26 shares 68% amino acid identity, CYP26 catalyses hydroxylation of all-*trans*-retinoic acid to its 4-hydroxy-, 4-oxo- and 18-hydroxy forms (White *et al.*, 1997a), and CYP26 mRNA expression in human LC-T, MCF-7, HB4 and HepG2 cells was strongly induced by retinoic acid. Ray *et al.* (1997) cloned CYP26 from human liver mRNA and found that 195 of 200 amino acids were identical to those of mouse CYP26. CYP26 is expressed in adult human liver, brain and placenta (Ray *et al.*, 1997) and also in fetal liver and brain (Trofimova-Griffin & Juchau, 1998). The highest levels of CYP26 transcription were observed in adult liver, heart, pituitary gland, adrenal gland, placenta and regions of the brain, whereas the fetal brain showed the highest level of expression, comparable to that of mRNA in adult tissues.

Sonneveld *et al.* (1998) demonstrated that CYP26 is induced within 1 h of all-*trans*-retinoic acid treatment in retinoic acid-sensitive T47-D human breast carcinoma cells but not in retinoic acid-resistant MDA-MB-231 human breast cancer cells or HCT 116 human colon cancer cells. Stable transfection of RARα and RARγ and to a lesser extent RARβ into HCT 116 cells showed that CYP26 induction is dependent on these retinoic acid nuclear receptors. Retinoic acid-induced CYP26 is highly specific for the hydroxylation of all-*trans*-retinoic acid and does not recognize either 13-*cis*- or 9-*cis*-retinoic acid.

Induction of oxidative metabolism of all-*trans*-retinoic acid in MCF-7 mammary carcinoma cells within 1 h of treatment with all-*trans*-retinoic acid at 10^{-9} to 10^{-6} mol/L was reported by Krekels *et al.* (1997). The apparent K_m value of the induced activity for all-*trans*-retinoic acid was 0.33 mmol/L, and the activity was observed after treatment of MCF-7 cells with 13-*cis*- and 9-*cis*-retinoic acid and several keto forms of retinoic acid.

all-*trans*-Retinoic acid induced its own oxidative metabolism in four of eight human squamous-cell carcinoma lines examined (Kim *et al.*, 1998). Induction was blocked by actinomycin D or cyclohexamide and was inhibited by the addition of ketoconazole, suggesting involvement of a CYP isozyme. The authors further reported that the metabolism was first detectable within 4 h of retinoic acid treatment and that 13-*cis*- and 9-*cis*-retinoic acid and all-*trans*-retinal also effectively induced CYP-mediated oxidative metabolism. Like Krekels *et al.* (1997), Kim *et al.* (1998) were probably exploring the actions of CYP26 or a closely related isoform.

A link between the CYP-catalysed oxidation of all-*trans*-retinoic acid and human disease was proposed by Rigas *et al.* (1993, 1996), who observed marked interindividual differences in the pharmacokinetics of all-*trans*-retinoic acid in patients with non-small-cell lung cancer. Initial studies indicated that patients who rapidly cleared all-*trans*-retinoic acid from their plasma also had significantly lower endogenous plasma concentrations of this compound than persons who cleared it from their circulation more slowly. Since administration of ketoconazole, a CYP inhibitor, attenuated all-*trans*-retinoic acid plasma clearance, these authors concluded that rapid plasma clearance was probably catalysed by a CYP-dependent oxidative pathway.

2.1.1.4 Other metabolism of all-trans-retinoic acid

Other metabolites of all-*trans*-retinoic acid generated *in vivo* include 13-*cis*-retinoic acid, 9-*cis*-retinoic acid, all-*trans*-retinoyl-β-glucuronide and all-*trans*-3,4-didehydroretinoic acid (Blaner & Olson, 1994). Some of these metabolites mediate retinoic acid function, whereas others are probably catabolic products destined for export from the body. This section focuses primarily on the conjugated metabolite all-*trans*-retinoyl-β-glucuronide, which is water-soluble and appears rapidly in the bile of animals given the parent compound, suggesting that it is a catabolic product of all-*trans*-retinoic acid destined for elimination from the body. all-*trans*-Retinoyl-β–glucuronide also induces retinoic acid-dependent differentiation of some human cell lines in culture. It is less toxic than the parent compound. Its synthesis appears to be catalysed by several distinct microsomal UDP-dependent glucuronyl transferases. As most tissues contain β-glucuronidases that can hydrolyse retinoyl-β-glucuronide to retinoic acid, the water-soluble all-*trans*-retinoyl-β-glu-

curonide may in some instances serve as a precursor for retinoic acid.

all-*trans*-Retinoyl-β-glucuronide is present in fasting human plasma at a concentration of 5–17 nmol/L (Barua & Olson, 1986). Eckhoff *et al.* (1991) reported the presence of both all-*trans*-4-oxoretinoic acid and 13-*cis*-4-oxo-retinoic acid in the plasma of volunteers given retinyl palmitate at 0.88 mmol/kg body weight orally for 20 days and showed that 4-oxygenated derivatives of retinoic acid were present in the human plasma before, during and after daily treatment. Similar observations were made after administration of 13-*cis*-retinoic acid (Creech Kraft *et al.*, 1991a).

Although some retinoyl-β-glucuronides are destined for excretion from the body, retinoyl-β-glucuronide can induce human promyelocytic HL-60 cell differentiation *in vitro* (Janick-Buckner *et al.*, 1991). Although it is a good inducer of cellular differentiation *in vitro* (Gallup *et al.*, 1987; Zile *et al.*, 1987; Janick-Buckner *et al.*, 1991) and *in vivo* (Sietsema & DeLuca, 1982), it does not bind to cellular retinoid-binding proteins or to nuclear retinoid receptors (Mehta *et al.*, 1992; Sani *et al.*, 1992). It is either hydrolysed to retinoic acid or induces differentiation by transferring its retinoyl moiety to a retinoid nuclear receptor (Olson *et al.*, 1992).

The metabolic basis of the limited toxicity of all-*trans*-retinoyl-β-glucuronide to the skin, to embryonic development and to cells in tissue culture in comparison with that of all-*trans*-retinoic acid may be due in part to its solubility in water (Janick-Buckner *et al.*, 1991; Gunning *et al.*, 1993). Whereas retinoyl-β-glucuronide undergoes slow hydrolysis *in vivo*, retinoyl-β-glucose, a synthetic conjugate, is hydrolysed rapidly to retinoic acid *in vivo* and is therefore both cytotoxic and teratogenic (Barua *et al.*, 1991; Janick-Buckner *et al.*, 1991). Thus, β-glycosidases appear to be less compartmentalized than β-glucuronidases.

2.1.1.5 Biosynthesis of 13-cis-retinoic acid

Figure 1 summarizes the hypothetical metabolic pathways that can give rise to 13-*cis*-retinoic acid. Since there is little evidence that 13-*cis*-retinol or 13-*cis*-retinal is present in tissues or cells, it is generally assumed that 13-*cis*-retinoic acid is formed from isomerization of all-*trans*-retinoic acid or 9-*cis*-retinoic acid. The absence of data on the biosynthesis of this compound cannot, however, be taken as evidence that it is formed only by isomerization of other retinoic acid isomers.

13-*cis*-Retinoic acid is formed in humans after consumption of vitamin A. The concentrations of all-*trans*-, 13-*cis*- and 13-*cis*-4-oxo-retinoic acid in the plasma of 20 volunteers after a single oral dose of retinyl palmitate at 0.87 mmol/kg body weight rose two- to four-fold, with maximal concentrations 1.5–6 h after dosing. When the volunteers were dosed daily for 20 days, the plasma concentrations of all-*trans*- and 13-*cis*-retinoic acid rose transiently but returned to the initial concentrations after 20 days, whereas the plasma concentrations of 13-*cis*-4-oxo-retinoic acid increased gradually over the 20-day period to a steady-state concentration which was approximately three times that present at day 0 (Eckhoff *et al.*, 1991). In human subjects given physiological or pharmacological doses of retinyl palmitate orally, the plasma concentrations of all-*trans*- and 13-*cis*-retinoic acid rose 1.3- and 1.9-fold, respectively (Tang & Russell, 1991).

2.1.1.6 Biosynthesis of 9-cis-retinoic acid

Any factor that influences the availability of 9-*cis*-retinoic acid to or within a cell affects retinoic acid signalling pathways and cellular responses. Little is known about how 9-*cis*-retinoid isomers are formed, although the mechanism of isomerization of all-*trans*-retinoids to 11-*cis*-retinoid isomers in the visual process is now well established to be catalysed by a specific enzyme. In the visual cycle, *trans* to 11-*cis* isomerization takes place at the level of retinal and not of retinaldehyde (Saari, 1994). Since the first reports in 1992 that 9-*cis*-retinoic acid is a ligand for the RXRs, possible pathways for 9-*cis*-retinoic acid formation have been explored, and three pathways have been proposed (Figure 2): isomerization of all-*trans*-retinoic acid, probably through non-enzymatic processes; enzymatic oxidation of 9-*cis*-retinol by a pathway similar to the oxidation of all-*trans*-retinol to all-*trans*-retinoic acid;

and cleavage of 9-*cis*-β-carotene or other 9-*cis*-carotenoids either to 9-*cis*-retinal and all-*trans*-retinal followed by oxidation or possibly directly to 9-*cis*-retinoic acid.

Humans appear to form 9-*cis*-retinoic acid after eating a meal rich in preformed vitamin A (Arnhold *et al.*, 1996). Significant quantities of both 9-*cis*-retinoic acid and 9,13,-di-*cis*-retinoic acid were present in the circulation after consumption of a retinoid-rich meal (Table 3). The mean maximum concentration at peak absorption (at 4 h) was 9 ± 3.7 nmol/L for 9-*cis*-retinoic acid and 57 ± 19 nmol/L for 9,13-di-*cis*-retinoic acid; the integrated area under the curve of concentration–time was 11 ± 3.4 ng-h/ml for 9-*cis*-retinoic acid and 68 ± 22 ng-h/ml for 9,13-di-*cis*-retinoic acid. Intravenous doses of 9,13-di-*cis*-retinoic acid substantially increase the concentration of 9-*cis*-retinoic acid in rats (see Handbook 3, section 3.2), which suggests that 9,13-di-*cis*-retinoic acid can serve as a precursor for 9-*cis*-retinoic acid rather than solely as a catabolic product destined for excretion from the body.

9-*cis*-Retinoic acid can be formed non-enzymatically in isolated human cells and homogenates from all-*trans*-retinoic acid. Lansink *et al.* (1997) studied the metabolism of this compound in primary cultures of human umbilical cord endothelial cells, primary human hepatocytes and human HepG2 hepatocytes and found that hepatocytes and HepG2 cells but not endothelial cells isomerized all-*trans*-retinoic acid to 9-*cis*-retinoic acid. Mertz *et al.* (1997) identified and cloned from a human mammary tissue an NAD+-dependent retinol dehydrogenase (9-*cis*-retinol dehydrogenase) which specifically oxidizes 9-*cis*-retinol and not all-*trans*-retinol. 9-*cis*-Retinol dehydrogenase, a member of the SCDR family, is expressed in adult human mammary tissue, kidney, liver, and testis and during the first trimester of pregnancy in several human embryonic tissues, including brain, kidney and adrenals.

9-*cis*-β-Carotene can be converted via 9-*cis*-retinal to 9-*cis*-retinoic acid (Ben-Amotz *et al.*, 1988; Levin & Mokady, 1994; Nagao & Olson, 1994; Hébuterne *et al.*, 1995). You *et al.* (1996) found that very little radiolabel from oral doses of [^{13}C]9-*cis*-β-carotene was present in

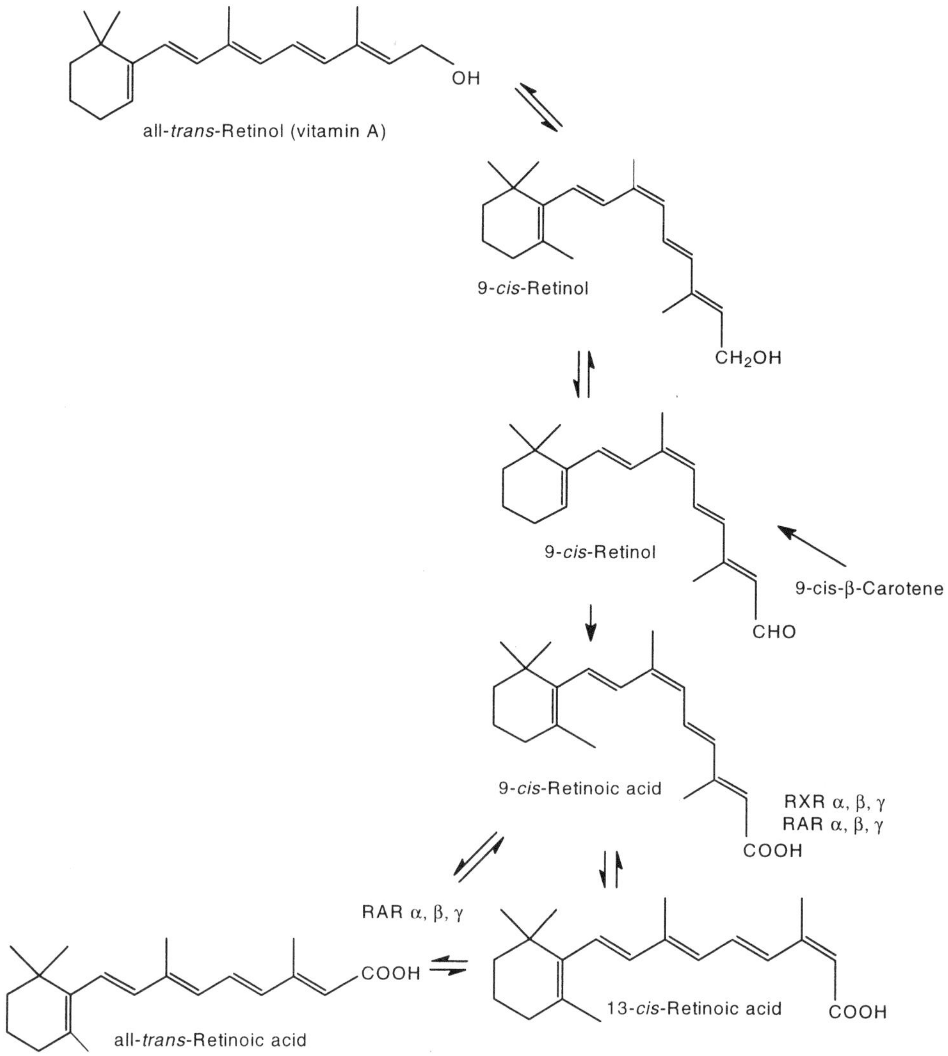

Figure 2. Hypothetical scheme for the synthesis of 9-*cis*-retinoic acid
As outlined in the text, three pathways have been proposed for the formation of 9-*cis*-retinoic acid: isomerization from all-*trans*-retinoic acid, oxidation of 9-*cis*-retinol and 9-*cis*-retinal and cleavage of 9-*cis*-β-carotene. It is not known to what extent each of these three routes contributes to 9-*cis*-retinoic acid formation in tissues.

postprandial plasma, and nearly all of the administered compound was found in the circulation as all-*trans*-β-carotene; *cis* to *trans* isomerization took place exclusively before uptake by the intestinal mucosa.

2.1.2 Plasma transport and kinetics
A small percentage of dietary vitamin A is converted to all-*trans*- and 13-*cis*-retinoic acid in the intestine and is absorbed through the portal system as retinoic acid bound to albumin

Table 3. Plasma retinoid concentrations after consumption of fried turkey liver by healthy male volunteers[a]

Retinoid	C_{end} (ng/mL)	C_{max} (ng/mL)	T_{max} (h)	$AUC_{0-24 h}$ (ng x h/mL)
Retinol	641 ± 99	800 ± 105*	9	16 822 ± 1982
Retinyl palmitate[b]	32.2 ±19.1	3540 ± 1736*	4	21 114 ± 7952
14-Hydroxy-4,14-retroretinol	[c]	3.7 ± 0.9	4	61.7 ± 9.0
all-*trans*-Retinoic acid	0.8 ± 0.2	2.0 ± 0.5*	2	19.7 ± 1.7
all-*trans*-4-Oxoretinoic acid	[c]	0.8 ± 0.2	10	14.7 ± 6.4
13-*cis*-Retinoic acid	1.1 ± 0.2	21.5 ± 4.3*	4	204 ± 35.3
13-*cis*-4-Oxoretinoic acid	2.4 ± 0.6	32.1 ± 4.9*	10	435 ± 68.5
9-*cis*-Retinoic acid	ND[d]	2.7 ± 1.1	4	10.7 ± 3.4
9,13-Di-*cis*-retinoic acid	ND[d]	17.1 ± 5.8	4	68.2 ± 21.6

From Arnhold *et al.* (1996)

[a] Value for C_{end}, C_{max} and $AUC_{0-24 h}$ are means ± SD; those for T_{max} ($n = 10$) are medians.

[b] Data calculated with $n = 9$ owing to one outlier (C_{max} = 14 106 ng/mL, and $AUC_{0-24 h}$ = 104 858 ng x h/mL).

[c] Endogenously detectable in three samples only; 1.3 ± 0.2 ng/mL (for 14-hydroxy-4,14-retroretinol) and 0.6 ± 0.3 ng/mL (for all-*trans*-4-oxo retinoic acid)

[d] Not detectable; detection limit; 0.3 ng/mL for 9-*cis*-retinoic acid and 0.5 ng/mL for 9,13-di-*cis*-retinoic acid

* Significantly greater than C_{end} ($p < 0.001$, Student's *t* test for paired data)

(Olson, 1990; Blaner & Olson, 1994). The plasma concentration of all-*trans*-retinoic acid in fasting humans is 4–14 nmol/L, which is 0.2–0.7% of the plasma concentration of retinol (De Leenheer *et al.*, 1982; Eckhoff & Nau, 1990). Retinoic acid can be taken up efficiently from the circulation by cells, although no specific cell surface receptor is known. all-*trans*-Retinoic acid is fully ionized in free solution at pH 7.4 but is uncharged in a lipid environment (Noy, 1992a,b). It can traverse cell membranes rapidly.

2.1.3 Tissue distribution and variations within human populations

Little information is available about the concentrations and distribution in human tissues of all-*trans*-, 13-*cis*- and 9-*cis*-retinoic acid, primarily because of the difficulty in measuring the relatively low concentrations of all-*trans*-retinoic acid in tissues. The extent to which diet, sex or other factors influence the physiological transport or metabolism of these compounds in humans is unclear. The work of Muindi *et al.* (1992) and Rigas *et al.* (1993, 1996) suggests that some cancer patients clear pharmacological doses of all-*trans*-retinoic acid from their circulation more rapidly than controls because of differences in the CYP-mediated oxidative metabolism of the retinoic acid.

2.2 Experimental models
2.2.1 Overview
Most studies of the transport and metabolism of retinoic acid have been carried out in rats; others have been carried out in mice, rabbits and primates. None of these animal models fully mimics the human situation.

2.2.2 Metabolism
Much of the early information on the enzymes responsible for retinol oxidation was obtained by studying enzymatic activity in tissue homogenates or fractionated homogenates or in cells in culture. Since 1990, an increasing

number of enzymes have been studied *in vitro* and proposed to act *in vivo* as retinol dehydrogenases. The increase is due in part to the development of cloning strategies based on searches for sequence homology to identify previously unknown retinol dehydrogenases. Because nearly all of the enzymes that have been identified by either classical or more modern approaches as retinol dehydrogenases do not show absolute substrate specificity for retinol, it is difficult to demonstrate unequivocally that a 'retinol dehydrogenase' actually catalyses retinol oxidation *in vivo*.

As only a few enzymes that catalyse the oxidation of retinal to retinoic acid have been described, there is generally greater agreement on their physiological significance in retinoic acid formation than is the case for retinol dehydrogenases.

The oxidative metabolism of retinoic acid was actively investigated nearly two decades ago, when many oxidative metabolites of retinoic acid were identified. Renewed interest in this area stems from the finding that the oxidative metabolism of retinoic acid plays an important role in strictly maintaining its tissue and blood concentrations. It is now believed that specific CYP isoenzymes are involved in the metabolism of retinoic acid and are important in maintaining it. Moreover, it is now generally assumed that the oxidative metabolism of retinoic acid is a significant factor in its chemopreventive activity.

2.2.2.1 Biosynthesis of all-*trans*-retinoic acid — Oxidation of retinol

Enzymes of two distinct families, the ADHs and the SCDRs, are considered to be important in catalysing the oxidation of retinol (see section 2.1.1.1).

Although the relatively nonspecific cytosolic ADH of liver can catalyse the oxidation of retinol to retinal (Zachman & Olson, 1961; Mezey & Holt, 1971), the physiological role of this enzyme in the conversion of retinol to retinoic acid is still debated (Duester, 1996; Napoli, 1996). Early research on retinol oxidation focused mainly on cytosolic retinol dehydrogenases, but by the mid-1980s microsomal retinol dehydrogenases were also being investigated (Frolik, 1984; Blaner & Olson, 1994). Leo and Lieber (1984) described a strain of deermice which genetically lack cytosolic ADH in the liver and testis and reported that cytosolic preparations from these organs were unable to oxidize retinol to retinal at a significant rate, even though the testes of these animals were morphologically normal and the animals could reproduce normally. Later studies by these investigators indicated that the livers of this strain have a microsomal retinol dehydrogenase (Leo *et al.*, 1987). When cytosolic fractions from the testis of these ADH-deficient animals were incubated with microsomal fractions of liver, all-*trans*-retinoic acid was formed from all-*trans*-retinol (Kim *et al.*, 1992), and retinal was shown to be an intermediate in this process. In contrast, Posch and Napoli (1992) found that cytosolic preparations from the testis of the deermice could convert all-*trans*-retinol into all-*trans*-retinoic acid. When these cytosolic preparations were fractionated by anion-exchange fast-proton liquid chromatography followed by size-exclusion fast-proton liquid chromatography, the peaks for retinol and retinal dehydrogenase activity co-migrated. Thus, the enzymes that can synthesize retinoic acid from exogenous retinol seemed to reside in a tightly bound protein–protein complex.

Because inhibitors of alcohol and acetaldehyde metabolism do not block retinoic acid synthesis from retinol in LLC-PK1 porcine kidney cells, Napoli (1986) concluded that the enzymes involved in the formation of retinoic acid in these cells are distinct from ADH, ALDH and aldehyde oxidase. Napoli and Race (1988) demonstrated the oxidation of free retinol (not bound to CRBP I) to retinal by cytosolic, but not by microsomal, preparations of rat liver and kidney. In soluble extracts of hairless-mouse epidermis, retinol is oxidized to retinoic acid in two steps, which are catalysed by two NAD^+-dependent enzymes (Connor & Smit, 1987). The retinol oxidizing enzyme had characteristics of a cytosolic ADH, whereas the retinaldehyde oxidizing activity was not further characterized. An $NADP^+$-dependent oxidase in rat liver microsomes converts retinol to retinal (Shih & Hill, 1991); this oxidase was induced by 3-methylcholanthrene and inhibited by citral, ketoconazole and α-naphthoflavone, but was unaffected by the dehydrogenase inhibitor pyrazole.

Several membrane-bound dehydrogenases catalyse this oxidation–reduction reaction in ocular tissue, and one such enzyme, present in the rod outer segments, catalyses the interconversion of all-*trans*-retinol and all-*trans*-retinal (Lion *et al.*, 1975; Blaner & Churchich, 1980; Nicotra & Livrea, 1982). In the retinal pigment epithelium, a different membrane-bound dehydrogenase was reported to catalyse the stereospecific interconversion of 11-*cis*-retinol and 11-*cis*-retinal (Lion *et al.*, 1975; Nicotra & Livrea, 1976), and 11-*cis*-retinal bound to cellular retinal-binding protein is reduced by this enzyme to 11-*cis*-retinol (Saari & Bredberg, 1982). Although soluble ADHs are present in the eye, they may not play a major role in retinoid metabolism (Nicotra & Livrea, 1976; Julia *et al.*, 1986). The eye needs 11-*cis*-retinal as the visual pigment and all-*trans*-retinoic acid to maintain normal retinoid-regulated gene expression. Cultured rabbit Müller cells can synthesize retinoic acid from [^{3}H]retinol (Edwards *et al.*, 1992). Thus, some cells of the adult vertebrate retina can synthesize retinoic acid from retinol and release retinoic acid into the extracellular environment.

(i) Cytosolic retinol dehydrogenases

In rat and mouse tissues, all-*trans*-retinol can be oxidized to all-*trans*-retinoic acid by multiple enzymes present in the cytosol or in microsomes (Duester, 1996; Napoli, 1996; see section 2.1.1.1), and it has been proposed that ADH4 contributes importantly to retinoic acid biosynthesis *in vivo*. Ang *et al.* (1996a,b) demonstrated in developing mouse embryos that the pattern of expression of ADH4 overlaps both temporally and spatially with the distribution of retinoic acid in the embryo. Investigations of the expression of ADH1 and ADH4 in developing mouse embryos demonstrated that both isoforms are present in day-11.5 adrenal blastemas (Haselbeck & Duester, 1998a). The presence of both ADH1 and ADH4 during the earliest stages of adrenal gland development and the observation of high con-

centrations of retinoic acid in embryonic adrenal glands (Haselbeck *et al.*, 1997) suggest that an early function of ADH1 and ADH4 is to provide an embryonic source of retinoic acid (Haselbeck & Duester, 1998a). Investigations with ADH4-*lacZ* transgenic mice showed that ADH4 expression is located in the brain and craniofacial region of the embryo as early as days 8.5–9.5, during neuroregulation. At day 8.5, ADH4-*lacZ* expression was seen in several dispersed regions throughout the head, but by day 9.5 expression was evident in regions that corresponded to the otic vesicles and migrating neural crest cells, particularly the mesencephalic, trigeminal, facial and olfactory neural crest (Haselbeck & Duester, 1998b).

(ii) Microsomal dehydrogenases

Oxidation of all-*trans*-retinol to all-*trans*-retinal is catalysed by microsomal enzymes that can use all-*trans*-retinol bound to CRBP I as a substrate. These microsomal enzymes are members of the SCDR family of enzymes (see above). Three retinol dehydrogenases, RoDH(I), RoDH(II) and RoDH(III), have been cloned and characterized from rat microsomes (Posch *et al.*, 1991; Boerman & Napoli, 1995; Chai *et al.*, 1995, 1996), each of which recognizes all-*trans*-retinol bound to CRBP I as a substrate. Since most retinol within cells is bound to CRBP I, this substrate specificity suggests that these enzymes are physiologically relevant for retinol oxidation. The three enzymes are 82% identical and very similar to other members of the SCDR family. Each requires NADP$^+$ and is expressed most prominently in liver. RoDH(I) is the best studied isoform and is present in kidney, brain, lung and testis but at concentrations less than 1% that in liver. RoDH(II) is also expressed in kidney, brain, lung and testis, at concentrations 25, 8, 4 and 3%, respectively, of that in liver, whereas RoDH(III) is expressed only in liver (Chai *et al.*, 1996). RoDH(I) does not use 9-*cis*-retinol as a substrate (Posch *et al.*, 1991; Boerman & Napoli, 1995); the substrate specificities of RoDH(II) and RoDH(III) for different retinol isomers have not been reported. These three enzymes are probably involved in the oxidation of all-*trans*-retinol to all-*trans*-retinal, the first step in retinoic acid formation.

Zhai *et al.* (1997) demonstrated that CRBP I mRNA and mRNA for RoDH(I) and RoDH(II) are co-expressed in adult rat hepatocytes and in the proximal tubules of rat renal cortex. CRBP I and RoDH(I) and RoDH(II) were also co-expressed in rat testicular Sertoli cells with weaker co-expression in spermatogonia and primary spermatocytes. Since CRBP I and RoDH(I) and/or RoDH(II) are expressed in the same cellular loci *in vivo*, the authors suggested that their data support the hypothesis that holo-CRBP I serves as a substrate for RoDH isozyme-catalysed retinoic acid synthesis.

Rat RoDH(II) has been characterized by Imaoka *et al.* (1998) as a binding protein that is associated with CYP2D1 in the liver. After isolating and cDNA cloning the protein, these workers purified the same protein described by Chai *et al.* (1995) and demonstrated that recombinant RoDH(II) binds tightly to CYP2D1 even in the presence of 1% sodium cholate. Since CYP2D1 contributes to steroid metabolism and can hydroxylate testosterone, oestrogen and cortisol, it was suggested that the binding of RoDH(II) to CYP2D1 is important in the metabolism of diverse bioactive substances including retinoids and steroids. Links between the metabolism of retinoids and steroids were first reported by Biswas and Russell (1997; see section 2.1.1.1).

Members of the ADH family can also catalyse both retinol and hydroxysteroid oxidation (Kedishvili *et al.*, 1997). cDNAs encoding for a class III ADH and a previously unknown ADH were cloned from chick embryo limb bud and heart RNA. The previously unknown ADH cDNA clone exhibited 67 and 68% sequence identity with chicken class I and III ADHs, respectively, and had less identity with mammalian class II and IV ADH isozymes. Expression of this cDNA yielded an active ADH species that was stereospecific for the 3β,5α-hydroxysteroids as opposed to 3β,5β-hydroxysteroids, and this cytosolic enzyme catalysed retinol oxidation with an apparent K_m of 56 mmol/L for all-*trans*-retinol, as compared with a K_m of 31 mmol/L for epiandrosterone. Thus, like members of the SCDR family, ADH enzymes can catalyse reactions involving both steroids and retinoids.

2.2.2.2 Biosynthesis of all-*trans*-*retinoic acid*— Oxidation of retinal

Moffa *et al.* (1970) partially purified an enzyme from intestinal mucosa that converted retinal to retinoic acid and found that it was stimulated by glutathione, NAD$^+$ and FADr$^+$; it had an apparent K_m of 0.3 mmol/L for retinal. Since cellular retinal concentrations are less than 0.1 mmol/L (McCormick & Napoli, 1982; Williams *et al.*, 1984), this enzyme may have limited physiological importance. Cytosols of rat kidney, testis and lung cells also can catalyse the oxidation of retinal to retinoic acid (Bhat *et al.*, 1988a,b). Leo *et al.* (1989a) demonstrated that a cytosolic NAD$^+$-utilizing aldehyde dehydrogenase activity in rat tissues catalysed the oxidation of retinal to retinoic acid. Hupert *et al.* (1991) reported that an enzyme present in rat liver cytosol is responsible for the formation of retinoic acid from retinal.

Lee *et al.* (1991) explored the ability of the 13 ALDHs in mouse tissues to catalyse oxidation of all-*trans*-retinal to all-*trans*-retinoic acid. Three of the six ALDHs present in mouse liver cytosol, ALDH-2, ALDH-7 and xanthine oxidase, catalysed this oxidation. ALDH-2 was estimated to catalyse about 95% of retinaldehyde oxidation to retinoic acid in the liver. The apparent K_m of ALDH-2 for all-*trans*-retinal was 0.7 mmol/L. Since none of the ALDH present in the particulate fractions of mouse liver could catalyse significant retinaldehyde oxidation, the authors concluded that the enzymes responsible for retinoic acid formation from retinal are cytosolic, NAD$^+$-linked, non-substrate-specific dehydrogenases.

Bhat *et al.* (1988a,b) and Labrecque *et al.* (1993, 1995) purified the cytosolic retinal dehydrogenase present in rat kidney. The purified enzyme (subunit relative molecular mass of 53 kDa) is NAD$^+$-dependent and catalyses the oxidation of both all-*trans*- and 9-*cis*-retinal to the corresponding retinoic acid isomer. The rat kidney cytosolic ALDH had typical Michaelis–Menten kinetics towards all-*trans*-retinal, with an apparent K_m of 8–10 mmol/L, whereas the apparent K_m for 9-*cis*-retinol is 5.7 mmol/L. The rat kidney ALDH was subsequently cloned by Bhat *et al.* (1995), who found that its amino acid sequence was very similar to those of other cytosolic ALDHs cloned from rat, mouse and human livers. The enzyme is also strongly expressed in rat lung, testis, intestine, stomach and trachea. Initially, the relevant cDNA was used to define the pattern of expression of this ALDH in fetal and adult rat kidney (Bhat *et al.*, 1998), but Bhat (1998) subsequently investigated its expression in the stomach and small intestine of rats during postnatal development and in vitamin A deficiency. Two days before birth, expression was high in the small intestine but was not detectable in the stomach, whereas after birth expression in the intestine decreased progressively, while expression in the stomach increased and reached its highest concentration at postnatal day 42. Vitamin A deficiency was found to upregulate enzyme expression in the stomach and small intestine while administration of retinoids downregulated expression in these tissues.

Two distinct ALDHs, ALDH-1 and ALDH-2, that can catalyse retinal oxidation have been purified from bovine kidney. They have relatively low apparent K_m values of 6.4 and 9.1 mmol/L, respectively, for all-*trans*-retinal (Bhat *et al.*, 1996). ALDH-1 is proposed to be the primary enzyme in the oxidation of retinal to retinoic acid in this tissue. A retinal dehydrogenase (designated RalDH(I)) purified from rat liver cytosol by Posch *et al.* (1992) and El Akawi and Napoli (1994) is the predominant ALDH isoform in rat liver, kidney and testis (Posch *et al.*, 1992). all-*trans*-Retinal concentrations greater than 6 mmol/L were reported to inhibit RalDH(I). RalDH(I) also recognizes all-*trans*-retinol bound to CRBP I as a substrate. El Akawi and Napoli (1994) demonstrated that RalDH(I) catalyses the oxidation of both all-*trans*- and 9-*cis*-retinal in an NAD+-dependent manner, but 13-*cis*-retinal was not an effective substrate. Oxidation of retinal was not inhibited by all-*trans*- or 9-*cis*-retinoic acid or by holo-CRBP I. RalDH(I) may serve as a common enzyme in the conversion of all-*trans*- and 9-*cis*-retinal into their acids.

Wang *et al.* (1996a) cloned another ALDH from rat testis and called it RalDH(II). The amino acid sequence of RalDH(II) from rat testis is 85% identical to that of RalDH(I), 85% identical to mouse AHD-2, 87% identical to human ALDH1 and 87% identical to bovine retina retinal dehydrogenase. Recombinant RalDH(II) recognizes as substrate both unbound all-*trans*-retinal and all-*trans*-retinal in the presence of CRBP I (Wang *et al.*, 1996a). In addition, RalDH(II) can use as a substrate all-*trans*-retinal generated *in situ* by the action of rat liver microsomal retinol dehydrogenase(s) from holo-CRBP I.

An ALDH present at high concentrations in the basal forebrain of mice catalyses the formation of retinoic acid (McCaffery & Dräger, 1995; Zhao *et al.*, 1996). This enzyme, now called RalDH-2, is expressed very early in embryonic development and at lower levels later in development (Niederreither *et al.*, 1997). Expression of this enzyme in mouse embryos given a teratogenic dose of all-*trans*-retinoic acid on day 8.5 results in downregulation of expression. Labrecque *et al.* (1993, 1995) purified a cytosolic retinal dehydrogenase from rat kidney which is NAD+-dependent and catalyses the oxidation of both all-*trans*- and 9-*cis*-retinal to the corresponding retinoic acid isomer. This retinal dehydrogenase is either identical or very similar to the retinal dehydrogenase partially purified from rat liver cytosol by El Akawi and Napoli (1994). Both enzymes catalyse the oxidation of all-*trans*- and 9-*cis*-retinaldehyde in an NAD+-dependent manner. The presence of CRBP I reduces the rate of all-*trans*-retinoic acid synthesis by rat liver retinaldehyde dehydrogenase. These and other studies (Blaner & Olson, 1994) strongly indicate that cytosolic retinaldehyde dehydrogenases play a role in the formation of retinoic acid *in vivo*. CYP1A2 and CYP3A6 from rabbit liver microsomes can oxidize retinaldehyde to retinoic acid (Roberts *et al.*, 1992).

2.2.2.3 Synthesis of all-*trans*-retinoic acid from β-carotene

A small percentage of the retinal formed from dietary β-carotene can be oxidized to all-*trans*-retinoic acid and taken into the circulation bound to albumin (Goodman & Blaner, 1984; Blaner & Olson, 1994; Wang *et al.*, 1996b). A large percentage of the retinoic acid of dietary origin appears to be removed from the circulation by tissues. Dietary intake of preformed vitamin A and/or provitamin A carotenoids can give rise to increased circulating concentrations of all-*trans*- and 13-*cis*-retinoic acid (Folman *et al.*, 1989; Tang *et al.*, 1995). Rabbits maintained for several weeks on a β-carotene-supplemented diet had a markedly higher plasma concentration of all-*trans*- and 13-*cis*-retinoic acid than rabbits maintained on a control diet (Folman *et al.*, 1989). Thus, dietary intake of β-carotene (and presumably other provitamin A carotenoids) contributes directly to the synthesis of all-*trans*-retinoic acid and consequently to the concentrations of all-*trans*- and 13-*cis*-retinoic acid in the circulation.

Cytosol preparations from rat tissues catalyse the formation of all-*trans*-retinoic acid from β-carotene (Napoli & Race, 1988). Retinol that was generated during β-carotene metabolism was not the major substrate, and all-*trans*-retinal was not detected as a free intermediate in this process. Thus, it might be tightly bound by the enzyme, or β-carotene might be oxidized to a 15,15′-enediol before dioxygenase cleavage, by analogy to the conversion of catechol to *cis,cis*-muconic acid. Homogenates of liver, lung, kidney and fat from monkeys, ferrets and rats incubated with β-carotene generate all-*trans*-retinoic acid (Wang *et al.*, 1991) through a biochemical process which does not involve all-*trans*-retinal as an intermediate (Wang *et al.*, 1992).

2.2.2.4 Oxidative metabolism of all-trans-retinoic acid

The most abundant oxidized metabolites produced from all-*trans*-retinoic acid are its 4-hydroxy and 4-oxo derivatives, with some all-*trans*-5,6-epoxy-retinoic acid.

(i) Metabolites

Roberts *et al.* (1979) demonstrated in hamster liver microsome preparations that all-*trans*-retinoic acid is first converted to all-*trans*-4-hydroxyretinoic acid, which in turn is oxidized to the 4-oxo derivative. The formation of 4-hydroxyretinoic acid required NADPH, whereas the subsequent formation of 4-oxoretinoic acid is NAD$^+$-dependent (Roberts *et al.*, 1980). Frolik *et al.* (1980) established that both all-*trans*-4-hydroxy- and all-*trans*-4-

oxoretinoic acid are formed *in vivo* after administration of all-*trans*-[^{3}H]retinoic acid to hamsters maintained on a control diet. Subsequent work by Leo *et al.* (1984, 1989b) and Roberts *et al.* (1992) demonstrated that CYP isoforms in rat and in human liver preparations promote conversion of all-*trans*-retinoic acid to its 4-hydroxy and 4-oxo-forms. Hence, the CYP system plays a role in the physiological formation of these 4-oxygenated retinoids.

Barua *et al.* (1991) found that rats given large oral doses of all-*trans*-retinoic acid had significant amounts of both all-*trans*-4-hydroxy- and all-*trans*-4-oxoretinoic acid in their serum, small intestine, liver, kidney and stomach contents within 60 min. The intestinal mucosa of vitamin A-deficient rats given all-*trans*-[^{3}H]retinoic acid formed 5,6-epoxyretinoic acid, which was shown to be a metabolite of retinoic acid *in vivo* (McCormick *et al.*, 1978). Napoli *et al.* (1982) showed that all-*trans*-5,6-epoxyretinoyl-β-glucuronide was also formed in the small intestinal mucosa of vitamin A-deficient rats given intrajugular doses of all-*trans*-[^{3}H]5,6-epoxyretinoic acid. This compound was found in significant concentrations in the liver, small intestinal mucosa and intestinal contents, but not in the kidney, of vitamin A-deficient rats. It was synthesized in the kidney of vitamin A-sufficient rats given physiological doses of [^{3}H]retinol, suggesting that both retinoic acid and all-*trans*-5,6-epoxyretinoic acid are formed endogenously from retinol under normal physiological conditions (McCormick & Napoli, 1982). Barua *et al.* (1991) also reported that all-*trans*-5,6-epoxyretinoic acid was present in the serum, small intestine, liver and kidney of control rats given a large oral dose of all-*trans*-retinoic acid.

(ii) Enzymes and enzyme systems

CYP isoenzymes appear to be important in the formation of oxidized metabolites of all-*trans*-retinoic acid, and a novel isoform, CYP26, has been implicated as a catalyser in the oxidative metabolism of all-*trans*-retinoic acid. Formation of polar metabolites of retinoic acid is catalysed by rat intestine and liver microsomes, the activity being attributed to members of a class of mixed-function oxidases containing

CYPs (Roberts *et al.*, 1979). This activity requires NADPH and oxygen and is strongly inhibited by carbon monoxide. Leo *et al.* (1984) reported that rats fed a diet containing a 100-fold excess of retinyl acetate for two to three weeks had an increased hepatic microsomal CYP content. Purified cyto-chromes P450f and P450b catalysed the conversion of retinoic acid to polar metabolites, including 4-hydroxy-retinoic acid. The P450 isozyme P450IIC8 in human liver microsomes was shown to be responsible for oxidizing all-*trans*-retinoic acid to all-*trans*-4-hydroxyretinoic acid and all-*trans*-4-oxoretinoic acid (Leo *et al.*, 1989b).

Many rabbit liver CYP isoforms, including 2A4, 1A2, 2E1, 2E2, 2C3, 2G1 and 3A6, catalyse the 4-hydroxylation of retinoic acid (Roberts *et al.*, 1992). These cytochromes also catalysed the 4-hydroxylation of retinol and retinal but not the conversion of 4-hydroxyretinoids to the corresponding 4-oxoretinoids. Van Wauwe *et al.* (1992) showed that oral administration of a dose of 40 mg/kg body weight of liarazole, which inhibits CYP activity, enhanced the endogenous plasma concentrations of retinoic acid from less than 1.7 to 10–15 nmol/L.

CYP26, which can metabolize retinoic acid, was cloned independently by several groups (White *et al.*, 1996; Fujii *et al.*, 1997; Ray *et al.*, 1997; White *et al.*, 1997a). Fujii *et al.* (1997) reported that expressed murine P450RA cDNA catalysed the oxidation of all-*trans*-retinoic acid to all-*trans*-5,6-epoxyretinoic acid. Both 13-*cis*- and 9-*cis*-retinoic acid were found to serve as substrates for P450RA. This isoform was expressed in a stage- and region-specific fashion during mouse development, but expression did not appear to be inducible after exposure of mouse embryos to excess retinoic acid. In adult mice, P450RA was expressed only in liver.

White *et al.* (1996) reported the isolation and characterization of a cDNA for CYP26 from zebrafish, which they called P450RAI. This iso-form was found to be expressed during gastru-lation. When the cDNA for P450RAI was expressed in COS-1 cells, all-*trans*-retinoic acid was rapidly metabolized to more polar metabo-lites including all-*trans*-4-oxoretinoic acid and all-*trans*-4-hydroxyretinoic acid. Thus, P450RAI, which is induced after exposure to retinoic acid, catalyses the oxidative metabolism of retinoic acid. White *et al.* (1997a) cloned the human homologue of zebrafish P450RAI, the enzyme that catalyses hydroxylation of all-*trans*-retinoic acid to its 4-hydroxy, 4-oxo and 18-hydroxy forms. Moreover, *P450RAI* mRNA expression was highly induced by treatment of human LC-T, MCF-7, HB4 and HepG2 cells with retinoic acid.

Abu-Abed *et al.* (1998) reported the cloning of the mouse homologue for P450RAI which catalyses metabolism of retinoic acid into 4-hydroxyretinoic acid, 4-oxoretinoic acid and 18-hydroxyretinoic acid. They observed a direct relationship between the level of retinoic acid metabolic activity and retinoic acid-induced P450RAI mRNA in wild-type F9 cells and deriv-atives lacking RARs and/or RXRs, and suggested that RARγ and RXRα mediate the induction of the expression of the *P450RAI* gene by retinoic acid.

Simultaneously, Ray *et al.* (1997) reported the cloning of CYP26 (identical to P450RA and P450RAI) from a mouse embryonic stem cell library. Expression of this isoform was limited in the adult to liver and brain and was detectable in mouse embryos as early as day 8.5. Moreover, *CYP26* mRNA was upregulated during the retinoic acid-induced neural differ-entiation of mouse embryonic stem cells *in vitro*. These authors also cloned human CYP26, in which 195 of 200 amino acids were identical to those of mouse CYP26. In human adults, CYP26 is expressed in liver, brain and placenta.

The total retinol concentrations in liver from aryl hydrocarbon receptor-null (AHR$^{-/-}$) mice are approximately threefold higher than those in wild-type mice (Andreola *et al.*, 1997). In addition, AHR$^{-/-}$ mice showed a reduced capacity to oxidize retinoic acid and signifi-cantly lower hepatic levels of mRNA for retinaldehyde dehydrogenase types 1 and 2, although expression of CYP26 was similar in the AHR-deficient and wild-type mice, in keep-ing with earlier observations that mice and rats given 2,3,7,8-tetrachlorodibenzo-*para*-dioxin show a rapid decline in total hepatic retinol concentrations (Brouwer *et al.*, 1985; Chen *et al.*, 1992a).

A direct role for cellular retinoic acid-binding protein, type I (CRABP I) in the oxidative metabolism of retinoic acid was proposed by Fiorella and Napoli (1991). When all-*trans*-retinoic acid is bound to CRABP I, microsomal enzymes of rat testes catalyse the conversion of retinoic acid to 3,4-didehydro-, 4-hydroxy-, 4-oxo-, 16-hydroxy-4-oxo- and 18-hydroxy-retinoic acids. Ketoconazole inhibited oxidation by testis microsomes of both free and CRABP I-bound retinoic acid, suggesting that CYP isozymes are involved in this metabolism. CRABP I may well play a direct role in the oxidative metabolism of all-*trans*-retinoic acid.

2.2.2.5 Other metabolism of all-trans-retinoic acid

When all-*trans*-retinoic acid is given orally to rats, all-*trans*-retinoyl-β-glucuronide is secreted into the bile (Dunagin et al., 1966; Swanson et al., 1981; Skare & DeLuca, 1983; Frolik, 1984). Retinoyl-β-glucuronide can be synthesized from all-*trans*-retinoic acid and UDP-glucuronic acid in the liver, intestine, kidney and other tissues by several members of the microsomal glucuronyl transferase family of enzymes (Lippel & Olson, 1968; Frolik, 1984). The intestinal mucosa seems to be the most active tissue in synthesizing and retaining retinoyl-β-glucuronide (Zile et al., 1982; McCormick et al., 1983; Cullum & Zile, 1985; Barua et al., 1991). After all-*trans*-retinoic acid was administered to rats, the all-*trans*-retinoyl-β-glucuronides were shown to consist of all-*trans*- and 13-*cis*-retinoyl-β-glucuronides in a ratio of 1.5 to 1.0 (Zile et al., 1982), but when 13-*cis*-retinoic acid was administered all-*trans*-retinoyl-β-glucuronide was a major metabolite in rats *in vivo* (McCormick et al., 1983; Meloche & Besner, 1986). Isomerization to all-*trans*-retinoic acid probably, but not necessarily, occurs before the conjugation reaction (McCormick et al., 1983).

all-*trans*-Retinoyl-β-glucuronide can be synthesized from retinoic acid and UDP-glucuronic acid by extracts of rat liver, intestine, kidney and other tissues (Barua & Olson, 1986; Barua, 1997). Genchi et al. (1996) demonstrated that the relative rates of retinoid-β-glucuronide formation from uninduced rat liver microsomes were: 9-*cis*-retinoic acid > 13-*cis*-retinoic acid > all-*trans*-4-oxoretinoic acid > all-*trans*-retinoic acid > 13-*cis*-retinol > 9-*cis*-retinol > all-*trans*-retinol. They concluded that the rates of glucuronidation of retinoids depend on both the isomeric state and the chemical structure of the retinoids and that different UDP-glucuronosyl transferases might act on different geometric isomers of retinoic acid.

A specific UDP-glucuronosyl transferase with all-*trans*-[³H]retinoic acid as a substrate was identified in rat liver microsomes by photoincorporation of both [³²P]5-azido-UDP-glucuronic acid and all-*trans*-[³H]retinoic acid into the 52-kDa microsomal protein. This enzyme (and possibly similar ones) plays a physiologically relevant role in hepatic synthesis of retinoyl-β-glucuronides (Little & Radominska, 1997). Recombinant rat UDP-glucuronosyl transferase 1.1 catalyses the glucuronidation of all-*trans*-retinoic acid with an apparent K_m of 59.1 ± 5.4 mmol/L. Micro-somes from the livers of Gunn rats, which lack this enzyme, still have significant all-*trans*-retinoic acid glucuronidating activity, suggesting that other hepatic UDP-glucuronosyltransferase isoforms also contribute to retinoic acid glucuronidation (Radominska et al., 1997).

Although retinoyl-β-glucuronides can be excreted into bile, they can also be hydrolysed to retinoic acid by enzymes present in rat liver, kidney and intestine (Kaul & Olson, 1998). The rates of hydrolysis were higher in tissue preparations from vitamin A-deficient rats than from controls, indicating that a regulatory mechanism may exist in vitamin A-deficiency that enhances the actions of tissue β-glucuronidases to increase the rate of retinoic acid formation from retinoyl-β-glucuronides.

About one-third of the retinoid-β-glucuronides excreted into the bile of rats is recycled back to the liver by enterohepatic circulation (Zachman et al., 1966; Swanson et al., 1981). Very little retinol, retinyl ester or retinoic acid is involved in the circulation, however, and the water-soluble retinyl-β-glucuronide and retinoyl-β-glucuronide are presumably reabsorbed by the portal rather than by the lymphatic route (Ribaya-Mercado et al., 1988).

2.2.2.6 Biosynthesis of 13-cis-retinoic acid

Cullum and Zile (1985) reported that 13-*cis*-retinoic acid is endogenous in the intestinal mucosa, intestinal muscle and plasma of vitamin A-sufficient rats. When 20 mg all-*trans*-[³H]retinyl acetate were administered to vitamin A-sufficient rats, 13-*cis*-retinoic acid appeared in the plasma and small intestine, and the authors concluded that 13-*cis*-retinoic acid is a naturally occurring metabolite of all-*trans*-retinyl acetate. Napoli *et al.* (1985) similarly demonstrated that 13-*cis*-retinoic acid is a naturally occurring form of retinoic acid in rat plasma, possibly arising from all-*trans*-retinoic acid.

Incubation of 13-*cis*-retinoic acid (0.83 mmol/L) with mouse liver microsomes in the presence of appropriate cofactors yielded all-*trans*-retinoic acid, 13-*cis*- and all-*trans*-4-hydroxyretinoic acid and 13-*cis*- and all-*trans*-4-oxoretinoic acid as the major metabolites. Metabolism of 13-*cis*-retinoic acid was not detectable in microsomal preparations from mouse skin, indicating that CYP isozymes in liver but not in skin are active towards 13-*cis*-retinoic acid (Oldfield, 1990).

Chen and Juchau (1997) reported that purified hepatic glutathione *S*-transferases from rats catalysed the isomerization of 13-*cis*-retinoic acid to all-*trans*-retinoic acid. The reaction was protein-dependent and independent of the presence of glutathione, indicating that the isomerization reaction is not linked to glutathione *S*-transferase activity. Chen and Juchau (1998) demonstrated that conversion of 13-*cis*- and 9-*cis*-retinoic acid to all-*trans*-retinoic acid can be catalysed by cell-free preparations from rat embryo tissue at day 12.5 of gestation. The isomerization was protein-dependent and showed substrate saturation kinetics.

When small doses of 13-*cis*-[³H]retinoic acid were administered to hamsters on a control diet, the major metabolite formed was 13-*cis*-4-oxoretinoic acid (Frolik *et al.*, 1980). A 10 000 x *g* supernatant from hamster liver homogenate exposed to 13-*cis*-[³H]retinoic acid similarily generated 13-*cis*-4-oxoretinoic acid as the major metabolite. 13-*cis*-4-Hydroxyretinoic acid, a putative metabolic precursor of 13-*cis*-4-oxoretinoic acid, was also identified in these experiments.

2.2.2.7 Biosynthesis of 9-cis-retinoic acid

As outlined in section 2.1.1.6., the 9-*cis*-isomer of retinoic acid may be formed directly from all-*trans*-retinoic acid or by an independent pathway. Membranes from bovine liver non-enzymatically catalyse the isomerization of all-*trans*-retinoic acid to 9-*cis*-retinoic acid due to the presence of free sulfhydryl groups (Urbach & Rando, 1994). Shih *et al.* (1997) also showed that interconversion of 9-*cis*-retinoic acid, all-*trans*-retinoic acid, 13-*cis*-retinoic acid and 9,13-di-*cis*-retinoic acid may be catalysed by sulfhydryl compounds of low relative molecular mass (including L-cysteine methyl ester, glutathione and N-acetyl-L-cysteine), and by proteins containing sulfhydryl groups (apoferritin, native microsomes and boiled microsomes). Sass *et al.* (1994) reported that both treated and untreated rat liver microsomes can catalyse the formation of 9-*cis*-retinoic acid and its glucuronide from all-*trans*- and 13-*cis*-retinoic acid.

Hébuterne *et al.* (1995) reported that 9-*cis*-β-carotene is a precursor for 9-*cis*-retinoic acid *in vivo* in perfused ferrets, but the significance of this pathway for the formation of 9-*cis*-retinoic acid has been questioned since the rate of cleavage of 9-*cis*-β-carotene in pigs is only 6–7% that of all-*trans*-β-carotene (Nagao & Olson, 1994). Furthermore, studies by You *et al.* (1996) in humans (see section 2.1.1) indicate that very little 9-*cis*-β-carotene is absorbed without undergoing isomerization to all-*trans*-β-carotene. Since rats and other animals maintained on carotenoid-free diets remain healthy, the conversion of 9-*cis*-β-carotene to 9-*cis*-retinoic acid cannot be essential for formation of this retinoic acid isomer. Labrecque *et al.* (1993, 1995) reported that the retinal dehydrogenase present in rat kidney can catalyse the oxidation of 9-*cis*-retinal to 9-*cis*-retinoic acid and suggested that a pathway starting with 9-*cis*-retinol may be important for 9-*cis*-retinoic acid formation. They demonstrated the presence of 9-*cis*-retinol in rat kidney at a concentration approximately 10% of that of all-*trans*-retinol.

An NAD⁺-dependent retinol dehydrogenase which specifically oxidizes 9-*cis*-retinol but not all-*trans*-retinol has been cloned from a human mammary tissue cDNA library (Mertz *et al.*, 1997; see section 2.1.1.6). Although it was suggested that the protein and mRNA of 11-*cis*-retinol dehydrogenase occur only in the retinal pigment epithelium (Simon *et al.*, 1995) and that the enzyme does not catalyse 9-*cis*-retinol oxidation (Suzuki *et al.*, 1993), this appears to be incorrect (Driessen *et al.*, 1998). The mouse homologue of 9-*cis*-retinol dehydrogenase is expressed in brain, liver, kidney and testis and at low concentrations in several other tissues and shows a marked substrate preference for 9-*cis*-retinol (Gamble *et al.*, 1999). 13-*cis*-Retinoic acid is a very potent inhibitor of 9-*cis*-retinol dehydrogenase activity. The enzyme is expressed in human and mouse kidney, tissues which have been reported to contain significant quantities of 9-*cis*-retinol and 9-*cis*-retinal dehydrogenase activity (Labrecque *et al.*, 1993, 1995).

A second *cis*-retinol dehydrogenase, also a member of the SCDR family, was described by Chai *et al.* (1997). The cDNA for this mouse liver enzyme, known as the *cis*-retinol/3α-hydroxy sterol short-chain dehydrogenase 1 (CRAD1), encodes an enzyme comprising 317 amino acids that recognizes 9-*cis*- and 11-*cis*-retinol, 5α-androstan-3α,17β-diol and 5α-androstan-3α-ol-17-one as substrates, although it has a greater affinity for sterol than for retinol substrates. The preferred cofactor of this mouse enzyme, which is closely homologous to mouse RoDH(I) (86%) and RoDH(II) isozymes (91%), is NAD⁺, and it is expressed in liver, kidney, small intestine, heart, retinal pigment epithelium, brain, spleen, testis and lung.

Su *et al.* (1998) cloned a second *cis*-retinol/3α-hydroxysteroid short-chain dehydrogenase isozyme (CRAD2) from a mouse embryonic cDNA library, which has 87% amino acid identity with CRAD1, recognizes both androgens and retinols as substrates and has cooperative kinetics for 5α-androstan-3α,17β-diol (3α-adiol) and testosterone but Michaelis–Menten kinetics for androsterone, all-*trans*-, 11-*cis*- and 9-*cis* retinols. *CRAD2* mRNA was highly expressed in mouse liver and at much lower levels in lung, eye, kidney and brain.

2.2.2.8 *Subsequent metabolism of 9-*cis*-retinoic acid*

Horst *et al.* (1995) reported that 9,13-di-*cis*-retinoic acid is the major endogenous circulating retinoic acid isomer in bovine plasma. After intravenous administration of this retinoic acid to rats, circulating 9-*cis*-retinoic acid was found at a concentration that was approximately 3% of that of 9,13-di-*cis*-retinoic acid. When 9-*cis*-retinoic acid was injected intramuscularly into rats, the peak plasma concentration of 9,13-di-*cis*-retinoic acid followed that of 9-*cis*-retinoic acid by about 1.5 h, and detectable concentrations were seen for at least 24 h, whereas the concentration of 9-*cis*-retinoic decreased below the limit of detection (< 1.7 nmol/L) by 12 h after injection.

2.2.3 *Plasma transport and kinetics*

The plasma of rats contains low concentrations of all-*trans*- and 13-*cis*-retinoic acid (Cullum & Zile, 1985; Napoli *et al.*, 1985). Plasma all-*trans*-retinoic acid may be an important source of this retinoid for some but not all tissues (Kurlandsky *et al.*, 1995).

2.2.3.1 *Plasma concentrations, transport and kinetics*

Plasma all-*trans*-retinoic acid may be derived from dietary sources and presumably from endogenous metabolism of retinol within tissues. all-*trans*-Retinoic acid appears in the circulation after intraduodenal, oral or intraperitoneal administration of radiolabelled all-*trans*-retinoic acid to experimental animals (Zachman *et al.*, 1966; Geison & Johnson, 1970; Ito *et al.*, 1974; Skare & DeLuca, 1983). In rats, retinoic acid is absorbed in the intestine, and about two-thirds of the absorbed dose is distributed as retinoic acid throughout the body (Smith *et al.*, 1973). Lehman *et al.* (1972) and Smith *et al.* (1973) demonstrated that circulating retinoic acid is bound to serum albumin but not to retinol-binding protein. When radiolabelled all-*trans*-retinoic acid was administered in dimethyl sulfoxide by intrajugular injection to rats, it was rapidly (< 2 min) taken up by the intestines and other tissues; subsequently, 13-*cis*-retinoic acid and uncharacterized polar metabolites appeared in plasma (Cullum & Zile, 1985).

Two further extracellular proteins, epididymal retinoic acid-binding protein (Newcomer & Ong, 1990) and β-trace (Eguchi *et al.*, 1997; Tanaka *et al.*, 1997), are reported to bind all-*trans*-retinoic acid with high affinity. These proteins, like plasma retinol-binding protein, are members of the lipocalin family of extracellular lipid-binding proteins (Flower, 1996). Both epididymal retinoic acid-binding protein and β-trace have been proposed to play a role in the extracellular transport and economy of all-*trans*-retinoic acid in the body (Newcomer & Ong, 1990; Eguchi *et al.*, 1997). Targeted disruption of the mouse *β-trace* gene results in a lack of tactile pain (Eguchi *et al.*, 1999).

Using a steady-state tracer kinetic approach, Kurlandsky *et al.* (1995) explored the contribution of plasma all-*trans*-retinoic acid to tissue pools of all-*trans*-retinoic acid in chow-fed male rats. More than 75% of the all-*trans*-retinoic acid present in liver and brain was derived from the circulation, while the results were 23% for seminal vesicles, 9.6% for epididymis, 33% for kidney, 30% for epididymal fat, 24% for perirenal fat, 19% for spleen and 27% for lungs. Only 2.3% of the retinoic acid present in the pancreas and 4.8% of that in the eyes was contributed by the circulation. The testis did not take up any (< 1%) all-*trans*-retinoic acid from the circulation. The fractional catabolic rate for this compound in plasma was 30 plasma pools per hour and the absolute catabolic rate was 640 pmol/h. These rates are much greater than those of all-*trans*-retinol, the only other naturally occurring form of vitamin A studied under normal physiological conditions (Lewis *et al.*, 1990). Very little 9-*cis*- or 13-*cis*-retinoic acid was detected in any of these tissues.

Kurlandsky *et al.* (1995) also assessed the rate of plasma clearance of all-*trans*-3-[³H]retinoic acid and [¹⁴C]oleic acid bound to albumin and given simultaneously to rats maintained on a control or a totally retinoid-free diet. The rats on the retinoid-free diet had a significantly greater fractional catabolic rate for all-*trans*-retinoic acid (23 ± 5.5 versus 12 ± 4.6 pools/h) than those on control diet. Moreover, the fraction catabolic rates for oleic acid in these rats were not affected by dietary retinoid intake (43 ± 6.0 pools/h for controls

and 38 ± 7.2 pools/h for the retinoid-free-group). Thus, dietary retinoid status influences all-*trans*-retinoic acid but not oleic acidturnover from the circulation The β-carotene content of the diet affected the serum concentrations of all-*trans*-retinoic acid in rabbits (Folman *et al.*, 1989).

2.2.3.2 Cellular uptake from plasma

Bovine serum albumin has three distinct binding sites for retinoic acid at mole ratios for retinoic acid:albumin of less than 1. Noy (1992a) reported that two of these binding sites correlated to two known binding sites for long-chain fatty acids, but one appeared to be a unique site for retinoic acid binding. Noy (1992b) found that the protonated (uncharged) form of retinoic acid, like other hydrophobic carboxylic acids (fatty acids and bile acids), was stabilized by incorporation into lipid bilayers. At physiological pH, uncharged retinoic acid crossed membranes rapidly and spontaneously. all-*trans*-Retinoic acid, although fully ionized in free solution at pH 7.4, is uncharged in a lipid environment (Noy, 1992a,b).

all-*trans*-Retinoic acid binds to the mannose-6-phosphate/insulin-like growth factor-II receptor on plasma membranes of rat cardiac myocytes (Kang *et al.*, 1998). The binding of all-*trans*-retinoic acid to this membrane receptor appears to be important in modulating the activity of cellular signal transduction pathways and cellular activity but not for facilitating its uptake from the circulation. Hodam and Creek (1996) showed that all-*trans*-[³H]retinoic acid was taken up rapidly by a culture medium containing human foreskin keratinocytes and converted to polar compounds that were subsequently excreted. In contrast, retinoic acid bound to albumin was taken up and metabolized slowly.

2.2.4 Tissue distribution

Cullum and Zile (1985) reported the endogenous concentrations of all-*trans*- and 13-*cis*-retinoic acid and retinoyl-β-glucuronide and a polar metabolite fraction consisting of all-*trans*-5,6-epoxy-retinoic acid, all-*trans*-4-oxoretinoic acid and other polar metabolites in rat intestinal mucosa, intestinal muscle, plasma, erythrocytes and bile (Table 4). Heyman *et al.* (1992) estimated that the endogenous concentrations of 9-*cis*-retinoic acid in mouse liver and kidney were 13 and 100 pmol/g tissue, respectively. Kurlandsky *et al.* (1995) reported the concentrations of all-*trans*-retinoic acid in eight tissues of rats (Table 5). They did not detect 9-*cis*-retinoic acid in liver, spleen, kidney, brain, adipose tissue, testis or muscle even though the limit of detection for 9-*cis*-retinoic acid was only 4 pmol/g of tissue. The concentrations of all-*trans*- and 13-*cis*-retinoic acid have also been determined in rat conceptuses (Creech Kraft & Juchau, 1992).

2.2.5 Intra- and inter-species variation
The metabolism of all-*trans*-, 13-*cis*- and 9-*cis*-retinoic acid differs between species in a number of significant ways. The pharmacokinetics and metabolic profiles of all-*trans*- and 13-*cis*-retinoic acid in mice, monkeys and humans vary widely (Creech Kraft *et al.*, 1991a,b). The predominant metabolite of all-*trans*-retinoic acid is all-*trans*-4-oxoretinoic acid in mice and all-*trans*-retinoyl-β-glucuronide in monkeys. The predominant metabolite of 13-*cis*-retinoic acid is 13-*cis*-retinoyl-β-glucuronide in mice and 13-*cis*-4-oxoretinoic acid in monkeys and humans, although the metabolite is much more predominant in humans than in monkeys. all-*trans*-Retinoic acid was more rapidly cleared than 13-*cis*-retinoic acid in monkeys, while the reverse was observed in mice.

Marchetti *et al.* (1997) found that all-*trans*-, 13-*cis*- and 9-*cis*-retinoic acid each underwent substantial isomerization to the other two in hepatic microsome preparations from male and female Sprague-Dawley and Hairless rats. The isomerization was independent of NADPH and dependent on the presence of microsomal protein. The 4-oxo metabolites of these retinoic acid isomers were formed to a lesser extent. The authors concluded that the metabolism of retinoic acid isomers is influenced by sex but not strain.

3. Molecular mechanisms of retinoid action

Retinoids are signalling molecules that act through interaction with two families of retinoid receptors, RARs α, β and γ and RXRs α, β and γ. These receptors belong to the super-

Table 4. Endogenous vitamin A compounds in plasma, erythrocytes, small intestine and bile of vitamin A-sufficient rats

Endogenous vitamin A compound	Concentration (ng/g tissue)				
	Intestinal mucosa	Intestinal muscle	Plasma	Erythrocytes	Bile
Retinyl stearate	3.5	7.2	ND	ND	ND
Retinyl palmitate	30	22	0.8	1.1	ND
Retinyl linoleate	19	7.7	ND	ND	ND
Retinol	47	7.4	400	28	31
all-*trans*-Retinoic acid	2.3	1.1	2.7	1.1	7.7
13-*cis*-Retinoic acid	1.0	0.2	0.9	0.6	6.1
Retinoyl-β-glucuronide	1.3	ND	ND	ND	19
all-*trans*-5,6-Epoxyretinoic acid + all-*trans*-4-oxoretinoic acid + polar metabolites	7.5	13	5.5	2.8	390
Total retinoids	110	59	410	34	450

From Cullum & Zile (1985). Values represent the rounded average of two determinations for samples obtained from four rats 48 h after feeding of retinyl acetate and 12 h after fasting. Bile was collected 2 h before sacrifice; ND, not detected

Table 5. Concentrations of all-*trans*-retinoic acid in various tissues of rats

Tissue	Concentration (pmol/g tissue)
Liver	11 ± 4.7
Brain	6.8 ± 3.3
Testis	11 ± 2.7
Seminal vesicle	12 ± 7.0
Epididymis	4.2 ± 1.6
Kidney	8.3 ± 4.0
Pancreas	29 ± 16
Epididymal fat	16 ± 12
Perirenal fat	13 ± 8.7
Spleen	13 ± 12
Eye	120 ± 37
Plasma	1.8 ± 0.7 pmol/ml

From Kurlandsky *et al.* (1995). Each value is the mean and standard deviation for separate measurements in eight 400–450-g male Sprague-Dawley rats.

family of nuclear receptors, comprising such diverse receptors as those for steroids and thyroid hormones, retinoids and vitamin D3, present in vertebrates, arthropods and nematodes. The members of this superfamily act both as ligand-modulated transcriptional activators and suppressors, while no ligands have yet been found for a large group of so-called 'orphan' nuclear receptors. Nuclear receptors may have acquired ligand-binding ability during evolution, suggesting that the ancestral nuclear receptor was an orphan (Escriva *et al.*, 1997).

Retinoid receptors regulate complex physiological events that trigger key steps in development, control maintenance of homeostasis and induce or inhibit cellular proliferation, differentiation and death. Retinoid receptors have strong differentiation and anti-proliferative activity. Each of the subtypes of retinoic acid comprises three isotypes designated α, β and γ localized to chromosomes 17q21, 3p24 and 12q13, respectively. The RXR α, β and γ genes have been mapped to chromosomes 9q34.3, 6p21.3 and 1q22-23, respectively (Chambon, 1996). The RARs bind both all-*trans*-retinoic acid and 9-*cis*-retinoic acid,

whereas the RXRs bind only 9-*cis*-retinoic acid. These receptors also bind a variety of synthetic retinoids, some of which show RAR or RXR selectivity or preferentially bind to specific RAR isotypes.

The genetic activities of retinoid receptors and other nuclear receptors result from both direct modulation of the activity of cognate gene programmes and mutual interference with the activity of other signalling pathways and regulatory events that occur at the post-transcriptional level (e.g. mRNA and protein stabilization or destabilization). More than 70 nuclear receptors have been identified. With the exception of some unusual nuclear receptors which appear to contain only regions homologous to the DNA- or ligand-binding domains, all have an identical structural organization, with an *N*-terminal region A/B followed by a DNA-binding domain comprised of two zinc fingers (region C), a linker region D and the ligand-binding domain. Some nuclear receptors contain a C-terminal region F of unknown function. Two autonomous *trans*-activation functions (AFs), a constitutively active AF-1 in region A/B and a ligand-dependent AF-2 in the ligand-binding domain, are responsible for the transcriptional activity of nuclear receptors (Gronemeyer & Laudet, 1995; Chambon, 1996). Figure 3 illustrates the canonical domain structure and associated functions of nuclear receptors.

For each RAR and RXR subtype, two to four isoforms (e.g. RARs β_1, β_2, β_3 and β_4) are generated by differential use of alternative promoters and alternative splicing; consequently, they differ in their A domain (Gronemeyer & Laudet, 1995; Chambon, 1996). Each receptor isoform may regulate a distinct subset of retinoid-responsive genes; these RARs have greater nucleotide sequence homology within single species (e.g. human RARα and human β), implying that RARs have distinct functions that have been conserved during evolution. Their expression is regulated spatio-temporally during embryonal development, and their expression patterns in certain adult tissues are distinct (Chambon, 1996). Studies with the embryonal carcinoma cell line F9, in which specific receptors have been disrupted by homologous

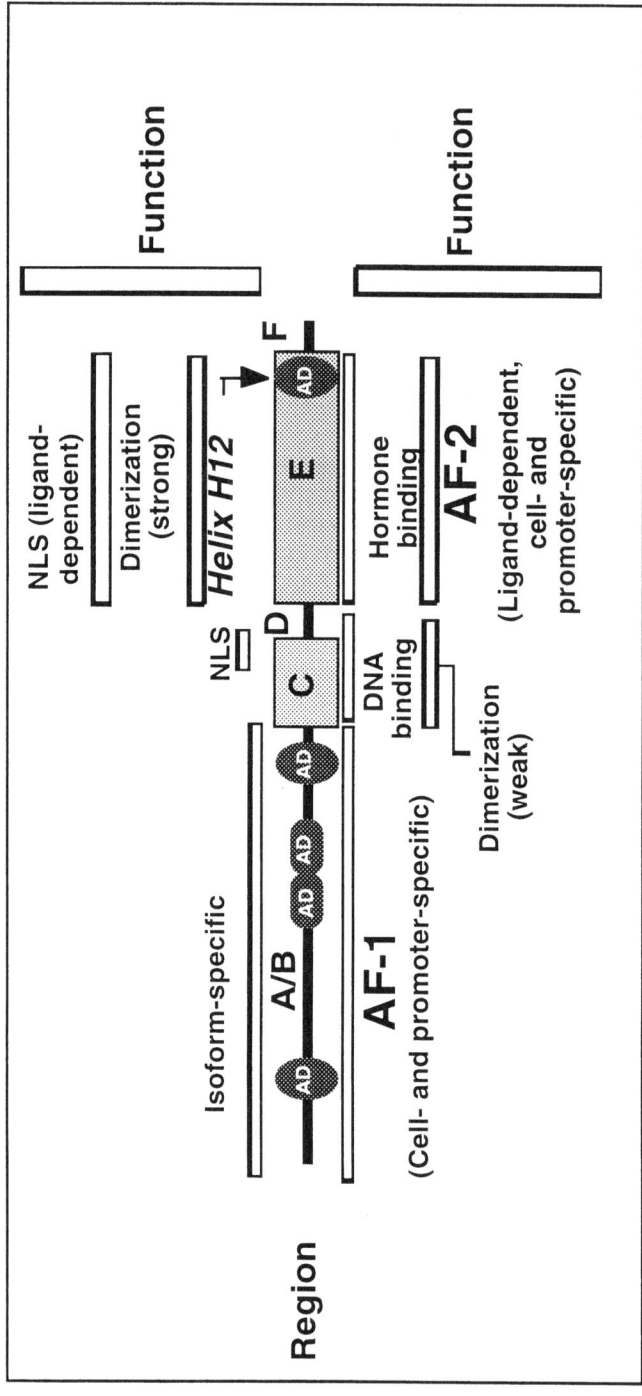

Figure 3. Schematic illustration of the structural and functional organization of nuclear receptors

The evolutionarily conserved regions C and E are indicated as boxes, and a black bar represents the divergent regions A/B, D and F. Note that region F may be absent in some receptors. Domain functions are depicted below and above the scheme; most were identified in structure–function studies of steroid, thyroid and retinoid receptors. Two transcription activation functions (AFs) have been described in several nuclear receptors: a constitutively active (only if taken out of the context of the full-length receptor) AF-1 in region A/B and a ligand-inducible AF-2 in region E. Within the AF-1s of some nuclear receptors, autonomous *trans*-activation domains (ADs) have been defined. At the C-terminal of the ligand-binding domain, the core of an activation domain, which is critical for AF-2 function, corresponds to the helix H12 in the three-dimensional structure of the ligand-binding domain. NLS, nuclear localization signal recombination, have indicated that RARα regulates the expression of CRABP-II and the homeobox gene *Hoxb-1*, whereas RARγ mediates the expression of the *Hoxa-1, Hoxa-3, laminin B1, collage IV (alpha-1)*, zinc finger transcription factor *GATA-4* and bone morphogenetic protein 2 (*BMP-2*) genes. Furthermore, RARα and RARγ were associated with opposite effects on the metabolism of all-*trans*-retinoic acid to more polar derivatives (Boylan *et al.*, 1995).

Nuclear receptors bind as homodimers (e.g. steroid receptors, RXR) and/or heterodimers (e.g. retinoic acid, thyroid and vitamin D receptors) with the promiscuous heterodimerization partner RXR to cognate response elements of target genes (Gronemeyer & Laudet, 1995; Chambon, 1996). Nuclear receptor activities are, however, not confined to cognate target genes; they can also 'cross-talk' in a ligand-dependent fashion with other signalling pathways, leading to mutual interference—positive or negative—with the *trans*-activation potentials of factors such as AP1 and NFκB (Pfahl, 1993; Göttlicher *et al.*, 1998). Other signalling pathways such as those operating through mitogen-activated protein kinase (Kato *et al.*, 1995; Hu *et al.*, 1996a) or cyclin-dependent kinase (CDK)7 (Rochette-Egly *et al.*, 1997) can target nuclear receptors directly and modify the activity of their AFs. For an illustration of the activities of nuclear receptors, see Figure 4.

Our understanding of nuclear receptor action at the molecular level has recently been enhanced dramatically due to progress in various domains, comprising:
- the identification and characterization of several novel classes of transcriptional mediators (transcription intermediary factors/co-regulators; co-activators and co-repressors) and the first steps towards the description of a plethora of interactions reported to occur between receptor, mediators, chromatin and the basal transcription machinery (Moras & Gronemeyer, 1998; Torchia *et al.*, 1998);
- the genetic analysis of receptor function (Beato *et al.*, 1995; Kastner *et al.*, 1995);
- the identification of novel (candidate) ligands for known and novel 'orphan' receptors (Mangelsdorf & Evans, 1995;

Forman *et al.*, 1998; Kliewer *et al.*, 1998);
- determination of the three-dimensional structures of the apo-, holo- and antagonist-bound ligand-binding domains of several nuclear receptors (Brzozowski *et al.*, 1997; Moras & Gronemeyer, 1998; Nolte *et al.*, 1998; Shiau *et al.*, 1998) and prediction of a common fold of all nuclear receptor ligand-binding domains (Wurtz *et al.*, 1996);
- crystallization of complexes between agonist-bound nuclear receptor ligand-binding domains and peptides derived from the nuclear receptor-binding surface of co-activators which revealed the structural basis of (one type of) antagonism; and
- the synthesis, characterization and analysis of the three-dimensional structure of isotype-selective nuclear receptor ligands, particularly for RARs and RXRs.

3.1 DNA recognition by nuclear receptors
3.1.1 Response elements of nuclear receptors: The common principle
All nuclear receptors recognize derivatives of the same hexameric DNA core motif, 5'-PuGGTCA (Pu = A or G; this sequence corresponds to a so-called 'half-site' of the everted repeat (ER) recognition sequence in Figure 5). Nevertheless, mutation, extension, duplication and distinct relative orientations of repeats of this motif generate response elements that are selective for a given class of receptors (Figure 5). Apparently co-evolutionarily, nuclear receptors devised mechanisms to interact with these sequences optimally: they either modified residues which establish contacts to the nucleotides that specify a given response element or generated response element-adapted homo- or heterodimerization interfaces.

3.1.2 Synthetic ligand response elements and spacer 'rules'
A simple rule has been proposed to describe the preference of the various direct repeat (DR)-recognizing receptors for elements with a certain spacer length (Umesono & Evans, 1989; Kliewer *et al.*, 1992). According to this rule, DRn elements with *n* spacer nucleotides have the following specifications:

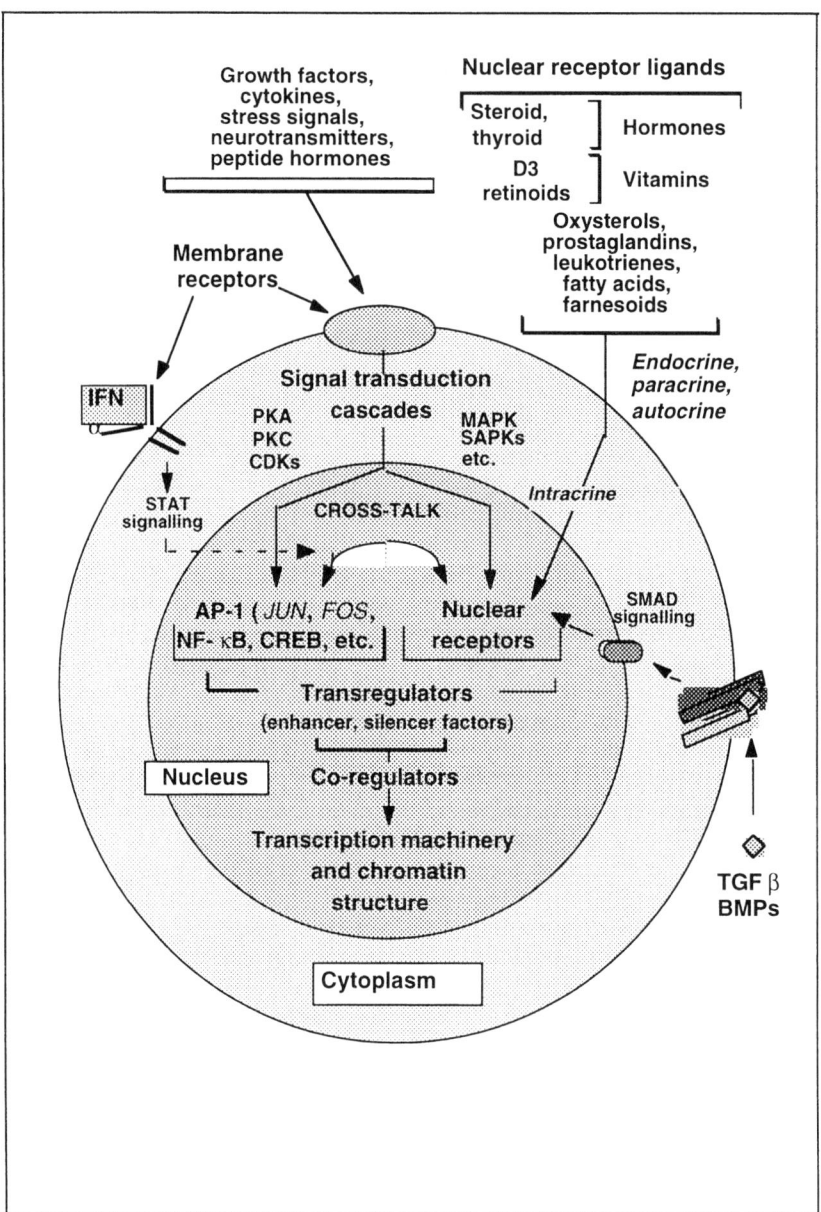

Figure 4. Schematic illustration of major signal transduction pathways involving membrane or nuclear receptors

Note the 'cross-talk' which gives rise to mutual interference between the various signalling cascades.
NR, nuclear receptor, IFN, interferon; PKA, protein kinase A; PKC, protein kinase C; CDK, cyclin-dependent kinase; MAPK, mitogen-activated protein kinase; SAPK, serum-activated protein kinase; STAT, signal transducer and activator of transcription; SMAD, mediator in transforming growth factor α (TGFα) signalling pathway; BMP, bone morphogenic protein

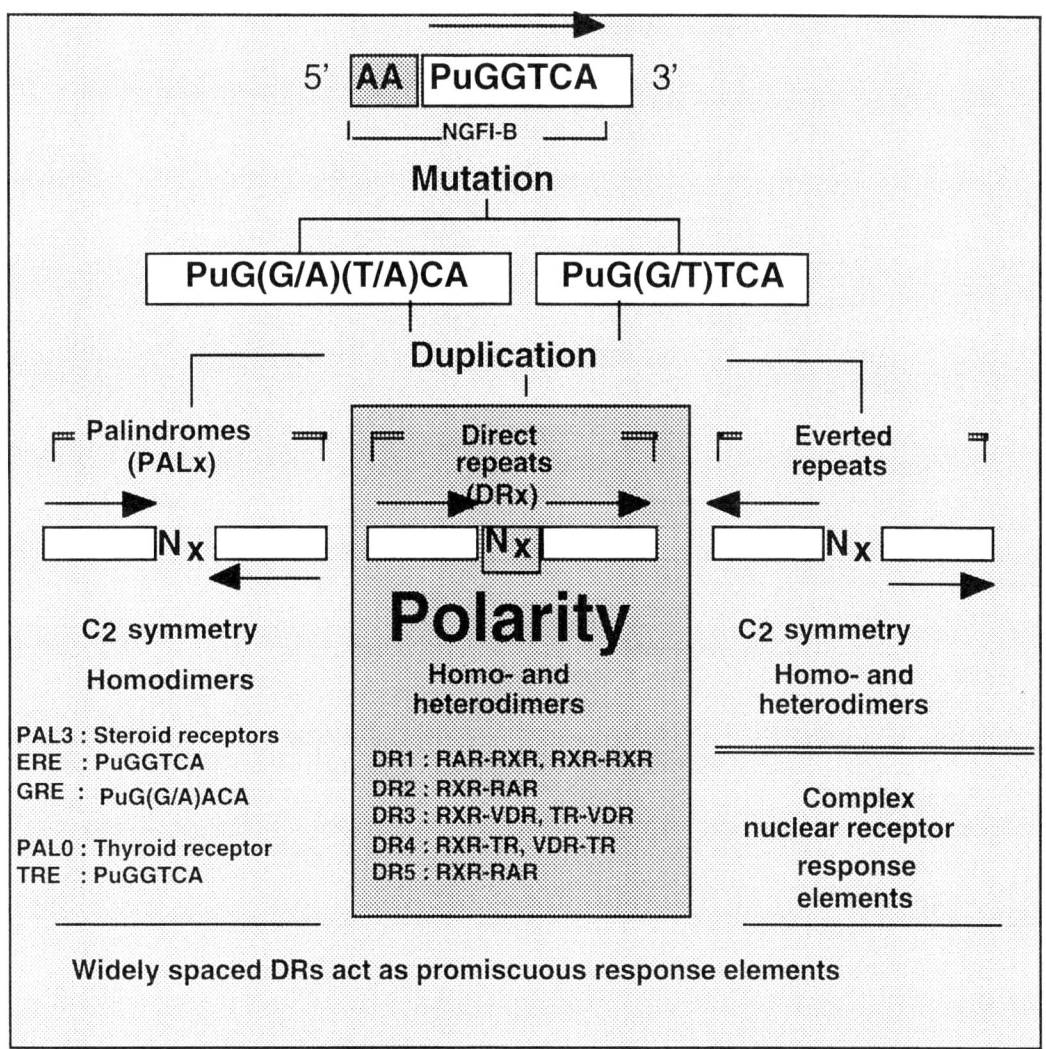

Figure 5. Response elements of nuclear receptors

The canonical core recognition sequence is 5'-PuGGTCA (arrows indicate the 5' to 3' direction) which, together with two 5' As, is a response element of the orphan receptor NGFI-B. Duplication of the core sequence generates symmetrical palindromes (PALx) and everted repeats (ERx), and polar direct repeats (DRx), with x bp separating the two half-sites. PAL3 is an oestrogen-response element (ERE), while PAL0 corresponds to a thyroid hormone-response element (TRE). A single alteration at position 4 of the core sequence from T to A leads to PAL3 response elements (GREs) recognized by the glucocorticoid receptor (and also androgen, progesterone and mineralocorticoid receptors). Note that most response elements are far from ideal; often one of the half-sites contains one or more mutations. Whereas PALs bind homodimers, DRs can bind homo- or heterodimers with the specificities shown in the dark box (polarity of the receptors on their cognate DRs: left, 5'; right, 3'). Note that the 3'-positioned receptor makes minor groove DNA contacts in the spacer. Some everted repeats are response elements for homo- or heterodimers of the thyroid or retinoid receptors. Response elements are known which are comprised of complex arrangements of the core motif. TR, thyroid receptor; VDR vitamin D receptor

n	Systematic name	Acronym	Receptor complex
1	DR1	RXRE	RXR–RXR
2	DR2	RARE	RAR–RXR
3	DR3	VDRE	VDR–RXR
4	DR4	TRE	TR–RXR
5	DR5	RARE	RAR–RXR

where TR is thyroid receptor and VDR is vitamin D receptor.

This rule does not take into consideration a number of important aspects of receptor–DNA interaction:

- It is unclear whether DR1 RXREs exist in natural genes.
- DR1 elements have been shown to act as RAREs (Durand *et al.*, 1992).
- Several orphan receptors bind as homo- (HNF4) or heterodimers (COUP-TF/arp-1) with RXR to certain DR elements which 'belong' to other receptors according to the above spacer rule.
- The rule does not distinguish between homo- and heterodimers that may bind to distinct DR options (DR3 and DR6 VDREs).
- The rule does not take into consideration the polarity of the receptor–DNA complexes.

Note that, in addition to DR elements, several other types of (more complex) response elements exist (Figure 5).

3.1.3 Variability of the binding motif, spacer sequence and flanking nucleotides

There is considerable degeneration in the sequence of half-site motifs of a given type of natural retinoid response element (see Figure 6), and the various receptors have distinct preferences for certain motifs. For example, the preference for the half-site motif 5'-PuGGTCA over 5'-GTTCA follows the order TR > RXR > RAR (Mader *et al.*, 1993). A receptor-specific preference for certain nucleotides in the DR spacer is also seen. A DNA binding site selection with RAR/RXR, TR/RXR and VDR/RXR heterodimers to identify the optimal 3'-positioned motif and spacer sequence has been reported (Kurokawa *et*

al., 1993) and is easily rationalized in the light of the crystallographic data (Rastinejad *et al.*, 1995).

3.1.4 Response elements for retinoids

The classical retinoic acid response element (RARE), which was found in the P2 promoter of the *RARβ* gene and gives rise to *RARβ2* mRNA, is a 5 base pair-spaced direct repeat 4 (generally referred to as DR5) of the motif 5'-PuGTTCA (Figure 6). In addition, response elements with a DR5 containing the motif 5'-PuGGTCA (also termed DR5G to distinguish it from the DR5T of the RARβ2 promoter) act as perfect RAREs (de Thé *et al.*, 1990; Hoffmann *et al.*, 1990; Sucov *et al.*, 1990), as do direct 5'-PuGGTCA repeats spaced by one base pair (DR1) or two base pairs (DR2) (Figures 5 and 6). RAR–RXR heterodimers bind to and activate transcription from these three types of RARE, provided the target cells express both RARs and RXRs. DR1 elements bind not only RAR–RXR heterodimers but also RXR homodimers *in vitro*, and RXRs can *trans*-activate target genes containing DR1 elements in response to a RXR ligand. The notion that DR1 elements can act as functional retinoid X-receptor response elements (RXREs) *in vivo* is supported by their activity in yeast cells (Heery *et al.*, 1994), in which any contribution of endogenous RAR by heterodimerization with RXR can be excluded. The only reported natural RXRE is a DR1-related element found in the rat CRBPII promoter (Mangelsdorf *et al.*, 1991). RXR-specific induction of this CRBPII promoter *in vivo* has not yet been demonstrated, and the lack of conservation of the CRBPII RXRE in the mouse homologue (Nakshatri & Chambon, 1994) casts some doubt on its physiological role as an RXRE.

Further examples of genes that have a DR5 response element and are induced by retinoids include RARα2 (Leroy *et al.*, 1991), RARγ2 (Lehmann *et al.*, 1992), the rat cellular retinoid binding protein I (cCRBPI) (Husmann *et al.*, 1992), the medium chain acyl-coenzyme A dehydrogenase gene (Raisher *et al.*, 1992), rat α-fetoprotein gene (Liu *et al.*, 1994), *Hoxb-1* (Marshall *et al.*, 1994), the human tissue-type plasminogen activator gene (Bulens *et al.*, 1995), intercellular adhesion molecule-1 gene

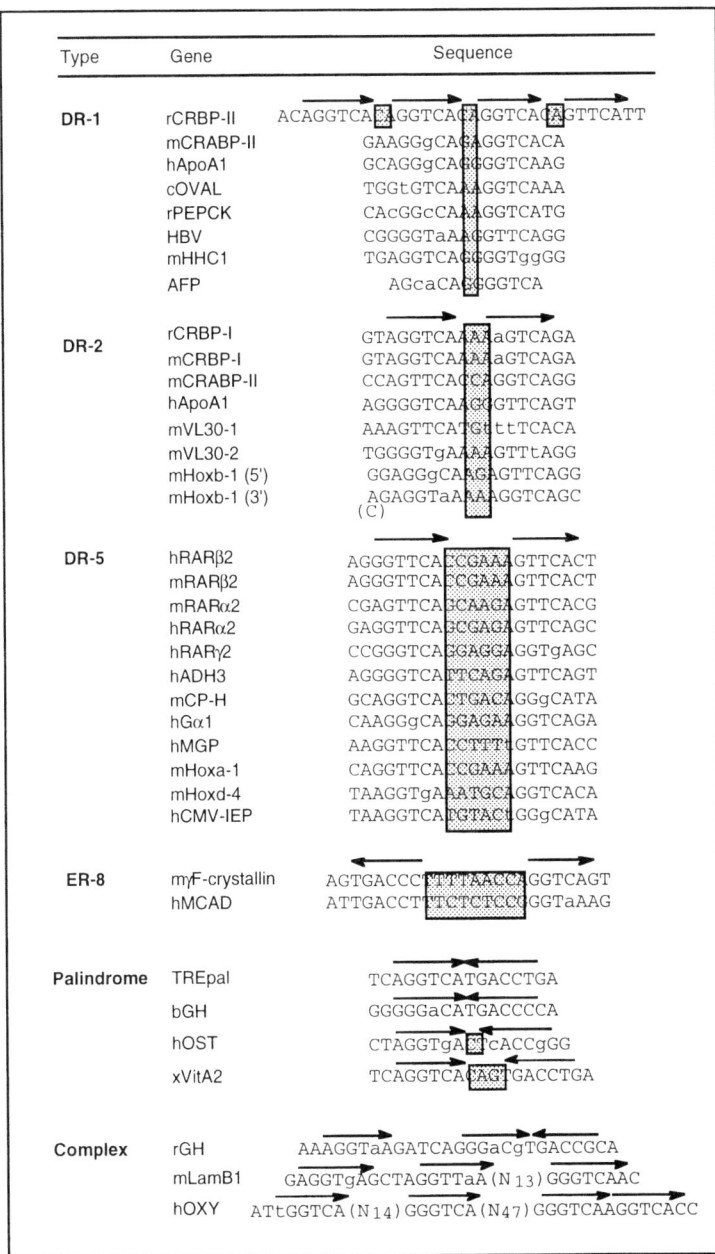

Figure 6. Natural retinoic acid response elements

Modified from Gronemeyer and Laudet (1995). Natural response elements that respond to retinoic acid are assembled into distinct direct-repeat (DR) groups and aligned according to their DR spacer (represented by a shaded box). The hexameric core motif and its orientation (compare with Figure 5) are indicated as an arrow. Non-consensus nucleotides are shown in small letters. ER, everted repeat

(Aoudjit *et al.*, 1995), the phosphoenolpyruvate carboxykinase gene (Scott *et al.*, 1996), the Pro alpha (I) collagen gene (Meisler *et al.*, 1997) and allelic human Pi class glutathione S-transferase gene (Lo & Ali-Osman, 1997).

In a few genes, RAREs have been found in the 3' flanking region rather than the 5' flanking region. These include the *Hox A* and *Hox B* homeobox gene cluster (Langston & Gudas, 1992; Langston *et al.*, 1997). A RARE was also found in the first intron of the human *CD38* gene (Kishimoto *et al.*, 1998).

In addition to RAR and RXR heterodimers, RXR homodimers may activate DR5 RARE such as the one in the RARβ promoter (Spanjaard *et al.*, 1995).

3.1.5 *DNA binding and receptor dimerization*
3.1.5.1 *Homo- and heterodimerization*
Nuclear receptors can bind their cognate response elements as monomers, homodimers or heterodimers with another family member (Glass, 1994). Dimerization is a general mechanism used to increase binding site affinity, specificity and diversity due to

*   cooperative DNA binding (an extreme case of cooperative binding is the existence, in solution, of stable dimers),
*   the lower frequency of two-hexamer rather than single-hexamer binding motifs separated by a defined spacer (statistically, a hexameric repeat like the oestrogen response element is 46 times less frequent than a single half-site motif) and
*   the existence of recognition sites in heterodimers that are distinct from those of homodimers.

Steroid hormone receptors generally bind as homodimers to their response elements, while RAR, RXR, TR and VDR can homo- and heterodimerize. RXRs play a central role in these signal transduction pathways, since they can both homodimerize and act as promiscuous heterodimerization partners for RAR, TR, VDR and some orphan receptors. Heterodimerization has a threefold effect: it leads to a novel response element repertoire, increases the efficiency of DNA binding relative to the corresponding homodimers, and allows two signalling inputs,

that of the ligands of RXR and its partner. A phenomenon called 'RXR subordination' maintains the identity of pathways for retinoic acid, thyroid and vitamin D signalling (see below). It is not clear whether some RXR complexes are permissive to RXR ligands in the absence of a ligand for the partner of RXR. Two dimerization interfaces can be distinguished in nuclear receptors, a weak one by the DNA-binding domains and a strong one by the ligand-binding domains. Ligand-binding domains dimerize in solution, while the interface of DNA-binding domains is apparently seen only when bound to DNA. The crystal structures of DNA-binding domain homo- and heterodimers and the RXR ligand-binding domain homodimer have defined the structures involved in dimerization (Gronemeyer & Moras, 1995). The response element repertoire described above for receptor homo- and heterodimers (Figure 5) is dictated by the DNA-binding domain, while the interface formed by the ligand-binding domains stabilizes the dimers but does not play any role in response element selection.

3.1.5.2 *Specificity of DNA recognition*
The specificity of the DNA response element (half-site sequence, spacing and orientation) is generated by recognition of the actual 'core' or 'half-site' motif and by the dimerization characteristics (mono-, homo- or heterodimerization; structure of the actual dimerization interface) of the receptor(s). The residues involved in distinguishing the hexameric half-site motives of oestrogen-response elements (5'-AGGTCA) and those recognized by glucocorticoid receptors (5'-AGAACA) were identified in a series of refined swapping experiments. Initially, DNA-binding domain swaps showed that specific half-site recognition depends on DNA-binding domain identity (Green & Chambon, 1987); subsequently, the N-terminal finger was found to differentiate between the two response elements (Green *et al.*, 1988). Three studies showed that two to three residues at the C-terminal 'knuckle' of the N-terminal finger, commonly referred to as the P-box (proximal box; see Figure 7), were responsible for the differentiation (Danielsen *et al.*, 1989; Mader *et al.*, 1989; Umesono & Evans, 1989).

A second region, the D-box (distal box; N-terminal 'knuckle' of the C-terminal finger; see Figure 7), was found to be involved in differentiating between binding to a three-base pair (characteristic of steroid receptor response elements) and a zero-base pair-spaced (one type of TRE) palindrome (Umesono & Evans, 1989). As was later confirmed by the crystal structures of GR and ER DNA-binding domains, this region does indeed contribute to the DNA-binding domain dimerization interface.

Two other boxes have been described within the DNA-binding domains of heterodimerizing receptors. The A-box was originally described as the sequence responsible for the recognition of two additional A nucleotides in the minor groove 5' of the hexameric core motif, thus generating an NGFI-B response element (NBRE; 5'-AAAGGTCA) (Wilson et al.,

1992). This A-box was later found to play a similar role in heterodimers such as 5'-RXR-TR on DR4 elements, where it specifies to some extent the spacer 5' of TR (Kurokawa et al., 1993) and sets minimal spacing by steric hindrance phenomena (Zechel et al., 1994). Interestingly, the A-box presents in the three-dimensional structure as a helix contacting the minor groove, and modelling indicates its role in setting a minimal distance between the half-sites (Rastinejad et al., 1995).

The T-box (Figure 7) was originally defined in RXRβ (then H-2RIIBP) as a sequence required for dimerization on a DR1 element (Wilson et al., 1992). Its role as a RXR homo- and heterodimerization surface has since been confirmed (Lee et al., 1993; Zechel et al., 1994).

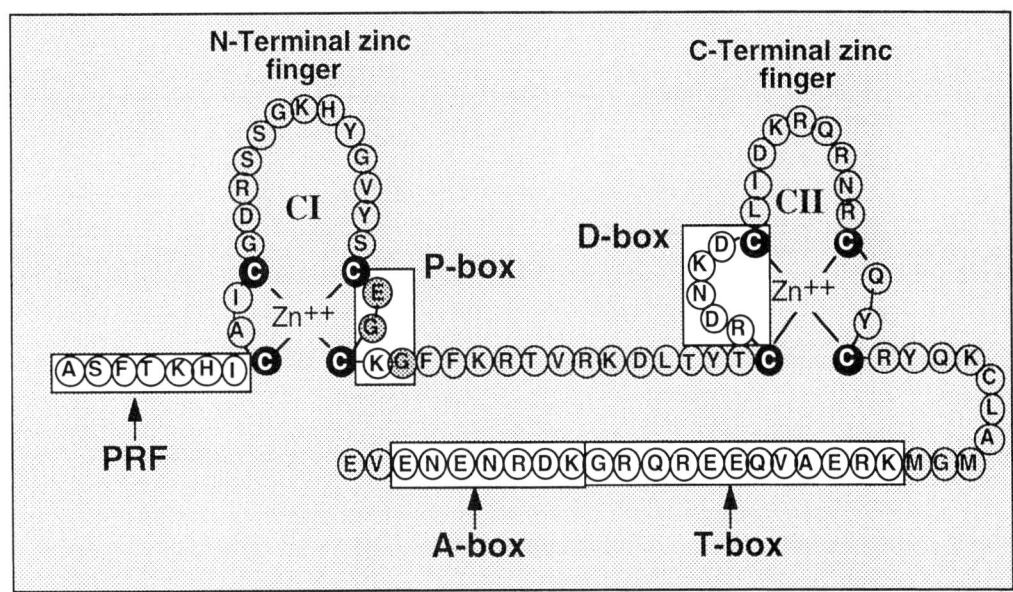

Figure 7. Schematic illustration of the retinoid X receptor DNA-binding domain

The boxes illustrate regions involved in response element selection. The P (proximal) box is part of the DNA recognition helix, and swapping of the EG. A residues (black circles, the sequence reads cEGckA) of the ER P-box with the corresponding GS..V residues of GR switches oestrogen-response element to that recognized by the glucocorticoid receptor. The D (distal) box is responsible for PAL3/PAL0 selection by oestrogen or thyroid hormone receptors and contributes to the homodimerization interfaces of ER and GR DNA-binding domains. The T-box region forms a helix and corresponds to a dimerization surface in RXR homodimers. The TR A-box forms a helix which makes DNA backbone and minor groove contacts and precludes the formation of RXR–TR complexes on direct repeats spaced by less than 4 base pairs. CI and CII are the two zinc-finger motifs; PRF, pre-finger region.

3.2 Structure of nuclear receptor ligand-binding domains

3.2.1 Canonical fold

The crystal structures of six nuclear receptor ligand-binding domains have been described so far: the dimeric apo-RXRα (Figures 8 and 9; Bourguet *et al.*, 1995), monomeric holo-RARγ (Figures 8 and 9; Renaud *et al.*, 1995; Klaholz *et al.*, 1998), monomeric holo-TRα (Wagner *et al.*, 1995), dimeric holo (oestradiol, diethylstilboestrol)- and antagonist (raloxifene, tamoxifen)-bound ERα (Brzozowski *et al.*, 1997; Shiau *et al.*, 1998; Tanenbaum *et al.*, 1998), dimeric holo (progesterone)-bound PR (Williams & Sigler, 1998) and apo- and holo (thiazolidinedione)-peroxisome proliferator-activated receptor (PPAR)γ (Nolte *et al.*, 1998). These nuclear receptor ligand-binding domains display a common fold, as originally predicted (Wurtz *et al.*, 1996), with 12 α-helices (H1–H12) and one β-turn arranged as an antiparallel α-helical 'sandwich' in a three-layer structure (Figures 8 and 9). Note that some variability exists; for example, no helix H2 was found in RARγ (Renaud *et al.*, 1995), while an additional short helix H2' is present in PPARγ (Shiau *et al.*, 1998).

3.2.2 The mouse-trap model

Comparison of the various apo- and holo-ligand-binding domain structures (Figures 8 and 9) suggested a common mechanism by which AF-2 becomes transcriptionally competent: after ligand binding, H11 is repositioned in the continuity of H10, and the concomitant swinging of H12 unleashes the W-loop which flips over underneath H6, carrying along the N-terminal part of H3. In its final position, H12 seals the ligand-binding cavity like a 'lid' and further stabilizes ligand binding (in some but not all nuclear receptors) by contributing additional ligand–protein interactions. It is a general and essential feature of the ligand 'activation' of nuclear receptors that the transconformation of H12 and additional structural changes such as bending of helix H3 create distinct surfaces on the apo- and holo-ligand-binding domains. The novel surfaces generated after agonist binding allow bona fide co-activators, such as members of the SRC-1/transcription intermediary

factor 2 family, to bind and recruit additional transcription factors (see below). Concomitantly, co-repressor proteins, which bind to presently unknown surface(s) of the apoligand-binding domain, dissociate after agonist but not necessarily antagonist binding (see below). Notably, certain antagonists 'force' H12 into a third position, distinct from the holo position whereby it impairs co-activator binding.

For a given receptor, the equilibrium between the apo and holo (or apo and antagonist) conformational states of a nuclear receptor ligand-binding domain can be affected through intramolecular interactions of H12, such as a salt bridge (holo-ligand-binding domain of RARγ, Figure 8; Renaud *et al.*, 1995) or hydrophobic contacts, as suggested for apo-ER (White *et al.*, 1997b). This implies that the apo conformation is not necessarily the default state, so that some nuclear receptors may be constitutive activators or repressors without possessing a cognate ligand. Moreover, an increase in co-activator concentration can generate a transcriptionally competent RAR under certain conditions (Voegel *et al.*, 1998), and the apo-ER conformation may be destabilized by phosphorylation (Weis *et al.*, 1996; White *et al.*, 1997b). Thus, overexpression of co-activators or receptor modification may generate ligand-independent receptors.

3.2.3 The dimer interface

Most studies of nuclear receptor co-regulator interactions consider only nuclear receptor monomers; however, heterodimers can have a very different gamut of co-regulator interactions. The roles of H1, H12 and (ligand-dependent) intradimeric allosteric effects must therefore be taken into account in order to have a comprehensive molecular view of nuclear receptor ligand-binding domain function.

As predicted from studies of mutagenesis, the homodimeric contacts involve helix H10. The three interfaces are very similar, as first seen in the crystal structure of apo-RXRα and now observed in ERα, PR and PPARγ. The key element that locks the dimer interface is H10, which can self-associate through hydrophobic

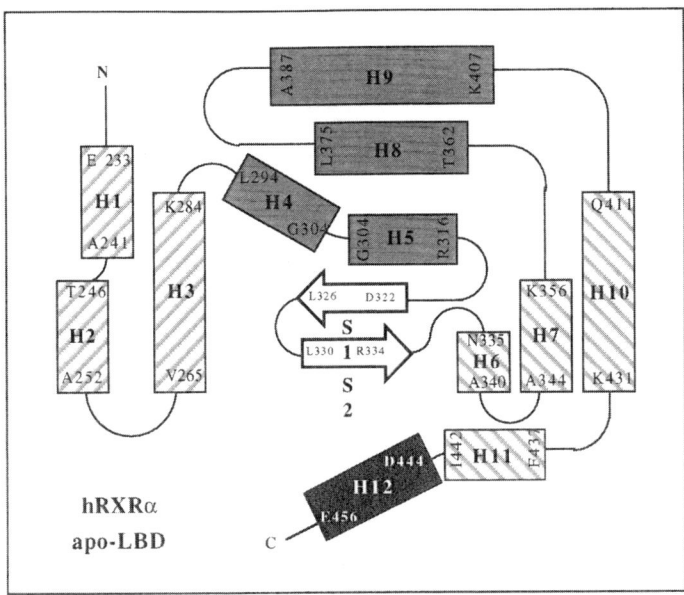

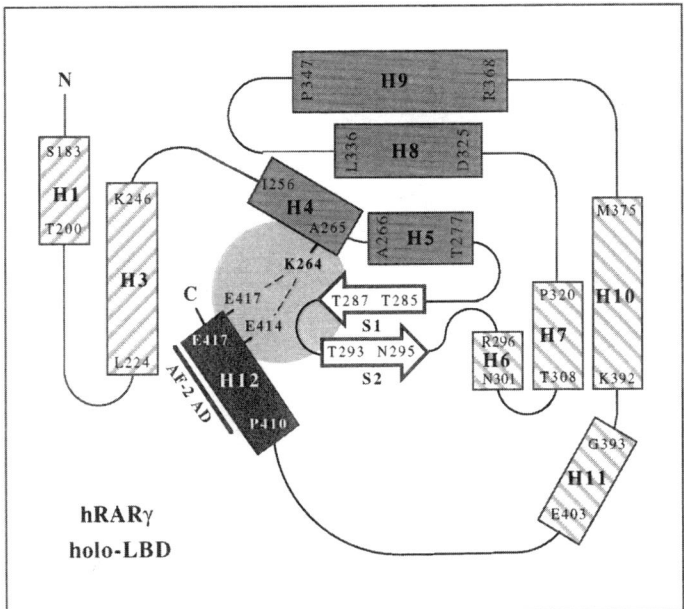

Figure 8. Topology of the apo-ligand-binding domain (LBD) of the retinoid X receptor (apo-RXRα) and the holo-LBD of the retinoic acid receptor (holo-RARγ).
Nuclear receptor ligand-binding domains form a β-helical sandwich with H4, H5, H8 and H9 (grey boxes) positioned between helices H1 to H3 and H6, H7, H10 (striped boxes). H12 (and to a lesser extent H11) undergoes major structural alteration ('*trans*-conformation') upon ligand binding. The N and C termini of the RXRα LBD are indicated, as well as the residues at the beginning and at the end of each α-helix or β-strand.

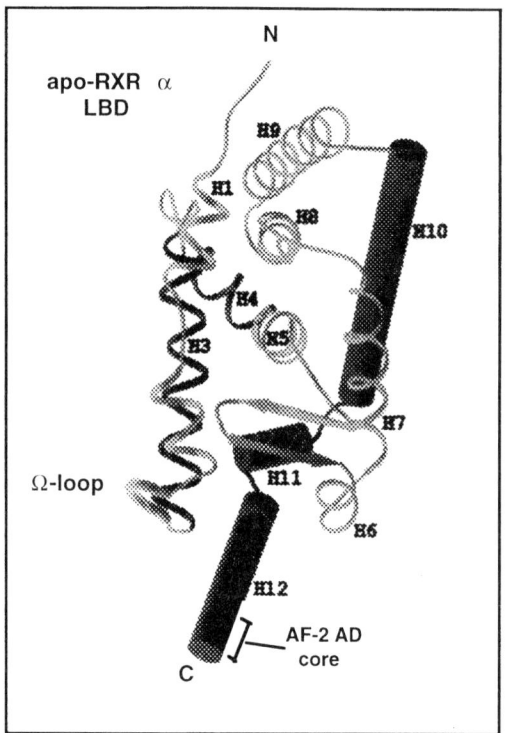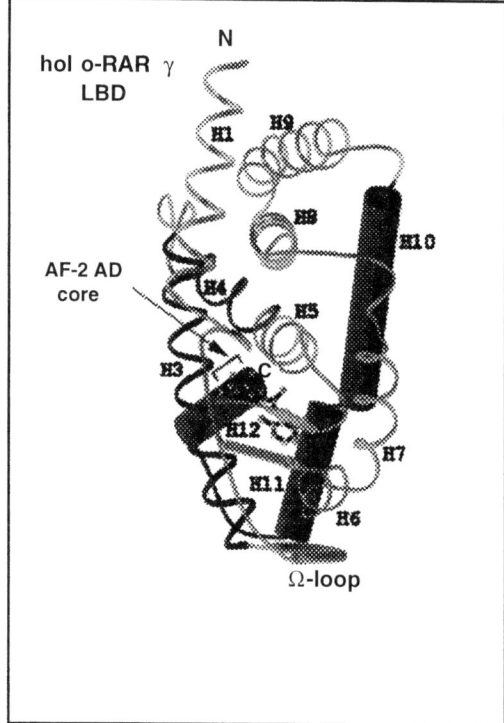

Figure 9. Three-dimensional structure of the apo-ligand-binding domain (LBD) of the retinoid X receptor (apo-RXRa) and the holo-LBD of the retinoic acid receptor (holo-RARγ)

The *trans*-conformation after ligand binding, which involves flipping of the W-loop, has been referred to as the 'mouse-trap mechanism' (see text and Renaud *et al.*, 1995). Note that these folds are prototypic folds which apply to the entire nuclear receptor superfamily (Wurtz *et al.*,1996). For illustration, helices H10, H11 and H12 are represented as black rods. The core of the activation func-

contacts, but helices H9 and H7 and the loops connecting H7 and H8 also contribute to dimer stability. The H12 of one subunit is proximal to H7 in the other, and this might provide the basis for allosteric cross-talk between subunits. If heterodimers were similarly associated, close proximity of H12 to the other subunit could play a significant role in the function of the nuclear receptor heterodimer, such as, for example, RXR subordination.

apo-RXR, in contrast to other apo-nuclear receptors, can form tetramers which dissociate after ligand binding (Kersten *et al.*, 1995, 1996; Chen *et al.*, 1998). These tetramers could be a storage form of this promiscuous heterodimerization partner.

3.2.4 The ligand-binding pocket

In all the crystal structures presently available, the ligand is embedded within the protein, with no clearly accessible entry or exit. PPARγ seems to be the only exception to that rule, since a potential access cleft to the ligand-binding protein was observed between H3 and the β-turn which could be of sufficient size to allow entry of small ligands without major adaptation. For all other receptors of known structure, significant conformational changes are necessary to generate potential entry sites. The mouse-trap model provides an easy solution to the problem: the mobility of H12 opens a channel by removing the 'lid' from the ligand pocket.

The ligand-binding pockets are lined with mostly hydrophobic residues. A few polar residues at the deep end of the pocket near the β-turn act as anchors for the ligand or play an essential role in the correct positioning and enforce the selectivity of the pocket. Most nuclear receptors contain a conserved arginine attached to H5 which points into this part of the cavity. These anchoring residues, conserved within a given subfamily, are indicative of the polar group characteristics of each family of ligands (i.e. carboxylate for retinoids and ketone for steroids).

3.2.5 Ligand selectivity

As shown in the cases of RARγ and TRβ, the shape of the ligand-binding pocket matches that of the ligand. The accordance of shape and volume maximize the number of mostly hydrophobic contacts, thus contributing to the stability of the complex and the selectivity of the pocket for the cognate ligand.

The RAR has a ligand-binding domain that can bind two chemically different ligands equally well: all-*trans*-retinoic acid and its 9-*cis* isomer. Crystallographic analysis of the two ligands in the RARγ ligand-binding domain showed that both adapt conformationally to the ligand-binding protein, which acts as a matrix (Klaholz et al., 1998). Moreover, the conformation of a RARγ-selective agonist was shown to match that of the natural ligands in their bound state. The adaptation of ligands to the protein leads to an optimal number of interactions for binding and selectivity and justifies modelling approaches for ligand design.

For steroid receptors, the volume of ligand-binding protein is significantly larger than that of the corresponding ligands, and the rigidity of the ligand does not allow adaptability. Therefore, selectivity cannot be driven by multiple hydrophobic contacts, which could not suffice to discriminate between small structurally similar ligands. Very large volumes of ligand-binding protein allow binding of multiple ligands with different stereochemistry, as in the case of PPAR (Nolte et al., 1998), often at the expense of lower binding affinities.

As in a structure-based sequence alignment, only three residues diverged in the ligand-binding proteins of RAR α, β and γ. It was predicted that these divergent residues were critically involved in differentiating between isotype-selective retinoids (Renaud et al., 1995). Indeed, swapping of these residues confirmed the hypothesis (Gehin et al., 1999) and also confirmed the agonistic/antagonistic response towards the ligand onto any other RAR isotype.

3.2.6 Molecular consequences of ligand binding

A model was proposed in which holo nuclear receptors transmitted their activity to the basal transcription machinery via transcription intermediary factors or co-regulators. This hypothesis was based on so-called 'squelching' experiments in which it was observed that overexpression of one receptor ('autosquelching'; Bocquel et al., 1989) or of a different receptor ('heterosquelching'; Meyer et al., 1989) inhibited agonist-induced *trans*-activation in a receptor dose- and ligand-dependent manner. These data were interpreted as the result of sequestration of transcription intermediary factors from the transcription initiation complex by either excess of the same or addition of another ligand-activated receptor.

3.3 Retinoid X receptor subordination

RXR cannot respond to RXR-selective agonists in the absence of an RAR ligand. This phenomenon is generally referred to as RXR 'subordination' or RXR 'silencing' by apoRAR. In the presence of an RAR agonist or certain RAR antagonists, RXR agonists further stimulate the transcriptional activity of RAR–RXR heterodimers synergistically (Figure 10; Chen et al., 1996). RXR subordination solves a potential problem that arises from the ability of RXR to act as a promiscuous heterodimerization partner for numerous nuclear receptors, compromising signalling pathway identity, since in the absence of subordination RXR ligands could simultaneously activate multiple heterodimeric receptors, such as RAR–RXR, TR–RXR and VDR–RXR and confuse retinoic acid, thyroid hormone and vitamin D3 signalling, respectively. Retinoic acid-deprived animals do not, however, have abnormalities that could readily be related to impaired thyroid hormone or vitamin D3 signalling. Moreover, RXR-selective ligands on their own could not trigger RXR–RAR heterodimer-mediated retinoic acid-induced events in various cell systems (Chen *et al.*, 1996; Clifford *et al.*, 1996; Taneja *et al.*, 1996). This is not due to an inability of the RXR partner to bind its cognate ligand in DNA-bound heterodimers, as was previously suggested (Kurokawa *et al.*, 1994), as RXR ligand binding has been demonstrated to occur in such complexes in several studies *in vitro*, and synergistic *trans*-activation induced by RAR- and RXR-selective ligands has been observed *in vivo* (Apfel *et al.*, 1995; Chen *et al.*, 1996, 1997; Clifford *et al.*, 1996; Kersten *et al.*, 1996; Taneja *et al.*, 1996; Li *et al.*, 1997; Minucci *et al.*, 1997). Thus, RAR apparently 'controls' the activity of RXR–RAR heterodimers in two ways: it induces transcription in response to its own ligand and silences RXR activity in the absence of an RAR ligand. Consequently, the only way for RXR to affect *trans*-activation in response to its ligand in RXR–RAR heterodimers is through synergy with RAR ligands (Figure 10). This concept of RXR silencing may not apply to all nuclear receptor partners, as the ligand-induced RXR activity was permissive in heterodimers with NGFI-B, leading even to a synergistic response (Forman *et al.*, 1995; Perlmann & Jansson, 1995). Neither the existence of an endogenous NGFI-B ligand nor weak constitutive activity of the NGFI-B AF-2 can be excluded; both could readily explain RXR activity and NGFI-B–RXR synergy due to the absence of RXR silencing.

3.4   Retinoid receptor cross-talk with other signalling pathways

Retinoid receptors can regulate gene expression by interacting directly, as homodimers and/or heterodimers, with cognate response elements in target gene promoters. At least three types of regulatory mechanism exist, by which several nuclear receptors, including retinoid receptors:

- can positively or negatively mutually interfere with gene activation in programmes of other signalling pathways (including so-called AP-1 *trans*-repression; Göttlicher *et al.*, 1998),
- act through the response elements of other

transcription factors in a ligand-dependent but DNA binding-independent fashion (Gaub *et al.*, 1990; Paech *et al.*, 1997),
- be affected by the activity of other signalling pathways, resulting for example in receptor phosphorylation and concomitant modification of its activity (Kato *et al.*, 1995; Hu *et al.*, 1996a; Rochette-Egly *et al.*, 1997).

Transcriptional interference is not restricted to AP-1 but can also involve factors such as NFκB1, STAT5, C/EBP and Oct-2A. Examples of genes that have been shown to be suppressed by all-*trans*-retinoic acid through antagonism of AP-1 include stromelysin (Nicholson *et al.*, 1990), collagenase (matrix metalloproteinase-1) (Schüle *et al.*, 1991; Schroen & Brinckerhoff, 1996; Guerin *et al.*, 1997), involucrin (Monzon *et al.*, 1996) and relaxin (Bernacki *et al.*, 1998).

all-*trans*-Retinoic acid can increase AP-1 activity, and this may be associated with cell differentiation in melanoma cells (Desai & Niles, 1997) or cell growth enhancement in a lung carcinoma cell line (Wan *et al.*, 1997). Whether all-*trans*-retinoic acid suppresses or increases AP-1 activity appears to be cell type-specific and may depend on the differentiation programme elicited and the abundance of co-factors.

3.4.1 Dissociation of trans-*activation and* AP-1 trans-*repression by synthetic retinoids*

Both RARs and RXRs (α, β and γ isotypes) can act as ligand-dependent *trans*-repressors of AP-1 (*c-Jun/c-Fos*) activity, and, reciprocally, AP-1 can inhibit *trans*-activation by RARs and RXRs. In the case of RAR, mutant analyses have shown that the integrity of both DNA and ligand-binding domains is required for efficient AP-1 repression. Notably, C-terminal truncation mutants lacking H12 fail to *trans*-repress, suggesting that H12 *trans*-conformation is involved in both *trans*-activation and *trans*-repression.

Several groups have generated ligands which are RAR isotype or RXR-selective agonists and antagonists and separate the *trans*-activation and *trans*-repression functions of

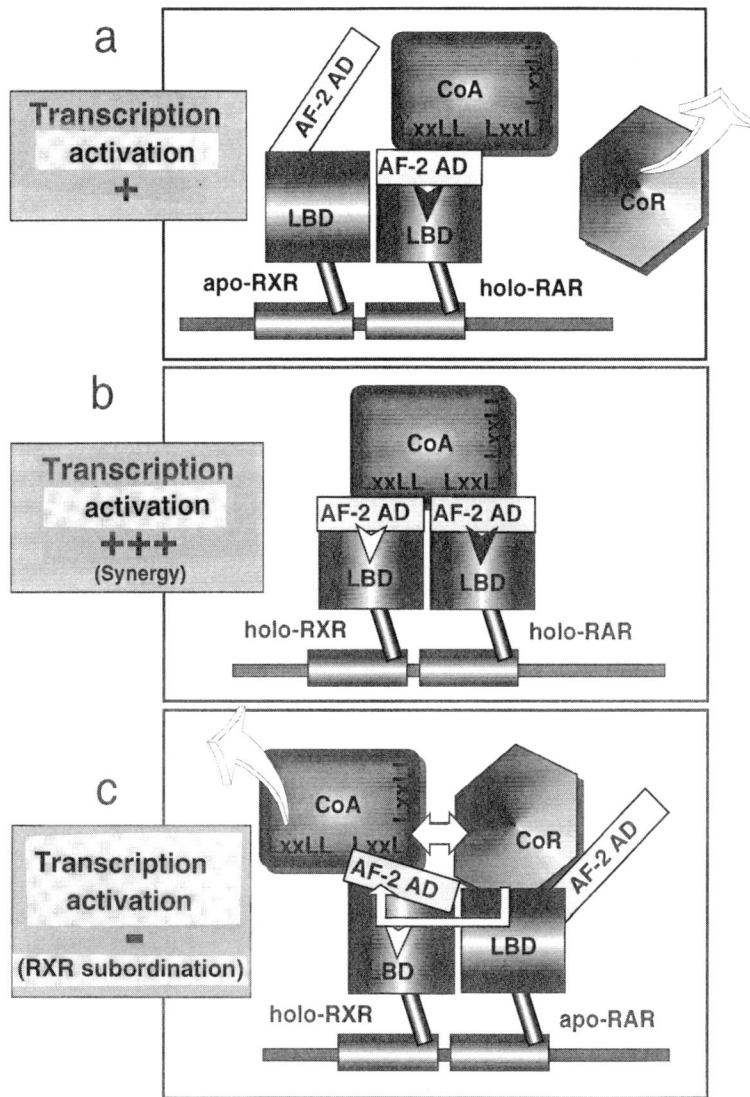

Figure 10. Model of retinoid X receptor (RXR) subordination by apo-retinoic acid receptor (RAR)

(a) In the presence of RAR agonists, co-repressor (CoR) dissociates from the RAR–RXR heterodimer and co-activator (CoA) is recruited and establishes a transcription activation-competent complex, probably through the RAR subunit. (b) Synergy between RAR and RXR agonists is due to cooperative binding of a co-activator through two of its LxxLL nuclear receptor boxes. (c) RXR ligand alone is unable to dissociate the co-repressor from the heterodimer but allows co-activator recruitment to the RXR subunit. Either allosteric or direct steric hindrance effects exerted by the co-repressor destabilize the co-activator complex, resulting in RXR subordination. LBD, ligand-binding protein retinoid receptors. The aim is to find ligands which are largely devoid of the side-effects of all-*trans*-retinoic acid and function as inducers of either apoptosis and/or differentiation or inhibitors of cell proliferation, preferably in a cell-specific manner. Both subunits of the RAR–RXR heterodimer contribute synergistically to differentiation and apoptosis in the model NB4 and HL60 acute promyelocytic leukaemia cell lines (Chen *et al.*, 1996; Kizaki *et al.*, 1996). Retinoids that can *trans*-repress AP-1 but are largely devoid of the ability to *trans*-activate cognate target genes can inhibit the growth of tumour cells (Chen *et al.*, 1995). Huang *et al.* (1997) suggested that the antitumour effect of synthetic retinoids requires the AP-1 repressive but not the 'classical' *trans*-activation ability of the cognate receptor, but HL60 cells differentiated and ceased proliferation in response to RAR–RXR agonists and not to a retinoid with anti-AP-1 activity that did not *trans*-activate target genes (Kizaki *et al.*, 1996). Similar AP-1 antagonism-independent antitumour effects of retinoids have been reported for neuroblastoma (Giannini *et al.*, 1997) and prostate cancer (de Vos *et al.*, 1997) cells. It may be possible to target the antitumour effect of retinoids to specific cell types or tissues by designing synthetic retinoids with a defined pattern of RAR isotype and RXR selectivity and *trans*-activation or *trans*-repression ability.

There may be insufficient experimental evidence to establish that 9-*cis*-retinoic acid is 'the' or 'a' physiological ligand for the RXR family of receptors. There is a considerable body of literature on the formation of 9-*cis*-retinoic acid within cells, tissues and organisms and on the actions of 9-*cis*-retinoic acid in living systems. Heyman *et al.* (1992) reported that the concentrations of 9-*cis*-retinoic acid in adult mouse liver and kidney are 13 and 100 pmol/g tissue, respectively, but Kurlandsky *et al.* (1995), who reported a limit of detection of only 4 pmol/g of tissue, were unable to detect this compound in adult rat liver, spleen, kidney, brain, adipose tissue, testis or muscle. Since no further reports of 9-*cis*-retinoic acid concentrations in tissues have appeared, it can only be considered a putative physiological ligand for RXRs.

The mechanisms by which nuclear receptors cross-talk with other signalling pathways remain elusive. Three models are being discussed, none of which comprehensively accounts for the observed phenomena.

(i) The CBP (a 265-kDa CREB-binding protein) sequestration model (Kamei *et al.*, 1996) is based on the assumption that both nuclear receptors and AP-1 compete for CBP/p300 as a common cofactor. The problem with this model is that receptor mutants (Heck *et al.*, 1994) and antagonists (Chen *et al.*, 1995; Vayssière *et al.*, 1997) exist which do not induce *trans*-activation and do not recruit co-activators but nevertheless are potent *trans*-repressors of AP-1 activity.

(ii) Interference with the Jun N-terminal kinase (JNK) signalling pathway, based on the blockade by hormone-activated nuclear receptors of c-Jun phosphorylation on Ser-63/73, is required to recruit the transcriptional co-activator CBP (Caelles *et al.*, 1997). A similar mechanism was observed in human bronchial epithelial cells where all-*trans*-retinoic acid decreased the amount and activation of AP-1 components. It inhibited JNK and, to a lesser extent, extracellular signal-regulated kinase activity and also reduced c-fos mRNA (Lee *et al.*, 1998). Pretreatment of human skin with all-*trans*-retinoic acid was found to inhibit induction of c-Jun protein by ultraviolet radiation and, consequently, AP-1 via a post-transcriptional mechanism, since all-*trans*-retinoic acid did not inhibit induction of c-Jun mRNA (Fisher *et al.*, 1998). This mechanism does not account for the inhibition of nuclear receptor activity by AP-1.

(iii) Disruption of c-Jun/c-Fos dimerization by retinoid receptors (Zhou *et al.*, 1999), observed in a mammalian two-hybrid system, could account for the finding that agonist-bound RAR can inhibit DNA binding by AP-1 *in vitro*. The mechanism does not, however, apply for the glucocorticoid receptor, as inhibition of AP-1 DNA binding by glucocorticoid receptor has been shown to be an artefact (König *et al.*, 1992).

3.4.2 Post-transcriptional mechanisms

Although transcriptional control is recognized as a major mechanism of regulation of gene expression during differentiation and development, alterations in gene expression through a post-transcriptional process are also an acknowledged mechanism for modulating important growth regulatory gene products. Through this mechanism, all-*trans*-retinoic acid can enhance or suppress the expression of genes that are already being actively transcribed rather than only inducing the expression of silent genes. A number of genes have been reported to be regulated by retinoic acid at the post-transcriptional level, but the mechanism is not clear. It has been proposed that all-*trans*-retinoic acid modulates RNA processing or transport out of the nucleus (Rosenbaum & Niles, 1992). In most studies, it was found that all-*trans*-retinoic acid stabilizes mRNA, and the stable mRNA levels of the oncogenes *p53* and *c-myc* were found to decrease in F9 embryonal carcinoma cells induced to differentiate into parietal endoderm by treatment with all-*trans*-retinoic acid and dibutyryl cyclic AMP. The decrease in *c-myc* was rapid (< 24 h), whereas the decrease in *p53* was observed after two to three days, and both were due to post-transcriptional regulation, as indicated by nuclear transcription assay *in vitro* (Dony *et al.*, 1985). Thus, in F9 embryonal carcinoma cells, some genes are regulated by all-*trans*-retinoic acid at the transcriptional level and others at the post-transcriptional level. Likewise, nuclear run-on transcriptional analysis showed no changes in the transcription rate of the four homeobox genes (*HOX-1*, *HOX-2*, *HOX-3* and *HOX-5*) in human embryonal carcinoma cells treated with all-*trans*-retinoic acid and induced to differentiate into several cell types. These data suggest that the activation of homeobox gene expression in retinoic acid-induced embryonal carcinoma cells is controlled, at least in part, by post-transcriptional mechanisms (Simeone *et al.*, 1989). Other genes shown to be up-regulated by mRNA stabilization include protein kinase C in melanoma cells (Rosenbaum & Niles, 1992), alkaline phosphatase in pre-osteoblastic cells (Zhou *et al.*, 1994), keratin 19 in squamous carcinoma cells (Crowe, 1993),

a secreted binding protein for fibroblast growth factors in squamous carcinoma cells (Liaudet-Coopman & Wellstein, 1996), connexin 43 in F9 embryonal carcinoma cells (Clairmont & Sies, 1997), Pbx protein (a heterodimerization partner of Hox proteins) in P19 embryonal carcinoma cells (Knoepfler & Kamps, 1997) and leukotriene C4 synthase in rat basophilic leukaemia cells (Hamasaki *et al.*, 1997). Although it is not clear how all-*trans*-retinoic acid stabilizes the mRNA of certain genes, it affects connexin 43 gene expression at the level of mRNA stability via elements located in the 3'-untranslated region (Clairmont & Sies, 1997). Another mechanism was suggested by studies on differentiation of the pre-osteoblastic cell line, UMR 201. In these cells, all-*trans*-retinoic acid caused a marked increase in the proficiency of post-transcriptional nuclear processing of alkaline phosphatase mRNA as a result of dephosphorylation of nuclear U1 70K spliceosome-component protein. A twofold decrease in mRNA expression of an isoform of alternative splicing factor that inhibits splicing was also observed (Manji *et al.*, 1999). Other mechanisms were described for the increased transcription of interleukin-1 β mRNA induced by all-*trans*-retinoic acid, although, unlike for other primary target genes, mRNA expression is regulated at pre-mRNA processing (Jarrous & Kaempfer, 1994).

A few studies have shown that all-*trans*-retinoic acid induces changes in protein stability. The half-life of bcl-2 protein was markedly shortened after treatment of blast stem cells of acute myeloblastic leukaemia with this compound (Hu *et al.*, 1996b). all-*trans*-Retinoic acid induced cyclin D1 proteolysis via proteasome in normal and immortalized human bronchial epithelial cells (Langenfeld *et al.*, 1997; Boyle *et al.*, 1999), and this effect may depend on retinoid receptors because retinoids that activated RARβ or RXR pathways preferentially led to a decrease in the amount of cyclin D1 protein (Boyle *et al.*, 1999). In contrast, all-*trans*-retinoic acid increased the stability of p53 protein in non-small cell lung cancer cells (Maxwell & Mukhopadhyay, 1994).

4.   Cellular biology of retinoids

Normal tissue homeostasis depends on coordinated regulation of cell proliferation, differentiation and apoptosis. The putative cancer-preventive effects of retinoids are thought to be associated with their ability to modulate the growth, differentiation and apoptosis of normal, premalignant and malignant cells *in vitro* and *in vivo*. Although cancer prevention occurs by definition *in vivo*, many fundamental concepts of the mechanisms of action of chemopreventive agents can be explored in studies with cells in monolayer culture, semisolid media, three-dimensional raft cultures and organ cultures. Retinoids exert pleiotropic effects on transformation of cells and tissues in culture. They suppress the transforming effects of carcinogens, inhibit the growth of immortalized 'premalignant' cells and suppress the transformed phenotype of fully malignant cells.

4.1   Effects of retinoids on cell transformation
The effects of retinoids on transformation of normal cells *in vitro* were examined in mouse embryonal cell, rat tracheal epithelial cell and human keratinocyte model systems. Certain retinoids inhibited transformation induced by carcinogens whether they were chemicals (Bertram, 1983; Langenfeld *et al.*, 1996), physical agents (Harisiadis *et al.*, 1978), viruses (Talmage & Lackey, 1992; Agarwal *et al.*, 1991; Khan *et al.*, 1993; Pomponi *et al.*, 1996) or oncogenes (Roberts *et al.*, 1985; Cox *et al.*, 1991).

Retinoids suppressed the growth of immortalized keratinocytes that mimic a carcinoma *in situ* in raft culture (Shindoh *et al.*, 1995; Eicher & Lotan, 1996). They also reversed histological changes induced by vitamin A deficiency in hamster trachea (Newton *et al.*, 1980; Chopra, 1983) and by exposure of mouse prostate to carcinogens in organ culture (Lasnitzki, 1976). Some of these systems (e.g. the hamster trachea system) have been used as preclinical screens for chemopreventive effects of retinoids (Newton *et al.*, 1980).

4.2   Effects of retinoids on cell proliferation
Investigations have been conducted with cells derived from normal tissues and cells immortalized with simian virus 40 large T antigen (Reddel *et al.*, 1988; Langenfeld *et al.*, 1996; Sun *et al.*, 1999a), human papillomavirus (HPV) E6/E7 (Khan *et al.*, 1993; Shindoh *et al.*, 1995) or Epstein-Barr virus (Pomponi *et al.*, 1996). Some of the latter cells were further transformed by exposure to carcinogens *in vitro* (Langenfeld *et al.*, 1997; Boyle *et al.*, 1999) or *in vivo* (Klein-Szanto *et al.*, 1992). The immortal and transformed cells provided an isogenic system of carcinogenesis *in vitro* in which the activities of chemopreventive agents could be compared (Sun *et al.*, 1999a; Boyle *et al.*, 1999). Retinoids were found to suppress the growth of certain cells. Human keratinocytes immortalized by HPV 16 DNA became more sensitive than normal keratinocytes to growth control by retinoids (Pirisi *et al.*, 1992). Treatment decreased the level of HPV E2/E5/6/E7 transcripts (Pirisi *et al.*, 1992; Khan *et al.*, 1993). Whereas early-passage HKc/HPV16 cells were very sensitive to growth inhibition by all-*trans*-retinoic acid, as the cells progressed in culture they lost their sensitivity to the retinoid (Creek *et al.*, 1995).

Most studies on the effects of retinoids on cells *in vitro* have been performed with cell lines derived from carcinogen-induced rodent tumours and spontaneous human cancers (Amos & Lotan, 1990; Gudas *et al.*, 1994). In most cells that are sensitive to the growth-inhibitory effects of retinoids in monolayer or suspension cultures, there are changes in cell cycle, most often an accumulation of cells in the G1 phase and a concomitant decrease in the numbers of cells in S and G2/M (Zhu *et al.*, 1997; Matsuo & Thiele, 1998). Growth inhibition is usually observed within 24–48 h of treatment and requires the continuous presence of retinoids, as the effects are usually reversible (except when apoptosis is induced, as described below). The concentrations of retinoids required to induce 50% growth inhibition (IC_{50}) relative to control cultures can range from nanomolar (physiological) to micromolar (pharmacological) concentrations. They depend on the solubility, hydro-phobicity and affinity for nuclear retinoid receptors of the retinoid and the rate of uptake, rate of catabolism of the retinoid, expression of cellular and nuclear retinoid-binding proteins and receptors and other factors related to the transcriptional machinery in the cell. The growth inhibitory effects of retinoids have been documented in a wide variety of tumour cell types, including melanoma, neuroblastoma, glioma, retinoblastoma, embryonal carcinoma, carcinomas of the lung, breast, prostate, bladder, colon, skin, head and neck and cervix and various types of sarcoma that grow as adherent monolayers on plastic tissue culture dishes, as well as in small-cell lung cancer cells isolated from pleural effusions and haematopoietic malignancies such as lymphomas, leukaemias, myelomas, premonocytic leukaemia and promyelocytic leukaemia which normally grow in suspension (Amos & Lotan, 1990; Gudas et al., 1994).

Retinoids also suppress the ability of certain malignant cells to form colonies in semisolid media, an anchorage-independence property that is a hallmark of transformed cells (Lotan et al., 1982; Amos & Lotan, 1990; Gudas et al., 1994). Tumour cells examined for response to retinoids in this assay are often more sensitive than in monolayer cultures (Lotan et al., 1982). Another advantage of the assay is that it has been adapted for analysis of the sensitivity to retinoids of tumour cells dissociated from fresh surgical specimens (Meyskens & Salmon, 1979; Meyskens et al., 1983; Cowan et al., 1983).

Natural and synthetic retinoids have been identified that are more effective in the various assays than all-trans-retinoic acid (Sun et al., 1997; 1999a). Some of these retinoids may pave the way towards the next generation of chemopreventive retinoids if they are found to have greater cell specificity and fewer side-effects than those currently in use.

4.3 Effects of retinoids on cell differentiation

HPV-transformed ectocervical cells were sensitive to the ability of retinoids to suppress squamous differentiation in monolayer cultures, which is also observed in normal cells (Agarwal et al., 1991). Many HPV-immortalized cell lines have shown greater sensitivity to sup-

pression of squamous differentiation by all-trans-retinoic acid than normal cells (Choo et al., 1995), but when HPV-immortalized keratinocytes derived in another laboratory were allowed to form three-dimensional organotypic raft cultures, they became less sensitive than normal cells to the suppressive effects of all-trans-retinoic acid on squamous differentiation (Merrick et al., 1993). all-trans-Retinoic acid enhanced mucin secretion by SPOC1 cells (rat tracheal cells immortalized by growth on tracheal grafts in vivo) during the early plateau stage of culture (Randell et al., 1996). Thus, it appears that all-trans-retinoic acid enhances the expression of the mucous phenotype while suppressing the squamous one.

Retinoids were found to modulate the differentiation of numerous types of cells derived from embryonal carcinoma, germ-cell tumour, choriocarcinoma, melanoma, neuroblastoma, astrocytoma, medulloblastoma, retinoblastoma, rhabdomyosarcoma, colon carcinoma, breast carcinoma, myeloid leukaemia, premonocytic leukaemia, erythroleukaemia and others (Lotan, 1995a). With the exception of normal and malignant keratinocytes, retinoids induced or enhanced the differentiation of these tumour cells (Gudas et al., 1994; Lotan, 1995a). In cultured keratinocytes and squamous-cell carcinomas, retinoids inhibited keratinizing squamous differentiation (Jetten et al., 1992; Lotan, 1993). Because in many tissues, such as buccal mucosa and bronchial epithelium, the keratinizing squamous differentiation of tumours derived from normally non-keratinizing epithelial cells is aberrant (i.e. it occurs during carcinogenesis or other pathological states), the inhibitory effect of retinoids on the expression of squamous differentiation markers can be viewed as restoration of the normal non-keratinizing phenotype (Lotan, 1993).

Although retinoids can induce many pathways of differentiation, extensive studies with cell lines derived from embryonal carcinoma, normal and malignant keratinocytes, premonocytic and myeloid leukaemias, neuroblastoma and melanoma indicate that they do not determine the pathway of differentiation but rather enhance predetermined programmes in cells that can undergo differentiation along one or more specific pathways. Notable examples are the P19 embryonal carcinoma cells, which can be induced to undergo either myogenic differentiation or neuronal differentiation, depending on the concentration of all-*trans*-retinoic acid used (McBurney *et al.*, 1982). In F9 embryonal carcinoma cells, all-*trans*-retinoic acid can induce parietal or visceral endodermal differentiation depending on whether the cells are grown in monolayer culture or as three-dimensional aggregates (Strickland *et al.*, 1980; Gudas, 1992). Furthermore, all-*trans*-retinoic acid induced three distinct differentiation pathways: ectodermal, mesodermal and endodermal in a developmentally pluripotent germ-cell tumour (Damjanov *et al.*, 1993). The potential of all-*trans*-retinoic acid may sometimes be restricted to a specific pathway, as in HL-60 myeloid leukaemia cells which can undergo both myeloid and monocytoid differentiation, even though retinoids can induce only the granulocytic pathway (Breitman *et al.*, 1980). Presumably, the effects of retinoids on the differentiation pathway depend on various cellular factors that are either expressed constitutively (e.g. certain transcription factors) or are induced by retinoic acid and then turn on a specific differentiation pathway, such as *Hox* genes (Boncinelli *et al.*, 1991) and AP-2 (Luscher *et al.*, 1989).

The induction of differentiation of tumour cells is not restricted to established cell lines, since fresh leukaemic cells in short-term culture were also responsive to treatment with retinoids (Imaizumi & Breitman, 1987). Because retinoids can enhance the differentiation of malignant cells, they have been developed for clinical trials of 'differentiation therapy' aimed at inducing the differentiation of tumour cells *in vivo* (see section 6). So far, reports on induction of differentiation of solid tumour cells *in vivo* are restricted to murine embryonal carcinoma cells injected into syngeneic mice. A significant degree of differentiation was observed in teratocarcinomas when retinoic acid was injected directly into the tumour (Speers & Altmann, 1984) or when several retinoids were administered in the diet (McCue *et al.*, 1988).

4.4   Effects of retinoids on apoptosis

Activation of apoptosis in cells at risk of undergoing neoplastic transformation may constitute a physiological anti-neoplastic mechanism. Apoptosis of DNA-damaged cells can protect the organism from cancer development by eliminating cells that might otherwise replicate the damaged DNA, a process that may lead to mutations and eventually to cancer. Agents that can induce or restore the ability to undergo apoptosis in premalignant and malignant cells are expected, therefore, to be effective in cancer prevention and treatment (Thompson *et al.*, 1992). In this context, it is of special interest that retinoids have been found to induce apoptosis in mesenchymal, neuroectodermal, haematopoietic and epithelial cells during normal development and in cultured untransformed and tumour cells (Davies *et al.*, 1992; Lotan, 1995b).

Different retinoids were found to induce distinct types of apoptosis. One type involves initial differentiation followed by 'physiological' apoptosis of the differentiated cells. This pathway is exemplified by HL-60 myeloid leukaemia cells, which undergo differentiation into granulocytes and subsequently apoptosis by a process that requires six to eight days of treatment with all-*trans*-retinoic acid (Martin *et al.*, 1990). A second type of apoptosis does not require induction of differentiation and is usually more rapid; it can be accomplished in HL-60 cells by treatment with 9-*cis*-retinoic acid or RXR-selective retinoids (Nagy *et al.*, 1995). In HL-60 cells, activation of RARs by an RAR-specific ligand is sufficient to induce differentiation, whereas activation of RXRs by their ligand is essential for the induction of apoptosis (Nagy *et al.*, 1995). A third pattern of apoptosis is one in which cells that are resistant to induction of differentiation become responsive to induction of apoptosis, as described for a subclone of NB4 cells (a t15;17 human promyelocytic leukaemia cell line). When the parental cells were treated with all-*trans*-retinoic acid or 9-*cis*-retinoic acid, they differentiated into granulocytes and eventually underwent apoptosis as mature cells; however, the differentiation-resistant subclone underwent apoptosis after 72 h of treatment with all-*trans*-retinoic acid (Bruel *et al.*, 1995). In these cells, apoptosis and differentiation may include events that cannot occur simultaneously. A fourth pattern of apoptosis was found in cultured PCC7-Mz1 embryonal carcinoma cells, which after exposure to all-*trans*-retinoic acid differentiated into neuronal, astroglial and fibroblast-like derivatives over several days. With the all-*trans*-retinoic acid concentrations that induce differentiation, apoptotic cells are detected as early as 10 h after exposure (Herget *et al.*, 1998).

Retinoids have also been found to protect cells from apoptosis. This phenomenon was described in the specific case of T cell receptor activation-induced T cell hybridoma death, which is mediated by the engagement of Fas by activation-up-regulated Fas ligand. Retinoic acids were found to suppress apoptosis by inhibiting the induction of Fas ligand expression (Yang *et al.*, 1993). Although 9-*cis*-retinoic acid was more effective than all-*trans*-retinoic acid, the effect required both nuclear retinoid receptors (RARs and RXRs) (Yang *et al.*, 1995).

An unusual induction of apoptosis was noted in SH SY 5Y human neuroblastoma cells which underwent apoptosis after treatment with 9-*cis*-retinoic acid for five days followed by incubation for four days without treatment. No apoptosis was observed when the cells were incubated under the same conditions with all-*trans*-retinoic acid or with LGD 1069, an RXR-selective retinoid or, surprisingly, when the cells were treated with 9-*cis*-retinoic acid for nine days continuously (Lovat *et al.*, 1997; Irving *et al.*, 1998). The mechanism of this effect remains to be explained.

Whereas all these studies were conducted with natural retinoic acids, several studies have demonstrated that some synthetic retinoids, such as *N*-(4-hydroxyphenyl)retinamide, are more potent than all-*trans*-retinoic acid or 9-*cis*-retinoic acid. *N*-(4-Hydroxyphenyl)retinamide induced apoptosis in all-*trans*-retinoic acid-resistant variant HL-60 cells and other leukaemia cells (Delia *et al.*, 1993), neuroblastoma cells (Ponzoni *et al.*, 1995), lung carcinoma (Kalemkerian *et al.*, 1995; Zou *et al.*, 1998), ovarian carcinoma (Supino *et al.*, 1996),

head-and-neck squamous cell carcinomas (Oridate *et al.*, 1996), breast carcinoma (Wang & Phang, 1996) and prostate carcinoma cells (Roberson *et al.*, 1997; Sun *et al.*, 1999b). *N*-(4-Hydroxyphenyl)retinamide did not induce differentiation of HL-60 cells (Delia *et al.*, 1993) or neuroblastoma cells (Ponzoni *et al.*, 1995). Because this compound induced apoptosis in cells that are resistant to all-*trans*-retinoic acid and other retinoids, it may exert its effect by a distinct mechanism. Indeed, it was able to induce reactive oxygen species in leukaemia cells (Delia *et al.*, 1997) and cervical cancer cells (Oridate *et al.*, 1997); however, a survey of 13 cell lines indicated that only about 20% had increased production of reactive oxygen species after exposure to *N*-(4-hydroxyphenyl)retinamide, suggesting that other mechanisms should be considered (Sun *et al.*, 1999b,c).

5. The role of retinoids in embryogenesis

5.1 Involvement of retinoids in embryonic development

The unique features of retinoids in embryos is that they are endogenous and are required for normal embryonic development.

5.1.1 Endogenous retinoids in the embryo

Endogenous retinoids such as retinol, didehydroretinol, all-*trans*-retinoic acid, 4-oxoretinoic acid and didehydroretinoic acid have been identified by high-performance liquid chromatography in the embryos of all species examined to date. These include birds (Thaller & Eichele, 1987, 1990; Scott *et al.*, 1994; Dong & Zile, 1995), rodents (Satre *et al.*, 1989; Collins *et al.*, 1994; Tzimas *et al.*, 1995), rabbits (Tzimas *et al.*, 1996a), primates, including humans (Creech Kraft *et al.*, 1993; Hummler *et al.*, 1994; Sass, 1994; Tzimas *et al.*, 1996b), *Xenopus* (Durston *et al.*, 1989) and zebrafish (Costaridis *et al.*, 1996). Furthermore, retinoic acid is differentially distributed within single embryonic regions such as the chick limb bud where it forms a concentration gradient across the anterior–posterior axis, with the highest concentrations posteriorly (Thaller & Eichele, 1987; Scott *et al.*, 1994). A similar gradient of all-*trans*-retinoic acid concentrations from the forebrain (lowest) to the spinal cord (highest) is found in the nervous system of early mouse embryos (Horton & Maden, 1995).

Transgenic mice carrying a reporter gene under the transcriptional control of a RARE (Rossant *et al.*, 1991; Mendelsohn *et al.*, 1991; Balkan *et al.*, 1992) and cell lines transfected with a retinoic acid-driven reporter gene (Chen *et al.*, 1992b; Wagner *et al.*, 1992; Chen *et al.*, 1994a) have been used to study the molecular basis of retinoid action. The response of the reporter system is assumed to reflect the presence of all-*trans*-retinoic acid and other active retinoids but cannot be considered to reflect the chemical identity of the retinoids conclusively. Despite this caveat, such methods demonstrate the existence of some 'hot spots' of embryonic retinoid concentrations which include the Hensen node of chicken embryos (Chen *et al.*, 1992b) and anterior–posterior gradients of retinoid concentrations in early neurula *Xenopus* embryos (Chen *et al.*, 1994a), the central nervous system tissue of rat embryos (Wagner *et al.*, 1992) and early chick embryos (Maden *et al.*, 1998).

5.1.2 Differential distribution of retinoid synthesizing enzymes

The enzymes that synthesize retinoic acid are distributed differentially in the embryo, a good example being the high level of activity of the enzyme retinaldehyde dehydrogenase(II) in mouse embryo spinal cord at the brachial and lumbar enlargements (McCaffery & Dräger, 1994). In each of these locations, there are more motor neurons than in the rest of the spinal cord. These neurons innervate the limbs which grow out at those two locations, and retinoic acid is required for motor neuron differentiation. Another example concerns the same enzyme, which is expressed in the mesenchyme of the early chick embryo (soon after gastrulation) in a domain that has an anterior border at the level of the second somite (Maden *et al.*, 1998).

5.1.3 Differential distribution of binding proteins and receptors

Retinoid cytoplasmic binding proteins and nuclear receptors are differently distributed in the embryo. The cytosolic binding proteins for retinoic acid and retinol (CRABPs and CRBPs, respectively) show very specific expression patterns within the embryo (Maden *et al.*, 1991; Gustafson *et al.*, 1993; Dekker *et al.*, 1994; Scott *et al.*, 1994). They may be involved in the metabolism of retinol to retinoic acid as well as in the control of local concentrations of 'free' all-*trans*-retinoic acid which is available for nuclear receptor binding. Indeed, CRBP occurs at relatively high concentrations in tissues sensitive to retinoid deficiency (such as embryonic heart), while CRABP occurs at high concentrations in tissues that are very sensitive to excess retinoic acid (such as the central nervous system). 'Knock-out' experiments have suggested, however, that these cytosolic binding proteins are 'dispensable' for embryonic development (Gorry *et al.*, 1994), as null mutant mice have no major developmental defects.

Studies of mouse embryos (Scott *et al.*, 1994) showed that the concentrations of all-*trans*-retinoic acid were much lower than those of its cellular binding protein CRABPI. In contrast, the whole-embryo concentration of retinol exceeded the concentration of its cellular binding protein CRBPI. Thus, it appears that all-*trans*-retinoic acid is predominantly bound to CRABPI in mouse embryos, while most of retinol remains unbound. CRABP can therefore function as a 'sink' for extensive accumulation of all-*trans*-retinoic acid in the embryo in the presence of low plasma concentrations (Tzimas *et al.*, 1996a).

The RARs and RXRs show very specific spatial and temporal distributions in the embryo (Dollé *et al.*, 1989, 1990; Ruberte *et al.*, 1990, 1991, 1993; Mangelsdorf *et al.*, 1994; Yamagata *et al.*, 1994). RARα is expressed ubiquitously throughout the embryo, while RARβ and RARγ show temporally and spatially restricted expression that is often mutually exclusive. For example, RARβ was found in the closed portion of the neural tube, while RARγ was present only in the open neural folds of the mouse embryo on day 8.5 of gestation (Dollé *et al.*, 1990; Ruberte *et al.*, 1991, 1993), suggesting a role for RARβ and RARγ in the formation and closure of the neural tube. By day 13.5 of gestation, RARβ was no longer expressed in the cartilagenous condensations of the limb but was found in the interdigital mesenchyme, whereas RARγ was strongly expressed in the digits (Dollé *et al.*, 1990). These distribution patterns suggest that RARβ and RARγ are involved in the formation of the digits, and interference with retinoid signalling may cause interdigital webbing. Of the RXR family, RXRβ showed the widest distribution pattern within the embryo, while RXRα and RXRγ had more restricted patterns of expression (Mangelsdorf *et al.*, 1994).

5.1.4 Retinol deficiency and embryogenesis
When the concentrations of retinol and its metabolites in the embryo are reduced substantially, increased embryonic death and terata occur, as shown classically by removing vitamin A from the diet of the mother. Hale (1933) found that frank vitamin A deficiency in pigs induced anophthalmia in their offspring. Subsequent experiments by Warkany (1945), Wilson *et al.* (1953) and Kalter and Warkany (1959) showed that rodent embryos born to vitamin A-deficient mothers were afflicted with anophthalmia, microphthalmia, defects of the retina, hydrocephalus, cleft palate, malformed hind legs, cryptorchidism, cardiovascular malformations and urogenital tract malformations. Major defects in the developing central nervous system of the embryo could also be induced (Maden *et al.*, 1996).

Administration of various retinoids during specific developmental periods showed the efficiency of 'rescue' of embryonic structures by particular retinoids (Dickman *et al.*, 1997; Wellik *et al.*, 1997; Zile, 1998). In vitamin A-deficient rats, all-*trans*-retinoic acid can substitute for vitamin A in all instances except for reproduction (spermatogenesis) and vision. The embryos of vitamin A-deficient dams which were 'rescued' with all-*trans*-retinoic acid developed normally but were blind and sterile. Retinoic acid cannot be reduced to retinal, and no cofactor for rhodopsin can be produced from exogenous retinoic acid. Furthermore,

retinoic acid cannot cross the blood–testis barrier (Kurlandsky *et al.*, 1995), and retinol is needed in the testis where it can be metabolized to retinoic acid.

It is clear, therefore, that any disturbance in the concentration of retinoids either by the provision of excess ligand or removal of ligand, disturbance of enzyme levels or removal of binding protein or receptors will result in terata. The terata are, as indicated above, remarkably uniform across all vertebrate species, although some differences between species are apparent. For example, at least in mammals, placental type may play a role. It is well established that rodents at different gestational ages have different types of placenta. In rats, the choriovitelline (yolk-sac) placenta is formed after angiogenesis of the chorionic placenta. An additional type of placenta, the chorioallantoic placenta, differentiates from day 11.5 of gestation and becomes functional from day 12 onwards (Beck, 1976; Jollie & Craig, 1979; Garbis-Berkvens & Peters, 1987). Most of the information on the transplacental distribution of retinoids in rodents is derived from studies performed on mid-organogenesis stages, such as day 11 in mice and day 12 in rats, thus prior to full development of the chorioallantoic placenta. In monkeys, development of the chorioallantoic placenta occurs much earlier during gestation and is already accomplished when embryonic retinoid concentrations can be measured (Beck, 1976).

Another factor is the presence of binding proteins in the embryo or the placenta. Harnish *et al.* (1992) found prolonged induction of CRABP II expression in mouse embryos after administration of teratogenic doses of retinoids. Increased CRABP II expression after exposure to all-*trans*-retinoic acid has also been observed in other systems and is compatible with the presence of a RARE and a RXRE in the promoter of the CRABP II gene (Durand *et al.*, 1992). In the presence of more CRABP II, more retinoic acid will be taken up by the embryo.

5.2 Molecular pathways for the teratogenicity of retinoids
During embryogenesis, the molecular code present in the genome is used to generate

mechanisms for the control of cell proliferation, differentiation and morphogenesis. Numerous processes must be strictly defined in developmental time and location to allow formation of the appropriate three-dimensional structure of the developing embryo during organogenesis and during all other developmental periods. Interference with such processes during organogenesis—when the most drastic structural defects can be induced—may be expected to be most efficient in altering gene expression. The complex retinoid signalling pathways, involving retinoid receptors, retinoid ligands and their strict spatio-temporal expression, are discussed in section 3. A major class of patterning genes which has been the subject of considerable research with regard to retinoids and teratogenesis are the *Hox* genes, many of which have retinoic acid response elements in their upstream sequences (Langston & Gudas, 1992; Pöpperl & Featherstone, 1993; Marshall *et al.*, 1994; Gould *et al.*, 1998; Packer *et al.*, 1998). Although the developing hindbrain of the central nervous system has been one focus of study, *Hox* genes are also expressed in other areas of the embryo, such as the limbs, the urogenital system, the genitalia and the gut, which helps to explain why retinoids have such pleiotropic effects.

5.3   New retinoids

New retinoids which can selectively activate individual RARs or RXRs may produce subsets of teratological defects in embryos. As the ability to bind the RARs decreases, so the teratogenicity of these retinoids decreases, such that RXR-selective compounds are not teratogenic *in vitro* or *in vivo* (Jiang *et al.*, 1994; Kochhar *et al.*, 1996). Thus, if RXR-selective compounds are found to be useful, they could eliminate the teratogenic side-effects of retinoid therapy.

6.   Differentiation therapy of cancer

The fact that cancer may be envisaged as a disorder of differentiation provides at least a theoretical basis for therapy (Lynch, 1995). The possible therapeutic effect of retinoids has been recognized in this context for some years

(Gudas, 1992; Smith *et al.*, 1992) and is considered to be strengthened by their ability to induce apoptosis (section 4.4). Uncontrolled proliferation of tumour cells may be due to the loss, altered expression or altered structure of particular gene products as a consequence of gene mutation or chromosomal translocation. The biology of leukaemia and a range of tumour types suggests that cancer may be understood as a disorder of differentiation. Thus, spontaneous differentiation of tumour cells has been described, specifically in teratocarcinoma (Pierce & Speers, 1988) and neuroblastoma.

The identification of *Patched*, a gene essential for the embryonic development of *Drosophila melanogaster*, as a tumour suppressor gene provides direct support for the understanding that tumorigenesis involves abnormalities of development (Gailani *et al.*, 1996). Genes that play a critical role in cell cycle regulation may function as tumour suppressor genes. Loss of the cyclin-dependent kinase inhibitors p15 and p16 is evident in some tumours (Hunter & Pines, 1994). In turn, cellular proliferation is influenced by differentiation and DNA repair, the complex interrelationships being mediated in part by *p53* (Vogelstein & Kinzler, 1992). Thus, in the lymphoid and myeloid lineages there is evidence that wild-type *p53* is associated with growth regulation and stage-specific differentiation (Shaulsky *et al.*, 1991; Zhang *et al.*, 1992).

The *p53* tumour suppressor gene also exemplifies the close relationship between cell cycle regulation, DNA repair and apoptosis. Most currently used anticancer drugs inhibit DNA replication or formation of the mitotic spindle, thereby causing cell cycle arrest and in many cases initiating DNA repair processes. Depending on the cell type, prolonged cell cycle arrest or persistent DNA damage may result in cell death by either apoptosis or mitotic catastrophe (King & Cidlowski, 1995), although the same cytotoxic agents have been shown to induce differentiation of many cell lines at low concentrations (Darzynkiewicz, 1995). For example, adriamycin and daunomycin may mediate differentiation of HL-60 cells (Yung *et al.*, 1992)

Most, if not all cytotoxic drugs mediate cell death by apoptosis (Hickman *et al.*, 1994). In some cell populations and in response to particular stimuli, differentiation and apoptosis may be regulated independently (Delia *et al.*, 1993; Ponzoni *et al.*, 1995). In many instances, however, a close relationship between differentiation and apoptosis has been observed. For example, apoptosis is observed in human HL-60 cells induced to differentiate by phorbol esters and etoposide (Solary *et al.*, 1994).

Sachs (1978) proposed that an impairment of the proliferation–differentiation balance occurs in malignancy, raising the possibility of characterizing differentiating agents that can modify the biological response. In contradistinction to cytotoxic therapy, differentiation therapy is specifically targeted to the transformed malignant cell which is induced to differentiate terminally and to lose self-renewal potential. Hence, inducing malignant cells to differentiate is an established approach to cancer therapy. As differentiation of tumour cells to cells incapable of further division is not necessarily accompanied by depletion of the tumour stem-cell pool, differentiation therapy may have to be combined with other cytotoxic or apoptotic strategies.

6.1 Retinoid differentiation therapy in acute promyelocytic leukaemia

Studies on myeloid leukaemic cell lines have played a pivotal role. The demonstration of terminal differentiation of HL-60 cell line in response to retinoic acid (Breitman *et al.*, 1980) led to the finding that cells from patients with acute promyelocytic leukaemia are terminally differentiated by retinoic acid both *in vitro* (Chomienne *et al.*, 1990) and *in vivo* (Castaigne *et al.*, 1990), resulting in complete remission in 90% of cases. Despite a growing number of differentiating agents, however, few have been effective in clinical trials in improving the chances of long-term survival. Other models for differentiation therapy have been studied, such as the use of G-CSF for acute myeloid leukaemia associated with the t(8;21) translocation (Da Silva *et al.*, 1997).

6.1.1 Molecular basis of acute promyelocytic leukaemia

Acute promyelocytic leukaemia accounts for approximately 10% of all cases of acute myeloid leukaemia. It is characterized morphologically by blast cells (differentiation block at the promyelocytic stage; Bennett *et al.*, 1976), the t(15;17) chromosomal translocation (Larson *et al.*, 1984) and coagulopathy (Dombret *et al.*, 1992). The breakpoint has been cloned and has revealed a fusion between the *RARα* (located on chromosome 17) and *PML* (for promyelocytic leukaemia, located on chromosome 15) genes, giving rise to a *PML/RARα* chimaera (de Thé *et al.*, 1991). *PML* belongs to a gene family which encodes nuclear proteins with a zinc finger DNA-binding domain characteristic of many transcription factors that have a 'leucine zipper' motif, which functions as a dimerization interface in certain proteins (Kakizuka *et al.*, 1991). Each acute promyelocytic leukaemia patient is characterized by a specific *PML/RARα* fusion transcript termed *bcr1*, *bcr2* or *bcr3* (Grignani *et al.*, 1994). A variant translocation t(11;17) in an acute myeloid leukaemia patient has been cloned and another transcription factor has been identified, called PLZF, fused to RARα (Chen *et al.*, 1993). There is evidence that both fusion proteins alter the DNA binding and *trans*-activation properties of the wild-type RARα receptor (de Thé *et al.*, 1991; Chen *et al.*, 1994b) and lead to differentiation block (Rousselot *et al.*, 1994). Normal PML and PLZF proteins are located in large nuclear bodies which in the fusion protein have a microspeckled pattern (Koken *et al.*, 1994; Reid *et al.*, 1995). Two other rare fusions have been cloned from acute myeloid leukaemia patients with t(5;17) and t(11;17) translocations involving, respectively, the nucleophosmin (*NPM*) and nuclear mitotic apparatus (*NuMA*) genes with RARα (Redner *et al.*, 1996; Wells & Kamel-Reid, 1996).

6.1.2 Retinoic acid differentiation of acute promyelocytic leukaemic cells

Acute promyelocytic leukaemia cells are successfully induced to differentiate *in vitro* to polymorphonuclear cells in the presence of retinoids, as demonstrated by morphology, nitroblue tetrazolium reduction assay and expression of differentiation antigens (CD11b, CD15). all-*trans*-Retinoic acid gave better results than the 13-*cis* isomer or 4-oxo metabolites, and a one-log difference in concentration for the same magnitude of effect was found (Chomienne *et al.*, 1989, 1990). The 9-*cis*-retinoic acid derivative gives results similar to those for all-*trans*-retinoic acid (Miller *et al.*, 1995). Cells that harbour chromosomal translocations resulting in rearrangements of the *RARα* gene but involving other fusion genes such as *PLZF* and *NPM* do not differentiate in the presence of all-*trans*-retinoic acid (Licht *et al.*, 1995).

6.1.3 all-*trans*-Retinoic acid differentiation therapy in acute promyelocytic leukaemia

The first clinical trial of all-*trans*-retinoic acid therapy in acute promyelocytic leukaemia was reported in 1988 from China (Huang *et al.*, 1988). About 90% of patients with newly diagnosed or first relapsed disease achieved complete remission with a dose of 45 mg/m^2 daily. When the data on 565 patients in studies conducted in China, France, Japan and the United States were combined, complete remission was found to have been achieved in 84%. Results for more than 1000 patients with acute promyelocytic leukaemia led to the conclusion that there was no resistance, the response was about 95% when the specific PML/RARα rearrangement was present, the differentiating effect was obtained without aplasia and coagulopathy rapidly improved (Warrell *et al.*, 1993). The major side-effect is the condition referred to as the 'all-*trans*-retinoic acid syndrome', sometimes associated with hyperleukocytosis and characterized by fever, respiratory distress, weight gain, pleural or pericardial effusion and sometimes renal failure (Frankel *et al.*, 1992). It occurs during the first month of treatment and can be prevented by giving chemotherapy when hyperleukocytosis occurs (Fenaux *et al.*, 1993). Steroids such as dexamethasone significantly reduce the severity and frequency of symptoms (Wiley & Firkin, 1995).

The shortness of the duration of complete remission after all-*trans*-retinoic acid therapy

alone and the weaker activity of subsequent treatment led to the identification of acquired resistance due to autoinduced catabolism of all-*trans*-retinoic acid, by the induction of 4-hydroxylase of CYP involved in plasma catabolism (Lippman & Meyskens, 1987). A European multicentre randomized trial of chemotherapy alone and of all-*trans*-retinoic acid followed by the same chemotherapy in newly diagnosed cases of acute promyelocytic leukaemia was performed between 1991 and 1992. The trial was terminated when event-free actuarial survival at three years was 76% in the group receiving chemotherapy and all-*trans*-retinoic acid and 53% in the group given chemotherapy alone (Fenaux *et al.*, 1993). Subsequent clinical trials have established the superiority of combined treatment based on all-*trans*-retinoic acid and cytotoxic chemotherapy for acute promyelocytic leukaemia (Tallman *et al.*, 1997).

Patients at high risk for relapse can be identified by a positive reaction in a reverse transcriptase polymerase chain reaction by amplification of the different PML/RARα transcripts resulting from the t(15;17) translocation (Fenaux & Chomienne, 1996). Patients defined as poor responders, less than 50% of whose cells differentiate after three days of culture in the presence of all-*trans*-retinoic acid, have low intracellular concentrations of all-*trans*-retinoic acid and a greater risk for relapse (Agadir *et al.*, 1995).

In primary cultures of acute promyelocytic leukaemia cells *in vitro*, other agents have been shown to be more effective than all-*trans*-retinoic acid. These include RARα agonists (Cassinat *et al.*, 1998) and the aromatic retinoid AM80, which was effective in resistant patients (Takeshita *et al.*, 1996). 9-*cis*-Retinoic acid, which is as effective *in vitro* as all-*trans*-retinoic acid, also had equivalent activity in inducing complete remission *in vivo*. It has the added advantage of not decreasing 9-*cis*-retinoic acid plasma concentrations during treatment. Longer follow-up will be required to determine if 9-*cis*-retinoic acid is more effective in eradicating the leukaemia clone than all-*trans*-retinoic acid (Miller *et al.*, 1995).

6.2 Retinoid therapy in other haematological disorders

Myelodysplastic disorders are lethal, as they involve a stem-cell defect that affects the control of myeloid differentiation and apoptosis. In one-third of cases, the cause of death is acute myeloid leukaemia. 13-*cis*-Retinoic acid and all-*trans*-retinoic acid have been used in randomized trials alone or in association with other drugs with no significant effect (Greenberg *et al.*, 1985; Clark *et al.*, 1987; Koeffler *et al.*, 1988; Aul *et al.*, 1993; Kurzrock *et al.*, 1993). Subtypes of myelodysplastic disorders with a proliferative disease such as chronic myelomonocytic leukaemia or juvenile chronic myeloid leukaemia appear to benefit more from the antiproliferative effect of retinoids. Preliminary results in cases of juvenile chronic myeloid leukaemia have shown that 13-*cis*-retinoic acid can reduce lymphocyte counts and organomegaly in one-half of patients (Castleberry *et al.*, 1994). These results prompted Cambier *et al.* (1996) to test the efficacy of all-*trans*-retinoic acid in adult chronic myelomonocytic leukaemia, as this disorder has many features in common with the juvenile disease. Of 10 patients with advanced adult chronic myelomonocytic leukaemia treated with all-*trans*-retinoic acid (45 mg/m² per day), two developed 'all-*trans*-retinoic acid syndrome' and four had a significant response; two of the latter had reduced transfusion requirement and two showed increased platelet counts. all-*trans*-Retinoic acid alone was not associated with a reduction in hepatosplenomegaly or leukocytosis. The improvement in cytopenia observed by Cambier *et al.* (1996) in four patients was not reported in the cases of juvenile chronic myeloid leukaemia. Whether those differences in response to retinoids in adult and juvenile disease are due to intrinsic biological differences between the two disorders or to different actions of 13-*cis*-retinoic acid and all-*trans*-retinoic acid remains to be clarified.

6.3 Retinoid therapy in solid tumours

The efficacy of retinoids in inhibiting malignant cell growth *in vitro* and, in some cases, inducing differentiation and/or apoptosis have led to trials of their use for the therapy of invasive and preinvasive tumours of epithelial origin, including skin cancers such as basal-cell carcinomas and advanced squamous-cell carcinomas (Lippman *et al.*, 1987, 1995), cutaneous T-cell lymphoma, mycosis fungoides (Molin *et al.*, 1985) and Kaposi sarcoma (Bonhomme *et al.*, 1991). Pilot studies have been conducted with 13-*cis*-retinoic acid and etretinate for bladder cancer, prostate cancer and central nervous system cancers (Lippman & Meyskens, 1987; Grunberg & Itri, 1987; Reynolds *et al.*, 1990; Lippman *et al.*, 1992; Cobleigh *et al.*, 1993; Reynolds *et al.*, 1994; Defer, 1996). A phase II clinical trial of all-*trans*-retinoic acid showed no significant antitumour activity in patients with chemotherapy-refractory germ-cell tumours (Moasser *et al.*, 1995). Further, the combination of all-*trans*-retinoic acid and interferon α-2a was inactive in patients with advanced carcinoma of the cervix (Castaigne *et al.*, 1990).

On the basis of a small number of patients, it was suggested that 13-*cis*-retinoic acid might be effective in the treatment of Ki-1 anaplastic large-cell lymphoma (Chou *et al.*, 1996). A phase II trial in children with recurrent neuroblastoma showed few responses, but the drug may be of more benefit in patients who have been treated by bone-marrow transplantation. It has been shown to be effective as a single agent in the treatment of squamous-cell carcinomas of the skin and mycosis fungoides (Villablanca *et al.*, 1995). In combination with interferon α-2a, 13-*cis*-retinoic acid was of benefit in the treatment of renal-cell carcinoma (Motzer *et al.*, 1995).

The lack of efficacy of retinoids against solid tumours is probably due to reduced accessibility, the heterogeneity of tumour cells and the lack of specific targeting of the retinoid to a tumour-specific retinoid receptor. In comparison with haematopoietic cells, which preferentially express the RARα receptor, a target for all-*trans*-retinoic acid, lung, nervous and thyroid cells express RARβ. In some of these tumours, RARβ expression is decreased or absent. *In vitro*, the response to retinoids has been shown to be linked to an increase in RARβ (Houle *et al.*, 1993; Lotan *et al.*, 1995; Carpentier *et al.*, 1997;

Schmutzler *et al.*, 1998). The general lack of efficacy, despite promising results in studies in cell lines, prompted trials with the more active receptor-targeted ligands such as targretin (RXR) (Miller *et al.*, 1997) and LGD 1550 (RAR).

7. Use of retinoids in the treatment of other conditions

7.1 Treatment of psoriasis

During the past decade, retinoids have been used increasingly for the treatment of psoriasis and other hyperkeratotic and parakeratotic skin diseases with or without dermal inflammation and as a standard treatment for severe acne and acne-related dermatoses (Peck *et al.*, 1982; Orfanos *et al.*, 1997). Vitamin A deficiency in experimental animals and humans is associated with xerosis, epithelial hyperkeratosis and squamous metaplasia of mucosal surfaces. Because these effects are reversible after intake of vitamin A and because of the similarity between certain disorders of keratinization and hypovitaminosis A, retinol and its esters were used in the treatment of psoriasis, ichthyoses and Darier disease in the 1940s. Topical all-*trans*-retinoic acid was later shown to have some activity in the treatment of psoriasis vulgaris. Later, etretinate was selected for clinical evaluation in psoriatic patients because of its favourable 'therapeutic index', which is 10 times better than that of all-*trans*-retinoic acid in animals.

Both etretinate and acitretin have been shown in extensive clinical trials to be effective in treating severe forms of psoriasis. The best responses are obtained in erythrodermic psoriasis and in localized or generalized pustular psoriasis, in which improvement has been reported in approximately 90% of all treated patients (Lowe *et al.*, 1988). Accordingly, retinoids have been used for topical and systemic treatment of psoriasis and other hyperkeratotic and parakeratotic skin disorders, keratotic genodermatoses and severe acne-related dermatoses (Bjerke & Geiger, 1989; Orfanos *et al.*, 1997). Etretinate was also used in the treatment of psoriatic arthritis, although its

efficacy failed to achieve statistical significance in a meta-analysis (Jones *et al.*, 1997).

In psoriatic skin, etretinate has strong keratinolytic activity, leading to restoration of the normal epidermis by causing reappearance of the granular layer, disappearance of parakeratosis and reduction of acanthosis. Autoradiographic studies have demonstrated a decrease in the labelling index for [^{3}H]thymidine incorporation and prolonged DNA synthesis in the affected and uninvolved epidermis of psoriatic patients. Clinical benefit after initiation of etretinate therapy for psoriasis occurs one to two weeks after desquamation begins, and healing may be seen after three weeks (Gollnick *et al.*, 1990).

Acitretin is very similar in efficacy to etretinate for the treatment of psoriasis. In several 8–12-week randomized, double-blind clinical trials (Lauharanta & Geiger, 1989; Lassus & Geiger, 1988), acitretin was as effective as etretinate in patients with erythrodermic and pustular psoriasis. It has been suggested that etretinate may be better tolerated than acitretin when tested at equivalent doses (Cunningham & Geiger, 1992; Koo *et al.*, 1997). Acitretin was tested at administered doses of 10–75 mg/day in more than 1000 patients with psoriasis between 1985 and 1992 (Pilkington & Brogden, 1992) in non-comparative and placebo-controlled, double-blind clinical trials ranging in length from six weeks to 12 months. In the non-comparative studies, in which 8–52 evaluable patients per study received the drug orally for periods up to six months, body surface involvement was reduced by 33–96%. In the placebo-controlled trials, involving similar treatment protocols, a dose-dependent improvement of 6–85% was seen. In these and related studies, acitretin at 10–25 mg/day resulted in responses equivalent to those of the placebo, whereas doses of 50–75 mg/day significantly improved the symptoms of psoriasis (Koo *et al.*, 1997).

The mode of action of acitretin in psoriasis is unknown. Since retinoids have immunomodulatory and anti-inflammatory effects in human peripheral blood lymphocytes and polymorphonuclear leukocytes, an immune mechanism might be involved. During therapy with acitretin and other agents, IgG-Fc receptor levels increase but do not reach those registered in normal controls, indicating an immunological defect that is not corrected by effective therapy (Bjerke *et al.*, 1994). Acitretin may mediate its effect on psoriasis through modification of cAMP-dependent protein kinases (Raynaud *et al.*, 1993).

Combination therapy involving acitretin and ultraviolet B radiation was of greater benefit to patients with plaque-type psoriasis than either treatment alone (Iest & Boer, 1989). Most of the trials lasted from 8 to 12 weeks and involved 34–88 patients taking 20–50 mg of acitretin per day alone or in combination with ultraviolet B radiation. With either monotherapy or combination therapy, 50% to over 90% of patients showed improvement (Koo *et al.*, 1997).

Acitretin is also effective in the treatment of psoriasis associated with HIV infection (Buccheri *et al.*, 1997). Etretinate has also been combined with other systemic treatments such as methotrexate, hydroxyurea and cyclosporine.

7.2   Other dermatological conditions

13-*cis*-Retinoic acid is regarded as an extremely effective drug when given systemically in the treatment of severe acne. Its efficacy is attributed to its ability to inhibit sebaceous gland activity. Orally administered retinoids such as etretinate and acitretin do not inhibit sebum production in humans and are ineffective against acne (Geiger, 1995).

Systemically administered retinoids such as etretinate and those given topically such as all-*trans*-retinoic acid are of benefit in the treatment of oral lichen planus (Lozada-Nur & Miranda, 1997). Acitretin has been used to treat skin complications in renal transplant recipients (Yuan *et al.*, 1995). Topical administration of all-*trans*-retinoic acid is useful for treating patients with dry eye disorders in which squamous metaplasia with keratinization of the ocular epithelium is present (Wright, 1985; Tseng, 1986; Murphy *et al.*, 1996). In addition, all-*trans*-retinoic acid can block the process of premature skin ageing induced by sunlight (Fisher *et al.*, 1997).

7.3   Other non-malignant conditions

The use of retinoids for a variety of conditions has been proposed on the basis of experimental observations. In a single case report, 13-*cis*-retinoic acid was of benefit in the treatment of thrombotic thrombocytopenic purpura (Raife *et al.*, 1998). Etretinate was proposed to be of benefit in the treatment of severe Reiter syndrome associated with HIV infection (Louthrenoo, 1993).

Studies of collagen production in human lung fibroblasts indicate that all-*trans*-retinoic acid inhibits the basal and transforming growth factor-β-stimulated production of types I and III collagen by these cells (Redlich *et al.*, 1995). In an isolated, spontaneously beating neonatal rat cardiac myocyte preparation, all-*trans*-retinoic acid (10–20 μmol/L) prevented arrhythmia induced by isoproterenol or lysophosphatidylcholine (Kang & Leaf, 1995).

Retinoids like retinol and retinyl esters, which must be activated to retinoic acid, are beneficial in the treatment of bronchopulmonary dysplasia in premature infants (Chytil, 1996). In rats, all-*trans*-retinoic acid reversed the effects of elastase-induced pulmonary emphysema, and the efficacy of all-*trans*-retinoic acid in the treatment of emphysema is being assessed in clinical trials (Massaro & Massaro, 1996, 1997).

all-*trans*-Retinoic acid was also reported to be effective in reducing neointimal mass and eliciting favourable remodelling of vessel walls after balloon-withdrawal injury to the common carotid artery in rats (Miano *et al.*, 1998). Thus, all-*trans*-retinoic acid may prove useful for preventing or treating restenosis in patients with cardiovascular disease. Similarly, retinoids may prove effective for treating non-insulin-dependent diabetes mellitus, as studies of RXR-selective retinoids in mouse models for this disease indicate that RXR agonists function as insulin sensitizers and can decrease hyperglycaemia, hypertriglycidaemia and hyperinsulinaemia (Mukherjee *et al.*, 1997). The treatment of experimental mouse models of arthritis with any of several retinoids significantly inhibited the severity and development of arthritis (Takaoka *et al.*, 1997; Nagai *et al.*, 1999).

References

Anonymous (1990) Nomenclature policy: Generic descriptors and trivial names for vitamins and related compounds. *J. Nutr.,* **120**, 12–19

Abu-Abed, S.S., Beckett, B.R., Chiba, H., Chithalen, J.V., Jones, G., Metzger, D., Chambon, P. & Petkovich, M. (1998) Mouse *P450RAI* (CYP26) expression and retinoic acid-inducible retinoic acid metabolism in F9 cells are regulated by retinoic acid receptor γ and retinoid X receptor α. *J. Biol. Chem.,* **273**, 2409–2415

Agadir, A., Cornic, M., Lefebvre, P., Gourmel, B., Jerome, M., Degos, L., Fenaux, P. & Chomienne, C. (1995) All-*trans*-retinoic acid pharmacokinetics and bioavailability in acute promyelocytic leukemia: Intracellular concentrations and biologic response relationship. *J. Clin. Oncol.,* **13**, 2517–2523

Agarwal, C., Rorke, E.A., Irwin, J.C. & Eckert, R.L. (1991) Immortalization by human papillomavirus type 16 alters retinoid regulation of human ectocervical epithelial cell differentiation. *Cancer Res.,* **51**, 3982–3989

Allali-Hassani, A., Peralba, J.M., Martras, S., Farres, J. & Pares, X. (1998) Retinoids, omega-hydroxyfatty acids and cytotoxic aldehydes as physiological substrates, and H2-receptor antagonists as pharmacological inhibitors, of human class IV alcohol dehydrogenase. *FEBS Lett.,* **426**, 362–366

Amos, B. & Lotan, R. (1990) Retinoid-sensitive cells and cell lines. In: Packer L., ed., *Methods in Enzymology: Retinoids.* Orlando, FL, Academic Press, pp. 217–225

Andreola, F., Fernandez Salguero, P.M., Chiantore, M.V., Petkovich, M.P., Gonzalez, F.J. & De Luca, L.M. (1997) Aryl hydrocarbon receptor knockout mice (AHR$^{-/-}$) exhibit liver retinoid accumulation and reduced retinoic acid metabolism. *Cancer Res.,* **57**, 2835–2838

Ang, H.L., Deltour, L., Zgombic, K.M., Wagner, M.A. & Duester, G. (1996a) Expression patterns of class I and class IV alcohol dehydrogenase genes in developing epithelia suggest a role for alcohol dehydrogenase in local retinoic acid synthesis. *Alcohol Clin. Exp. Res.,* **20**, 1050–1064

Ang, H.L., Deltour, L., Hayamizu, T.F., Zgombic-Knight, M. & Duester, G. (1996b) Retinoic acid synthesis in mouse embryos during gastrulation and craniofacial development linked to class IV alcohol dehydrogenase gene expression. *J. Biol. Chem.,* **271**, 9526–9534

Aoudjit, F., Brochu, N., Morin, N., Poulin, G., Stratowa, C. & Audette, M. (1995) Heterodimeric retinoic acid receptor-β and retinoid X receptor-α complexes stimulate expression of the intercellular adhesion molecule-1 gene. *Cell Growth Differ.,* **6**, 515–521

Apfel, C.M., Kamber, M., Klaus, M., Mohr, P., Keidel, S. & LeMotte, P.K. (1995) Enhancement of HL-60 differentiation by a new class of retinoids with selective activity on retinoid X receptor. *J. Biol. Chem.,* **270**, 30765–30772

Arnhold, T., Tzimas, G., Wittfoht, W., Plonait, S. & Nau, H. (1996) Identification of 9-*cis*-retinoic acid, 9,13-di-*cis*-retinoic acid, and 14-hydroxy-4,14-*retro*-retinol in human plasma after liver consumption. *Life Sci.,* **59**, L169–L177

Aul, C., Runde, V. & Gattermann, N. (1993) all-*trans*-Retinoic acid in patients with myelodysplastic syndromes: Results of a pilot study. *Blood,* **82**, 2967–2974

Baker, M.E. (1994) Sequence analysis of steroid- and prostaglandin-metabolizing enzymes: Application to understanding catalysis. *Steroids,* **59**, 248–258

Baker, M.E. (1998) Evolution of mammalian 11β- and 17β-hydroxysteroid dehydrogenases-type 2 and retinol dehydrogenases from ancestors in *Caenorhabditis elegans* and evidence for horizontal transfer of a eukaryote dehydrogenase to *E. coli. J. Steroid Biochem. Mol. Biol.,* **66**, 355–363

Balkan, W., Colbert, M., Bock, C. & Linney, E. (1992) Transgenic indicator mice for studying activated retinoic acid receptors during development. *Proc. Natl Acad. Sci. USA,* **89**, 3347–3351

Barua, A.B. (1997) Retinoyl β-glucuronide: A biologically active form of vitamin A. *Nutr. Rev.,* **55**, 259–267

Barua, A.B. & Olson, J.A. (1986) Retinoyl β-glucuronide: An endogenous compound of human blood. *Am. J. Clin. Nutr.,* **43**, 481–485

Barua, A.B., Gunning, D.B. & Olson, J.A. (1991) Metabolism *in vivo* of all-*trans*-[11-^{3}H]retinoic acid after an oral dose in rats. Characterization of retinoyl β-glucuronide in the blood and other tissues. *Biochem. J.,* **277**, 527–531

Beato, M., Herrlich, P. & Schütz, G. (1995) Steroid hormone receptors: Many actors in search of a plot. *Cell,* **83**, 851–857

Beck, F. (1976) Comparative placental morphology and function. *Environ. Health Perspect.,* **18**, 5–12

Ben-Amotz, A., Mokady, S. & Avron, M. (1988) The β-carotene-rich alga *Dunaliella bardawil* as a source of retinol in a rat diet. *Br. J. Nutr.,* **59**, 443–449

Bennett, J.M., Catovsky, D., Daniel, M.T., Flandrin, G., Galton, D.A., Gralnick, H.R. & Sultan, C. (1976) Proposals for the classification of the acute leukaemias. French– American– British (FAB) co-operative group. *Br. J. Haematol.,* **33**, 451–458

Bernacki, S.H., Medvedev, A., Holloway, G., Dawson, M., Lotan, R. & Jetten, A.M. (1998) Suppression of relaxin gene expression by retinoids in squamous differentiated rabbit tracheal epithelial cells. *Mol. Cell. Endocrinol.,* **138**, 115–125

Bertram, J.S. (1983) Inhibition of neoplastic transformation in vitro by retinoids. *Cancer Surv.,* **2**, 243–262

Bhat, P.V. (1998) Retinal dehydrogenase gene expression in stomach and small intestine of rats during postnatal development and in vitamin A deficiency. *FEBS Lett.,* **426**, 260–262

Bhat, P.V. & Samaha, H. (1999) Kinetic properties of the human liver cytosolic aldehyde dehydrogenase for retinal isomers. *Biochem. Pharmacol.,* **57**, 195–197

Bhat, P.V., Poissant, L., Falardeau, P. & Lacroix, A. (1988a) Enzymatic oxidation of all-*trans* retinal to retinoic acid in rat tissues. *Biochem. Cell. Biol.,* **66**, 735–740

Bhat, P.V., Poissant, L. & Lacroix, A. (1988b) Properties of retinal-oxidizing enzyme activity in rat kidney. *Biochim. Biophys. Acta,* **967**, 211–217

Bhat, P.V., Labrecque, J., Boutin, J.M., Lacroix, A. & Yoshida, A. (1995) Cloning of a cDNA encoding rat aldehyde dehydrogenase with high activity for retinal oxidation. *Gene,* **166**, 303–306

Bhat, P.V., Poissant, L. & Wang, X.L. (1996) Purification and partial characterization of bovine kidney aldehyde dehydrogenase able to oxidize retinal to retinoic acid. *Biochem. Cell. Biol.,* **74**, 695–700

Bhat, P.V., Marcinkiewicz, M., Li, Y. & Mader, S. (1998) Changing patterns of renal retinal dehydrogenase expression parallel nephron development in the rat. *J. Histochem. Cytochem.,* **46**, 1025–1032

Biswas, M.G. & Russell, D.W. (1997) Expression cloning and characterization of oxidative 17β- and 3α-hydroxysteroid dehydrogenases from rat and human prostate. *J. Biol. Chem.,* **272**, 15959–15966

Bjerke, J.R. & Geiger, J.M. (1989) Acitretin versus etretinate in severe psoriasis. A double-blind randomized Nordic multicenter study in 168 patients. *Acta Derm. Venereol. Suppl. Stockh.,* **146**, 206–207

Bjerke, J.R., Tigalonova, M., Jensen, T.S. & Matre, R. (1994) Fcγ-receptors in skin and serum from patients with psoriasis, before and after therapy. *Acta Derm. Venereol. Suppl. Stockh.,* **186**, 141–142

Blaner, W.S. & Churchich, J.E. (1980) The membrane bound retinol dehydrogenase from bovine rod outer segments. *Biochem. Biophys. Res. Commun.,* **94**, 820–826

Blaner, W.S. & Olson, J.A. (1994) Retinol and retinoic acid metabolism. In: Sporn, M.B., Roberts, A.B. & Goodman, D.S., eds, *The Retinoids: Biology, Chemistry, and Medicine,* 2nd ed. New York, Raven Press, pp. 229–255

Bocquel, M.T., Kumar, V., Stricker, C., Chambon, P. & Gronemeyer, H. (1989) The contribution of the N- and C-terminal regions of steroid receptors to activation of transcription is both receptor and cell-specific. *Nucleic Acids Res.,* **17**, 2581–2595

Boerman, M.H. & Napoli, J.L. (1995) Characterization of a microsomal retinol dehydrogenase: A short-chain alcohol dehydrogenase with integral and peripheral membrane forms that interacts with holo-CRBP (type I). *Biochemistry,* **34**, 7027–7037

Boleda, M.D., Saubi, N., Farres, J. & Pares, X. (1993) Physiological substrates for rat alcohol dehydrogenase classes: Aldehydes of lipid peroxidation, omega-hydroxyfatty acids, and retinoids. *Arch. Biochem. Biophys.,* **307**, 85–90

Bollag, W. & Holdener, E.E. (1992) Retinoids in cancer prevention and therapy. *Ann. Oncol.,* **3**, 513–526

Boncinelli, E., Simeone, A., Acampora, D. & Mavilio, F. (1991) *HOX* gene activation by retinoic acid. *Trends Genet.,* **7**, 329–334

Bonhomme, L., Fredj, G., Averous, S., Szekely, A.M., Ecstein, E., Trumbic, B., Meyer, P., Lang, J.M., Misset, J.L. & Jasmin, C. (1991) Topical treatment of epidemic Kaposi's sarcoma with all-*trans*-retinoic acid. *Ann. Oncol.*, **2**, 234–235

Bourguet, W., Ruff, M., Chambon, P., Gronemeyer, H. & Moras, D. (1995) Crystal structure of the ligand-binding domain of the human nuclear receptor RXR-α. *Nature*, **375**, 377–382

Boylan, J.F., Lufkin, T., Achkar, C.C., Taneja, R., Chambon, P. & Gudas, L.J. (1995) Targeted disruption of retinoic acid receptor α (RARα) and RARγ results in receptor-specific alterations in retinoic acid-mediated differentiation and retinoic acid metabolism. *Mol. Cell. Biol.*, **15**, 843–851

Boyle, J.O., Langenfeld, J., Lonardo, F., Sekula, D., Reczek, P., Rusch, V., Dawson, M.I. & Dmitrovsky, E. (1999) Cyclin D1 proteolysis: A retinoid chemoprevention signal in normal, immortalized, and transformed human bronchial epithelial cells. *J. Natl Cancer Inst.*, **91**, 373–379

Breitman, T.R., Selonick, S.E. & Collins, S.J. (1980) Induction of differentiation of the human promyelocytic leukemia cell line (HL-60) by retinoic acid. *Proc. Natl Acad. Sci. USA*, **77**, 2936–2940

Brouwer, A., van den Berg, K.J. & Kukler, A. (1985) Time and dose responses of the reduction in retinoid concentrations in C57BL/Rij and DBA/2 mice induced by 3,4,3',4'-tetrachlorobiphenyl. *Toxicol. Appl. Pharmacol.*, **78**, 180–189

Bruel, A., Benoit, G., De-Nay, D., Brown, S. & Lanotte, M. (1995) Distinct apoptotic responses in maturation sensitive and resistant t(15;17) acute promyelocytic leukemia NB4 cells. 9-cis Retinoic acid induces apoptosis independent of maturation and Bcl-2 expression. *Leukemia*, **9**, 1173–1184

Brzozowski, A.M., Pike, A.C., Dauter, Z., Hubbard, R.E., Bonn, T., Engstrom, O., Ohman, L., Greene, G.L., Gustafsson, J.A. & Carlquist, M. (1997) Molecular basis of agonism and antagonism in the oestrogen receptor. *Nature*, **389**, 753–758

Buccheri, L., Katchen, B.R., Karter, A.J. & Cohen, S.R. (1997) Acitretin therapy is effective for psoriasis associated with human immunodeficiency virus infection. *Arch. Dermatol.*, **133**, 711–715

Bulens, F., Ibanez-Tallon, I., Van Acker, P., De Vriese, A., Nelles, L., Belayew, A. & Collen, D. (1995) Retinoic acid induction of human tissue-type plasminogen activator gene expression via a direct repeat element (DR5) located at –7 kilobases. *J. Biol. Chem.*, **270**, 7167–7175

Caelles, C., González-Sancho, J.M. & Muñoz, A. (1997) Nuclear hormone receptor antagonism with AP-1 by inhibition of the JNK pathway. *Genes Dev.*, **11**, 3351–3364

Cambier, N., Wattel, E., Menot, M.L., Guerci, A., Chomienne, C. & Fenaux, P. (1996) All-*trans* retinoic acid in adult chronic myelomonocytic leukemia: Results of a pilot study. *Leukemia*, **10**, 1164–1167

Carpentier, A., Balitrand, N., Rochette-Egly, C., Shroot, B., Degos, L. & Chomienne, C. (1997) Distinct sensitivity of neuroblastoma cells for retinoid receptor agonists: Evidence for functional receptor heterodimers. *Oncogene*, **15**, 1805–1813

Cassinat, B., Balitrand, N., Zassadowski, F., Barbey, C., Delva, L., Bastie, J.N., Rain, J.D., Degos, L., Fenaux, P. & Chomienne, C. (1998) Combination of ATRA with G-CSF or RARα agonists enhances differentiation induction of fresh APL cells. *Blood*, **92** (Suppl. 1), 596a

Castaigne, S., Chomienne, C., Daniel, M.T., Ballerini, P., Berger, R., Fenaux, P. & Degos, L. (1990) All-*trans*-retinoic acid as a differentiation therapy for acute promyelocytic leukemia. I. Clinical results. *Blood*, **76**, 1704–1709

Castleberry, R.P., Emanuel, P.D., Zuckerman, K.S., Cohn, S., Strauss, L., Byrd, R.L., Homans, A., Chaffee, S., Nitschke, R. & Gualtieri, R.J. (1994) A pilot study of isotretinoin in the treatment of juvenile chronic myelogenous leukemia. *N. Engl. J. Med.*, **331**, 1680–1684

Chai, X., Zhai, Y., Popescu, G. & Napoli, J.L. (1995) Cloning of a cDNA for a second retinol dehydrogenase type II. Expression of its mRNA relative to type I. *J. Biol. Chem.*, **270**, 28408–28412

Chai, X., Zhai, Y. & Napoli, J.L. (1996) Cloning of a rat cDNA encoding retinol dehydrogenase isozyme type III. *Gene*, **169**, 219–222

Chai, X., Zhai, Y. & Napoli, J.L. (1997) cDNA cloning and characterization of a *cis*-retinol/3α-hydroxysterol short-chain dehydrogenase. *J. Biol. Chem.*, **272**, 33125–33131

Chambon, P. (1996) A decade of molecular biology of retinoic acid receptors. *FASEB J.,* **10**, 940–954

Chen, H. & Juchau, M.R. (1997) Glutathione S-transferases act as isomerases in isomerization of 13-*cis*-retinoic acid to all-*trans*-retinoic acid in vitro. *Biochem.J.,* **327**, 721–726

Chen, H. & Juchau, M.R. (1998) Biotransformation of 13-*cis*- and 9-*cis*-retinoic acid to all-*trans*-retinoic acid in rat conceptal homogenates. Evidence for catalysis by a conceptal isomerase. *Drug Metab. Dispos.,* **26**, 222–228

Chen, L.C., Berberian, I., Koch, B., Mercier, M., Azais, B., V, Glauert, H.P., Chow, C.K. & Robertson, L.W. (1992a) Polychlorinated and polybrominated biphenyl congeners and retinoid levels in rat tissues: Structure–activity relationships. *Toxicol. Appl. Pharmacol.,* **114**, 47–55

Chen, Y., Huang, L., Russo, A.F. & Solursh, M. (1992b) Retinoic acid is enriched in Hensen's node and is developmentally regulated in the early chicken embryo. *Proc. Natl Acad. Sci. USA,* **89**, 10056–10059

Chen, Z., Brand, N.J., Chen, A., Chen, S.J., Tong, J.H., Wang, Z.Y., Waxman, S. & Zelent, A. (1993) Fusion between a novel *Krüppel*-like zinc finger gene and the retinoic acid receptor-α locus due to a variant t(11;17) translocation associated with acute promyelocytic leukaemia. *EMBO J.,* **12**, 1161–1167

Chen, Y., Huang, L. & Solursh, M. (1994a) A concentration gradient of retinoids in the early *Xenopus laevis* embryo. *Dev. Biol.,* **161**, 70–76

Chen, Z., Guidez, F., Rousselot, P., Agadir, A., Chen, S.J., Wang, Z.Y., Degos, L., Zelent, A., Waxman, S. & Chomienne, C. (1994b) PLZF-RARα fusion proteins generated from the variant t(11;17)(q23;q21) translocation in acute promyelocytic leukemia inhibit ligand-dependent transactivation of wild-type retinoic acid receptors. *Proc. Natl Acad. Sci. USA,* **91**, 1178–1182

Chen, J.Y., Penco, S., Ostrowski, J., Balaguer, P., Pons, M., Starrett, J.E., Reczek, P., Chambon, P. & Gronemeyer, H. (1995) RAR-specific agonist/antagonists which dissociate transactivation and AP1 transrepression inhibit anchorage-independent cell proliferation. *EMBO J.,* **14**, 1187–1197

Chen, J.Y., Clifford, J., Zusi, C., Starrett, J., Tortolani, D., Ostrowski, J., Reczek, P.R., Chambon, P. & Gronemeyer, H. (1996) Two distinct actions of retinoid-receptor ligands. *Nature,* **382**, 819–822

Chen, H., Lin, R.J., Schiltz, R.L., Chakravarti, D., Nash, A., Nagy, L., Privalsky, M.L., Nakatani, Y. & Evans, R.M. (1997) Nuclear receptor coactivator ACTR is a novel histone acetyltransferase and forms a multimeric activation complex with P/CAF and CBP/p300. *Cell,* **90**, 569–580

Chen, Z.P., Iyer, J., Bourguet, W., Held, P., Mioskowski, C., Lebeau, L., Noy, N., Chambon, P. & Gronemeyer, H. (1998) Ligand- and DNA-induced dissociation of RXR tetramers. *J. Mol. Biol.,* **275**, 55–65

Chomienne, C., Ballerini, P., Balitrand, N., Amar, M., Bernard, J.F., Boivin, P., Daniel, M.T., Berger, R., Castaigne, S. & Degos, L. (1989) Retinoic acid therapy for promyelocytic leukaemia. *Lancet,* **2**, 746–747

Chomienne, C., Ballerini, P., Balitrand, N., Daniel, M.T., Fenaux, P., Castaigne, S. & Degos, L. (1990) All-*trans* retinoic acid in acute promyelocytic leukemias. II. In vitro studies: Structure–function relationship. *Blood,* **76**, 1710–1717

Choo, C.K., Rorke, E.A. & Eckert, R.L. (1995) Retinoid regulation of cell differentiation in a series of human papillomavirus type 16-immortalized human cervical epithelial cell lines. *Carcinogenesis,* **16**, 375–381

Chopra, D.P. (1983) Retinoid reversal of squamous metaplasia in organ cultures of tracheas derived from hamsters fed on vitamin A-deficient diet. *Eur. J. Cancer Clin. Oncol.,* **19**, 847–857

Chou, W.C., Su, I.J., Tien, H.F., Liang, D.C., Wang, C.H., Chang, Y.C. & Cheng, A.L. (1996) Clinicopathologic, cytogenetic, and molecular studies of 13 Chinese patients with Ki-1 anaplastic large cell lymphoma. Special emphasis on the tumor response to 13-*cis*-retinoic acid. *Cancer,* **78**, 1805–1812

Chytil, F. (1996) Retinoids in lung development. *FASEB J.,* **10**, 986–992

Clairmont, A. & Sies, H. (1997) Evidence for a posttranscriptional effect of retinoic acid on connexin43 gene expression via the 3'-untranslated region. *FEBS Lett.,* **419**, 268–270

Clark, R.E., Jacobs, A., Lush, C.J. & Smith, S.A. (1987) Effect of 13-*cis*-retinoic acid on survival of patients with myelodysplastic syndrome. *Lancet*, **i**, 763–765

Clifford, J., Chiba, H., Sobieszczuk, D., Metzger, D. & Chambon, P. (1996) RXRα-null F9 embryonal carcinoma cells are resistant to the differentiation, anti-proliferative and apoptotic effects of retinoids. *EMBO J.*, **15**, 4142–4155

Cobleigh, M.A., Dowlatshahi, K., Deutsch, T.A., Mehta, R.G., Moon, R.C., Minn, F., Benson, A.B., Rademaker, A.W., Ashenhurst, J.B., Wade, J.L. & Wolter, J. (1993) Phase I/II trial of tamoxifen with or without fenretinide, an analog of vitamin A, in women with metastatic breast cancer. *J. Clin. Oncol.*, **11**, 474–477

Collins, M.D., Tzimas, G., Hummler, H., Burgin, H. & Nau, H. (1994) Comparative teratology and transplacental pharmacokinetics of all-*trans*-retinoic acid, 13-*cis*-retinoic acid, and retinyl palmitate following daily administrations in rats. *Toxicol. Appl. Pharmacol.*, **127**, 132–144

Connor, M.J. & Smit, M.H. (1987) Terminal-group oxidation of retinol by mouse epidermis. Inhibition in vitro and in vivo. *Biochem.J.*, **244**, 489–492

Costaridis, P., Horton, C., Zeitlinger, J., Holder, N. & Maden, M. (1996) Endogenous retinoids in the zebrafish embryo and adult. *Dev. Dyn.*, **205**, 41–51

Cowan, J.D., Von Hoff, D.D., Dinesman, A. & Clark, G. (1983) Use of a human tumor cloning system to screen retinoids for antineoplastic activity. *Cancer*, **51**, 92–96

Cox, L.R., Motz, J., Troll, W. & Garte, S.J. (1991) Effects of retinoic acid on NIH3T3 cell transformation by the H-*ras* oncogene. *J. Cancer Res. Clin. Oncol.*, **117**, 102–108

Creech Kraft, J. & Juchau, M.R. (1992) Conceptual biotransformation of 4-oxo-all-*trans*-retinoic acid, 4-oxo-13-*cis*-retinoic acid and all-*trans*-retinoyl-β-glucuronide in rat whole embryo culture. *Biochem.Pharmacol.*, **43**, 2289–2292

Creech Kraft, J., Slikker, W., Bailey, J.R., Roberts, L.G., Fischer, B., Wittfoht, W. & Nau, H. (1991a) Plasma pharmacokinetics and metabolism of 13-*cis*- and all-*trans*-retinoic acid in the cynomolgus monkey and the identification of 13-*cis*- and all-*trans*-retinoyl-β-glucuronides. A comparison to one human case study with isotretinoin. *Drug Metab. Dispos.*, **19**, 317–324

Creech Kraft, J., Eckhoff, C., Kochhar, D.M., Bochert, G., Chahoud, I. & Nau, H. (1991b) Isotretinoin (13-*cis*-retinoic acid) metabolism, *cis-trans* isomerization, glucuronidation, and transfer to the mouse embryo: Consequences for teratogenicity. *Teratog. Carcinog. Mutag.*, **11**, 21–30

Creech Kraft, J., Shepard, T. & Juchau, M.R. (1993) Tissue levels of retinoids in human embryos/fetuses. *Reprod. Toxicol.*, **7**, 11–15

Creek, K.E., Geslani, G., Batova, A. & Pirisi, L. (1995) Progressive loss of sensitivity to growth control by retinoic acid and transforming growth factor-beta at late stages of human papillomavirus type 16-initiated transformation of human keratinocytes. *Adv. Exp. Med. Biol.*, **375**, 117–135

Crowe, D.L. (1993) Retinoic acid mediates post-transcriptional regulation of keratin 19 mRNA levels. *J. Cell Sci.*, **106**, 183–188

Cullum, M.E. & Zile, M.H. (1985) Metabolism of all-*trans*-retinoic acid and all-*trans*-retinyl acetate. Demonstration of common physiological metabolites in rat small intestinal mucosa and circulation. *J. Biol. Chem.*, **260**, 10590–10596

Cunningham, W.J. & Geiger, J.M. (1992) Practical use of retinoids in psoriasis. *Semin. Dermatol.*, **11**, 291–301

Damjanov, I., Horvat, B. & Gibas, Z. (1993) Retinoic acid-induced differentiation of the developmentally pluripotent human germ cell tumor-derived cell line, NCCIT. *Lab. Invest.*, **68**, 220–232

Danielsen, M., Hinck, L. & Ringold, G.M. (1989) Two amino acids within the knuckle of the first zinc finger specify DNA response element activation by the glucocorticoid receptor. *Cell*, **57**, 1131–1138

Darzynkiewicz, Z. (1995) Apoptosis in antitumor strategies: Modulation of cell cycle or differentiation. *J. Cell Biochem.*, **58**, 151–159

Da Silva, N., Meyer-Monard, S., Menot, M.L., Degos, L., Baruchel, A., Dombret, H. & Chomienne, C. (1997) G-CSF activates STAT pathways in Kasumi-1 myeloid leukemic cells with the t(8;21) translocation: Basis for potential therapeutic efficacy. *Cytokines Cell. Mol. Ther.*, **3**, 75–80

Davies, P.J., Stein, J.P., Chiocca, E.A., Basilon, I.P., Gentile, V., Thomazy, V. & Fesus, L. (1992) Retinoid-regulated expression of transglutaminases: Links to the biochemistry of programmed cell death. In: Morriss-Kay, G., ed., *Retinoids in Normal Development and Teratogenesis.* Oxford, Oxford University Press, pp. 249–263

Defer, G. (1996) Retinoids and glial tumors. A new therapeutic approach? *Rev. Neurol. Paris*, **152**, 653–657

Dekker, E.J., Vaessen, M.J., van den Berg, C., Timmermans, A., Godsave, S., Holling, T., Nieuwkoop, P., Geurts-van, K.A. & Durston, A. (1994) Overexpression of a cellular retinoic acid binding protein (xCRABP) causes antero-posterior defects in developing Xenopus embryos. *Development*, **120**, 973–985

De Leenheer, A.P., Lambert, W.E. & Claeys, I. (1982) All-*trans*-retinoic acid: Measurement of reference values in human serum by high performance liquid chromatography. *J. Lipid Res.*, **23**, 1362–1367

Delia, D., Aiello, A., Lombardi, L., Pelicci, P.G., Grignani, F., Formelli, F., Ménard, S., Costa, A., Veronesi, U. & Pierotti, M.A. (1993) N-(4-Hydroxyphenyl)retinamide induces apoptosis of malignant hemopoietic cell lines including those unresponsive to retinoic acid. *Cancer Res.*, **53**, 6036–6041

Delia, D., Aiello, A., Meroni, L., Nicolini, M., Reed, J.C. & Pierotti, M.A. (1997) Role of antioxidants and intracellular free radicals in retinamide-induced cell death. *Carcinogenesis*, **18**, 943–948

Desai, S.H. & Niles, R.M. (1997) Characterization of retinoic acid-induced AP-1 activity in B16 mouse melanoma cells. *J. Biol. Chem.*, **272**, 12809–12815

Dickman, E.D., Thaller, C. & Smith, S.M. (1997) Temporally-regulated retinoic acid depletion produces specific neural crest, ocular and nervous system defects. *Development*, **124**, 3111–3121

Dollé, P., Ruberte, E., Kastner, P., Petkovich, M., Stoner, C.M., Gudas, L.J. & Chambon, P. (1989) Differential expression of genes encoding α, β and γ retinoic acid receptors and CRABP in the developing limbs of the mouse. *Nature*, **342**, 702–705

Dollé, P., Ruberte, E., Leroy, P., Morriss-Kay, G. & Chambon, P. (1990) Retinoic acid receptors and cellular retinoid binding proteins. I. A systematic study of their differential pattern of transcription during mouse organogenesis. *Development*, **110**, 1133–1151

Dombret, H., Sutton, L., Duarte, M., Daniel, M.T., Leblond, V., Castaigne, S. & Degos, L. (1992) Combined therapy with all-*trans*-retinoic acid and high-dose chemotherapy in patients with hyperleukocytic acute promyelocytic leukemia and severe visceral hemorrhage. *Leukemia*, **6**, 1237–1242

Dong, D. & Zile, M.H. (1995) Endogenous retinoids in the early avian embryo. *Biochem. Biophys. Res. Commun.*, **217**, 1026–1031

Dony, C., Kessel, M. & Gruss, P. (1985) Post-transcriptional control of myc and p53 expression during differentiation of the embryonal carcinoma cell line F9. *Nature*, **317**, 636–639

Driessen, C.A., Winkens, H.J., Kuhlmann, E.D., Janssen, A.P., van-Vugt, A.H., Deutman, A.F. & Janssen, J.J. (1998) The visual cycle retinol dehydrogenase: Possible involvement in the 9-*cis*-retinoic acid biosynthetic pathway. *FEBS Lett.*, **428**, 135–140

Duell, E.A., Kang, S. & Voorhees, J.J. (1996) Retinoic acid isomers applied to human skin *in vivo* each induce a 4-hydroxylase that inactivates only *trans*-retinoic acid. *J. Invest. Dermatol.*, **106**, 316–320

Duester, G. (1996) Involvement of alcohol dehydrogenase, short-chain dehydrogenase/reductase, aldehyde dehydrogenase, and cytochrome P450 in the control of retinoid signaling by activation of retinoic acid synthesis. *Biochemistry*, **35**, 12221–12227

Dunagin, P.E.Jr., Zachman, R.D. & Olson, J.A. (1966) The identification of metabolites of retinal and retinoic acid in rat bile. *Biochim. Biophys. Acta*, **124**, 71–85

Durand, B., Saunders, M., Leroy, P., Leid, M. & Chambon, P. (1992) All-*trans*- and 9-*cis*-retinoic acid induction of CRABPII transcription is mediated by RAR–RXR heterodimers bound to DR1 and DR2 repeated motifs. *Cell*, **71**, 73–85

Durston, A.J., Timmermans, J.P., Hage, W.J., Hendriks, H.F., de Vries, N.J., Heideveld, M. & Nieuwkoop, P.D. (1989) Retinoic acid causes an anteroposterior transformation in the developing central nervous system. *Nature*, **340**, 140–144

Eckhoff, C. & Nau, H. (1990) Identification and quantitation of all-*trans*- and 13-*cis*-retinoic acid and 13-*cis*-4-oxoretinoic acid in human plasma. *J. Lipid Res.*, **31**, 1445–1454

Eckhoff, C., Collins, M.D. & Nau, H. (1991) Human plasma all-*trans*-, 13-*cis*- and 13-*cis*-4-oxoretinoic acid profiles during subchronic vitamin A supplementation: Comparison to retinol and retinyl ester plasma levels. *J. Nutr.*, **121**, 1016–1025

Edwards, R.B., Adler, A.J., Dev, S. & Claycomb, R.C. (1992) Synthesis of retinoic acid from retinol by cultured rabbit Müller cells. *Exp. Eye Res.*, **54**, 481–490

Eguchi, Y., Eguchi, N., Oda, H., Seiki, K., Kijima, Y., Matsu, U.Y., Urade, Y. & Hayaishi, O. (1997) Expression of lipocalin-type prostaglandin D synthase (beta-trace) in human heart and its accumulation in the coronary circulation of angina patients. *Proc. Natl Acad. Sci. USA*, **94**, 14689–14694

Eguchi, N., Minami, T., Shirafuji, N., Kanaoka, Y., Tanaka, T., Nagata, A., Yoshida, N., Urade, Y., Ito, S. & Hayaishi, O. (1999) Lack of tactile pain (allodynia) in lipocalin-type prostaglandin D synthase-deficient mice. *Proc. Natl Acad. Sci. USA*, **96**, 726–730

Eicher, S.A. & Lotan, R. (1996) Differential effects of retinoic acid and N-(4-hydroxyphenyl)retinamide on head and neck squamous cell carcinoma cells. *Laryngoscope*, **106**, 1471–1475

El Akawi, Z. & Napoli, J.L. (1994) Rat liver cytosolic retinal dehydrogenase: Comparison of 13-*cis*-, 9-*cis*-, and all-*trans*-retinal as substrates and effects of cellular retinoid-binding proteins and retinoic acid on activity. *Biochemistry*, **33**, 1938–1943

Escriva, H., Safi, R., Hänni, C., Langlois, M.C., Saumitou-Laprade, P., Stehelin, D., Capron, A., Pierce, R. & Laudet, V. (1997) Ligand binding was acquired during evolution of nuclear receptors. *Proc. Natl Acad. Sci. USA*, **94**, 6803–6808

Fenaux, P. & Chomienne, C. (1996) Biology and treatment of acute promyelocytic leukemia. *Curr. Opin. Oncol.*, **8**, 3–12

Fenaux, P., Le Deley, M.C., Castaigne, S., Archimbaud, E., Chomienne, C., Link, H., Guerci, A., Duarte, M., Daniel, M.T., Bowen, D., Huebner, G., Bauters, F., Fegueux, N., Fey, M., Sanz, M., Lowenberg, B., Maloisel, F., Auzanneau, G., Sadoun, A., Gardin, C., Bastion, Y., Ganser, A., Jacky, E., Dombret, H., Chastang, C. & Degos, L. (1993) Effect of all-*trans*-retinoic acid in newly diagnosed acute promyelocytic leukemia. Results of a multicenter randomized trial. European APL 91 Group. *Blood*, **82**, 3241–3249

Fiorella, P.D. & Napoli, J.L. (1991) Expression of cellular retinoic acid binding protein (CRABP) in *Escherichia coli*. Characterization and evidence that holo-CRABP is a substrate in retinoic acid metabolism. *J. Biol. Chem.*, **266**, 16572–16579

Fisher, G.J., Wang, Z.Q., Datta, S.C., Varani, J., Kang, S. & Voorhees, J.J. (1997) Patho-physiology of premature skin aging induced by ultraviolet light. *N. Engl. J. Med.*, **337**, 1419–1428

Fisher, G.J., Talwar, H.S., Lin, J., Lin, P., McPhillips, F., Wang, Z., Li, X., Wan, Y., Kang, S. & Voorhees, J.J. (1998) Retinoic acid inhibits induction of c-Jun protein by ultraviolet radiation that occurs subsequent to activation of mitogen-activated protein kinase pathways in human skin in vivo. *J. Clin. Invest.*, **101**, 1432–1440

Flower, D.R. (1996) The lipocalin protein family: Structure and function. *Biochem. J.*, **318**, 1–14

Folman, Y., Russell, R.M., Tang, G.W. & Wolf, D.G. (1989) Rabbits fed on beta-carotene have higher serum levels of all-*trans*-retinoic acid than those receiving no beta-carotene. *Br. J. Nutr.*, **62**, 195–201

Forman, B.M., Umesono, K., Chen, J. & Evans, R.M. (1995) Unique response pathways are established by allosteric interactions among nuclear hormone receptors. *Cell*, **81**, 541–550

Forman, B.M., Tzameli, I., Choi, H.S., Chen, J., Simha, D., Seol, W., Evans, R.M. & Moore, D.D. (1998) Androstane metabolites bind to and deactivate the nuclear receptor CAR-β. *Nature*, **395**, 612–615

Frankel, S.R., Eardley, A., Lauwers, G., Weiss, M. & Warrell, R.P.J. (1992) The 'retinoic acid syndrome' in acute promyelocytic leukemia. *Ann. Intern. Med*, **117**, 292–296

Frolik, C.A. (1984) Metabolism of retinoids. In: Sporn, M.B., Roberts, A.B., & Goodman, D.S., eds, *The Retinoids*. Orlando, FL, Academic Press, pp. 177-208

Frolik, C.A., Roller, P.P., Roberts, A.B. & Sporn, M.B. (1980) *In vitro* and *in vivo* metabolism of all-*trans*- and 13-*cis*-retinoic acid in hamsters. Identification of 13-*cis*-4-oxoretinoic acid. *J. Biol. Chem.*, **255**, 8057–8062

Fujii, H., Sato, T., Kaneko, S., Gotoh, O., Fujii-Kuriyama, Y., Osawa, K., Kato, S. & Hamada, H. (1997) Metabolic inactivation of retinoic acid by a novel P450 differentially expressed in developing mouse embryos. *EMBO J.*, **16**, 4163–4173

Gailani, M.R., Stahle-Backdahl, M., Leffell, D.J., Glynn, M., Zaphiropoulos, P.G., Pressman, C., Unden, A.B., Dean, M., Brash, D.E., Bale, A.E. & Toftgard, R. (1996) The role of the human homologue of *Drosophila patched* in sporadic basal cell carcinomas. *Nat. Genet.*, **14**, 78–81

Gallup, J.M., Barua, A.B., Furr, H.C. & Olson, J.A. (1987) Effects of retinoid beta-glucuronides and N-retinoyl amines on the differentiation of HL-60 cells in vitro. *Proc. Soc. Exp. Biol. Med.*, **186**, 269–274

Gamble, M.V., Shang, E., Piantedosi, R., Mertz, J.R., Wolgemuth, D.J. & Blaner, W.S. (1999) Biochemical properties, tissue expression, and gene structure of a short chain dehydrogenase/reductase able to catalyze *cis*-retinol oxidation. *J. Lipid Res.*, **40**, pp. 2279–2292

Garbis-Berkvens, J.M. & Peters, P.W.J. (1987) Comparative morphology and physiology of embryonic and fetal membranes. In: Nau H. & Scott W.J.J., eds, *Pharmacokinetics in Teratogenesis*. Boca Raton, FL, CRC Press, pp. 13–44

Gaub, M.P., Bellard, M., Scheuer, I., Chambon, P. & Sassone-Corsi, P. (1990) Activation of the ovalbumin gene by the estrogen receptor involves the fos-jun complex. *Cell*, **63**, 1267–1276

Gehin, M., Vivat, V., Wurtz, J.M., Losson, R., Chambon, P., Moras, D. & Gronemeyer, H. (1999) Structural basis for engineering of retinoic acid receptor isotype-selective agonists and antagonists. *Chem. Biol.*, **6**, 519–529

Geiger, J.M. (1995) Retinoids and sebaceous gland activity. *Dermatology*, **191**, 305–310

Geison, R.L. & Johnson, B.C. (1970) Studies on the in vivo metabolism of retinoic acid in the rat. *Lipids*, **5**, 371–378

Genchi, G., Wang, W., Barua, A., Bidlack, W.R. & Olson, J.A. (1996) Formation of β-glucuronides and of β-galacturonides of various retinoids catalyzed by induced and noninduced microsomal UDP-glucuronosyltransferases of rat liver. *Biochim. Biophys. Acta*, **1289**, 284–290

Giannini, G., Dawson, M.I., Zhang, X. & Thiele, C.J. (1997) Activation of three distinct RXR/RAR heterodimers induces growth arrest and differentiation of neuroblastoma cells. *J. Biol. Chem.*, **272**, 26693–26701

Glass, C.K. (1994) Differential recognition of target genes by nuclear receptor monomers, dimers, and heterodimers. *Endocr. Rev.*, **15**, 391–407

Gollnick, H., Ehlert, R., Rinck, G. & Orfanos, C.E. (1990) Retinoids: An overview of pharmacokinetics and therapeutic value. *Methods Enzymol.*, **190**, 291–304

Goodman, D.S. & Blaner, W.S.(1984) Biosynthesis, absorption, and hepatic metabolism of retinol. In: Sporn, M.B., Roberts, A.B. & Goodman, D.S., eds, *The Retinoids*. New York, Academic Press, pp. 1–39

Gorry, P., Lufkin, T., Dierich, A., Rochette-Egly, C., Decimo, D., Dollé, P., Mark, M., Durand, B. & Chambon, P. (1994) The cellular retinoic acid binding protein I is dispensable. *Proc. Natl Acad. Sci. USA*, **91**, 9032–9036

Göttlicher, M., Heck, S. & Herrlich, P. (1998) Transcriptional cross-talk, the second mode of steroid hormone receptor action. *J. Mol. Med.*, **76**, 480–489

Gough, W.H., VanOoteghem, S., Sint, T. & Kedishvili, N.Y. (1998) cDNA cloning and characterization of a new human microsomal NAD·-dependent dehydrogenase that oxidizes all-*trans*-retinol and 3α-hydroxysteroids. *J. Biol. Chem.*, **273**, 19778–19785

Gould, A., Itasaki, N. & Krumlauf, R. (1998) Initiation of rhombomeric Hoxb4 expression requires induction by somites and a retinoid pathway. *Neuron*, **21**, 39–51

Green, S. & Chambon, P. (1987) Oestradiol induction of a glucocorticoid-responsive gene by a chimaeric receptor. *Nature*, **325**, 75–78

Green, S., Kumar, V., Theulaz, I., Wahli, W. & Chambon, P. (1988) The N-terminal DNA-binding 'zinc finger' of the oestrogen and glucocorticoid receptors determines target gene specificity. *EMBO J.*, **7**, 3037–3044

Greenberg, B.R., Durie, B.G., Barnett, T.C. & Meyskens, F.L.J. (1985) Phase I–II study of 13-*cis*-retinoic acid in myelodysplastic syndrome. *Cancer Treat. Rep.*, **69**, 1369–1374

Grignani, F., Fagioli, M., Alcalay, M., Longo, L., Pandolfi, P.P., Donti, E., Biondi, A., Lo Coco, F. & Pelicci, P.G. (1994) Acute promyelocytic leukemia: From genetics to treatment. *Blood,* **83**, 10–25

Gronemeyer, H. & Laudet, V. (1995) Transcription factors 3: Nuclear receptors. *Protein Profile,* **2**, 1173–1308

Gronemeyer, H. & Moras, D. (1995) Nuclear receptors. How to finger DNA. *Nature,* **375**, 190–191

Grunberg, S.M. & Itri, L.M. (1987) Phase II study of isotretinoin in the treatment of advanced non-small cell lung cancer. *Cancer Treat. Rep.,* **71**, 1097–1098

Gudas, L.J. (1992) Retinoids, retinoid-responsive genes, cell differentiation, and cancer. *Cell Growth Differ.,* **3**, 655–662

Gudas, L.J., Sporn, M.B. & Roberts, A.B. (1994) Cellular biology and biochemistry of the retinoids. In: Sporn M.B., Roberts A.B. & Goodman D.S., eds, *The Retinoids. Biology, Chemistry and Medicine,* 2nd Ed. New York, Raven Press, pp. 443–520

Guerin, E., Ludwig, M.G., Basset, P. & Anglard, P. (1997) Stromelysin-3 induction and interstitial collagenase repression by retinoic acid. Therapeutic implication of receptor-selective retinoids dissociating transactivation and AP-1-mediated transrepression. *J. Biol. Chem.,* **272**, 11088–11095

Gunning, D.B., Barua, A.B. & Olson, J.A. (1993) Comparative teratogenicity and metabolism of all-*trans*-retinoic acid, all-*trans*-retinoyl beta-glucose, and all-*trans*-retinoyl beta-glucuronide in pregnant Sprague-Dawley rats. *Teratology,* **47**, 29–36

Gustafson, A.L., Dencker, L. & Eriksson, U. (1993) Non-overlapping expression of CRBP I and CRABP I during pattern formation of limbs and craniofacial structures in the early mouse embryo. *Development,* **117**, 451–460

Haeseleer, F., Huang, J., Lebioda, L., Saari, J.C. & Palczewski, K. (1998) Molecular characterization of a novel short-chain dehydrogenase/reductase that reduces all-*trans*-retinal. *J. Biol. Chem.,* **273**, 21790–21799

Hale, F. (1933) Pigs born without eye balls. *J. Hered.,* **24**, 105–106

Hamasaki, Y., Murakami, M., Kudo, I. & Miyazaki, S. (1997) Post-transcriptional regulation of LTC4 synthase activity by retinoic acid in rat basophilic leukemia cells. *Biochim. Biophys. Acta,* **1347**, 205–211

Han, I.S. & Choi, J.H. (1996) Highly specific cytochrome P450-like enzymes for all-*trans*-retinoic acid in T47D human breast cancer cells. *J. Clin. Endocrinol. Metab.,* **81**, 2069–2075

Harisiadis, L., Miller, R.C., Hall, E.J. & Borek, C. (1978) A vitamin A analogue inhibits radiation-induced oncogenic transformation. *Nature,* **274**, 486–487

Harnish, D.C., Soprano, K.J. & Soprano, D.R. (1992) Mouse conceptuses have a limited capacity to elevate the mRNA level of cellular retinoid binding proteins in response to teratogenic doses of retinoic acid. *Teratology,* **46**, 137–146

Haselbeck, R.J. & Duester, G. (1998a) ADH1 and ADH4 alcohol/retinol dehydrogenases in the developing adrenal blastema provide evidence for embryonic retinoid endocrine function. *Dev. Dyn.,* **213**, 114–120

Haselbeck, R.J. & Duester, G. (1998b) ADH4-lacZ transgenic mouse reveals alcohol dehydrogenase localization in embryonic midbrain/hindbrain, otic vesicles, and mesencephalic, trigeminal, facial, and olfactory neural crest. *Alcohol Clin. Exp. Res.,* **22**, 1607–1613

Haselbeck, R.J., Ang, H.L. & Duester, G. (1997) Class IV alcohol/retinol dehydrogenase localization in epidermal basal layer: Potential site of retinoic acid synthesis during skin development. *Dev. Dyn.,* **208**, 447–453

Hébuterne, X., Wang, X.D., Johnson, E.J., Krinsky, N.I. & Russell, R.M. (1995) Intestinal absorption and metabolism of 9-*cis*-β-carotene in vivo: Biosynthesis of 9-*cis*-retinoic acid. *J. Lipid Res.,* **36**, 1264–1273

Heck, S., Kullmann, M., Gast, A., Ponta, H., Rahmsdorf, H.J., Herrlich, P. & Cato, A.C. (1994) A distinct modulating domain in glucocorticoid receptor monomers in the repression of activity of the transcription factor AP-1. *EMBO J.,* **13**, 4087–4095

Heery, D.M., Pierrat, B., Gronemeyer, H., Chambon, P. & Losson, R. (1994) Homo- and heterodimers of the retinoid X receptor (RXR) activated transcription in yeast. *Nucleic Acids Res.,* **22**, 726–731

Herget, T., Specht, H., Esdar, C., Oehrlein, S.A. & Maelicke, A. (1998) Retinoic acid induces apoptosis-associated neural differentiation of a murine teratocarcinoma cell line. *J. Neurochem.*, **70**, 47–58

Heyman, R.A., Mangelsdorf, D.J., Dyck, J.A., Stein, R.B., Eichele, G., Evans, R.M. & Thaller, C. (1992) 9-*cis*-Retinoic acid is a high affinity ligand for the retinoid X receptor. *Cell*, **68**, 397–406

Hickman, J.A., Potten, C.S., Merritt, A.J. & Fisher, T.C. (1994) Apoptosis and cancer chemotherapy. *Phil. Trans. R. Soc. Lond. B Biol. Sci.*, **345**, 319–325

Hodam, J.R. & Creek, K.E. (1996) Uptake and metabolism of [³H]retinoic acid delivered to human foreskin keratinocytes either bound to serum albumin or added directly to the culture medium. *Biochim. Biophys. Acta*, **1311**, 102–110

Hoffmann, B., Lehmann, J.M., Zhang, X.K., Hermann, T., Husmann, M., Graupner, G. & Pfahl, M. (1990) A retinoic acid receptor-specific element controls the retinoic acid receptor-β promoter. *Mol. Endocrinol.*, **4**, 1727–1736

Hofmann, C. & Eichele, G.(1994) Retinoids in development. In: Sporn, M.B., Roberts, A.B., & Goodman, D.S., eds, *The Retinoids. Biology, Chemistry and Medicine*, 2nd Ed. New York, Raven Press, pp. 387-441

Horst, R.L., Reinhardt, T.A., Goff, J.P., Nonnecke, B.J., Gambhir, V.K., Fiorella, P.D. & Napoli, J.L. (1995) Identification of 9-*cis*,13-*cis*-retinoic acid as a major circulating retinoid in plasma. *Biochemistry*, **34**, 1203–1209

Horton, C. & Maden, M. (1995) Endogenous distribution of retinoids during normal development and teratogenesis in the mouse embryo. *Dev. Dyn.* , **202**, 312–323

Houle, B., Rochette-Egly, C. & Bradley, W.E. (1993) Tumor-suppressive effect of the retinoic acid receptor β in human epidermoid lung cancer cells. *Proc. Natl Acad. Sci. USA*, **90**, 985–989

Hu, E., Kim, J.B., Sarraf, P. & Spiegelman, B.M. (1996a) Inhibition of adipogenesis through MAP kinase-mediated phosphorylation of PPARγ. *Science,* **274**, 2100–2103

Hu, Z.B., Minden, M.D. & McCulloch, E.A. (1996b) Post-transcriptional regulation of bcl-2 in acute myeloblastic leukemia: Significance for response to chemotherapy. *Leukemia*, **10**, 410–416

Huang, C., Ma, W.Y., Dawson, M.I., Rincon, M., Flavell, R.A. & Dong, Z. (1997) Blocking activator protein-1 activity, but not activating retinoic acid response element, is required for the antitumor promotion effect of retinoic acid. *Proc. Natl Acad. Sci. USA*, **94**, 5826–5830

Huang, M.E., Ye, Y.C., Chen, S.R., Chai, J.R., Lu, J.X., Zhoa, L., Gu, L.J. & Wang, Z.Y. (1988) Use of all-*trans*-retinoic acid in the treatment of acute promyelocytic leukemia. *Blood*, **72**, 567–572

Hummler, H., Hendrickx, A.G. & Nau, H. (1994) Maternal toxicokinetics, metabolism, and embryo exposure following a teratogenic dosing regimen with 13-*cis*-retinoic acid (isotretinoin) in the cynomolgus monkey. *Teratology*, **50**, 184–193

Hunter, T. & Pines, J. (1994) Cyclins and cancer. II: Cyclin D and CDK inhibitors come of age. *Cell*, **79**, 573–582

Hupert, J., Mobarhan, S., Layden, T.J., Papa, V.M. & Lucchesi, D.J. (1991) In vitro formation of retinoic acid from retinal in rat liver. *Biochem. Cell. Biol.*, **69**, 509–514

Husmann, M., Hoffmann, B., Stump, D.G., Chytil, F. & Pfahl, M. (1992) A retinoic acid response element from the rat CRBPI promoter is activated by an RAR/RXR heterodimer. *Biochem. Biophys. Res. Commun.*, **187**, 1558–1564

IARC (1997) *IARC Handbooks of Cancer Prevention*, Vol. 1, *Non-steroidal Anti-inflammatory Drugs*, Lyon, International Agency for Research on Cancer, 202 pp.

IARC (1998a) *IARC Handbooks of Cancer Prevention*, Vol. 2, *Carotenoids*, Lyon, International Agency for Research on Cancer, 326 pp.

IARC (1998b) *IARC Handbooks of Cancer Prevention*, Vol. 3, *Vitamin A*, Lyon, International Agency for Research on Cancer, 261 pp.

Iest, J. & Boer, J. (1989) Combined treatment of psoriasis with acitretin and UVB phototherapy compared with acitretin alone and UVB alone. *Br. J. Dermatol.*, **120**, 665–670

Imaizumi, M. & Breitman, T.R. (1987) Retinoic acid-induced differentiation of the human promyelocytic leukemia cell line, HL-60, and fresh human leukemia cells in primary culture: A model for differentiation inducing therapy of leukemia. *Eur. J. Haematol.*, **38**, 289–302

Imaoka, S., Wan, J., Chow, T., Hiroi, T., Eyanagi, R., Shigematsu, H. & Funae, Y. (1998) Cloning and characterization of the CYP2D1-binding protein, retinol dehydrogenase. *Arch. Biochem. Biophys.*, **353**, 331–336

Irving, H., Lovat, P.E., Campbell Hewson, Q., Malcolm, A.J., Pearson, A.D. & Redfern, C.P. (1998) Retinoid-induced differentiation of neuroblastoma: Comparison between LG69, an RXR-selective analogue and 9-*cis*-retinoic acid. *Eur. J. Cancer*, **34**, 111–117

Ito, Y., Zile, M., DeLuca, H.F. & Ahrens, H.M. (1974) Metabolism of retinoic acid in vitamin A-deficient rats. *Biochim. Biophys. Acta*, **369**, 338–350

IUPAC Commission on the Nomenclature of Biological Chemistry (1960) Definitive rules for the nomenclature of amino acids, steroids, vitamins, and carotenoids. *J. Am. Chem. Soc.*, **82**, 5575–5584

IUPAC–IUB Commission on Biochemical Nomenclature (1966) IUPAC–IUB Commission on Biochemical Nomenclature. Trivial names of miscellaneous compounds of importance in biochemistry. *J. Biol. Chem.*, **241**, 2987–2988

IUPAC–IUB Joint Commission on Biochemical Nomenclature (1983) IUPAC–IUB Joint Commission on Biochemical Nomenclature (JCBN). Nomenclature of Retinoids. Recom-mendations 1981. *J. Biol. Chem.*, **258**, 5329–5333

IUPAC–IUB Joint Commission on Biochemical Nomenclature (1998) IUPAC–IUBMB Joint Commission on Biochemical Nomenclature (JCBN) and Nomenclature Committee of IUBMB (NC–IUBMB). Newsletter 1996. *J. Mol. Biol.*, **275**, 527–537

Janick-Buckner, D., Barua, A.B. & Olson, J.A. (1991) Induction of HL-60 cell differentiation by water-soluble and nitrogen-containing conjugates of retinoic acid and retinol. *FASEB J.*, **5**, 320–325

Jarrous, N. & Kaempfer, R. (1994) Induction of human interleukin-1 gene expression by retinoic acid and its regulation at processing of precursor transcripts. *J. Biol. Chem.*, **269**, 23141–23149

Jetten, A.M., Nervi, C. & Vollberg, T.M. (1992) Control of squamous differentiation in tracheobronchial and epidermal epithelial cells: Role of retinoids. *Natl Cancer Inst. Monogr.*, 93–100

Jiang, H., Gyda, M., Harnish, D.C., Chandraratna, R.A., Soprano, K.J., Kochhar, D.M. & Soprano, D.R. (1994) Teratogenesis by retinoic acid analogs positively correlates with elevation of retinoic acid receptor-beta 2 mRNA levels in treated embryos. *Teratology*, **50**, 38–43

Jollie, W.P. & Craig, S.S. (1979) The fine structure of placental junctional zone cells during prolonged pregnancy in rats. *Acta Anat. Basel*, **105**, 386–400

Jones, G., Crotty, M. & Brooks, P. (1997) Psoriatic arthritis: A quantitative overview of therapeutic options. The Psoriatic Arthritis Meta-analysis Study Group. *Br. J. Rheumatol.*, **36**, 95–99

Jörnvall, H. & Höög, J.O. (1995) Nomenclature of alcohol dehydrogenases. *Alcohol Alcohol.*, **30**, 153–161

Jörnvall, H., Persson, B., Krook, M., Atrian, S., Gonzalez, D.R., Jeffery, J. & Ghosh, D. (1995) Short-chain dehydrogenases/reductases (SDR). *Biochemistry*, **34**, 6003–6013

Julia, P., Farres, J. & Pares, X. (1986) Ocular alcohol dehydrogenase in the rat: Regional distribution and kinetics of the ADH-1 isoenzyme with retinol and retinal. *Exp. Eye Res.*, **42**, 305–314

Kakizuka, A., Miller, W.H.J., Umesono, K., Warrell, R.P.J., Frankel, S.R., Murty, V.V., Dmitrovsky, E. & Evans, R.M. (1991) Chromosomal translocation t(15;17) in human acute promyelocytic leukemia fuses RARα with a novel putative transcription factor, PML. *Cell*, **66**, 663–674

Kalemkerian, G.P., Slusher, R., Ramalingam, S., Gadgeel, S. & Mabry, M. (1995) Growth inhibition and induction of apoptosis by fenretinide in small-cell lung cancer cell lines. *J. Natl Cancer Inst.*, **87**, 1674–1680

Kalter, H. & Warkany, J. (1959) Experimental production of congenital malformations in mammals by metabolic procedure. *Physiol. Rev.*, **39**, 69–115

Kamei, Y., Xu, L., Heinzel, T., Torchia, J., Kurokawa, R., Gloss, B., Lin, S.C., Heyman, R.A., Rose, D.W., Glass, C.K. & Rosenfeld, M.G. (1996) A CBP integrator complex mediates transcriptional activation and AP-1 inhibition by nuclear receptors. *Cell*, **85**, 403–414

Kang, J.X. & Leaf, A. (1995) Protective effects of all-*trans*-retinoic acid against cardiac arrhythmias induced by isoproterenol, lysophosphatidylcholine or ischemia and reperfusion. *J. Cardiovasc. Pharmacol.,* **26,** 943–948

Kang, J.X., Li, Y. & Leaf, A. (1998) Mannose-6-phosphate/insulin-like growth factor-II receptor is a receptor for retinoic acid. *Proc. Natl Acad. Sci. USA,* **95,** 13671–13676

Kastner, P., Mark, M. & Chambon, P. (1995) Nonsteroid nuclear receptors: What are genetic studies telling us about their role in real life? *Cell,* **83,** 859–869

Kato, S., Endoh, H., Masuhiro, Y., Kitamoto, T., Uchiyama, S., Sasaki, H., Masushige, S., Gotoh, Y., Nishida, E., Kawashima, H., Metzger, D. & Chambon, P. (1995) Activation of the estrogen receptor through phosphorylation by mitogen-activated protein kinase. *Science,* **270,** 1491–1494

Kaul, S. & Olson, J.A. (1998) Effect of vitamin A deficiency on the hydrolysis of retinoyl beta-glucuronide to retinoic acid by rat tissue organelles in vitro. *Int. J. Vitam. Nutr. Res.,* **68,** 232–236

Kedishvili, N.Y., Gough, W.H., Chernoff, E.A., Hurley, T.D., Stone, C.L., Bowman, K.D., Popov, K.M., Bosron, W.F. & Li, T.K. (1997) cDNA sequence and catalytic properties of a chick embryo alcohol dehydrogenase that oxidizes retinol and 3β,5α-hydroxysteroids. *J. Biol. Chem.,* **272,** 7494–7500

Kedishvili, N.Y., Gough, W.H., Davis, W.I., Parsons, S., Li, T.K. & Bosron, W.F. (1998) Effect of cellular retinol-binding protein on retinol oxidation by human class IV retinol/alcohol dehydrogenase and inhibition by ethanol. *Biochem. Biophys. Res. Commun.,* **249,** 191–196

Kersten, S., Kelleher, D., Chambon, P., Gronemeyer, H. & Noy, N. (1995) Retinoid X receptor α forms tetramers in solution. *Proc. Natl Acad. Sci. USA,* **92,** 8645–8649

Kersten, S., Dawson, M.I., Lewis, B.A. & Noy, N. (1996) Individual subunits of heterodimers comprised of retinoic acid and retinoid X receptors interact with their ligands independently. *Biochemistry,* **35,** 3816–3824

Khan, M.A., Jenkins, G.R., Tolleson, W.H., Creek, K.E. & Pirisi, L. (1993) Retinoic acid inhibition of human papillomavirus type 16-mediated transformation of human keratinocytes. *Cancer Res.,* **53,** 905–909

Kim, C.I., Leo, M.A. & Lieber, C.S. (1992) Retinol forms retinoic acid via retinal. *Arch. Biochem. Biophys.,* **294,** 388–393

Kim, S.Y., Han, I.S., Yu, H.K., Lee, H.R., Chung, J.W., Choi, J.H., Kim, S.H., Byun, Y., Carey, T.E. & Lee, K.S. (1998) The induction of P450-mediated oxidation of all-*trans*-retinoic acid by retinoids in head and neck squamous cell carcinoma cell lines. *Metabolism,* **47,** 955–958

King, K.L. & Cidlowski, J.A. (1995) Cell cycle and apoptosis: Common pathways to life and death. *J. Cell Biochem.,* **58,** 175–180

Kishimoto, H., Hoshino, S., Ohori, M., Kontani, K., Nishina, H., Suzawa, M., Kato, S. & Katada, T. (1998) Molecular mechanism of human CD38 gene expression by retinoic acid. Identification of retinoic acid response element in the first intron. *J. Biol. Chem.,* **273,** 15429–15434

Kizaki, M., Dawson, M.I., Heyman, R., Elster, E., Morosetti, R., Pakkala, S., Chen, D.L., Ueno, H., Chao, W., Morikawa, M., Ikeda, Y., Heber, D., Pfahl, M. & Koeffler, H.P. (1996) Effects of novel retinoid X receptor-selective ligands on myeloid leukemia differentiation and proliferation in vitro. *Blood,* **87,** 1977–1984

Klaholz, B.P., Renaud, J.P., Mitschler, A., Zusi, C., Chambon, P., Gronemeyer, H. & Moras, D. (1998) Conformational adaptation of agonists to the human nuclear receptor RARγ. *Nat. Struct. Biol.,* **5,** 199–202

Klein-Szanto, A.J., Iizasa, T., Momiki, S., Garcia, P., I, Caamano, J., Metcalf, R., Welsh, J. & Harris, C.C. (1992) A tobacco-specific N-nitrosamine or cigarette smoke condensate causes neoplastic transformation of xenotransplanted human bronchial epithelial cells. *Proc. Natl Acad. Sci. USA,* **89,** 6693–6697

Kliewer, S.A., Umesono, K., Heyman, R.A., Mangelsdorf, D.J., Dyck, J.A. & Evans, R.M. (1992) Retinoid X receptor-COUP-TF interactions modulate retinoic acid signaling. *Proc. Natl Acad. Sci. USA,* **89,** 1448–1452

Kliewer, S.A., Moore, J.T., Wade, L., Staudinger, J.L., Watson, M.A., Jones, S.A., McKee, D.D., Oliver, B.B., Willson, T.M., Zetterström, R.H., Perlmann, T. & Lehmann, J.M. (1998) An orphan nuclear receptor activated by pregnanes defines a novel steroid signaling pathway. *Cell,* **92,** 73–82

Knoepfler, P.S. & Kamps, M.P. (1997) The Pbx family of proteins is strongly upregulated by a post- transcriptional mechanism during retinoic acid-induced differentiation of P19 embryonal carcinoma cells. *Mech. Dev.*, **63**, 5–14

Kochhar, D.M., Jiang, H., Penner, J.D., Beard, R.L. & Chandraratna, R.A. (1996) Differential teratogenic response of mouse embryos to receptor selective analogs of retinoic acid. *Chem. Biol. Interact.*, **100**, 1–12

Koeffler, H.P., Heitjan, D., Mertelsmann, R., Kolitz, J.E., Schulman, P., Itri, L., Gunter, P. & Besa, E. (1988) Randomized study of 13-*cis* retinoic acid *v* placebo in the myelodysplastic disorders. *Blood*, **71**, 703–708

Koken, M.H., Puvion-Dutilleul, F., Guillemin, M.C., Viron, A., Linares-Cruz, G., Stuurman, N., de Jong, L., Szostecki, C., Calvo, F., Chomienne, C., Degos, L., Puvion, E. & de Thé, H. (1994) The t(15;17) translocation alters a nuclear body in a retinoic acid-reversible fashion. *EMBO J.*, **13**, 1073–1083

König, H., Ponta, H., Rahmsdorf, H.J. & Herrlich, P. (1992) Interference between pathway-specific transcription factors: Glucocorticoids antagonize phorbol ester-induced AP-1 activity without altering AP-1 site occupation *in vivo*. *EMBO J.*, **11**, 2241–2246

Koo, J., Nguyen, Q. & Gambla, C. (1997) Advances in psoriasis therapy. *Adv. Dermatol.*, **12**, 47–73

Krekels, M.D., Verhoeven, A., van Dun, J., Cools, W., Van Hove, C., Dillen, L., Coene, M.C. & Wouters, W. (1997) Induction of the oxidative catabolism of retinoid acid in MCF-7 cells. *Br. J. Cancer*, **75**, 1098–1104

Kurlandsky, S.B., Gamble, M.V., Ramakrishnan, R. & Blaner, W.S. (1995) Plasma delivery of retinoic acid to tissues in the rat. *J. Biol. Chem.*, **270**, 17850–17857

Kurokawa, R., Yu, V.C., Näär, A., Kyakumoto, S., Han, Z., Silverman, S., Rosenfeld, M.G. & Glass, C.K. (1993) Differential orientations of the DNA-binding domain and carboxy-terminal dimerization interface regulate binding site selection by nuclear receptor heterodimers. *Genes Dev.*, **7**, 1423–1435

Kurokawa, R., DiRenzo, J., Boehm, M., Sugarman, J., Gloss, B., Rosenfeld, M.G., Heyman, R.A. & Glass, C.K. (1994) Regulation of retinoid sig-nalling by receptor polarity and allosteric control of ligand binding. *Nature,* **371**, 528–531

Kurzrock, R., Estey, E. & Talpaz, M. (1993) All-*trans*-retinoic acid: Tolerance and biologic effects in myelodysplastic syndrome. *J. Clin. Oncol.*, **11**, 1489–1495

Labrecque, J., Bhat, P.V. & Lacroix, A. (1993) Purification and partial characterization of a rat kidney aldehyde dehydrogenase that oxidizes retinal to retinoic acid. *Biochem. Cell. Biol.*, **71**, 85–89

Labrecque, J., Dumas, F., Lacroix, A. & Bhat, P.V. (1995) A novel isoenzyme of aldehyde dehydrogenase specifically involved in the biosynthesis of 9-*cis* and all-*trans* retinoic acid. *Biochem. J.*, **305**, 681–684

Langenfeld, J., Lonardo, F., Kiyokawa, H., Passalaris, T., Ahn, M.J., Rusch, V. & Dmitrovsky, E. (1996) Inhibited transformation of immortalized human bronchial epithelial cells by retinoic acid is linked to cyclin E down-regulation. *Oncogene*, **13**, 1983–1990

Langenfeld, J., Kiyokawa, H., Sekula, D., Boyle, J. & Dmitrovsky, E. (1997) Posttranslational regulation of cyclin D1 by retinoic acid: A chemoprevention mechanism. *Proc. Natl Acad. Sci. USA*, **94**, 12070–12074

Langston, A.W. & Gudas, L.J. (1992) Identification of a retinoic acid responsive enhancer 3' of the murine homeobox gene *Hox-1.6*. *Mech. Dev.*, **38**, 217–227

Langston, A.W., Thompson, J.R. & Gudas, L.J. (1997) Retinoic acid-responsive enhancers located 3' of the *Hox A* and *Hox B* homeobox gene clusters. Functional analysis. *J. Biol. Chem.*, **272**, 2167–2175

Lansink, M., Van Bennekum, A.M., Blaner, W.S. & Kooistra, T. (1997) Differences in metabolism and isomerization of all-*trans*-retinoic acid and 9-*cis*-retinoic acid between human endothelial cells and hepatocytes. *Eur. J. Biochem.*, **247**, 596–604

Larson, R.A., Kondo, K., Vardiman, J.W., Butler, A.E., Golomb, H.M. & Rowley, J.D. (1984) Evidence for a 15;17 translocation in every patient with acute promyelocytic leukemia. *Am. J. Med.*, **76**, 827–841

Lasnitzki, I. (1976) Reversal of methylcholanthrene-induced changes in mouse prostates *in vitro* by retinoic acid and its analogues. *Br. J. Cancer*, **34**, 239–248

Lassus, A. & Geiger, J.M. (1988) Acitretin and etretinate in the treatment of palmoplantar pustulosis: A double-blind comparative trial. *Br. J. Dermatol.*, **119**, 755–759

Lauharanta, J. & Geiger, J.M. (1989) A double-blind comparison of acitretin and etretinate in combination with bath PUVA in the treatment of extensive psoriasis. *Br. J. Dermatol.*, **121**, 107–112

Lee, M.O., Manthey, C.L. & Sladek, N.E. (1991) Identification of mouse liver aldehyde dehydrogenases that catalyze the oxidation of retinaldehyde to retinoic acid. *Biochem. Pharmacol.*, **42**, 1279–1285

Lee, M.S., Kliewer, S.A., Provencal, J., Wright, P.E. & Evans, R.M. (1993) Structure of the retinoid X receptor α DNA binding domain: A helix required for homodimeric DNA binding. *Science,* **260**, 1117–1121

Lee, H.Y., Walsh, G.L., Dawson, M.I., Hong, W.K. & Kurie, J.M. (1998) All-*trans*-retinoic acid inhibits Jun N-terminal kinase-dependent signaling pathways. *J. Biol. Chem.*, **273**, 7066–7071

Lehman, E.D., Spivey, H.O., Thayer, R.H. & Nelson, E.C. (1972) The binding of retinoic acid to serum albumin in plasma. *Fed. Proc. Am. Soc. Exp. Biol.*, **31**, A672–A672

Lehmann, J.M., Zhang, X.K. & Pfahl, M. (1992) RARγ2 expression is regulated through a retinoic acid response element embedded in Sp1 sites. *Mol. Cell. Biol.*, **12**, 2976–2985

Leo, M.A. & Lieber, C.S. (1984) Normal testicular structure and reproductive function in deermice lacking retinol and alcohol dehydrogenase activity. *J. Clin. Invest.*, **73**, 593–596

Leo, M.A., Iida, S. & Lieber, C.S. (1984) Retinoic acid metabolism by a system reconstituted with cytochrome P-450. *Arch. Biochem. Biophys.*, **234**, 305–312

Leo, M.A., Kim, C.I. & Lieber, C.S. (1987) NAD+-dependent retinol dehydrogenase in liver microsomes. *Arch. Biochem. Biophys.*, **259**, 241–249

Leo, M.A., Kim, C.I., Lowe, N. & Lieber, C.S. (1989a) Increased hepatic retinal dehydrogenase activity after phenobarbital and ethanol administration. *Biochem. Pharmacol.*, **38**, 97–103

Leo, M.A., Lasker, J.M., Raucy, J.L., Kim, C.I., Black, M. & Lieber, C.S. (1989b) Metabolism of retinol and retinoic acid by human liver cytochrome P450IIC8. *Arch. Biochem. Biophys.*, **269**, 305-312

Leroy, P., Nakshatri, H. & Chambon, P. (1991) Mouse retinoic acid receptor alpha 2 isoform is transcribed from a promoter that contains a retinoic acid response element. *Proc. Natl Acad. Sci. USA*, **88**, 10138–10142

Levin, G. & Mokady, S. (1994) 9-*cis*-β-Carotene as a precursor of retinol isomers in chicks. *Int. J. Vitam. Nutr. Res.*, **64**, 165–169

Lewis, K.C., Green, M.H., Green, J.B. & Zech, L.A. (1990) Retinol metabolism in rats with low vitamin A status: A compartmental model. *J. Lipid Res.*, **31**, 1535–1548

Li, C., Schwabe, J.W., Banayo, E. & Evans, R.M. (1997) Coexpression of nuclear receptor partners increases their solubility and biological activities. *Proc. Natl Acad. Sci. USA*, **94**, 2278–2283

Liaudet-Coopman, E.D.E. & Wellstein, A. (1996) Regulation of gene expression of a binding protein for fibroblast growth factors by retinoic acid. *J. Biol. Chem.*, **271**, 21303–21308

Licht, J.D., Chomienne, C., Goy, A., Chen, A., Scott, A.A., Head, D.R., Michaux, J.L., Wu, Y., DeBlasio, A., Miller, W.H.J., Zelenetz, A.D., Willman, C.L., Chen, Z., Chen, S.J., Zelent, A., Macintyre, E., Veil, A., Cortes, J., Kantarjian, H. & Waxman, S. (1995) Clinical and molecular characterization of a rare syndrome of acute promyelocytic leukemia associated with translocation (11;17). *Blood,* **85**, 1083–1094

Lion, F., Rotmans, J.P., Daemen, F.J. & Bonting, S.L. (1975) Biochemical aspects of the visual process. XXVII. Stereospecificity of ocular retinol dehydrogenases and the visual cycle. *Biochim. Biophys. Acta ,* **384**, 283–292

Lippel, K. & Olson, J.A. (1968) Biosynthesis of beta-glucuronides of retinol and of retinoic acid in vivo and in vitro. *J. Lipid Res.*, **9**, 168–175

Lippman, S.M. & Meyskens, F.L.Jr. (1987) Treatment of advanced squamous cell carcinoma of the skin with isotretinoin. *Ann. Intern. Med,* **107**, 499–502

Lippman, S.M., Kessler, J.F. & Meyskens, F.L.J. (1987) Retinoids as preventive and therapeutic anticancer agents (Part II). *Cancer Treat. Rep.*, **71**, 493–515

Lippman, S.M., Kavanagh, J.J., Paredes-Espinoza, M., Delgadillo-Madrueno, F., Paredes-Casillas,

P., Hong, W.K., Holdener, E. & Krakoff, I.H. (1992) 13-*cis*-Retinoic acid plus interferon α-2a: Highly active systemic therapy for squamous cell carcinoma of the cervix. *J. Natl Cancer Inst.*, **84**, 241–245

Lippman, S.M., Heyman, R.A., Kurie, J.M., Benner, S.E. & Hong, W.K. (1995) Retinoids and chemoprevention: Clinical and basic studies. *J. Cell Biochem. Suppl.*, **22**, 1–10

Little, J.M. & Radominska, A. (1997) Application of photoaffinity labeling with [11,12-^{3}H]all-*trans*-retinoic acid to characterization of rat liver microsomal UDP-glucuronosyltransferase(s) with activity toward retinoic acid. *Biochem. Biophys. Res. Commun.*, **230**, 497–500

Liu, Y., Chen, H. & Chiu, J.F. (1994) Identification of a retinoic acid response element upstream of the rat alpha-fetoprotein gene. *Mol. Cell. Endocrinol.*, **103**, 149–156

Lo, H.W. & Ali-Osman, F. (1997) Genomic cloning of hGSTP1*C, an allelic human Pi class glutathione S-transferase gene variant and functional characterization of its retinoic acid response elements. *J. Biol. Chem.*, **272**, 32743–32749

Lotan, R.(1993) Retinoids and squamous cell differentiation. In: Hong, W.K. & Lotan, R., eds, *Retinoids in Oncolog.*, New York, Marcel Dekker, pp. 43–72

Lotan, R. (1995a) Cellular biology of the retinoids. In: Degos L. & Parkinson D.R., eds, *Retinoids in Oncology*. Berlin, Springer Verlag, pp. 27–42

Lotan, R. (1995b) Retinoids and apoptosis: Implications for cancer chemoprevention and therapy. *J. Natl Cancer Inst.*, **87**, 1655–1657

Lotan, R., Lotan, D. & Kadouri, A. (1982) Comparison of retinoic acid effects on anchorage-dependent growth, anchorage-independent growth and fibrinolytic activity of neoplastic cells. *Exp. Cell Res.*, **141**, 79–86

Lotan, R., Dawson, M.I., Zou, C.C., Jong, L., Lotan, D. & Zou, C.P. (1995) Enhanced efficacy of combinations of retinoic acid- and retinoid X receptor-selective retinoids and α-interferon in inhibition of cervical carcinoma cell proliferation. *Cancer Res.*, **55**, 232–236

Louthrenoo, W. (1993) Successful treatment of severe Reiter's syndrome associated with human immunodeficiency virus infection with etretinate. Report of 2 cases. *J. Rheumatol.*, **20**, 1243–1246

Lovat, P.E., Irving, H., Annicchiarico-Petruzzelli, M., Bernassola, F., Malcolm, A.J., Pearson, A.D., Melino, G. & Redfern, C.P. (1997) Retinoids in neuroblastoma therapy: Distinct biological properties of 9-*cis*- and all-*trans*-retinoic acid. *Eur. J. Cancer*, **33**, 2075–2080

Lowe, N.J., Lazarus, V. & Matt, L. (1988) Systemic retinoid therapy for psoriasis. *J. Am. Acad. Dermatol.*, **19**, 186–191

Lozada-Nur, F. & Miranda, C. (1997) Oral lichen planus: Topical and systemic therapy. *Semin. Cutan. Med. Surg.*, **16**, 295–300

Luscher, B., Mitchell, P.J., Williams, T. & Tjian, R. (1989) Regulation of transcription factor AP-2 by the morphogen retinoic acid and by second messengers. *Genes Dev.*, **3**, 1507–1517

Lynch, R.G. (1995) Differentiation and cancer: The conditional autonomy of phenotype. *Proc. Natl Acad. Sci. USA*, **92**, 647–648

Maden, M., Hunt, P., Eriksson, U., Kuroiwa, A., Krumlauf, R. & Summerbell, D. (1991) Retinoic acid-binding protein, rhombomeres and the neural crest. *Development*, **111**, 35–43

Maden, M., Gale, E., Kostetskii, I. & Zile, M. (1996) Vitamin A-deficient quail embryos have half a hindbrain and other neural defects. *Curr. Biol.*, **6**, 417–426

Maden, M., Sonneveld, E., van der Saag, P.T. & Gale, E. (1998) The distribution of endogenous retinoic acid in the chick embryo: Implications for developmental mechanisms. *Development*, **125**, 4133–4144

Mader, S., Kumar, V., de Verneuil, H. & Chambon, P. (1989) Three amino acids of the oestrogen receptor are essential to its ability to distinguish an oestrogen from a glucocorticoid-responsive element. *Nature*, **338**, 271–274

Mader, S., Chen, J.Y., Chen, Z., White, J., Chambon, P. & Gronemeyer, H. (1993) The patterns of binding of RAR, RXR and TR homo- and heterodimers to direct repeats are dictated by the binding specificites of the DNA binding domains. *EMBO J.*, **12**, 5029–5041

Mangelsdorf, D.J. & Evans, R.M. (1995) The RXR heterodimers and orphan receptors. *Cell*, **83**, 841–850

Mangelsdorf, D.J., Umesono, K., Kliewer, S.A., Borgmeyer, U., Ong, E.S. & Evans, R.M. (1991)

A direct repeat in the cellular retinol-binding protein type II gene confers differential regulation by RXR and RAR. *Cell,* **66,** 555–561

Mangelsdorf, D.J., Umesono, K. & Evans, R.M. (1994) The retinoid receptors. In: Sporn M.B., Roberts A.B. & Goodman D.S., eds, *The Retinoids: Biology, Chemistry, and Medicine,* 2nd Ed. New York, Raven Press, pp. 319–350

Manji, S.S., Pearson, R.B., Pardee, M., Paspaliaris, V., d'Apice, A., Martin, T.J. & Ng, K.W. (1999) Dual posttranscriptional targets of retinoic acid-induced gene expression. *J. Cell Biochem.,* **72,** 411–422

Marchetti, M.N., Sampol, E., Bun, H., Scoma, H., Lacarelle, B. & Durand, A. (1997) *In vitro* metabolism of three major isomers of retinoic acid in rats. Intersex and interstrain comparison. *Drug Metab. Dispos.,* **25,** 637–646

Marshall, H., Studer, M., Pöpperl, H., Aparicio, S., Kuroiwa, A., Brenner, S. & Krumlauf, R. (1994) A conserved retinoic acid response element required for early expression of the homeobox gene *Hoxb-1. Nature,* **370,** 567–571

Martin, S.J., Bradley, J.G. & Cotter, T.G. (1990) HL-60 cells induced to differentiate towards neutrophils subsequently die via apoptosis. *Clin. Exp. Immunol.,* **79,** 448–453

Massaro, G.D. & Massaro, D. (1996) Postnatal treatment with retinoic acid increases the number of pulmonary alveoli in rats. *Am. J. Physiol.,* **270,** L305–L310

Massaro, G.D. & Massaro, D. (1997) Retinoic acid treatment abrogates elastase-induced pulmonary emphysema in rats. *Nat. Med.,* **3,** 675–677

Matsuo, T. & Thiele, C.J. (1998) p27Kip1: A key mediator of retinoic acid induced growth arrest in the SMS-KCNR human neuroblastoma cell line. *Oncogene,* **16,** 3337–3343

Maxwell, S.A. & Mukhopadhyay, T. (1994) Transient stabilization of p53 in non-small cell lung carcinoma cultures arrested for growth by retinoic acid. *Exp. Cell Res.,* **214,** 67–74

McBurney, M.W., Jones-Villeneuve, E.M., Edwards, M.K. & Anderson, P.J. (1982) Control of muscle and neuronal differentiation in a cultured embryonal carcinoma cell line. *Nature,* **299,** 165–167

McCaffery, P. & Dräger, U.C. (1994) Hot spots of retinoic acid synthesis in the developing spinal cord. *Proc. Natl Acad. Sci. USA,* **91,** 7194–7197

McCaffery, P. & Dräger, U.C. (1995) Retinoic acid synthesizing enzymes in the embryonic and adult vertebrate. *Adv. Exp. Med. Biol.,* **372,** 173–183

McCormick, A.M. & Napoli, J.L. (1982) Identification of 5,6-epoxyretinoic acid as an endogenous retinol metabolite. *J. Biol. Chem.,* **257,** 1730–1735

McCormick, A.M., Napoli, J.L., Schnoes, H.K. & DeLuca, H.F. (1978) Isolation and identification of 5,6-epoxyretinoic acid: A biologically active metabolite of retinoic acid. *Biochemistry,* **17,** 4085–4090

McCormick, A.M., Kroll, K.D. & Napoli, J.L. (1983) 13-*cis*-Retinoic acid metabolism *in vivo.* The major tissue metabolites in the rat have the all-*trans* configuration. *Biochemistry,* **22,** 3933–3940

McCue, P.A., Thomas, R.S., Schroeder, D., Gubler, M.L. & Sherman, M.I. (1988) Effects of dietary retinoids upon growth and differentiation of tumors derived from several murine embryonal carcinoma cell lines. *Cancer Res.,* **48,** 3772–3779

Mehta, R.G., Barua, A.B., Moon, R.C. & Olson, J.A. (1992) Interactions between retinoid-β-glucuronides and cellular retinol- and retinoic acid-binding proteins. *Int. J. Vitam. Nutr. Res.,* **62,** 143–147

Meisler, N.T., Parrelli, J., Gendimenico, G.J., Mezick, J.A. & Cutroneo, K.R. (1997) All-*trans*-retinoic acid inhibition of Pro alpha1(I) collagen gene expression in fetal rat skin fibroblasts: Identification of a retinoic acid response element in the Pro alpha1(I) collagen gene. *J. Invest. Dermatol.,* **108,** 476–481

Meloche, S. & Besner, J.G. (1986) Metabolism of isotretinoin. Biliary excretion of isotretinoin glucuronide in the rat. *Drug Metab. Dispos.,* **14,** 246–249

Mendelsohn, C., Ruberte, E., LeMeur, M., Morriss Kay, G. & Chambon, P. (1991) Developmental analysis of the retinoic acid-inducible RAR-β2 promoter in transgenic animals. *Development,* **113,** 723–734

Merrick, D.T., Gown, A.M., Halbert, C.L., Blanton, R.A. & McDougall, J.K. (1993) Human papillomavirus-immortalized keratinocytes are resistant to the effects of retinoic acid on terminal differentiation. *Cell Growth Differ.,* **4,** 831–840

Mertz, J.R., Shang, E., Piantedosi, R., Wei, S., Wolgemuth, D.J. & Blaner, W.S. (1997) Identification and characterization of a stereo-specific human enzyme that catalyzes 9-*cis*-retinol oxidation. A possible role in 9-*cis*-retinoic acid formation. *J. Biol. Chem.*, **272**, 11744–11749

Meyer, M.E., Gronemeyer, H., Turcotte, B., Bocquel, M.T., Tasset, D. & Chambon, P. (1989) Steroid hormone receptors compete for factors that mediate their enhancer function. *Cell*, **57**, 433–442

Meyskens, F.L., Jr & Salmon, S.E. (1979) Inhibition of human melanoma colony formation by retinoids. *Cancer Res.*, **39**, 4055–4057

Meyskens, F.L., Jr, Alberts, D.S. & Salmon, S.E. (1983) Effect of 13-*cis*-retinoic acid and 4-hydroxyphenyl-all-*trans*-retinamide on human tumor colony formation in soft agar. *Int. J. Cancer*, **32**, 295–299

Mezey, E. & Holt, P.R. (1971) The inhibitory effect of ethanol on retinol oxidation by human liver and cattle retina. *Exp. Mol. Pathol.*, **15**, 148–156

Miano, J.M., Kelly, L.A., Artacho, C.A., Nuckolls, T.A., Piantedosi, R. & Blaner, W.S. (1998) all-*trans*-Retinoic acid reduces neointimal formation and promotes favorable geometric remodeling of the rat carotid artery after balloon withdrawal injury. *Circulation*, **98**, 1219–1227

Miller, W.H.J., Jakubowski, A., Tong, W.P., Miller, V.A., Rigas, J.R., Benedetti, F., Gill, G.M., Truglia, J.A., Ulm, E., Shirley, M. & Warrell, R.P.J. (1995) 9-*cis*-Retinoic acid induces complete remission but does not reverse clinically acquired retinoid resistance in acute promyelocytic leukemia. *Blood*, **85**, 3021–3027

Miller, V.A., Benedetti, F.M., Rigas, J.R., Verret, A.L., Pfister, D.G., Straus, D., Kris, M.G., Crisp, M., Heyman, R., Loewen, G.R., Truglia, J.A. & Warrell, R.P.J. (1997) Initial clinical trial of a selective retinoid X receptor ligand, LGD1069. *J. Clin. Oncol.*, **15**, 790–795

Minucci, S., Leid, M., Toyama, R., Saint Jeannet, J.P., Peterson, V.J., Horn, V., Ishmael, J.E., Bhattacharyya, N., Dey, A., Dawid, I.B. & Ozato, K. (1997) Retinoid X receptor (RXR) within the RXR-retinoic acid receptor heterodimer binds its ligand and enhances retinoid-dependent gene expression. *Mol. Cell. Biol.*, **17**, 644–655

Moasser, M.M., Motzer, R.J., Khoo, K.S., Lyn, P., Murphy, B.A., Bosl, G.J. & Dmitrovsky, E. (1995) all-*trans*-Retinoic acid for treating germ cell tumors. In vitro activity and results of a phase II trial. *Cancer,* **76**, 680–686

Moffa, D.J., Lotspeich, F.J. & Krause, R.F. (1970) Preparation and properties of retinal-oxidizing enzyme from rat intestinal mucosa. *J. Biol. Chem.*, **245**, 439–447

Molin, L., Thomsen, K., Volden, G. & Lange Wantzin, G. (1985) Retinoid dermatitis mimicking progression in mycosis fungoides: A report from the Scandinavian Mycosis Fungoides Group. *Acta Derm. Venereol.*, **65**, 69–71

Monzon, R.I., LaPres, J.J. & Hudson, L.G. (1996) Regulation of involucrin gene expression by retinoic acid and glucocorticoids. *Cell Growth Differ.*, **7**, 1751–1759

Moras, D. & Gronemeyer, H. (1998) The nuclear receptor ligand-binding domain: Structure and function. *Curr. Opin. Cell Biol.*, **10**, 384–391

Motzer, R.J., Schwartz, L., Law, T.M., Murphy, B.A., Hoffman, A.D., Albino, A.P., Vlamis, V. & Nanus, D.M. (1995) Interferon alfa-2a and 13-*cis*-retinoic acid in renal cell carcinoma: Antitumor activity in a phase II trial and interactions in vitro. *J. Clin. Oncol.*, **13** , 1950–1957

Muindi, J.R., Frankel, S.R., Huselton, C., DeGrazia, F., Garland, W.A., Young, C.W. & Warrell,R.P., Jr (1992) Clinical pharmacology of oral all-*trans*-retinoic acid in patients with acute promyelocytic leukemia. *Cancer Res.*, **52**, 2138–2142

Mukherjee, R., Davies, P.J., Crombie, D.L., Bischoff, E.D., Cesario, R.M., Jow, L., Hamann, L.G., Boehm, M.F., Mondon, C.E., Nadzan, A.M., Paterniti, J.R., Jr & Heyman, R.A. (1997) Sensitization of diabetic and obese mice to insulin by retinoid X receptor agonists. *Nature,* **386**, 407–410

Murphy, P.T., Sivakumaran, M., Fahy, G. & Hutchinson, R.M. (1996) Successful use of topical retinoic acid in severe dry eye due to chronic graft-versus-host disease. *Bone Marrow Transplant.*, **18**, 641–642

Nagai, H., Matsuura, S., Bouda, K., Takaoka, Y., Wang, T., Niwa, S. & Shudo, K. (1999) Effect of Am-80, a synthetic derivative of retinoid, on experimental arthritis in mice. *Pharmacology,* **58**, 101–112

Nagao, A. & Olson, J.A. (1994) Enzymatic formation of 9-*cis*, 13-*cis*, and all-*trans*-retinals from isomers of β-carotene. *FASEB J.*, **8**, 968–973

Nagy, L., Thomazy, V.A., Shipley, G.L., Fesus, L., Lamph, W., Heyman, R.A., Chandraratna, R.A. & Davies, P.J. (1995) Activation of retinoid X receptors induces apoptosis in HL-60 cell lines. *Mol. Cell. Biol.*, **15**, 3540–3551

Nakshatri, H. & Chambon, P. (1994) The directly repeated RG(G/T)TCA motifs of the rat and mouse cellular retinol-binding protein II genes are promiscuous binding sites for RAR, RXR, HNF-4, and ARP-1 homo- and heterodimers. *J. Biol. Chem.*, **269**, 890–902

Napoli, J.L. (1986) Retinol metabolism in LLC-PK1 Cells. Characterization of retinoic acid synthesis by an established mammalian cell line. *J. Biol. Chem.*, **261**, 13592–13597

Napoli, J.L. (1996) Retinoic acid biosynthesis and metabolism. *FASEB J.*, **10**, 993–1001

Napoli, J.L. & Race, K.R. (1988) Biogenesis of retinoic acid from β-carotene. Differences between the metabolism of β-carotene and retinal. *J. Biol. Chem.*, **263**, 17372–17377

Napoli, J.L., Khalil, H. & McCormick, A.M. (1982) Metabolism of 5,6-epoxyretinoic acid in vivo: Isolation of a major intestinal metabolite. *Biochemistry*, **21**, 1942–1949

Napoli, J.L., Pramanik, B.C., Williams, J.B., Dawson, M.I. & Hobbs, P.D. (1985) Quantification of retinoic acid by gas–liquid chromatography–mass spectrometry: total versus all-*trans*-retinoic acid in human plasma. *J. Lipid Res.*, **26**, 387–392

Newcomer, M.E. & Ong, D.E. (1990) Purification and crystallization of a retinoic acid-binding protein from rat epididymis. Identity with the major androgen-dependent epididymal proteins. *J. Biol. Chem.*, **265**, 12876–12879

Newton, D.L., Henderson, W.R. & Sporn, M.B. (1980) Structure–activity relationships of retinoids in hamster tracheal organ culture. *Cancer Res.*, **40**, 3413–3425

Nicholson, R.C., Mader, S., Nagpal, S., Leid, M., Rochette-Egly, C. & Chambon, P. (1990) Negative regulation of the rat stromelysin gene promoter by retinoic acid is mediated by an AP1 binding site. *EMBO J.*, **9**, 4443–4454

Nicotra, C. & Livrea, M.A. (1976) Alcohol dehydrogenase and retinol dehydrogenase in bovine retinal pigment epithelium. *Exp. Eye Res.*, **22**, 367–376

Nicotra, C. & Livrea, M.A. (1982) Retinol dehydrogenase from bovine retinal rod outer segments. Kinetic mechanism of the solubilized enzyme. *J. Biol. Chem.*, **257**, 11836–11841

Niederreither, K., McCaffery, P., Dräger, U.C., Chambon, P. & Dollé, P. (1997) Restricted expression and retinoic acid-induced downregulation of the retinaldehyde dehydrogenase type 2 (RALDH-2) gene during mouse development. *Mech. Dev.*, **62**, 67–78

Nierenberg, D.W. (1984) Determination of serum and plasma concentrations of retinol using high-performance liquid chromatography. *J. Chromatogr.*, **311**, 239–248

Nolte, R.T., Wisely, G.B., Westin, S., Cobb, J.E., Lambert, M.H., Kurokawa, R., Rosenfeld, M.G., Willson, T.M., Glass, C.K. & Milburn, M.V. (1998) Ligand binding and co-activator assembly of the peroxisome proliferator-activated receptor-γ. *Nature,* **395**, 137–143

Noy, N. (1992a) The ionization behavior of retinoic acid in aqueous environments and bound to serum albumin. *Biochim. Biophys. Acta,* **1106**, 151–158

Noy, N. (1992b) The ionization behavior of retinoic acid in lipid bilayers and in membranes. *Biochim. Biophys. Acta,* **1106**, 159–164

Oldfield, N. (1990) The metabolic fate of 13-*cis*-retinoic acid in mouse skin microsomal preparations. *Drug Metab. Dispos.*, **18**, 1105–1107

Olson, J.A.(1990) Vitamin A. In: Machlin, L.J., ed., *Handbook of Vitamins.* New York, Marcel Dekker, pp. 1–57

Olson, J.A., Moon, R.C., Anders, M.W., Fenselau, C. & Shane, B. (1992) Enhancement of biological activity by conjugation reactions. *J. Nutr.*, **122**, 615–624

Orfanos, C.E., Zouboulis, C.C., Almond-Roesler, B. & Geilen, C.C. (1997) Current use and future potential role of retinoids in dermatology. *Drugs*, **53**, 358–388

Oridate, N., Lotan, D., Xu, X.C., Hong, W.K. & Lotan, R. (1996) Differential induction of apoptosis by all-*trans*-retinoic acid and *N*-(4-hydroxyphenyl)retinamide in human head and neck squamous cell carcinoma cell lines. *Clin. Cancer Res.*, **2**, 855–863

Oridate, N., Suzuki, S., Higuchi, M., Mitchell, M.F., Hong, W.K. & Lotan, R. (1997) Involvement of reactive oxygen species in *N*-(4-hydroxyphenyl)-retinamide-induced apoptosis in cervical carcinoma cells. *J. Natl Cancer Inst.,* **89**, 1191–1198

Packer, A.I., Crotty, D.A., Elwell, V.A. & Wolgemuth, D.J. (1998) Expression of the murine Hoxa4 gene requires both autoregulation and a conserved retinoic acid response element. *Development,* **125**, 1991–1998

Paech, K., Webb, P., Kuiper, G.G., Nilsson, S., Gustafsson, J., Kushner, P.J. & Scanlan, T.S. (1997) Differential ligand activation of estrogen receptors ERα and ERβ at AP1 sites. *Science,* **277**, 1508–1510

Peck, G.L., Gross, E.G., Butkus, D. & DiGiovanna, J.J. (1982) Chemoprevention of basal cell carcinoma with isotretinoin. *J. Am. Acad. Dermatol.,* **6**, 815–823

Perlmann, T. & Jansson, L. (1995) A novel pathway for vitamin A signaling mediated by RXR heterodimerization with NGFI-B and NURR1. *Genes Dev.,* **9**, 769–782

Pfahl, M. (1993) Nuclear receptor/AP-1 interaction. *Endocr. Rev.,* **14**, 651–658

Pierce, G.B. & Speers, W.C. (1988) Tumors as caricatures of the process of tissue renewal: Prospects for therapy by directing differentiation. *Cancer Res.,* **48**, 1996–2004

Pilkington, T. & Brogden, R.N. (1992) Acitretin. A review of its pharmacology and therapeutic use. *Drugs,* **43**, 597–627

Pirisi, L., Batova, A., Jenkins, G.R., Hodam, J.R. & Creek, K.E. (1992) Increased sensitivity of human keratinocytes immortalized by human papillomavirus type 16 DNA to growth control by retinoids. *Cancer Res.,* **52**, 187–193

Pomponi, F., Cariati, R., Zancai, P., De Paoli, P., Rizzo, S., Tedeschi, R.M., Pivetta, B., De Vita, S., Boiocchi, M. & Dolcetti, R. (1996) Retinoids irreversibly inhibit in vitro growth of Epstein-Barr virus-immortalized B lymphocytes. *Blood,* **88**, 3147–3159

Ponzoni, M., Bocca, P., Chiesa, V., Decensi, A., Pistoia, V., Raffaghello, L., Rozzo, C. & Montaldo, P.G. (1995) Differential effects of *N*-(4-hydroxyphenyl)retinamide and retinoic acid on neuroblastoma cells: Apoptosis *versus* differentiation. *Cancer Res.,* **55**, 853–861

Pöpperl, H. & Featherstone, M.S. (1993) Identification of a retinoic acid response element upstream of the murine *Hox-4.2* gene. *Mol. Cell. Biol.,* **13**, 257–265

Posch, K.C. & Napoli, J.L. (1992) Multiple retinoid dehydrogenases in testes cytosol from alcohol dehydrogenase negative or positive deermice. *Biochem.Pharmacol.,* **43**, 2296–2298

Posch, K.C., Boerman, M.H., Burns, R.D. & Napoli, J.L. (1991) Holocellular retinol binding protein as a substrate for microsomal retinal synthesis. *Biochemistry,* **30**, 6224–6230

Posch, K.C., Burns, R.D. & Napoli, J.L. (1992) Biosynthesis of all-trans-retinoic acid from retinal. Recognition of retinal bound to cellular retinol binding protein (type I) as substrate by a purified cytosolic dehydrogenase. *J. Biol. Chem.,* **267**, 19676–19682

Radominska, A., Little, J.M., Lehman, P.A., Samokyszyn, V., Rios, G.R., King, C.D., Green, M.D. & Tephly, T.R. (1997) Glucuronidation of retinoids by rat recombinant UDP: Glucuronosyltransferase 1.1 (bilirubin UGT). *Drug Metab. Dispos.,* **25**, 889–892

Raife, T.J., McArthur, J., Peters, C., Kisker, C.T. & Lentz, S.R. (1998) Remission after 13-*cis*-retinoic acid in thrombotic thrombocytopenic purpura. *Lancet,* **352**, 454–455

Raisher, B.D., Gulick, T., Zhang, Z., Strauss, A.W., Moore, D.D. & Kelly, D.P. (1992) Identification of a novel retinoid-responsive element in the promoter region of the medium chain acyl-coenzyme A dehydrogenase gene. *J. Biol. Chem.,* **267**, 20264–20269

Randell, S.H., Liu, J.Y., Ferriola, P.C., Kaartinen, L., Doherty, M.M., Davis, C.W. & Nettesheim, P. (1996) Mucin production by SPOC1 cells—An immortalized rat tracheal epithelial cell line. *Am. J. Respir. Cell. Mol. Biol.,* **14**, 146–154

Rastinejad, F., Perlmann, T., Evans, R.M. & Sigler, P.B. (1995) Structural determinants of nuclear receptor assembly on DNA direct repeats. *Nature,* **375**, 203–211

Ray, W.J., Bain, G., Yao, M. & Gottlieb, D.I. (1997) CYP26, a novel mammalian cytochrome P450, is induced by retinoic acid and defines a new family. *J. Biol. Chem.,* **272**, 18702–18708

Raynaud, F., Gerbaud, P., Bouloc, A., Gorin, I., Anderson, W.B. & Evain, B.D. (1993) Rapid effect of treatment of psoriatic erythrocytes with the synthetic retinoid acitretin to increase 8-azido cyclic AMP binding to the RI regulatory subunit. *J. Invest. Dermatol.,* **100,** 77–81

Reddel, R.R., Ke, Y., Gerwin, B.I., McMenamin, M.G., Lechner, J.F., Su, R.T., Brash, D.E., Park, J.B., Rhim, J.S. & Harris, C.C. (1988) Transformation of human bronchial epithelial cells by infection with SV40 or adenovirus-12 SV40 hybrid virus, or transfection via strontium phosphate coprecipitation with a plasmid containing SV40 early region genes. *Cancer Res.,* **48,** 1904–1909

Redlich, C.A., Delisser, H.M. & Elias, J.A. (1995) Retinoic acid inhibition of transforming growth factor-β-induced collagen production by human lung fibroblasts. *Am. J. Respir. Cell. Mol. Biol.,* **12,** 287–295

Redner, R.L., Rush, E.A., Faas, S., Rudert, W.A. & Corey, S.J. (1996) The t(5;17) variant of acute promyelocytic leukemia expresses a nucleophosmin-retinoic acid receptor fusion. *Blood,* **87,** 882–886

Reid, A., Gould, A., Brand, N., Cook, M., Strutt, P., Li, J., Licht, J., Waxman, S., Krumlauf, R. & Zelent, A. (1995) Leukemia translocation gene, *PLZF,* is expressed with a speckled nuclear pattern in early hematopoietic progenitors. *Blood,* **86,** 4544–4552

Renaud, J.P., Rochel, N., Ruff, M., Vivat, V., Chambon, P., Gronemeyer, H. & Moras, D. (1995) Crystal structure of the RAR-γ ligand-binding domain bound to all-*trans*-retinoic acid. *Nature,* **378,** 681–689

Reynolds, C.P., Matthay, K. & Crouse, K. (1990) Response of neuroblastoma bone marrow metastases to 13-*cis*-retinoic acid. *Proc. Am. Soc. Clin. Oncol.,* **9,** 54–54

Reynolds, C.P., Schindler, P.F., Jones, D.M., Gentile, J.L., Proffitt, R.T. & Einhorn, P.A. (1994) Comparison of 13-*cis*-retinoic acid to *trans*-retinoic acid using human neuroblastoma cell lines. *Prog. Clin. Biol. Res.,* **385,** 237–244

Ribaya-Mercado, J.D., Kassarjian, Z. & Russell, R.M. (1988) Quantitation of the enterohepatic circulation of retinol in the rat. *J. Nutr.,* **118,** 33–38

Rigas, J.R., Francis, P.A., Muindi, J.R., Kris, M.G., Huselton, C., DeGrazia, F., Orazem, J.P., Young, C.W. & Warrell-RP, J. (1993) Constitutive variability in the pharmacokinetics of the natural retinoid, all-*trans*-retinoic acid, and its modulation by ketoconazole. *J. Natl Cancer Inst.,* **85,** 1921–1926

Rigas, J.R., Miller, V.A., Zhang, Z.F., Klimstra, D.S., Tong, W.P., Kris, M.G. & Warrell, R.P. (1996) Metabolic phenotypes of retinoic acid and the risk of lung cancer. *Cancer Res.,* **56,** 2692–2696

Roberson, K.M., Penland, S.N., Padilla, G.M., Selvan, R.S., Kim, C.S., Fine, R.L. & Robertson, C.N. (1997) Fenretinide: Induction of apoptosis and endogenous transforming growth factor beta in PC-3 prostate cancer cells. *Cell Growth Differ.,* **8,** 101–111

Roberts, A.B., Nichols, M.D., Newton, D.L. & Sporn, M.B. (1979) *In vitro* metabolism of retinoic acid in hamster intestine and liver. *J. Biol. Chem.,* **254,** 6296–6302

Roberts, A.B., Lamb, L.C. & Sporn, M.B. (1980) Metabolism of all-*trans*-retinoic acid in hamster liver microsomes: Oxidation of 4-hydroxy- to 4-keto-retinoic acid. *Arch. Biochem. Biophys.,* **199,** 374–383

Roberts, A.B., Roche, N.S. & Sporn, M.B. (1985) Selective inhibition of the anchorage-independent growth of *myc*-transfected fibroblasts by retinoic acid. *Nature,* **315,** 237–239

Roberts, E.S., Vaz, A.D. & Coon, M.J. (1992) Role of isozymes of rabbit microsomal cytochrome P-450 in the metabolism of retinoic acid, retinol, and retinal. *Mol. Pharmacol.,* **41,** 427–433

Rochette-Egly, C., Adam, S., Rossignol, M., Egly, J.M. & Chambon, P. (1997) Stimulation of RARα activation function AF-1 through binding to the general transcription factor TFIIH and phosphorylation by CDK7. *Cell,* **90,** 97–107

Rosenbaum, S.E. & Niles, R.M. (1992) Regulation of protein kinase C gene expression by retinoic acid in B16 mouse melanoma cells. *Arch. Biochem. Biophys.,* **294,** 123–129

Rossant, J., Zirngibl, R., Cado, D., Shago, M. & Giguère, V. (1991) Expression of a retinoic acid response element-*hsplacZ* transgene defines specific domains of transcriptional activity during mouse embryogenesis. *Genes Dev.*, 5, 1333–1344

Rousselot, P., Hardas, B., Patel, A., Guidez, F., Gaken, J., Castaigne, S., Dejean, A., de Thé, H., Degos, L., Farzaneh, F. & Chomienne, C. (1994) The PML-RARα gene product of the t(15;17) translocation inhibits retinoic acid-induced granulocytic differentiation and mediated transactivation in human myeloid cells. *Oncogene*, 9, 545–551

Ruberte, E., Dollé, P., Krust, A., Zelent, A., Morriss, K.G. & Chambon, P. (1990) Specific spatial and temporal distribution of retinoic acid receptor gamma transcripts during mouse embryogenesis. *Development*, 108, 213–222

Ruberte, E., Dollé, P., Chambon, P. & Morriss, K.G. (1991) Retinoic acid receptors and cellular retinoid binding proteins. II. Their differential pattern of transcription during early morphogenesis in mouse embryos. *Development*, 111, 45–60

Ruberte, E., Friederich, V., Chambon, P. & Morriss, K.G. (1993) Retinoic acid receptors and cellular retinoid binding proteins. III. Their differential transcript distribution during mouse nervous system development. *Development*, 118, 267–282

Saari, J.C. (1994) Retinoids in photosensitive systems. In: Sporn, M.B., Roberts, A.B., & Goodman, D.S., eds, *The Retinoids: Biology, Chemistry, and Medicine,* 2nd Ed. New York, Raven Press, pp. 351–385

Saari, J.C. & Bredberg, L. (1982) Enzymatic reduction of 11-*cis*-retinal bound to cellular retinal-binding protein. *Biochim. Biophys. Acta*, 716, 266–272

Sachs, L. (1978) Control of normal cell differentiation and the phenotypic reversion of malignancy in myeloid leukaemia. *Nature*, 274, 535–539

Sani, B.P., Barua, A.B., Hill, D.L., Shih, T.W. & Olson, J.A. (1992) Retinoyl beta-glucuronide: Lack of binding to receptor proteins of retinoic acid as related to biological activity. *Biochem. Pharmacol.*, 43, 919–922

Sass, J.O. (1994) 3,4-Didehydroretinol may be present in human embryos/fetuses. *Reprod. Toxicol.*, 8, 191–191

Sass, J.O., Forster, A., Bock, K.W. & Nau, H. (1994) Glucuronidation and isomerization of all-*trans*- and 13-*cis*-retinoic acid by liver microsomes of phenobarbital- or 3-methylcholanthrene-treated rats. *Biochem. Pharmacol.*, 47, 485–492

Satre, M.A., Penner, J.D. & Kochhar, D.M. (1989) Pharmacokinetic assessment of teratologically effective concentrations of an endogenous retinoic acid metabolite. *Teratology*, 39, 341–348

Schmutzler, C., Brtko, J., Winzer, R., Jakobs, T.C., Meissner-Weigl, J., Simon, D., Goretzki, P.E. & Kohrle, J. (1998) Functional retinoid and thyroid hormone receptors in human thyroid-carcinoma cell lines and tissues. *Int. J. Cancer*, 76, 368–376

Schroen, D.J. & Brinckerhoff, C.E. (1996) Inhibition of rabbit collagenase (matrix metalloproteinase-1; MMP-1) transcription by retinoid receptors: Evidence for binding of RARs/RXRs to the –77 AP-1 site through interactions with c-Jun. *J. Cell Physiol.*, 169, 320–332

Schüle, R., Rangarajan, P., Yang, N., Kleiwer, S., Ransone, L.J., Bolado, J., Verma, I.M. & Evans, R.M. (1991) Retinoic acid is a negative regulator of AP-1-responsive genes. *Proc. Natl Acad. Sci. USA*, 88, 6092–6096

Scott, W.J., Jr, Walter, R., Tzimas, G., Sass, J.O., Nau, H. & Collins, M.D. (1994) Endogenous status of retinoids and their cytosolic binding proteins in limb buds of chick vs mouse embryos. *Dev. Biol.*, 165, 397–409

Scott, D.K., Mitchell, J.A. & Granner, D.K. (1996) Identification and characterization of the second retinoic acid response element in the phosphoenolpyruvate carboxykinase gene promoter. *J. Biol. Chem.*, 271, 6260–6264

Shaulsky, G., Goldfinger, N., Peled, A. & Rotter, V. (1991) Involvement of wild-type p53 in pre-B-cell differentiation *in vitro*. *Proc. Natl Acad. Sci. USA*, 88, 8982–8986

Shiau, A.K., Barstad, D., Loria, P.M., Cheng, L., Kushner, P.J., Agard, D.A. & Greene, G.L. (1998) The structural basis of estrogen receptor/coactivator recognition and the antagonism of this interaction by tamoxifen. *Cell*, 95, 927–937

Shih, T.W. & Hill, D.L. (1991) Conversion of retinol to retinal by rat liver microsomes. *Drug Metab. Dispos.*, 19, 332–335

Shih, T.W., Lin, T.H., Shealy, Y.F. & Hill, D.L. (1997) Nonenzymatic isomerization of 9-*cis*-retinoic acid catalyzed by sulfhydryl compounds. *Drug Metab. Dispos.*, 25, 27–32

Shindoh, M., Sun, Q., Pater, A. & Pater, M.M. (1995) Prevention of carcinoma in situ of human papillomavirus type 16-immortalized human endocervical cells by retinoic acid in organotypic raft culture. *Obstet. Gynecol.*, **85**, 721–728

Sietsema, W.K. & DeLuca, H.F. (1982) A new vaginal smear assay for vitamin A in rats. *J. Nutr.*, **112**, 1481–1489

Simeone, A., Acampora, D., D'Esposito, M., Faiella, A., Pannese, M., Scotto, L., Montanucci, M., D'Alessandro, G., Mavilio, F. & Boncinelli, E. (1989) Posttranscriptional control of human homeobox gene expression in induced NTERA-2 embryonal carcinoma cells. *Mol. Reprod. Dev.*, **1**, 107–115

Simon, A., Hellman, U., Wernstedt, C. & Eriksson, U. (1995) The retinal pigment epithelial-specific 11-*cis* retinol dehydrogenase belongs to the family of short chain alcohol dehydrogenases. *J. Biol. Chem.*, **270**, 1107–1112

Skare, K.L. & DeLuca, H.F. (1983) Biliary metabolites of all-*trans*-retinoic acid in the rat. *Arch. Biochem. Biophys.*, **224**, 13–18

Smith, J.E., Milch, P.O., Muto, Y. & Goodman, D.S. (1973) The plasma transport and metabolism of retinoic acid in the rat. *Biochem. J.*, **132**, 821–827

Smith, M.A., Parkinson, D.R., Cheson, B.D. & Friedman, M.A. (1992) Retinoids in cancer therapy. *J. Clin. Oncol.*, **10**, 839–864

Solary, E., Bertrand, R. & Pommier, Y. (1994) Apoptosis of human leukemic HL-60 cells induced to differentiate by phorbol ester treatment. *Leukemia*, **8**, 792–797

Sonneveld, E., van den Brink, C.E., van der Leede, B.M., Schulkes, R.K., Petkovich, M., van der Burg, B. & van der Saag, P.T. (1998) Human retinoic acid (RA) 4-hydroxylase (CYP26) is highly specific for all-*trans*-RA and can be induced through RA receptors in human breast and colon carcinoma cells. *Cell Growth Differ.*, **9**, 629–637

Spanjaard, R.A., Sugawara, A., Ikeda, M. & Chin, W.W. (1995) Evidence that retinoid X receptors mediate retinoid-dependent transcriptional activation of the retinoic acid receptor beta gene in S91 melanoma cells. *J. Biol. Chem.*, **270**, 17429–17436

Speers, W.C. & Altmann, M. (1984) Chemically induced differentiation of murine embryonal carcinoma *in vivo*: Transplantation of differentiated tumors. *Cancer Res.*, **44**, 2129–2135

Strickland, S., Smith, K.K. & Marotti, K.R. (1980) Hormonal induction of differentiation in teratocarcinoma stem cells: Generation of parietal endoderm by retinoic acid and dibutyryl cAMP. *Cell*, **21**, 347–355

Su, J., Chai, X., Kahn, B. & Napoli, J.L. (1998) cDNA cloning, tissue distribution, and substrate characteristics of a *cis*-retinol/3α-hydroxysterol short-chain dehydrogenase isozyme. *J. Biol. Chem.*, **273**, 17910–17916

Sucov, H.M., Murakami, K.K. & Evans, R.M. (1990) Characterization of an autoregulated response element in the mouse retinoic acid receptor type β gene. *Proc. Natl Acad. Sci. USA*, **87**, 5392–5396

Sun, S.Y., Yue, P., Dawson, M.I., Shroot, B., Michel, S., Lamph, W.W., Heyman, R.A., Teng, M., Chandraratna, R.A., Shudo, K., Hong, W.K. & Lotan, R. (1997) Differential effects of synthetic nuclear retinoid receptor-selective retinoids on the growth of human non-small cell lung carcinoma cells. *Cancer Res.*, **57**, 4931–4939

Sun, S.Y., Kurie, J.M., Yue, P., Dawson, M.I., Shroot, B., Chandraratna, R.A., Hong, W.K. & Lotan, R. (1999a) Differential responses of normal, premalignant, and malignant human bronchial epithelial cells to receptor-selective retinoids. *Clin. Cancer Res.*, **5**, 431–437

Sun, S.Y., Yue, P. & Lotan, R. (1999b) Induction of apoptosis by *N*-(4-hydroxyphenyl)retinamide and its association with reactive oxygen species, nuclear retinoic acid receptors, and apoptosis-related genes in human prostate carcinoma cells. *Mol. Pharmacol.*, **55**, 403–410

Sun, S.Y., Li, W., Yue, P., Lippman, S.M., Hong, W.K. & Lotan, R. (1999c) Mediation of N-(4-hydroxyphenyl) retinamide-induced apoptosis in human cancer cells by different mechanisms. *Cancer Res.*, **59**, 2493–2498

Supino, R., Crosti, M., Clerici, M., Warlters, A., Cleris, L., Zunino, F. & Formelli, F. (1996) Induction of apoptosis by fenretinide (4HPR) in human ovarian carcinoma cells and its association with retinoic acid receptor expression. *Int. J. Cancer*, **65**, 491–497

Suzuki, Y., Ishiguro, S. & Tamai, M. (1993) Identification and immunohistochemistry of retinol dehydrogenase from bovine retinal pigment epithelium. *Biochim. Biophys. Acta*, **1163**, 201–208

Swanson, B.N., Frolik, C.A., Zaharevitz, D.W., Roller, P.P. & Sporn, M.B. (1981) Dose-dependent kinetics of all-*trans*-retinoic acid in rats. Plasma levels and excretion into bile, urine, and faeces. *Biochem. Pharmacol.*, **30**, 107–113

Takaoka, Y., Nagai, H., Mori, H. & Tanahashi, M. (1997) The effect of TRK-530 on experimental arthritis in mice. *Biol. Pharm. Bull.*, **20**, 1147–1150

Takeshita, A., Shibata, Y., Shinjo, K., Yanagi, M., Tobita, T., Ohnishi, K., Miyawaki, S., Shudo, K. & Ohno, R. (1996) Successful treatment of relapse of acute promyelocytic leukemia with a new synthetic retinoid, Am80. *Ann. Intern. Med*, **124**, 893–896

Tallman, M.S., Andersen, J.W., Schiffer, C.A., Appelbaum, F.R., Feusner, J.H., Ogden, A., Shepherd, L., Willman, C., Bloomfield, C.D., Rowe, J.M. & Wiernik, P.H. (1997) All-*trans*-retinoic acid in acute promyelocytic leukemia. *N. Engl. J. Med.*, **337**, 1021–1028

Talmage, D.A. & Lackey, R.S. (1992) Retinoic acid receptor α suppresses polyomavirus transformation and c-*fos* expression in rat fibroblasts. *Oncogene*, **7**, 1837–1845

Tanaka, T., Urade, Y., Kimura, H., Eguchi, N., Nishikawa, A. & Hayaishi, O. (1997) Lipocalin-type prostaglandin D synthase (β-trace) is a newly recognized type of retinoid transporter. *J. Biol. Chem.*, **272**, 15789–15795

Taneja, R., Roy, B., Plassat, J.L., Zusi, C.F., Ostrowski, J., Reczek, P.R. & Chambon, P. (1996) Cell-type and promoter-context dependent retinoic acid receptor (RAR) redundancies for *RARβ 2* and *Hoxa-1* activation in F9 and P19 cells can be artefactually generated by gene knockouts. *Proc. Natl Acad. Sci. USA*, **93**, 6197–6202

Tanenbaum, D.M., Wang, Y., Williams, S.P. & Sigler, P.B. (1998) Crystallographic comparison of the estrogen and progesterone receptor's ligand binding domains. *Proc. Natl Acad. Sci. USA*, **95**, 5998–6003

Tang, G.W. & Russell, R.M. (1990) 13-*cis*-Retinoic acid is an endogenous compound in human serum. *J. Lipid Res.*, **31**, 175–182

Tang, G. & Russell, R.M. (1991) Formation of all-*trans*-retinoic acid and 13-*cis*-retinoic acid from all-*trans*-retinyl palmitate in humans. *J. Nutr. Biochem.*, **2**, 210–213

Tang, G., Shiau, A., Russell, R.M. & Mobarhan, S. (1995) Serum retinoic acid levels in patients with resected benign and malignant colonic neoplasias on β-carotene supplementation. *Nutr. Cancer*, **23**, 291–298

Thaller, C. & Eichele, G. (1987) Identification and spatial distribution of retinoids in the developing chick limb bud. *Nature*, **327**, 625–628

Thaller, C. & Eichele, G. (1990) Isolation of 3,4-didehydroretinoic acid, a novel morphogenetic signal in the chick wing bud. *Nature*, **345**, 815–819

de Thé, H., Vivanco-Ruiz, M.M., Tiollais, P., Stunnenberg, H. & Dejean, A. (1990) Identification of a retinoic acid responsive element in the retinoic acid receptor β gene. *Nature*, **343**, 177–180

de Thé, H., Lavau, C., Marchio, A., Chomienne, C., Degos, L. & Dejean, A. (1991) The PML-RARα fusion mRNA generated by the t(15;17) translocation in acute promyelocytic leukemia encodes a functionally altered RAR. *Cell*, **66**, 675–684

Thompson, H.J., Strange, R. & Schedin, P.J. (1992) Apoptosis in the genesis and prevention of cancer. *Cancer Epidemiol. Biomarkers. Prev.*, **1**, 597–602

Torchia, J., Glass, C. & Rosenfeld, M.G. (1998) Co-activators and co-repressors in the integration of transcriptional responses. *Curr. Opin. Cell Biol.*, **10**, 373–383

Trofimova-Griffin, M.E. & Juchau, M.R. (1998) Expression of cytochrome P450RAI (CYP26) in human fetal hepatic and cephalic tissues. *Biochem. Biophys. Res. Commun.*, **252**, 487–491

Tseng, S.C. (1986) Topical tretinoin treatment for severe dry-eye disorders. *J. Am. Acad. Dermatol.*, **15**, 860–866

Tzimas, G., Collins, M.D. & Nau, H. (1995) Developmental stage-associated differences in the transplacental distribution of 13-*cis*- and all-*trans*-retinoic acid as well as their glucuronides in rats and mice. *Toxicol. Appl. Pharmacol.*, **133**, 91–101

Tzimas, G., Collins, M.D., Bürgin, H., Hummler, H. & Nau, H. (1996a) Embryotoxic doses of vitamin A to rabbits result in low plasma but high embryonic concentrations of all-*trans*-retinoic acid: Risk of vitamin A exposure in humans. *J. Nutr.*, **126**, 2159–2171

Tzimas, G., Nau, H., Hendrickx, A.G., Peterson, P.E. & Hummler, H. (1996b) Retinoid metabolism and transplacental pharmacokinetics in the cynomolgus monkey following a nonteratogenic dosing regimen with all-*trans*-retinoic acid. *Teratology,* **54**, 255–265

Umesono, K. & Evans, R.M. (1989) Determinants of target gene specificity for steroid/thyroid hormone receptors. *Cell,* **57**, 1139–1146

Urbach, J. & Rando, R.R. (1994) Isomerization of all-*trans*-retinoic acid to 9-*cis*-retinoic acid. *Biochem. J.,* **299**, 459–465

Van Wauwe, J., Van-Nyen, G., Coene, M.C., Stoppie, P., Cools, W., Goossens, J., Borghgraef, P. & Janssen, P.A. (1992) Liarozole, an inhibitor of retinoic acid metabolism, exerts retinoid-mimetic effects in vivo. *J. Pharmacol. Exp. Ther.,* **261**, 773–779

Vayssière, B.M., Dupont, S., Choquart, A., Petit, F., Garcia, T., Marchandeau, C., Gronemeyer, H. & Resche-Rigon, M. (1997) Synthetic glucocorticoids that dissociate transactivation and AP-1 transrepression exhibit antiinflammatory activity in vivo. *Mol. Endocrinol.,* **11**, 1245–1255

Villablanca, J.G., Khan, A.A., Avramis, V.I., Seeger, R.C., Matthay, K.K., Ramsay, N.K. & Reynolds, C.P. (1995) Phase I trial of 13-*cis*-retinoic acid in children with neuroblastoma following bone marrow transplantation. *J. Clin. Oncol.,* **13**, 894–901

Voegel, J.J., Heine, M.J., Tini, M., Vivat, V., Chambon, P. & Gronemeyer, H. (1998) The coactivator TIF2 contains three nuclear receptor-binding motifs and mediates transactivation through CBP binding-dependent and -independent pathways. *EMBO J.,* **17**, 507–519

Vogelstein, B. & Kinzler, K.W. (1992) p53 Function and dysfunction. *Cell,* **70**, 523–526

de Vos, S., Dawson, M.I., Holden, S., Le, T., Wang, A., Cho, S.K., Chen, D.L. & Koeffler, H.P. (1997) Effects of retinoid X receptor-selective ligands on proliferation of prostate cancer cells. *Prostate,* **32**, 115–121

Wagner, M., Han, B. & Jessell, T.M. (1992) Regional differences in retinoid release from embryonic neural tissue detected by an in vitro reporter assay. *Development,* **116**, 55–66

Wagner, R.L., Apriletti, J.W., McGrath, M.E., West, B.L., Baxter, J.D. & Fletterick, R.J. (1995) A structural role for hormone in the thyroid hormone receptor. *Nature,* **378**, 690–697

Wan, H., Dawson, M.I., Hong, W.K. & Lotan, R. (1997) Enhancement of Calu-1 human lung

carcinoma cell growth in serum-free medium by retinoids: Dependence on AP-1 activation, but not on retinoid response element activation. *Oncogene,* **15**, 2109–2118

Wang, T.T. & Phang, J.M. (1996) Effect of *N*-(4-hydroxyphenyl)retinamide on apoptosis in human breast cancer cells. *Cancer Lett.,* **107**, 65–71

Wang, X.D., Tang, G.W., Fox, J.G., Krinsky, N.I. & Russell, R.M. (1991) Enzymatic conversion of beta-carotene into beta-apo-carotenals and retinoids by human, monkey, ferret, and rat tissues. *Arch. Biochem. Biophys.,* **285**, 8–16

Wang, X.D., Krinsky, N.I., Tang, G.W. & Russell, R.M. (1992) Retinoic acid can be produced from excentric cleavage of beta-carotene in human intestinal mucosa. *Arch. Biochem. Biophys.,* **293**, 298–304

Wang, X., Penzes, P. & Napoli, J.L. (1996a) Cloning of a cDNA encoding an aldehyde dehydrogenase and its expression in *Escherichia coli*. Recognition of retinal as substrate. *J. Biol. Chem.,* **271**, 16288–16293

Wang, X.D., Russell, R.M., Liu, C., Stickel, F., Smith, D.E. & Krinsky, N.I. (1996b) Beta-oxidation in rabbit liver in vitro and in the perfused ferret liver contributes to retinoic acid biosynthesis from beta-apocarotenoic acids. *J. Biol. Chem.,* **271**, 26490–26498

Warkany, J. (1945) Manifestations of prenatal nutritional deficiency. *Vitam. Hormones,* **3**, 73–103

Warrell, R.P., Jr, de Thé, H., Wang, Z.Y. & Degos, L. (1993) Acute promyelocytic leukemia. *N. Engl. J. Med.,* **329**, 177–189

Weis, K.E., Ekena, K., Thomas, J.A., Lazennec, G. & Katzenellenbogen, B.S. (1996) Constitutively active human estrogen receptors containing amino acid substitutions for tyrosine 537 in the receptor protein. *Mol. Endocrinol.,* **10**, 1388–1398

Wellik, D.M., Norback, D.H. & DeLuca, H.F. (1997) Retinol is specifically required during midgestation for neonatal survival. *Am. J. Physiol.,* **272**, E25–E29

Wells, R.A. & Kamel-Reid, S. (1996) NuMA-RARα, a new gene fusion in acute promyelocytic leukaemia. *Blood,* **88** (Suppl. 1), 365a

White, J.A., Guo, Y.D., Baetz, K., Beckett-Jones, B., Bonasoro, J., Hsu, K.E., Dilworth, F.J., Jones, G. & Petkovich, M. (1996) Identification of the retinoic acid-inducible all-*trans*-retinoic acid 4-hydroxylase. *J. Biol. Chem.*, **271**, 29922–29927

White, J.A., Beckett-Jones, B., Guo, Y.D., Dilworth, F.J., Bonasoro, J., Jones, G. & Petkovich, M. (1997a) cDNA cloning of human retinoic acid-metabolizing enzyme (hP450RAI) identifies a novel family of cytochromes P450. *J. Biol. Chem.*, **272**, 18538–18541

White, R., Sjöberg, M., Kalkhoven, E. & Parker, M.G. (1997b) Ligand-independent activation of the oestrogen receptor by mutation of a conserved tyrosine. *EMBO J.*, **16**, 1427–1435

Wiley, J.S. & Firkin, F.C. (1995) Reduction of pulmonary toxicity by prednisolone prophylaxis during all-*trans*-retinoic acid treatment of acute promyelocytic leukemia. Australian Leukaemia Study Group. *Leukemia, 9*, 774–778

Williams, S.P. & Sigler, P.B. (1998) Atomic structure of progesterone complexed with its receptor. *Nature, 393*, 392–396

Williams, J.B., Pramanik, B.C. & Napoli, J.L. (1984) Vitamin A metabolism: Analysis of steady-state neutral metabolites in rat tissues. *J. Lipid Res.*, **25**, 638–645Wilson, J.G., Roth, B. & Warkany, J. (1953) An analysis of the syndrome of malformations induced by maternal vitamin A deficiency. Effects of restoration of vitamin A at various times during gestation. *Am. J. Anat., 92*, 189–217

Wilson, T.E., Paulsen, R.E., Padgett, K.A. & Milbrandt, J. (1992) Participation of non-zinc finger residues in DNA binding by two nuclear orphan receptors. *Science, 256*, 107–110

Wright, P. (1985) Topical retinoic acid therapy for disorders of the outer eye. *Trans. Ophthalmol. Soc. UK*, **104**, 869–874

Wurtz, J.M., Bourguet, W., Renaud, J.P., Vivat, V., Chambon, P., Moras, D. & Gronemeyer, H. (1996) A canonical structure for the ligand-binding domain of nuclear receptors. *Nat. Struct. Biol.*, **3**, 87–94

Yamagata, T., Momoi, M.Y., Yanagisawa, M., Kumagai, H., Yamakado, M. & Momoi, T. (1994) Changes of the expression and distribution of retinoic acid receptors during neurogenesis in mouse embryos. *Brain Res. Dev. Brain Res.*, **77**, 163–176

Yang, Y., Vacchio, M.S. & Ashwell, J.D. (1993) 9-*cis*-Retinoic acid inhibits activation-driven T-cell apoptosis: Implications for retinoid X receptor involvement in thymocyte development. *Proc. Natl Acad. Sci. USA*, **90**, 6170–6174

Yang, Z.N., Davis, G.J., Hurley, T.D., Stone, C.L., Li, T.K. & Bosron, W.F. (1994) Catalytic efficiency of human alcohol dehydrogenases for retinol oxidation and retinal reduction. *Alcohol Clin. Exp. Res.*, **18**, 587–591

Yang, Y., Minucci, S., Ozato, K., Heyman, R.A. & Ashwell, J.D. (1995) Efficient inhibition of activation-induced Fas ligand up-regulation and T cell apoptosis by retinoids requires occupancy of both retinoid X receptors and retinoic acid receptors. *J. Biol. Chem.*, **270**, 18672–18677

You, C.S., Parker, R.S., Goodman, K.J., Swanson, J.E. & Corso, T.N. (1996) Evidence of *cis–trans* isomerization of 9-*cis*-β-carotene during absorption in humans. *Am. J. Clin. Nutr.*, **64**, 177–183

Yuan, Z.F., Davis, A., Macdonald, K. & Bailey, R.R. (1995) Use of acitretin for the skin complications in renal transplant recipients. *N. Z. Med. J.*, **108**, 255–256

Yung, B.Y., Luo, K.J. & Hui, E.K. (1992) Interaction of antileukemia agents adriamycin and daunomycin with sphinganine on the differentiation of human leukemia cell line HL-60. *Cancer Res.*, **52**, 3593–3597

Zachman, R.D. & Olson, J.A. (1961) A comparison of retinene reductase and alcohol dehydrogenase of rat liver. *J. Biol. Chem.*, **236**, 2309–2313

Zachman, R.D., Dunagin, P.E., Jr & Olson, J.A. (1966) Formation and enterohepatic circulation of metabolites of retinol and retinoic acid in bile duct-cannulated rats. *J. Lipid Res.*, **7**, 3–9

Zechel, C., Shen, X.Q., Chen, J.Y., Chen, Z.P., Chambon, P. & Gronemeyer, H. (1994) The dimerization interfaces formed between the DNA binding domains of RXR, RAR and TR determine the binding specificity and polarity of the full-length receptors to direct repeats. *EMBO J.*, **13**, 1425–1433

Zhai, Y., Higgins, D. & Napoli, J.L. (1997) Coexpression of the mRNAs encoding retinol dehydrogenase isozymes and cellular retinol-binding protein. *J. Cell Physiol.*, **173**, 36–43

Zhang, W., Hu, G., Estey, E., Hester, J. & Deisseroth, A. (1992) Altered conformation of the p53 protein in myeloid leukemia cells and mitogen-stimulated normal blood cells. *Oncogene*, **7**, 1645–1647

Zhao, D., McCaffery, P., Ivins, K.J., Neve, R.L., Hogan, P., Chin, W.W. & Dräger, U.C. (1996) Molecular identification of a major retinoic-acid-synthesizing enzyme, a retinaldehyde-specific dehydrogenase. *Eur. J. Biochem.*, **240**, 15–22

Zhou, H., Manji, S.S., Findlay, D.M., Martin, T.J., Heath, J.K. & Ng, K.W. (1994) Novel action of retinoic acid. Stabilization of newly synthesized alkaline phosphatase transcripts. *J. Biol. Chem.*, **269**, 22433–22439

Zhou, X.F., Shen, X.Q. & Shemshedini, L. (1999) Ligand-activated retinoic acid receptor inhibits AP-1 transactivation by disrupting c-Jun/c-Fos dimerization. *Mol. Endocrinol.*, **13**, 276–285

Zhu, W.Y., Jones, C.S., Kiss, A., Matsukuma, K., Amin, S. & De-Luca, L.M. (1997) Retinoic acid inhibition of cell cycle progression in MCF-7 human breast cancer cells. *Exp. Cell Res.*, **234**, 293–299

Zile, M.H. (1998) Vitamin A and embryonic development: aAn overview. *J. Nutr.*, **128**, 455S–458S

Zile, M.H., Inhorn, R.C. & DeLuca, H.F. (1982) Metabolism in vivo of all-trans-retinoic acid. Biosynthesis of 13-*cis*-retinoic acid and all-*trans*- and 13-*cis*-retinoyl glucuronides in the intestinal mucosa of the rat. *J. Biol. Chem.*, **257**, 3544–3550

Zile, M.H., Cullum, M.E., Simpson, R.U., Barua, A.B. & Swartz, D.A. (1987) Induction of differentiation of human promyelocytic leukemia cell line HL-60 by retinoyl glucuronide, a biologically active metabolite of vitamin A. *Proc. Natl Acad. Sci. USA*, **84**, 2208–2212

Zou, C.P., Kurie, J.M., Lotan, D., Zou, C.C., Hong, W.K. & Lotan, R. (1998) Higher potency of N-(4-hydroxyphenyl)retinamide than all-*trans*-retinoic acid in induction of apoptosis in non-small cell lung cancer cell lines. *Clin. Cancer Res.*, **4**, 1345–1355

Handbook 1

all-*trans*-Retinoic acid

1. Chemical and Physical Characteristics

1.1 Nomenclature
See General Remarks, section 1.4

1.2 Name: all-*trans*-Retinoic acid
Chemical Abstracts Services Registry Number
302-79-4

IUPAC Systematic Name
(all-*E*)-9,13-Dimethyl-7(1,1,5-trimethylcyclohex-5-en-6-yl)nona-7,9,11,13-tetraen-15-oic acid (see 1.3), or (all-*E*)-3,7-dimethyl-9-(2,2,6-trimethylcy-clohex-1-en-1-yl)nona-2,4,6,8-tetraen-1-oic acid

Synonyms
Vitamin A acid, vitamin A_1 acid, *trans*-retinoic acid, tretinoin; Retin-A, Aberel, Airol, Aknoten, Atra, Cordes Vas, Dermairol, Epi-Aberol, Eudyna, Vesanoid.

1.3 Structural and molecular formulae and relative molecular mass

Composition: $C_{20}H_{28}O_2$
Relative molecular mass: 300.45

1.4 Physical and chemical properties

Description
Yellow crystals from ethanol

Melting-point
180–182°C (Budavari *et al.*, 1996)

Solubility
Soluble in most organic solvents, fats and oils; sparingly soluble in water (0.21 mmol/L) (Szuts & Harosi, 1991).

Spectroscopy
UV and visible: λ_{max} 350 (ethanol), $E_{1\ cm}^{1\%}$ 1510, E_M 45 300 (Frickel, 1984; Barua & Furr, 1998).

Nuclear magnetic resonance
^{1}H-NMR (CDCl$_3$, 220 MHz): δ 1.02 (1-CH$_3$), 1.47 (2-CH$_2$), 1.62 (3-CH$_2$), 1.72 (5-CH$_3$), 2.01 (9-CH$_3$), 2.02 (4-CH$_2$), 2.37 (13-CH$_3$), 5.79 (14-H), 6.14 (8-H), 6.15 (10-H), 6.29 (7-H), 6.31 (12-H), 7.03 (11-H); $J_{7,8}$ (16 Hz), $J_{10,11}$ (11.5 Hz), $J_{11,12}$ (15 Hz) (Schweiter *et al.*, 1969; Vetter *et al.*, 1971; Frickel, 1984; Barua & Furr, 1998).

^{13}C-NMR (CDCl$_3$, 68 MHz) δ 12.9 (9-CH$_3$), 13.9 (13-CH$_3$), 19.5 (3-C), 21.6 (5-CH$_3$), 29.0 (1,1-CH$_3$), 33.3 (4-C), 34.5 (1-C), 40.0 (2-C), 118.5 (14-C), 128.7 (7-C), 129.8 (5-C, 10-C), 131.1 (11-C), 135.5 (12-C), 137.6 (8-C), 138.0 (6-C), 139.3 (9-C), 153.2 (13-C), 168.6 (15-C) (Englert, 1975; Frickel, 1984; Barua & Furr, 1998).

Resonance Raman, infrared and mass spectrometry
(Frickel, 1984; Barua & Furr, 1998).

X-Ray analysis
(Stam & MacGillavry, 1963; Frickel, 1984).

Stability
Unstable to light, oxygen and heat, protected in solution by the presence of antioxidants, such as butylated hydroxytoluene and pyrogallol. A variety of factors influence the stability of all-*trans*-retinoic acid in tissue culture media. Degradation and isomerization are minimized by storing under an inert gas, e.g. argon, at –20 °C or lower temperatures in the dark (Frickel, 1984; Barua & Furr, 1998).

2. Occurrence, Production, Use, Human Exposure and Analysis

2.1 Occurrence

The concentration of all-*trans*-retinoic acid in the plasma of fasting individuals is 4–14 nmol/L (Blaner & Olson, 1994). Most other tissues of the body also contain all-*trans*-retinoic acid, at concentrations of 40–6000 pmol/g wet weight (Napoli, 1994; Zhuang *et al.*, 1995). The concentration of all-*trans*-retinoic acid is < 1% that of all-*trans*-retinol in human plasma and < 5% that of total vitamin A in the tissues of healthy animals and humans, and all-*trans*-retinoic acid is present only in traces in plants, if at all. Thus, all-*trans*-retinoic acid is a very minor constituent of the diet. Some foods, such as dairy products, sugar and comestible oils, have been fortified with vitamin A but not with all-*trans*-retinoic acid, which, unlike vitamin A and carotenoids, is not available as a dietary supplement.

2.2 Production

Attempts to synthesize retinol were initiated soon after its structure was determined by von Euler and Karrer in 1931. all-*trans*-Retinoic acid was synthesized by Arens and van Dorp in 1946. The first successful industrial synthesis of all-*trans*-retinol was devised by Isler in 1947 with the Lindlar catalyst. In the 1960s, Pommer and his colleagues used the Wittig reaction involving phosphonium salts to devise an elegant new industrial method for the synthesis of retinol, retinoic acid and β-carotene in the 1960s. In the early 1970s, Julia and Arnoud devised an effective synthesis of all-*trans*-retinoic acid by using the C-15 sulfone as an intermediate (Frickel, 1984). Other synthetic procedures have since been developed which have been used in the formation of a large number of related compounds (Frickel, 1984; Dawson & Hobbs, 1994).

2.3 Use

all-*trans*-Retinoic acid is used primarily for treating dermatological disorders (Peck & DiGiovanna, 1994; Vahlquist, 1994), but it has also been used to treat several types of human cancer (Hong & Itri, 1994), both in experimental animals and in humans, and to reduce elastase-induced emphysema in rats (Massaro & Massaro, 1997).

The skin disorders that have been treated with all-*trans*-retinoic acid are listed in Table 1. The most efficacious oral doses are 1–2 mg/kg bw per day (Peck & DiGiovanna, 1994; Vahlquist, 1994), although such doses often induce adverse side-effects, as discussed in section 2.4. Daily topical doses of up to 0.1% all-*trans*-retinoic acid in creams or gels are effective in treating acne and photoageing, but adverse side-effects are again common. Both the efficacy of all-*trans*-retinoic acid and the incidence of side-effects are dose-dependent. Thus, retinoids with therapeutic efficacy but little if any toxicity are being sought avidly.

Some of the precancerous conditions and cancers treated with all-*trans*-retinoic acid are summarized in Table 2. Oral doses of 0.5–2 mg/kg bw per day have commonly been used, but oral doses of 5–10 mg/day have also been given. all-*trans*-Retinoic acid has been approved for use in the treatment of acute promyelocytic leukaemia at a dose of 45 mg/m² per day, and patients with cervical dysplasia were treated topically with 0.37% all-*trans*-retinoic acid in a sponge or gel (Hong & Itri, 1994).

Table 1. Some skin disorders treated with all-*trans*-retinoic acid [a]

Acne vulgaris
Cystic acne
Keloids
Lichen planus
Photoaged skin
Psoriasis

[a] Modified from Vahlquist (1994) and from Peck & DiGiovanna (1994)

Table 2. Some precancerous conditions and cancers treated with all-*trans*-retinoic acid[a]

Actinic keratosis
Acute promyelocytic leukemia
Basal-cell carcinoma
Cervical dysplasia
Oral leukoplakia

[a] Cited by Hong & Itri (1994)

2.4 Human exposure

As indicated above, the amount of retinoic acids in the diet is very small, probably in the range of 10–100 µg/day. Because all-*trans*-retinoic acid is rapidly metabolized in the body and is not stored in the liver or other organs, it does not accumulate over time (Blaner & Olson, 1994). The amount of all-*trans*-retinoic acid ingested in the diet therefore poses neither a benefit nor a risk. As a consequence, exposure to all-*trans*-retinoic acid is limited, for all practical purposes, to the oral or topical treatment of medical disorders. As indicated in section 2.3, the maximum oral dose is approximately 2 mg/kg bw per day. The many adverse side-effects observed at such doses (Kamm *et al.*, 1984; Armstrong *et al.*, 1994) are described in section 7.1.

Topical treatment of acne and photoaged skin with creams or gels containing up to 0.1% all-*trans*-retinoic acid is common (Peck & DiGiovanna, 1994; Vahlquist, 1994). Previously, higher concentrations (0.3–0.4%) were used.

2.5 Analysis

all-*trans*-Retinoic acid in plasma and tissues is commonly measured by high-performance liquid chromatography (HPLC) (Barua & Furr, 1998). The plasma is collected in heparinized tubes, and either plasma or a tissue homogenate is acidified and then extracted several times with a suitable volume of an organic solvent, such as chloroform and methanol, diethyl ether, dichloromethane, acetonitrile, 2-propanol or ethyl acetate. After the combined extract has been dried with anhydrous sodium sulfate, the solvent is evaporated to dryness under yellow light (to avoid isomerization) in nitrogen or argon. The dried powder is immediately dissolved in the HPLC solvent and injected onto the HPLC column. In some cases, a solid-phase extraction or elution step is introduced to remove contaminants.

A reversed-phase C18 column is usually used for the separation, and the compound is usually detected by measuring the absorption at 350 nm and quantified by measuring the area under the absorption peak with an integrator. A known amount of a reference standard, usually all-*trans*-retinyl acetate, is added to the tissue, plasma or serum sample to correct for losses during extraction and analysis. An antioxidant such as butylated hydroxytoluene is also added at the outset to minimize oxidation of the retinoids.

A large number of chromatographic systems have been devised for the separation and quantification of all-*trans*-retinoic acid (Frolik & Olson, 1984; Furr *et al.*, 1992, 1994; Barua & Furr, 1998; Barua *et al.*, 1999).

all-*trans*-Retinoic acid can also be separated as its methyl or pentafluorobenzyl ester by gas–liquid or liquid–liquid chromatography and quantified by mass spectrometry. New ionization methods and tandem mass spectrometry have further enhanced the sensitivity and selectivity with which retinoic acid can be measured (Barua *et al.*, 1999).

3. Metabolism, Kinetics and Genetic Variation

Information on the metabolism, plasma transport and tissue distribution of all-*trans*-retinoic acid in humans and animal models after administration of pharmacological doses is summarized below. More information is given in the General Remarks on the endogeneous (physiological) metabolism of all-*trans*-retinoic acid.

3.1 Humans

3.1.1 Metabolism

Muindi *et al.* (1992) studied the metabolism of all-*trans*-retinoic acid in 13 patients with acute promyelocytic leukaemia who were receiving the drug orally at a dose of 45 mg/m². The only metabolite of all-*trans*-retinoic acid measured in plasma before treatment was all-*trans*-4-oxo-retinoic acid, which accounted for < 10% of the circulating all-*trans*-retinoic acid. The urine of these patients was found to contain all-*trans*-4-oxo-retinoyl-β-glucuronide, but urinary excretion of this compound accounted for < 1% of the administered dose. No drug was found in the cerebrospinal fluid.

3.1.2 Kinetics

Muindi *et al.* (1992) also assessed the pharmacokinetics of all-*trans*-retinoic acid. The peak plasma concentration (347 ± 266 ng/ml) was reached 1–2 h after ingestion of the drug, and this decayed in a mono-exponential fashion with a half-life of 0.8 ± 0.1 h. Continued oral administration of all-*trans*-

retinoic acid for an additional 2–6 weeks was associated with a significant decrease in both the peak plasma concentration and the integrated area under the curve of concentration–time (AUC). For a subset of the patients, this decrease occurred within the first 7 days after the start of treatment. The decrease was associated with a 10-fold increase in urinary excretion of all-*trans*-4-oxoretinoyl-β-glucuronide, suggesting that the accelerated clearance of all-*trans*-retinoic acid from plasma was associated with increased drug catabolism.

In patients with either squamous- or large-cell carcinomas of the lung, the mean plasma AUC value calculated after administration of a single oral dose of 45 mg/m² was significantly lower than that of patients with adenocarcinomas ($p = 0.0001$) or control subjects ($p = 0.01$). Individuals with an AUC value < 250 ng-h/mL had a greater likelihood of having squamous- or large-cell carcinoma (odds ratio = 5.9) (Rigas *et al.*, 1996). [It is unclear from these studies whether the phenotype for rapid clearance of all-*trans*-retinoic acid is a cause or an effect of the squamous- or large-cell lung cancer.]

After administration of all-*trans*-retinoic acid at a dose of 30 mg/m² to four children with acute promyelocytic leukaemia, the peak plasma concentration was 20–741 ng/mL and was reached within 60–120 min of administration. The patient with the lowest peak plasma concentration did not achieve complete remission and had a much higher concentration of all-*trans*-4-oxoretinoic acid in plasma than the other three children, who underwent remission. The authors concluded that accelerated metabolism of all-*trans*-retinoic acid to all-*trans*-4-oxoretinoic acid plays an important role in its failure to induce remission in cancer patients (Takitani *et al.*, 1995a,b).

3.1.3   Tissue distribution
No information was available on the tissue distribution of all-*trans*-retinoic acid in humans after its administration as a drug.

3.1.4   Variations within human populations
The studies of Rigas *et al.* (1996) and Takitani *et al.* (1995a,b) suggest that healthy individuals and patients with various types of cancers may have different capacities for the metabolism and plasma clearance of all-*trans*-retinoic acid. No information

was available about variations in the metabolism and/or plasma clearance of all-*trans*-retinoic acid in other human populations.

3.2   Experimental models
3.2.1   Metabolism
After female cynomolgus monkeys were given all-*trans*-retinoic acid orally at a dose of 6.7 µmol/kg bw per day for 10 days, the concentration of all-*trans*-retinoyl-β-glucuronide in the plasma rose to a maximum of 231 nmol/L (Creech Kraft *et al.*, 1991a). When 13-*cis*-retinoic acid was similarly administered, the maximal concentration of 13-*cis*-retinoyl-β-glucuronide was 42 nmol/L. The two isomers also partly interconverted, e.g. all-*trans*-retinoic acid to 13-*cis*-retinoic acid and to 13-*cis*-retinoyl-β-glucuronide and 13-*cis*-retinoic acid to all-*trans*-retinoic acid (Creech Kraft *et al.*, 1991b). Creech Kraft *et al.* (1991a) indicated that the extent of retinoyl-β-glucuronide formation from retinoic acid, as assessed pharmacokinetically, is dependent both on the isomer administered and the species studied.

In pregnant females of most but not all species, all-*trans*-retinoyl-β-glucuronide is a major metabolite in the plasma after administration of all-*trans*-retinoic acid (Creech Kraft *et al.*, 1987, 1991b; Eckhoff & Nau, 1990; Eckhoff *et al.*, 1991). In pregnant mice treated with 13-*cis*-retinoic acid, 13-*cis*-retinoyl-β-glucuronide was the most abundant plasma metabolite (Creech Kraft *et al.*, 1991b). In this study, all-*trans*-retinoic acid was transferred to the embryo 10 times more efficiently than 13-*cis*-retinoic acid and 100 times more efficiently than 13-*cis*-retinoyl-β-glucuronide. When retinoids were injected into the amnion of rat embryos on day 10 of gestation, the concentrations of all-*trans*-4-oxoretinoic acid, 13-*cis*-4-oxoretinoic acid and all-*trans*-retinoyl-β-glucuronide required to produce the same dysmorphogenic effects as all-*trans*-retinoic acid (250 ng/mL) were twofold, 10-fold and 16-fold higher, respectively (Creech Kraft & Juchau, 1992). The lack of teratogenicity of all-*trans*-retinoyl-β-glucuronide after oral administration of very high doses to pregnant rats seems to be due to its relatively slow absorption from the intestine, its slow hydrolysis to all-*trans*-retinoic acid, its relatively inefficient transfer across the placenta and its inherently low toxicity (Gunning *et al.*, 1993). all-*trans*-Retinoyl-β-glucuronide was more teratogenic at equimolar doses than all-*trans*-retinoic acid after subcutaneous application to mice on day 11 of gestation. This effect appears to be due to the extensive hydrolysis of all-*trans*-retinoyl-β-glucuronide after subcutaneous and intravenous administration, suggesting that it is a precursor of all-*trans*-retinoic acid when administered by these routes (Nau et al., 1996).

3.2.2   Kinetics

After intravenous administration of all-*trans*-retinoic acid to male DBA mice at a dose of 10 mg/kg bw, the serum concentrations showed a distribution phase that decreased rapidly over 30 min and was followed by a non-exponential phase. The mean serum concentration of all-*trans*-retinoic acid was 17 ± 1.1 μg/mL 5 min after treatment and < 0.1 μg/mL 6 h after injection. The concentrations of all-*trans*-retinoic acid in liver, kidney, lung, brain and small intestine were generally higher than those in serum throughout the study. By 8 h after injection, the brain still contained relatively high concentrations of all-*trans*-retinoic acid (1.8 ± 0.2 μg/g tissue), even though the dose had been effectively cleared from the circulation (Wang et al., 1980).

Fasted female B6D2F$_1$ mice received all-*trans*-retinoic acid intragastrically at a dose of 10 mg/kg bw, and clearance was followed for up to 12 h. all-*trans*-Retinoic acid was detected in the plasma by a more sensitive HPLC procedure within 30 min of administration; the plasma concentration was essentially constant for the first 4 h but decreased exponentially from 5–9 h after dosing. Subsequently, the compound was not detected at concentrations higher than those present endogenously in mouse plasma. The authors estimated that the half-life of all-*trans*-retinoic acid was 0.5 h (McPhillips et al., 1987).

In a study of the effects of pretreatment of male BDF$_1$ mice with phenobarbital (80 mg/kg bw intraperitoneally for 3 days), 3-methylcholanthrene (40 mg/kg intraperitoneally for 3 days) or all-*trans*-retinoic acid (10 mg/kg intragastrically for 3 days) on the disposition of an orally administered dose of 10 mg/kg bw of all-*trans*-retinoic acid, the AUC values for serum and for liver, lung, small intestine, kidney, spleen, large intestine, fat, heart, brain, muscle, testis and bladder were reduced relative to those of controls by an average of 54% after pretreatment with all-*trans*-retinoic acid and by 37% after phenobarbital. Pretreatment with 3-methylcholanthrene did not affect the disposition of all-*trans*-retinoic acid (Kalin et al., 1984) .

A dose of 25 mg of all-*trans*-retinoic acid was administered by intravenous infusion over 30 s into the cephalic vein of four anaesthetized male dogs with bile-duct cannulae. The concentration of all-*trans*-retinoic acid in blood over time was biphasic, with an estimated elimination half-life of 4.5 h, an apparent volume of distribution of 1 L/kg bw and a blood clearance rate of 23 mL/min. The mean AUC was 1190 ± 330 μg-min/mL. At 4 h after administration, only 0.63% of the dose was recovered in the bile, about 25% of which was unconjugated, the remainder occurring as a conjugated derivative. Only 0.04% of the dose was recovered in the bile as 13-*cis*-retinoic acid in the 4 h after infusion of all-*trans*-retinoic acid (Patel *et al.*, 1982).

Cynomolgus monkeys were given all-*trans*-retinoic acid at doses of 2 or 10 mg/kg bw for 10 days. The maximum mean plasma concentration of animals receiving 2 mg/kg bw was 420 ± 100 ng/ml on day 1 and 210 ± 10 ng/ml on day 10, while that of animals receiving 10 mg/kg bw was 1200 ± 345 ng/ml on day 1 and 460 ± 125 ng/ml on day 10. The mean plasma AUC value was 928 ± 233 ng-h/mL on day 1 and 432 ± 196 ng-h/mL by day 10 in animals at 2 mg/kg bw and 4607 ± 1194 ng-h/mL on day 1 and 1557 ± 484 ng-h/mlL on day 10 for animals given 10 mg/kg bw. Thus, the AUC values were proportional to the dose administered (Creech Kraft *et al.*, 1991a).

3.2.3   Tissue distribution

In mice, significant quantities of all-*trans*-retinoic acid were observed in all tissues examined (liver, kidney, lung, brain, testis and small intestine) after administration of 10 mg/kg bw intravenously. The highest concentrations were found in liver at each time studied between 5 and 480 min, followed by kidney, in which the concentrations were about 70% of those in liver. The testis took up the least, accounting for 5–15% of the concentration observed in liver (Wang et al., 1980).

The AUC values in mice after an oral dose of all-*trans*-retinoic acid were reported for liver, lung, small intestine, kidney, spleen, large intestine, fat, heart, brain, muscle, testis and urinary bladder. All tissues took up the retinoid (Kalin et al., 1984).

3.2.4 Intra- and inter-species variation

As discussed in section 3.2.1, different species have very different capacities for the metabolism and clearance of pharmacological doses of all-*trans*-retinoic acid. No one species appears to reflect the situation in humans.

4. Cancer-preventive Effects

4.1 Humans
4.1.1 Epidemiological studies
No data were available to the Working Group.

4.1.2 Intervention trials
No data were available to the Working Group.

4.1.3 Intermediate end-points
4.1.3.1 Skin
The use of all-*trans*-retinoic acid and etretinate was studied in the treatment of patients who had received renal transplants and who had more than 50 skin lesions, consisting of actinic keratosis, squamous-call carcinomas of the skin and warts. Seven patients received all-*trans*-retinoic acid topically plus etretinate systemically (10 mg/day), and four patients received it alone. After three months of therapy, six of seven patients receiving all-*trans*-retinoic acid plus etretinate and three of four of those receiving all-*trans*-retinoic acid alone showed clinical improvement, on the basis of at least a 25% decrease in the number of apparent actinic keratoses and a reduction in the size of warts. After six months of therapy, three of four evaluable patients receiving the two retinoids and two of three receiving all-*trans*-retinoic acid alone showed at least a 50% decrease in the number of lesions or in the number of new actinic keratoses or squamous-call carcinomas of the skin (Rook *et al.*, 1995). [The Working Group noted that no control group was included and that actinic keratoses may regress spontaneously.]

Two randomized trials were conducted of the use of topical all-*trans*-retinoic acid to reverse actinic keratoses. In both studies, patients were assigned randomly to the retinoid or to the vehicle, and treatment was continued for six months. In one study, 266 patients were given 0.05% all-*trans*-retinoic acid and compared with 261 patients given the vehicle; in the second study, 226 patients were given 0.1% all-*trans*-retinoic acid and 229

received the vehicle. Treatment with 0.05% retinoid resulted in a rate of regression of 42%, whereas the rate in the controls was 34% (not significant). At the higher dose, a statistically significantly higher rate of regression of lesions was seen among patients receiving all-*trans*-retinoic acid (55%) than among those given the vehicle (41%; $p < 0.001$) (Kligman & Thorne, 1991). [The Working Group noted the inadequate reporting of the study, that the rate of spontaneous regression in the control group was high and that actinic keratoses may regress spontaneously.]

The effects of all-*trans*-retinoic acid in patients with dysplastic naevi have been evaluated in two studies. In one trial (Edwards & Jaffe, 1990), eight patients were randomly assigned to topical treatment with 0.05% all-*trans*-retinoic acid and 13 received placebo. Five treated patients and 11 given placebo completed the four-month intervention, and their lesions were biopsied. The authors reported marked changes in the clinical and histological appearance of naevi in three of the five evaluable treated patients and in none of the 11 controls ($p < 0.001$). [The Working Group noted that losses from the treatment group and the unspecified methods of statistical analyses complicate interpretation of this report].

A second trial (Halpern *et al.*, 1994) involved five male patients with multiple dysplastic naevi who received applications of a 0.005% solution of all-*trans*-retinoic acid on the right or left half of the back, the side being chosen at random. Treatment was continued for six months, at which time all naevi were assessed clinically and four naevi were excised from each side and examined for histological appearance. A statistically significant ($p < 0.0001$) improvement in the clinical appearance of naevi on the treated side of the back was reported. Four of the 16 excised treated and 13 of the 16 untreated naevi met histological criteria for dysplasia. The histological results for naevi from one patient who did not finish the course of treatment were not reported.

4.1.3.2 Uterine cervix
In a randomized trial, all-*trans*-retinoic acid or placebo was given topically to 301 patients with moderate cervical intra-epithelial neoplasia ($n = 151$), or severe cervical intra-epithelial neoplasia or dysplasia ($n = 150$) as a 0.372% solution on a collagen sponge in a cervical cap daily for four days and

then daily for two days after three and six months. The patients were evaluated by serial colposcopy, cytology and cervical biopsy. The dose, schedule and delivery system were determined in prior single-arm phase I and II trials (Meyskens *et al.*, 1983; Graham *et al.*, 1986). A total of 52 patients were lost to follow-up. Among the 141 patients with moderate dysplasia, a higher rate of complete response was observed in those receiving all-*trans*-retinoic acid (43%) than in the group given placebo (27%; *p* = 0.041). No significant difference in the rates of regression of dysplasia were seen among treated and untreated patients with severe dysplasia. Signs of acute toxicity were infrequent, mild and reversible, consisting primarily of local (vaginal and vulvar) irritation and occurring in less than 5% of treated subjects (Meyskens *et al.*, 1994). [The Working Group noted the uncertain compliance of the patients lost to follow-up, which limits the interpretation of the results of this trial.]

4.2   Experimental models
4.2.1   Cancer and preneoplastic lesions
These studies are summarized in Table 3.

4.2.1.1   Skin
Female Swiss albino mice weighing 20–22 g were treated with 150 µg of 7,12-dimethylbenz[*a*]-anthracene (DMBA) by local application for initiation of skin papillomas. After three weeks, croton oil (0.5 mg in acetone) was applied twice weekly for three to eight months as a promoter. This treatment induced four to eight papillomas per mouse. all-*trans*-Retinoic acid was given at a dose of 200 or 400 mg/kg bw by intraperitoneal injection or gavage once a week for two weeks. The sum of the diameters of the papilloma was determined for each mouse and the average value calculated for each group. Treatment with all-*trans*-retinoic acid reduced the average of the papilloma diameters per animal from 25 to 16 mm and from 22 to 11 mm at the two doses, respectively (*p* < 0.05, Student's *t* test) (Bollag, 1974).

Groups of 25 female Sencar mice, seven to eight weeks of age, were treated topically with 5 µg of DMBA for initiation and two weeks later received either basal diet (controls) or a diet supplemented with 40 mg/kg all-*trans*-retinoic acid. The tumour incidence 30 weeks after initiation was 4% in controls and 68% with all-*trans*-retinoic acid (*p* < 0.01,

log rank analysis). In the same study, 25 mice received all-*trans*-retinoic acid topically at a concentration of 30 nmol twice weekly for 28 weeks. The incidence of papillomas was enhanced from 4% in controls to 58% (*p* < 0.01, log rank analysis) (McCormick *et al.*, 1987).

Groups of 30 male and 30 female hairless albino mutant mice received daily topical treatment with 0.001% or 0.01% all-*trans*-retinoic acid from 7 to 30 weeks of age. From day 15 of treatment, the mice were exposed daily for 2 h to simulated sunlight from a 6000-W Xenon-arc lamp for 28 weeks. At the end of the experiment at 55 weeks, the tumour multiplicity was 1.2 carcinomas per mouse in controls and 6.1 and 10 in the two groups given all-*trans*-retinoic acid. The cumulative tumour incidence (% tumour-bearing animals) was 45% in controls, 100% at the low dose and 94% at the high dose (Forbes *et al.*, 1979). [The Working Group noted the lack of statistical analysis.]

Groups of 30 female Sencar mice, six weeks of age, received a single topical application of 10 nmol/L DMBA in acetone, a dose that does not induce skin papillomas. Subsequently, the mice received twice weekly applications of 2 µg of 12-*O*-tetradecanoylphorbol 13-acetate (TPA) and all-*trans*-retinoic acid at doses of 1 and 10 µg for the remainder of the experiment of 18 weeks. The incidence of papillomas was 100% in controls and 76% and 50% at the low and high doses of all-*trans*-retinoic acid, respectively. The multiplicity of papillomas was reduced from 7.4 per mouse in controls to 3.5 and 1.4 per mouse, respectively. In a second part of the study, all-*trans*-retinoic acid had no effect on two-stage tumour promotion, tested by treating initiated skin with 2 µg of TPA twice a week for two weeks and subsequently with 2 µg of mezerein twice a week for 18 weeks. The mice receiving both TPA and mezerein had a papilloma incidence of 92%, with 4.2 papillomas per mouse. Treatment with 10 µg of all-*trans*-retinoic acid during TPA application (stage I promotion) had little or no effect (88% papilloma incidence and 4 papillomas per mouse), whereas treatment with all-*trans*-retinoic acid during mezerein application (stage II promotion) inhibited papilloma development (34% papilloma incidence and 0.8 papillomas per mouse) (Slaga *et al.*, 1980). [The Working Group noted that no statistical analysis was given.]

Table 3. Effects of all-*trans*-retinoic acid on carcinogenesis in animals

Cancer site	Species, sex, age at carcinogen treatment	No. of animals per group	Carcinogen, dose, route	all-*trans*-Retinoic acid dose, route	Duration in relation to carcinogen	Incidence Control	Incidence Treated	Multiplicity Control	Multiplicity Treated	Efficacy	Reference
Skin	Swiss albino mice, female	11	150 µg DMBA + 0.5 µg croton oil 2 x wk for 3–8 months	200 mg/kg bw, i.p. 400 mg/kg bw, orally	For 2 wks after papillomas developed	100	100	NA	NA	Reduced tumour size	Bollag (1974)
Skin	Hairless albino mice, male and female	60	2 h/day UVR exposure for 28 wks	0.001%, 0.01% topically	–2 to +30 wks	45	100	1.2	6.1	Tumour enhancing effect	Forbes et al. (1979)
						45	94	1.2	10.0		
Skin	SENCAR mice, female, 6 wks	30	10 nmol DMBA + TPA for 18 wks	1 µg	+1 wk to end	100	76	7.4	3.5	Effective	Slaga et al. (1980)
			TPA (2 wks) + mezerein 18 wks	10 µg	+1 wk to +3	100	50	7.4	1.4	Effective	
				10 µg		92	90	4.2	4.5	Ineffective	
			TPA (2 wks) + mezerein 16 wks	10 µg topically	+3 wks to end	92	38	4.2	1.0	Effective	
Skin	SENCAR mice, female, 7 wks	30	10 nmol DMBA + 2 µg TPA 3 x/wk/13 wks	5 µg 20 µg topically	+1 wk to end	100	90	10.0	6*	Effective	Fischer et al. (1985)
						100	90	10.0	6	Effective	
		30	10 nmol DMBA	5 µg 20 µg topically	+2 to 24 wks	0	25	0	0.5	Tumour enhancing effect	
						0	50	0	0.9		
		30	10 nmol DMBA	5 µg + 2 µg mezerein	+1 to 3 wks	17	37	0.3	1.3	Tumour enhancing effect	
				10 µg + 2 µg mezerein	+1 to 3 wks	17	43	0.3	1.6		
Skin	CD-1, female, 5–7 wks	30	200 nmol DMBA + 444 nmol anthralene daily/32 wks	1.7 nmol 17 nmol 170 nmol for 32 wks	+2 wks to end	64	41*	1.5	NA	Effective	Dawson et al. (1987)
						64	34*	1.5	NA	Effective	
						64	28*	1.5	NA	Effective	

Table 3 (contd)

Cancer site	Species, sex, age at carcinogen treatment	No. of animals per group	Carcinogen, dose, route	all-*trans*-Retinoic acid dose, route	Duration in relation to carcinogen	Incidence Control	Incidence Treated	Multiplicity Control	Multiplicity Treated	Efficacy	Reference
Skin	SENCAR mice, female, 7–8 wks	25	5 µg DMBA	40 mg/kg diet	+ 2 wks to end	4	68*	NA	NA	Tumour enhancing effect	McCormick et al. (1987)
				30 nmol topically 2 × wk	+ 2 wks to end	4	58*	NA	NA	Tumour enhancing effect	
Skin	SENCAR mice, female, 6 wks	24	20 nmol DMBA + 3.3 nmol TPA 2 wks + 2 mmol diacyl-glycerol for 17 wks	17 nmol topical	+ 2 wks to end	67	38*	5.3	0.7*	Effective as inhibitor of 2nd-stage promotion	Verma (1988)
Skin	SENCAR mice, 3 wks, male and female	30–40	20 µg DMBA + TPA 2 µg once a wk for 20 wks	3 µg/kg diet	0 to 45 wks	50		0.7		Effective**	Chen et al. (1994)
				30 µg/kg diet		18.5		0.2*			
				3/30 µg/kg diet		23.1		0.2*			
				30/3 µg/kg diet		23.1		0.2*			
Liver	B6D2F₁/Hsd mice, female, 4 wks	35	50 mg NDEA ip	30 mg/kg diet	+ 1 week to end at 6 mths	37	86	NA	NA	Tumour enhancing effect	McCormick et al. (1990)
			100 mg NDEA ip			44	90	NA	NA		
Mammary gland	Srague-Dawley rats, female, 50 days	12–24	MNU 50 mg/kg bw	60 mg/kg diet	+ 1 to 4.5 mths	100	91	3.6	3.3	Ineffective	Anzano et al. (1994)
				120 mg/kg diet		100	83	3.6	2.8		

wk, week; DMBA, 7,12-dimethylbenz[a]anthracene; TPA, 12-*O*-tetradecanoylphorbol 13-acetate; NDEA, *N*-nitrosodiethylamine; ip, intraperitoneal; NA, not available; MNU, *N*-methyl-*N*-nitrosourea

* Statistically significant (see text)

** Conversion of papilloma to carcinoma was inhibited.

In similar studies, Sencar mice received topical applications of a single dose of 10 nmol/L DMBA and then 5 or 20 µg of all-*trans*-retinoic acid simultaneously with 2 µg of TPA thrice weekly for 13 weeks. Both doses of all-*trans*-retinoic acid reduced the tumour yield, from approximately 10 per mouse in controls to 6 per mouse, and the papilloma incidence was 100% and 90%, respectively. The authors reported that papilloma development was delayed in the animals given all-*trans*-retinoic acid. In the same series of experiments, all-*trans*-retinoic acid was applied instead of TPA to the skin of Sencar mice initiated with 10 nmol/L DMBA. After 24 weeks, the papilloma yield was about 0.5 papillomas per mouse at 5 µg of all-*trans*-retinoic acid and 0.9 papillomas per mouse at 20 µg, with tumour incidences of about 50% and 25%, respectively. In another experiment, 2 µg of mezerein were applied to the skin of mice initiated with 10 nmol/L DMBA both as a first-stage promoter three times per week for two weeks and as a second-stage promoter three times per week for the subsequent 15–18 weeks. The papilloma yield per mouse was 0.3, and the papilloma incidence was 17%. When 10 µg of all-*trans*-retinoic acid were applied instead of mezerein during the first stage of promotion, the papilloma yield was 1.6 per mouse and the incidence was 43% per mouse (Fischer *et al.*, 1985). [The Working Group noted that no statistics were given, and the papilloma yields and incidences were gleaned from graphs.]

In another two-stage tumour promotion study in female SENCAR mice initiated with DMBA, TPA was applied as a stage-I promoter and L-α-dioctanoylglycerol (a protein kinase C inducer) as a stage-II promoter. all-*trans*-Retinoic acid (17 nmol/L) was topically applied 1 h before L-α-dioctanoylglycerol. The papilloma incidence at 17 weeks was 67% in controls and 38% in mice given all-*trans*-retinoic acid [no statistics given], and the tumour multiplicity was 5.3 and 0.3, respectively ($p < 0.01$ [method not given]) (Verma, 1988).

Groups of 30 female CD-1 mice, five to seven weeks of age, were treated topically with 200 nmol/L DMBA in acetone; two weeks later, the mice were treated with 444 nmol/L anthralene alone or with 1.7, 17 or 170 nmol/L all-*trans*-retinoic acid for 32 weeks. The incidences of skin papillomas were 64% in the control group and 41%, 34% and 28% at the low, intermediate and high doses of all-*trans*-retinoic acid ($p < 0.01$, Student's *t* test) (Dawson *et al.*, 1987).

Pregnant Sencar mice were placed on diets containing all-*trans*-retinoic acid at 3 or 30 µg/g of diet. Their pups were raised on the same diets, were initiated with a single dose of 20 µg DMBA at three weeks of age and promoted with 2 µg of TPA once a week for 20 weeks. At that time, half of the animals given the diet containing all-*trans*-retinoic acid at 3 µg/g were switched to the diet containing 30 µg/g, and half of those given 30 µg/g were switched to the diet containing 3 µg/g. The papilloma incidences in the four groups were not significantly different, but the carcinoma incidence and yield were significantly lower in the three groups that were maintained either continuously or for some period on the diet containing all-*trans*-retinoic acid at 30 µg/g ($p < 0.05$, Fisher's exact test). When the animals were 26 weeks of age, 27–40 in each group were still alive; the experiment was terminated when they were 45 weeks old. The cumulative carcinoma incidence was 50% in animals maintained continuously on the diet with the low concentration of all-*trans*-retinoic acid and 18–23% in animals kept continuously or for some period on the diet with the high concentration. The carcinoma yield was 0.68 in the mice maintained continuously at the low dose and 0.19–0.23 in animals maintained continuously or intermittently at the high dose (Chen *et al.*, 1994).

4.2.1.2 Liver

Groups of 35 female B6D2F$_1$/hsd, mice, four weeks of age, received intraperitoneal injections of 50 or 100 mg *N*-nitrosodiethylamine (NDEA) and dietary supplements of 0.1 mmol of all-*trans*-retinoic acid per kg of diet beginning one week after carcinogen treatment until the end of the study at six months. The combined incidence of benign and malignant liver tumours in animals given the low dose of NDEA was 37% in controls and 86% in those given all-*trans*-retinoic acid ($p < 0.05$; χ^2 test). The incidence of hepatocellular carcinoma in animals at the high dose of NDEA was 44% in controls and 90% with all-*trans*-retinoic acid ($p < 0.01$; χ^2 test). Since all-*trans*-retinoic acid alone did not induce any liver tumours, these results suggest that it enhanced the hepatocarcinogenicity of NDEA (McCormick *et al.*, 1990).

4.2.1.3 Mammary gland

Groups of 24 control and 12 treated female Sprague-Dawley rats, 50 days of age, received intravenous injections of 50 mg/kg bw N-methyl-N-nitrosourea and, one week later, all-*trans*-retinoic acid at 60 or 120 mg/kg of diet for 4.5 months. The incidences of mammary adenocarcinoma were 100% in controls and 83% and 91% at the high and low concentrations of all-*trans*-retinoic acid, respectively. The tumour multiplicity was 3.6 in controls and 3.3 and 2.8 with all-*trans*-retinoic acid, respectively. The differences were not statistically significant (Anzano *et al.*, 1994).

4.2.2 Intermediate biomarkers

Ornithine decarboxylase is considered to be a useful biomarker in experimental studies of skin carcinogenesis. Mice were given 0.2 mmol of DMBA in 0.2 mL of acetone as an initiator followed by twice weekly applications of 17 nmol/L TPA topically 1 h after application of 1.7 or 17 nmol of all-*trans*-retinoic acid in 0.2 ml of acetone. The mice were killed 4.5 h after the last of seven treatments with TPA, and ornithine decarboxylase was measured. all-*trans*-Retinoic acid suppressed the TPA-induced ornithine decarboxylase activity almost completely (Verma *et al.*, 1979).

4.2.3 In-vitro models

4.2.3.1 Models of carcinogenesis

Studies with cells in culture have provided important information on the pleiotropic effects of all-*trans*-retinoic acid that may be relevant for understanding the mechanisms of its chemopreventive effects. The types of cell that have been used to study the effects of retinoids include normal cells in short-term culture, cells immortalized spontaneously or by viral genes such as HPV 16 E6 and SV40 large T antigen or oncogenes such as H-ras, and cells derived from solid tumours or haematological malignancies and used in primary cultures or established as cell lines. Although some important information was gained from each of these cell systems, that obtained with non-malignant cells is more relevant to chemoprevention of cancer. A wide range of concentrations (10^{-11}–10^{-4} mol/L) was used in these studies.

Normal epithelial cells can be maintained in culture for a limited number of cell divisions, as they usually senesce and die. Specific media, which are often serum-free, have been developed to culture epithelial cells and exclude mesenchymal (stromal) cells. Investigations of the effects of retinoids on normal cells included studies on changes in cell growth and differentiation and on the prevention of malignant transformation. Because many of the cells in epithelial tissues *in vivo* are quiescent, adaptation of culture conditions to maximize cell proliferation may select for cells of higher proliferative capacity or allow the cells to exhibit an acquired proliferative potential. Proliferating normal cells in culture can be considered to be hyperplastic cells.

(a) Inhibition of carcinogen-induced neoplastic transformation

In studies with immortalized murine C3H/10 T1/2 murine fibroblasts, all-*trans*-retinoic acid inhibited 3-methylcholanthrene-induced neoplastic transformation when it was added to the medium seven days after removal of the carcinogen and weekly treatments were given for the four-week duration of the experiment. Activity was thus expressed in the promotion phase of transformation and required a concentration of about 10^{-6} mol/L (Bertram, 1980). The low activity was explained by the finding that these cells rapidly catabolized all-*trans*-retinoic acid. When this was blocked by liarazole, an inhibitor of a cytochrome P450 4-hydroxylase, all-*trans*-retinoic acid inhibited transformation at concentrations as low as 10^{-10} mol/L, in the absence of cytoxicity (Acevedo & Bertram, 1995).

(b) Rat tracheal epithelial cells

Primary rat tracheal epithelial cells grown in an air–liquid interface in the presence of all-*trans*-retinoic acid differentiate into normal mucociliary epithelium and produce large amounts of mucin glycoproteins (Kaartinen *et al.*, 1993). The differentiated cultures were shown to express the mucin genes *MUC1* and *MUC5* (Guzman *et al.*, 1996). After removal of all-*trans*-retinoic acid from the medium, the cells assumed a stratified squamous morphology and developed a cornified apical layer. Biochemical analysis revealed loss of expression of transglutaminase type II, keratin 18 and both *MUC1* and *MUC5* and aberrant expression of the squamous markers transglutaminase type I and keratin 13 (Kaartinen *et al.*, 1993; Guzman *et al.*,

1996). Addition of all-*trans*-retinoic acid to squamous differentiated rat tracheal epithelial cultures resulted in a rapid (24 h) down-regulation of prostaglandin H synthase-1 (*PGHS-1*) mRNA expression and a slower (three days) up-regulation of the expression of cytosolic phospholipase A2 and *PGHS-2* genes coincident with re-differentiation of the culture to a mucociliary phenotype (Hill *et al.*, 1996).

The rat tracheal epithelial cell system is useful for identifying potential chemopreventive agents because the cells can be transformed by exposure to chemical carcinogens such as the directly acting N-methyl-N'-nitro-N-nitrosoguanidine (MNNG). Exposure of primary rat tracheal epithelial cells *in vitro* to MNNG led to the appearance of initiated stem cells that grew under selective conditions in culture and differed from normal stem cells in that their probability of self-renewal was increased (Nettesheim *et al.*, 1987). When all-*trans*-retinoic acid was included in the medium for only three days at concentrations that did not affect cell survival (3–33 nmol/L), it inhibited transformation by 65–75% in a dose-dependent manner. Longer treatment at higher concentrations caused more than 90% inhibition, with no cytotoxicity. When treatment was delayed for three weeks after exposure to MNNG, 60% inhibition of transformation frequency was still achieved. all-*trans*-Retinoic acid inhibited the growth of normal rat tracheal epithelial cells. It was suggested that the mechanism of the preventive effect of all-*trans*-retinoic acid on tracheal cell transformation was inhibition of cell proliferation. Exposure of the rat tracheal epithelial cells to MNNG for more than five weeks resulted in loss of sensitivity to the growth inhibitory effect of all-*trans*-retinoic acid. This was deduced from the finding that the concentration of all-*trans*-retinoic acid required to cause 50% inhibition of colony formation increased from 0.1–0.3 nmol/L for cells isolated from 3–5-week-old transformed colonies to over 100-times higher concentrations for cells isolated from 12-week-old cultures. Rat tracheal epithelial cell lines established from cells in advanced stages of transformation also showed increased resistance to all-*trans*-retinoic acid, and two of five cell lines even formed more colonies in its presence (Fitzgerald *et al.*, 1986). In this model, cells in early stages of transformation retain responsiveness to factors that constrain proliferation, and most of their descendants differentiate and do not express transformed charactcristics. These are the cells that respond to all-*trans*-retinoic acid. Progression of the MNNG-initiated cells to the second stage of transformation, when the cells are immortalized, is accompanied by loss of responsiveness to the growth inhibitory effects of all-*trans*-retinoic acid. In this model, early stages of transformation are likely to respond better than later stages (Fitzgerald *et al.*, 1986; Nettesheim *et al.*, 1987).

Rat tracheal epithelial cells can also be transformed by benzo[*a*]pyrene. Inhibition of transformation by this carcinogen was developed as an assay for screening chemopreventive agents that act by altering metabolism or by inhibiting early stages of carcinogenesis. all-*trans*-Retinoic acid was active in this assay when added simultaneously with benzo[*a*]pyrene, due either to increased cytochrome P450 activity or restoration of differentiation (Steele *et al.*, 1990).

Immortalized rat tracheal epithelial 2C5 cells cultured in serum-free medium undergo squamous differentiation after the addition of serum. Concentrations of 0.1–1 nmol/L all-*trans*-retinoic acid inhibited this differentiation, as evidenced by suppression of several markers, including cross-linked envelope formation and keratin K13 expression (Denning & Verma, 1994).

(c)   *Immortalized and transformed human bronchial epithelial cells*

Normal bronchial epithelial cells were immortalized by SV40 large T antigen by Reddel *et al.* (1988) and designated BEAS-2B cells. The cells were then used to develop transformed and tumorigenic derivatives by culturing them on de-epithelialized rat tracheas, transplanting them into rats and exposing the rats to cigarette smoke condensate. Cell lines were derived from tumours which developed in the transplanted tissue in some animals. Certain cell lines were considered to be premalignant, while others, such as 1170-I cells, were tumorigenic and considered to be malignant (Klein-Szanto *et al.*, 1992). The effects of retinoids were compared in primary cultures of normal bronchial epithelial cells, the immortalized BEAS-2B cell line and premalignant and malignant cell lines in a model of multistage tracheobronchial carcinogenesis. The sensitivity to the growth inhibitory effects of all-*trans*-retinoic acid diminished with progression in this cell system: the most advanced cell line 1170-I was resistant, whereas the growth of normal and immortalized cells was inhibited (Kim *et al.*, 1995; Lee *et al.*, 1997).

In another model for carcinogen-induced transformation *in vitro* (Langenfeld *et al.*, 1996), SV40-T-immortalized human bronchial epithelial BEAS-2B cells are exposed to the carcinogenic agents present in cigarette smoke condensate or to the purified tobacco carcinogen N-nitrosamino-4-(methylnitrosamino)-1-(3-pyridyl)-1-butanone (NNK), and transformation is scored as increased anchorage-independent growth or acquired tumorigenicity in immune-compromised mice. When the BEAS-2B cells were treated with all-*trans*-retinoic acid during exposure to the transforming agents, the ability of the cells to form colonies in semi-solid media and to form tumours was inhibited. all-*trans*-Retinoic acid inhibited DNA synthesis in immortalized BEAS-2B cells and in their carcinogen-transformed derivative BEAS-2BNNK (Boyle *et al.*, 1999).

In human tracheal gland epithelial cells immortalized by adenovirus 12-simian virus 40 (Ad12-SV40) hybrid, all-*trans*-retinoic acid inhibited both cell proliferation and anchorage-independent growth in a dose-dependent manner when applied at concentrations of 1 nmol/L to 1 µmol/L. all-*trans*-Retinoic acid up-regulated *p53* but had no effect on the expression of *TGF-α* or *TGF-β 1* genes. These results suggest that all-*trans*-retinoic acid regulates the growth of human tracheal gland epithelial cells by up-regulating the expression of *p53* (Joiakim & Chopra, 1993).

[The Working Group noted that the relevance of these cell culture models is uncertain, since the original immortalizing agent, SV40 large T antigen, is not an etiological agent for human lung cancer. Since one of the main effects of the large T antigen is to decrease *p53* levels, the findings may be relevant only to carcinogenesis that involves defects in the *p53* pathway. The immortalized cells expressed only low levels of wild-type *p53* and not mutated *p53* as many human lung cancers do.]

(d)   Mouse epidermal keratinocytes

A cell culture model system analogous to initiated mouse epidermis was established by exposing cells of the keratinocyte cell line 308, derived from adult mouse skin, to DMBA. These cells behaved like initiated cells in that they formed papillomas when grafted onto the backs of athymic mice. Normal keratinocytes can normally inhibit the colony-forming ability of these cells in a medium containing a high concentration of Ca^{++}, but exposure to TPA for several weeks allowed initiated colonies to form. This action of TPA could be blocked by all-*trans*-retinoic acid at 10^{-6} mol/L (Hennings *et al.*, 1990).

In another model, treatment of the murine epidermal cell line JB6 with the tumour promoter TPA resulted in transformation into anchorage-independent tumorigenic cells, which was blocked by all-*trans*-retinoic acid at doses of 10^{-10}–10^{-6} mol/L (De Benedetti *et al.*, 1991).

(e)   Human papillomavirus type 16-immortalized human epidermal keratinocytes

The transforming ability of human papillomavirus (HPV) type 16 (HPV16), which has been implicated in the development of cervical cancer, resides in the oncogenes *E6* and *E7*. HPV-16 DNA was used to transfect human foreskin epidermal keratinocytes and thus obtain several immortalized cell lines. Treatment of normal keratinocytes with all-*trans*-retinoic acid at 1 nmol/L, during or immediately after transfection with HPV-16 DNA, inhibited immortalization by about 95% (Khan *et al.*, 1993). If the cells were first immortalized, all-*trans*-retinoic acid inhibited their growth by reducing the expression of the HPV-16 early genes (*E2*, *E5*, *E6* and *E7*) at the level of mRNA and protein (Pirisi *et al.*, 1992; Khan *et al.*, 1993). The HPV-16-immortalized cells were about 100 times more sensitive than their normal counterparts to growth inhibition by all-*trans*-retinoic acid in both clonal and mass culture growth assays. They were also more sensitive to modulation of keratin expression than normal cells.

This model was developed further to include more advanced stages of transformation by continuous culture, which resulted in the selection of variants that acquired independence from epidermal growth factor and growth factors present in bovine pituitary extract, which are required at early stages of transformation. The advanced stage cells could be transformed into tumorigenic cells by transfection with viral Harvey *ras* or herpes simplex virus type II DNA. all-*trans*-Retinoic acid inhibited the early stages of this progression, but the cells lost their sensitivity as they progressed in culture (Creek *et al.*, 1995). all-*trans*-Retinoic acid induced TGFβ1 and β2 expression in these cells. TGFβ was a potent inhibitor of the growth of early stages of progression in this model but the later-stage cells were resistant to this negative growth factor, which the authors concluded is the basis for the accompanying loss of response to all-*trans*-retinoic acid.

(f) Spontaneously immortalized human keratinocytes and their ras-transformed derivatives

Although spontaneous immortalization is a rare event, it occurred in a human keratinocyte culture which gave rise to a cell line designated HaCaT. These cells have been also transformed with *c-Ha-ras* oncogene, and benign and malignant clones have been isolated. The various cell types have maintained their ability to differentiate into stratified epithelium and in their response to regulation of keratins by all-*trans*-retinoic acid. The immortalized and *ras*-transformed cells expressed keratins K1 and K10 in medium depleted of retinoids, but the expression of these keratins was fully suppressed when the concentration of all-*trans*-retinoic acid was increased (Breitkreutz *et al.*, 1993). Lotan (1993) suggested that all-*trans*-retinoic acid can regulate differentiation of normal, premalignant and malignant human keratinocytes and can suppress the expression of squamous differentiation markers in malignant squamous-cell carcinomas.

(g) Human papillomavirus-immortalized human cervical cells

Because 90% of human cervical tumours contain HPV DNA, it is assumed that the virus plays a role in the development of this cancer, especially since the DNA can immortalize epithelial cells *in vitro* through the *E6* and *E7* oncogenes. In several immortalized ectocervical epithelial cell lines derived with HPV-16 DNA, all-*trans*-retinoic acid and other retinoids suppressed the expression of squamous differentiation markers like keratins (Agarwal *et al.*, 1991). all-*trans*-Retinoic acid inhibited the growth of the immortalized cells, although it had no effect on the growth of normal ectocervical cells (Sizemore & Rorke, 1993). It suppressed the differentiation markers keratins K5 and K16 and transglutaminase type 1 more effectively in HPV-immortalized cells than in normal ectocervical cells (Choo *et al.*, 1995).

HPV-immortalized keratinocytes can grow in organotypic cultures on a collagen gel substratum that contains fibroblasts, and a three-dimensional tissue-like growth is obtained, which can be viewed as a cervical carcinoma *in situ*. In such cultures, the expression of squamous markers can be suppressed by all-*trans*-retinoic acid, although higher concentrations of all-*trans*-retinoic acid were required to block terminal differentiation in these cultures than in control organotypic cultures of normal cells in which 30 times higher concentrations were required to suppress *K1* mRNA (Merrick *et al.*, 1993). The reason for the difference between the normal and immortalized cells is unknown, nor is it known why in another laboratory (Agarwal *et al.*, 1991, 1996) the immortalized cells were more sensitive than normal cells to all-*trans*-retinoic acid. [The Working Group noted that the two groups of investigators used different culture methods.]

In HPV-16-immortalized endocervical cell lines grown in organotypic culture, all-*trans*-retinoic acid prevented the dysplastic morphology and cytokeratin differentiation markers of carcinoma *in situ* (Shindoh *et al.*, 1995). Tumorigenic variants of HPV-immortalized cervical cells derived by treatment with cigarette smoke condensate were less sensitive to all-*trans*-retinoic acid than normal and immortalized non-tumorigenic cells. They formed organotypic epithelium resembling severe dysplasia which was persistent even in the presence of all-*trans*-retinoic acid, whereas the immortalized cells formed only a thin epithelium. The investigators predicted that similar resistance to all-*trans*-retinoic acid may occur clinically (Sarma *et al.*, 1996).

In a comparison of the sensitivity of cell lines derived from cervical intraepithelial neoplasia (CIN), HPV DNA-transfected cell lines and cervical carcinoma cell lines to all-*trans*-retinoic acid, the retinoid had comparable effects on growth, detected as a decrease in DNA synthesis, in all but two carcinoma cell lines, which were resistant. all-*trans*-Retinoic acid inhibited growth in cervical neoplastic cell lines, including cervical carcinoma cells (Behbakht *et al.*, 1996).

[See the comment of the Working Group in section (c), above.]

4.2.3.2 Effects on differentiation of normal cells

(a)   Normal human tracheobronchial epithelial cells

Normal human tracheobronchial epithelial cells cultured on collagen gels in medium containing all-*trans*-retinoic acid and triiodothyronine expressed a mucociliary phenotype. Removal of the retinoid from the medium caused the cultures to differentiate into a squamous epithelium, accompanied by decreased mucin secretion and reduced expression of the mucin genes *MUC2* and *MUC5AC*, indicating that all-*trans*-retinoic acid plays a major role in differentiation of the mucociliary epithelium (Yoon *et al.*, 1997). In normal human tracheobronchial epithelial cell cultures, all-*trans*-retinoic acid down-regulated the squamous marker cornifin α and upregulated *MUC2*, *MUC5AC* and *MUC5B* mRNAs sequentially at 24, 48 and 72 h, respectively (Koo *et al.*, 1999a). It has been suggested that nuclear RARα and, to a lesser extent, RARγ play a role in the control of mucin gene expression, since RARα- and RARγ-selective agonists strongly induced mucin mRNAs in a dose-dependent manner, whereas an RARβ-selective retinoid only weakly induced mucin gene expression at the high concentration of 1 μmol/L. Furthermore, an RARα antagonist inhibited mucin gene induction and mucous cell differentiation caused by all-*trans*-retinoic acid and by RARα- and, surprisingly, by RARγ–selective retinoids (Koo *et al.*, 1999b).

Treatment of primary cultures of human bronchial epithelial cells with all-*trans*-retinoic acid caused accumulation of cells in the G1 phase of the cell cycle and inhibition of DNA synthesis (Boyle *et al.*, 1999). all-*trans*-Retinoic acid also suppressed epidermal growth factor signalling in normal human tracheobronchial epithelial cells grown on collagen gels (Moghal & Neel, 1998).

(b)   Hamster trachea explants

Explants of hamster trachea prepared from vitamin A-deficient animals have been used to measure the ability of retinoids to prevent the squamous metaplasia which normally results when this tissue is cultured in the absence of vitamin A. all-*trans*-Retinoic acid dissolved in dimethyl sulfoxide inhibited metaplasia, with a median effective dose (ED_{50}) of 3×10^{-11} mol/L when applied over a 10-day period. Control cultures showed over 90% metaplasia (Newton *et al.*, 1980).

4.2.3.3 Cell lines established from tumours

The effects of all-*trans*-retinoic acid have been studied in numerous cell lines established from various malignancies. Many of these cancer cell lines maintained responsiveness to some of the pleiotropic effects of retinoids, including suppression of proliferation in monolayer culture, inhibition of colony formation in semi-solid media and induction of differentiation, sometimes including complete suppression of tumorigenic potential. The results of many of these studies have been reviewed (Gudas *et al.*, 1994; Lotan, 1995; and General Remarks to this volume). They are not included here because their relevance to cancer prevention is indirect.

4.2.3.4 Antimutagenicity in short-term tests for mutagenicity

Although most studies have focused on the role of all-*trans*-retinoic acid in the promotion and progression of cancer, the results of a few studies have indicated that it may sometimes act as an anti-initiator. It has been shown to modulate chemically-induced genotoxicity in a number of short-term assays, in both bacteria (Table 4) and mammalian cells (Table 5). [The Working Group noted that many of the reports do not give the isomer designation for the retinoic acid used. When the source of the retinoic acid was shown, the company was contacted and asked about the availability of different isomers at different times; for example, retinoic acid obtained from Sigma before 1988 was all-*trans*-retinoic acid, since it was the only form available at that time. In other cases, the author was contacted.]

(a)   Salmonella typhimurium

Of the studies in which the ability of all-*trans*-retinoic acid to inhibit the action of standard mutagens was tested in *Salmonella typhimurium* (Table 4), only one examined indirect DNA damage by assaying *umu* C gene expression in *S. typhimurium* TA1535/pSK1002; the others followed the standard assay of Ames. all-*trans*-Retinoic acid

Table 4. Inhibition by all-*trans*-retinoic acid of standard mutagens in the *Salmonella*/microsome test

Retinoid (tested dose)[a]	Mutagen (tested dose)[a]	*S. typhimurium* strain	S9 mix	Result[b]	LED/HID[c]	Reference
all-*trans*-RA (0.0003–300 µmol/plate)	3-Amino-3,4-dimethyl-5*H*-pyrido[4,3-*b*]indole (Trp-P-1) (0.2 µg/ml)	TA1535/pSK1002	+	+	0.54 µmol/plate (ID$_{50}$)	Okai *et al.* (1996)
all-*trans*-RA (0.003–30 µmol/plate)	Adriamycin (3 µg/ml)	TA1535/pSK1002	–	–	30 µmol/plate	Okai *et al.* (1996)
all-*trans*-RA (0.003–30 (µmol/plate)	Mitomycin C (0.3 µg/ml)	TA1535/pSK1002	–	–	30 µmol/plate	Okai *et al.* (1996)
RA (Sigma)[d] (0.1–10 µmol/plate)	Hydrogen peroxide (5 µmol/plate)	TA104	–	–	10 µmol/plate	Han (1992)
all-*trans*-RA (25–500 nmol/plate)	Cigarette smoke condensate (100–400 µg/plate)	TA98	+	–	500 nmol/plate	Wilmer & Spit (1986)
RA (Sigma)[e] (2.5–40 µg/plate)	Benzo[*a*]pyrene (5 µg/plate)	TA98	+	–	40 µg/plate	Qin & Huang (1985)
RA (Sigma)[e] (2.5–40 µg/plate)	Aflatoxin B$_1$ (0.5 µg/plate)	TA98	+	+	2.5 µg/plate	Qin & Huang (1985)
all-*trans*-RA (0.26–2600 nmol/plate)	Aflatoxin B$_1$ (50 ng/plate)	TA98	+	+	26 nmol/plate LED; 860 nmol/plate; 55% decrease in revertants	Whong *et al.* (1988)
RA (Sigma)[e] (0.2–2000 nmol/plate)	Aflatoxin B$_1$ (200 ng/plate)	TA98	+	+	0.2 nmol/plate; 70% decrease in revertants	Raina & Gurtoo (1985)
RA (Sigma)[e] (0.2–2000 nmol/plate)	Aflatoxin B$_1$ (200 ng/plate)	TA100	+	–	2000 nmol/plate	Raina & Gurtoo (1985)
RA (Sigma)[e] (0.1, 0.5 µmol/plate)	Aflatoxin B$_1$ (400 ng/plate)	TA100	+	+	0.1 µmol/plate; 50% decrease in revertants	Bhattacharya *et al.* (1987)

RA, retinoic acid; S9 mix, 9000 x *g* microsomal fraction used as exogenous metabolic system; ID$_{50}$ = dose of retinol required to inhibit *umu* C gene expression by 50%
[a] Doses of retinoids and mutagens are given as reported by the authors.
[b] +, inhibition of genotoxicity; –, no inhibition of genotoxicity
[c] LED, lowest effective (inhibitory) dose; HID, highest ineffective dose
[d] Probably all-*trans*-RA but could be 13-*cis*-RA, since, 13-*cis*-RA was listed in Sigma catalogue from 1988 and 9-*cis*-RA from 1996.
[e] Presumed to be all-*trans*-RA since 13-*cis*-RA was listed in Sigma catalogue only from 1988 and 9-*cis*-RA from 1996.

Table 5. Inhibition by all-*trans*-retinoic acid of genetic and related effects in cultured mammalian cells

Retinoid (tested dose)[a]	Genotoxic agent (tested dose)[a]	Cells/system	Investigated effect	Result[b]	LED/HID[c]	Reference
all-*trans*-RA (0.25–4 µg/ml)	Mitomycin C (0.03 µg/ml)	Chinese hamster V79 cells	Sister chromatid exchange	–	4 µg/ml	Sirianni *et al.* (1981)
all-*trans*-RA[d] (25–50 nmol/ml)	Cyclophosphamide (1 mmol/plate)	Chinese hamster epithelial liver cells	Sister chromatid exchange	+	(25 nmol/ml)	Cozzi *et al.* (1990)
all-*trans*-RA[d] (25–50 nmol/ml)	7,12-Dimethylbenz-[*a*]anthracene (0.078 µmol/plate)	Chinese hamster epithelial liver cells	Sister chromatid exchange	+	37 nmol/ml	Cozzi *et al.* (1990)
all-*trans*-RA (0.2–0.8 µg/ml)	Aqueous extract of *pan masala* (13.5, 12.5 µg/ml water-soluble *masala* with and without tobacco, respectively)	Chinese hamster ovary cells	Sister chromatid exchange	+	0.2 µg/ml	Patel *et al.* (1998)
all-*trans*-RA (0.2–0.8 µg/ml)	Aqueous extract of *pan masala* (13.5, 12.5 µg/ml water-soluble *masala* with and without tobacco, respectively)	Chinese hamster ovary cells	Chromosomal aberrations	+	0.4 µg/ml	Patel *et al.* (1998)
all-trans-RA[d] (0.1–10 mol/ml)	None	C127 mouse cells transformed by bovine papilloma-virus DNA	Chromosomal instability (chromatid bridges and fragments)	+	5 nmol/ml	Stich *et al.* (1990)
RA (Sigma)[e] (1–25 nmol/ml)	Ethyl methane-sulfonate (100 µg/ml)	Chinese hamster ovary cells	*Hprt* mutation	+	25 nmol/ml	Budroe *et al.* (1988)
RA (Sigma)[e] (1–25 nmol/ml)	7,12-Dimethylbenz-[*a*]anthracene (1.25–5 µg/ml)	Chinese hamster ovary cells	*Hprt* mutation	–	5 nmol/ml	Budroe *et al.* (1988)
RA (Sigma)[e] (1–50 nmol/ml)	Ethyl methanesul-fonate (200 µg/ml)	Rat primary hepatocytes	Unscheduled DNA synthesis	–	50 nmol/ml	Budroe *et al.* (1987)
RA (Sigma)[e] (1–25 nmol/ml)	Ultraviolet light (32 J/m^2)	Rat primary hepatocytes	Unscheduled DNA synthesis	–	25 nmol/ml	Budroe *et al.* (1987)
RA (Sigma)[e] (1–50 nmol/ml)	7,12-Dimethyl-benz[*a*]anthracene (2.5, 5 µg/ml)	Rat primary hepatocytes	Unscheduled DNA synthesis	+	1 nmol/ml	Budroe *et al.* (1987)
all-*trans*-RA (1–100 µg/ml)	Dimethylbenz[*a*]-anthracene (71 nmol/ml)	Mouse epidermal cells	Binding to DNA *in vitro*	+	10 µg/ml 22% decrease	Shoyab (1981)

Table 5. (contd)

Retinoid (tested dose)[a]	Genotoxic agent (tested dose)[a]	Cells/system	Investigated effect	Result[b]	LED/HID[c]	Reference
all-*trans*-RA (50,100 µg/ml)	³H-Benzo[*a*]pyrene	Cultured human bronchial explants	Binding to DNA	+	100 µg/ml; decreased binding	Bodo *et al.* (1989)
all-*trans*-RA (≤ 500 nmol/ml)	Aflatoxin B₁ (2 nmol/ml)	None	Binding to calf thymus DNA in presence of micro-somes	+	60 nmol/ml; 50% inhibition	Firozi *et al.* (1987) (see also Bhattacharya *et al.*, 1984)
all-*trans*-RA (≤ 500 nmol/ml)	Aflatoxin B₁ (43 nmol/ml)	None	Metabolism of aflatoxin B₁ to Tris-diol complex in presence of microsomes	+	75 nmol/ml; 50% inhibition	Firozi *et al.*, (1987)
all-*trans*-RA (≤ 200 nmol/ml)	Benzo[*a*]pyrene (60 nmol/ml)	None	Binding to calf thymus DNA	+	84 nmol/ml; 50% inhibition	Shah *et al.* (1992)
all-*trans*-RA ≤ 200 nmol/ml	Benzo[*a*]pyrene (60 nmol/ml)	None	B[a]P-7,8-diol formation	–	200 nmol/ml;	Shah *et al.* (1992)
all-*trans*-RA (0.1–30 nmol/ml)	None	Primary rat hepatocytes	Cytochrome p450C7 mRNA expression	#	0.1 nmol/ml	Westin *et al.* (1993)
all-*trans*-RA (40 nmol/ml)	None	Primary rat hepatocytes	Cytochrome P450 RNA activity			Jurima-Romet *et al.* (1997)
			Cyp1A1	#	40 nmol/ml	
			Cyp1A2	–	40 nmol/ml	
			Cyp3A	#	40 nmol/ml	

RA, retinoic acid; B[*a*]P, benzo[*a*]pyrene
[a] Doses of retinoids and mutagens are given as reported by the authors.
[b] +, inhibition of the investigated end-point; –, no effect on the investigated end-point; #, enhancement of the investigated end-point
[c] LED, lowest effective dose that inhibits or enhances the investigated effect; HID, highest ineffective dose
[d] Personal communication from author
[e] Presumed to be all-*trans*-RA since 13-*cis*-RA was listed in Sigma catalogue only from 1988 and 9-*cis*-RA from 1996

inhibited the induction of the *umu* C gene by the heterocyclic amine 3-amino-3,4-dimethyl-5*H*-pyrido[4,3-*b*]indole (Trp-P-1) in the presence of hepatic metabolizing enzymes derived from a 9000 x *g* liver supernatant (S9), but it did not prevent the induction of *umu* C expression by two directly acting mutagens, adriamycin and mitomycin C (Okai *et al.*, 1996).

Four of the studies conducted with the standard Ames' *Salmonella*/microsome test tested the ability of all-*trans*-retinoic acid to inhibit the effects of directly acting mutagens. It did not prevent the induction of reverse mutation by hydrogen peroxide in *S. typhimurium* TA104, a strain sensitive to oxidative mutagens (Han, 1992), and it had no effect on the mutagenic action of MNNG in strain TA100 or of 4-nitroquinoline 1-oxide in strain TA98 (Shetty *et al.*, 1988; Camoirano *et al.*, 1994). It significantly inhibited the mutagenicity of three nitroarenes: 2-nitrofluorene, 3-nitrofluoranthene and 1-nitropyrene in *S. typhimurium* TA98 (Tang & Edenharder, 1997).

The other studies, conducted with compounds and mixtures that require the presence of S9, showed mixed results. all-*trans*-Retinoic acid did not affect the mutagenicity of unfractionated cigarette smoke (Camoirano *et al.*, 1994) or of cigarette-smoke condensate in *S. typhimurium* TA98 (Wilmer & Spit, 1986) and did not affect the induction of mutation by benzo[*a*]pyrene, but it significantly reduced reverse mutation induced by aflatoxin B$_1$ in the same tester strain (Qin & Huang, 1985). The ability of all-*trans*-retinoic acid to inhibit aflatoxin B$_1$-induced mutation in strain TA98 has been reported in two other studies (Whong *et al.*, 1988; Raina & Gurtoo, 1985), while contradictory results were reported with TA100, one showing a protective effect (Bhattacharya *et al.*, 1987) and the other no inhibition (Raina & Gurtoo, 1985). [The Working Group noted that the protocol used by Raina and Gurtoo was different from that in the other five studies with Ames' test, in that a 5-min preincubation assay was used rather than the standard plate incorporation approach as described by Maron and Ames (1983). In addition, the S9 mixtures were prepared from the livers of C57BL/6Ha mice or Wistar rats without pretreatment, whereas in the other studies S9 liver fractions were prepared from Arochlor 1254-induced rats.]

(b)   *Mammalian cells*

The ability of all-*trans*-retinoic acid to inhibit sister chromatid exchange and chromosomal breakage has been tested in carcinogen-treated cultures of mammalian cells (Table 5). all-*trans*-Retinoic acid did not affect the induction of sister chromatid exchange by the directly acting carcinogen mitomycin C in Chinese hamster V79 cells (Sirianni *et al.*, 1981). [The Working Group noted that the retinoid was not present concomitantly with the carcinogen in this study but was added after the carcinogen.], whereas another study showed that all-*trans*-retinoic acid protected against the induction of sister chromatid exchange when present at the same time as cyclophosphamide or DMBA, which are indirect mutagens or carcinogens. In the latter study an epithelial liver cell line of Chinese hamster cells was used which is known to activate promutagens and procarcinogens (Cozzi *et al.*, 1990). In Chinese hamster ovary cells exposed to aqueous extracts of *pan masala*, a complex mixture of areca nut, catechu, lime and cardamom, with or without tobacco, a lower frequency of sister chromatid exchange was observed in the presence of all-*trans*-retinoic acid. The frequencies of chromatid-type and chromosome-type aberrations were also reduced (Patel *et al.*, 1998).

C127 mouse cell lines created by transformation with bovine papillomavirus DNA carry 20–160 copies of the DNA and increased frequencies of chromatid bridges and fragments (27–59%) and of micronuclei (6.6–35%). Three-day exposure to all-*trans*-retinoic acid significantly reduced this instability, but the effect was transient since the instability reappeared after cessation of treatment with the retinoid (Stich *et al.*, 1990).

The effect of all-*trans*-retinoic acid on mutation in mammalian cells has been addressed in only one study. It had no effect on cytotoxicity or mutation expression at the hypoxanthine-guanine phosphoribosyl transferase (*Hprt*) locus in Chinese hamster ovary cells exposed to the directly acting mutagen ethyl methanesulfonate, but it significantly reduced DMBA-induced cytotoxicity and mutation when metabolic activation was provided by either uninduced Sprague rat liver S9, Arochlor 1254-induced Sprague-Dawley rat liver S9 or co-cultivation with primary Sprague-Dawley rat hepatocytes (Budroe *et al.*, 1988). This retinoid also inhibited unscheduled DNA synthesis in primary rat hepatocytes induced by the procarcinogen DMBA, but not that induced by two directly acting mutagens, ethyl methanesulfonate and ultraviolet light. The inhibitory effect on DMBA activity occurred at nontoxic concentrations, and the authors hypothesized that the effect was due to a reduction in DMBA-induced DNA damage through alterations of the DNA adduct load in cells treated concurrently with retinoid and carcinogen (Budroe et al., 1987).

This hypothesis is supported by the results of five studies of the effect of all-trans-retinoic acid on the formation of carcinogen–DNA adducts. Three were carried out with cultured cells and the remaining two with calf thymus DNA co-incubated with rat liver microsomes (Table 5). When murine epidermal cells from newborn NIH Swiss mouse skin were exposed to [^{3}H]DMBA in the presence of all-trans-retinoic acid, a significant reduction was observed in the binding of the carcinogen to DNA, in the absence of a significant effect on the number of cells. This finding was particularly striking because the actual uptake of the radiolabelled carcinogen was higher in retinoid-treated cultures (Shoyab, 1981). In a similar study of the uptake and binding of [^{3}H]benzo[a]pyrene to DNA in cultured bronchial mucosa explants from 10 patients (all smokers) with bronchial cancer, the amount of DNA-bound carcinogen was significantly reduced when all-trans-retinoic acid was added. As in the previous study, binding to DNA was decreased even though the actual uptake of the carcinogen was increased in retinoid-treated cells. The authors concluded that since incorporation of [^{3}H]thymidine into DNA (as an index of the number of cells) did not change during treatment with the retinoid and the carcinogen, the increased cellular uptake of the carcinogen was not due to an increase in the number of cells in the explants (Bodo et al., 1989). [The Working Group noted that incorporation of [^{3}H]thymidine into DNA was found to be altered in other studies with retinoids.]

The ability of all-trans-retinoic acid to potentiate the action of the chemotherapeutic drug, cisplatin, was assessed in human ovarian carcinoma cell lines. The number of DNA adducts formed was increased in NIHOVCAR$_3$ cells, a line known to be sensitive to all-trans-retinoic acid, but not in IGROV1 cells, which are insensitive to this retinoid (Caliaro et al., 1997).

Both of the studies of the effect of all-trans-retinoic acid on the binding of carcinogens to calf thymus DNA showed a protective effect. Binding of [^{3}H]aflatoxin B$_1$ to calf thymus DNA, activated by liver microsomes from phenobarbital-induced Wistar rats, was significantly reduced by all-trans-retinoic acid. This effect was ascribed to a reduction in the formation of the reactive intermediate aflatoxin B$_1$-8,9-epoxide in the presence of the retinoid, measured by quantifying its hydrolysis product aflatoxin B$_1$-8,9-dihydrodiol as Tris-diol complex in the reaction mixtures (Firozi et al., 1987). all-trans-Retinoic acid suppressed the formation of adducts on calf thymus DNA by the carcinogen benzo[a]pyrene in a reaction catalysed by liver microsomes from Arochlor 1254-treated rats. The inhibitory effect did not appear to be associated with the enzymatic activation step (i.e. generation and further activation of the proximate carcinogen, benzo[a]pyrene-7,8-diol in reaction mixtures). Instead, the retinoid accelerated the rate at which the ultimate carcinogenic metabolite, benzo[a]pyrene-7,8-diol-9,10-epoxide, disappeared from the reaction mixture containing all-trans-retinoic acid (Shah et al., 1992).

In studies of the role of all-trans-retinoic acid in controlling the expression of genes involved in metabolism, a 19-fold induction of cytochrome P450 (CYP) 2C7 mRNA levels was found in primary rat hepatocytes exposed to all-trans-retinoic acid, this effect being exerted at the transcriptional level, as shown in nuclear run-on experiments (Westin et al., 1993). In a similar study, CYP3A mRNA levels were shown to increase by approximately eightfold in primary hepatocytes exposed to all-trans-retinoic acid. The levels of CYP1A1 in messenger RNA were nonsignificantly increased, whereas no effect was observed on CYP1A2 levels (Jurima-Romet et al., 1997).

(c)   Experimental animals

These studies are summarized in Table 6.

In rats, the activity of enzymes involved in the metabolism of N-acetylaminofluorene and N-hydroxyacetylaminofluorene was enhanced by feeding all-trans-retinoic acid. The glucuronyl transferase activity in microsomal preparations prepared from the livers of treated animals was enhanced by 37%, thus increasing detoxification of the carcinogen, and the activity of para-nitro-

Table 6. Effect of exposure to all-*trans*-retinoic acid on metabolic activity in rodents *in vivo*

Retinoid (tested dose and administration route)[a]	Carcinogen (tested dose and administration route)[a]	Animal strain and species	Investigated effect	Result[b]	LED/HID[c]	Reference
RA (0.25% in diet for 3 days)[d]	Acetylaminofluorene or N-hydroxyacetyl-aminofluorene (17 mg/kg bw ip for 3 days)	Sprague-Dawley rats	Liver enzyme activity: • glucuronyltransferase • sulfotransferase • AAF-deacylase	# + –	37% increase 50% decrease No effect	Daoud & Griffin (1978)
			AAF-deacylase			
all-*trans*-RA (30 mg/kg bw per day by gavage for 4 days)	None	Male Sprague-Dawley rats	Liver cytochrome P450 levels CYP1A2 CYP2B1/2 CYP2C11 CYP2E CYP3A CYP4A P450 metabolism Glucuronidation	– – + + – – (+) +		Howell *et al.* (1998)
all-*trans*-RA (single topical dose of 0.1% applied to skin)	None	Human	P450-mediated mediated metabolism of all-*trans*-RA to 4-hydroxyretinoic acid	#	0.1% (4.5-fold increase)	Duell *et al.* (1992)
all-*trans*-RA (single topical dose of 0.05% applied to skin)	None	Human	Basal P4501A1 expression	+	0.05% (68% decrease in P4501A1 mRNA levels; 75% decrease in P4501A1 protein levels)	Li *et al.* (1995)
all-*trans*-RA (single topical dose of 0.05% applied to skin)	None	Human	Basal P4501A2 expression	+	0.05% (93% reduction in P4501A2 mRNA levels)	Li *et al.* (1995)
all-*trans*-RA (single topical dose of 0.05% applied to skin)	10% crude coal-tar	Human	Induced P4501A1 expression	+	0.05% (46% decrease in P4501A1 mRNA levels)	Li *et al.* (1995)
all-*trans*-RA (single topical dose of 0.05% applied to skin)	0.025% clobetasol propionate	Human	Induced P4501A1 expression	+	0.05% (69% decrease in P4501A1 mRNA levels)	Li *et al.* (1995)

RA, retinoic acid; ip, intraperitoneally; AAF, acetylaminofluorene

[a] Doses of retinoids and carcinogens and routes of administration are given as reported by the authors.

[b] +, inhibition of the investigated end-point; (+), weak inhibition of the investigated end-point, not significantly different; –, no effect on the investigated end-point, #, enhancement of investigated end-point; (#) enhancement but statistically only approaching significance, $p < 0.06$

[c] LED, lowest effective dose that inhibits or enhances the investigated effect; HID, highest ineffective dose

[d] Source and type not given; presumed to be all-*trans*-RA because of date

phenol-sulfotransferase, the enzyme involved in activation of N-acetylaminofluorene and N-hydroxy-acetylaminofluorene to reactive states, was inhibited; however, it had no effect on N-acetylamino-fluorene-deacylase activity (Daoud & Griffin, 1978).

In a comprehensive study of the effect of five retinoids, one of which was all-*trans*-retinoic acid, on hepatic microsomal metabolism and CYP activity in Sprague-Dawley rats, the animals received daily oral doses of 30 mg/kg bw for 4 days, and liver microsomes were prepared on day 5. The activity of CYP isoenzymes was assayed by western blot immunoanalysis. The activities of CYP1A2, CYP2B1/2 and CYP3A were reduced by roughly 27%, 20% and 27% respectively, in animals receiving all-*trans*-retinoic acid, although these effects were not statistically significant. The activity of CYP2E was reduced by 30% and that of CYP2C11 by 40% (both $p < 0.05$), whereas that of CYP4A remained unchanged. The effect of this drug on metabolic activity was limited to a study of its own phase I and II metabolism. A decrease was observed in the CYP-mediated metabolism of all-*trans*-retinoic acid by microsomal preparations from treated animals, although the effect only approached significance ($p = 0.06$). In contrast, a significant decrease was found in the glucuronidation capacity of the microsomal preparation. The authors noted that the patterns of alterations in metabolism and isozyme profiles differed significantly among the retinoids studied and suggested that the effect could be related to binding selectivity of the different retinoids for either RAR or RXR receptors, although the data are not conclusive (Howell *et al.*, 1998).

Retinoids may also modulate the metabolism of carcinogens in CYP-independent pathways. In a study of the effect of all-*trans*-retinoic acid on DNA adduct formation, female CD-1 mice were given a topical application of the proximate carcinogen (7S,8S)-dihydroxy-7,8-dihydrobenzo[a]pyrene ((+)-BP-7,8-diol), which is further metabolized by epoxidation to 7,8-dihyroxy-9,10-epoxy-7,8,9,10 tetrahydrobenzo[a]pyrene (BPDE). When the BP-7,8-diol was applied by itself to the animals, it was metabolized mainly by CYP systems, resulting in (+)-*syn*-BPDE–DNA adducts; however, when the animals were pretreated with TPA 24 h before administration of TPA and (+)-BP-7,8-diol, the pattern of adducts changed to include (–)-*anti*-BPDE

adducts, thought to be derived from a CYP-independent pathway that probably involves peroxyl radical-dependent epoxidation. When all-*trans*-retinoic acid was administered with the second TPA treatment, formation of the (–)-*anti*-BPDE-DNA adducts was significantly inhibited. Administration of the retinoid with the first TPA treatment had no effect. The authors speculated that the first TPA dose recruited neutrophils to the treatment site and the second dose triggered the release of oxidants from these neutrophils. They further suggested that the retinoic acid acts as a radical scavenger, thus preventing peroxyl radical-dependent epoxidation (Marnett & Ji, 1994).

There have been few studies of the effect of all-*trans*-retinoic acid on metabolism in humans, but there is some indication that metabolic activity and the CYP enzyme profiles in tissues are altered by all-*trans*-retinoic acid. A single topical dose of 0.1% all-*trans*-retinoic acid cream or cream vehicle was applied to adult human skin and the region was occluded for four days with Saranwrap. After four days, the test area was washed and sliced off, and microsomal fractions were prepared and assayed for their capacity to metabolize [³H]all-*trans*-retinoic acid *in vitro*. Microsomes from treated sites had a 4.5-fold increase in their capacity to form 4-hydroxyretinoic acid in comparison with microsomes from vehicle-treated sites. This metabolism appeared to be CYP-mediated since the inclusion of ketoconazaole, an inhibitor of CYP-mediated activity, in the reaction mixtures resulted in inhibition of metabolism in microsomal fractions isolated from retinoic acid-treated sites (Duell *et al.*, 1992). In a similar study, the basal level of expression of CYP1A1 and CYP1A2 was quantified in skin samples from volunteers receiving topical 0.05% all-*trans*-retinoic acid in cream or cream without retinoic acid. The authors also examined the effect of all-*trans*-retinoic acid on the expression of these two isoenzymes in patients receiving the cream with either 10% crude coal-tar or 0.025% clobetasol proprionate, a potent glucocorticoid. all-*trans*-Retinoic acid reduced the basal activities of CYP1A1 mRNA and protein by 68% and 75% respectively, and the basal activity of CYP1A2 mRNA by 93%. Coal-tar and clobetasol increased the activity of CYP1A1 but not that of CYP1A2 mRNA expression. all-*trans*-Retinoic acid inhibited the CYP1A1 mRNA expression induced by coal-tar by 46% and that induced by clobetasol by 69% (Li *et al.*, 1995).

4.3 Mechanisms of cancer prevention

all-*trans*-Retinoic acid may prevent or delay carcinogenesis by several mechanisms, which depend on the cell type used *in vitro*, on the carcinogen and animal strain *in vivo* and on the tissue affected. Most of the studies indicate that retinoids inhibit the promotion step of the multistage carcinogenesis process, although there are indications that it also affects initiation. Several reports described in section 4.2.3.2 support the hypothesis that retinoids such as all-*trans*-retinoic acid can inhibit initiation induced by carcinogens that require metabolic activation, whereas they have little effect on directly acting carcinogens. The mechanisms of the suppression of initiation include: induction of the transcription of certain CYP enzymes that can detoxify carcinogens, decreased binding of carcinogens to DNA and decreased carcinogen-induced DNA damage. The activity of several CYP enzymes was found to be regulated at the level of transcription by direct binding of nuclear RARs to retinoic acid response elements in the gene promoters, as shown for CYP1A1 (Vecchini *et al.*, 1994).

Most studies on the effects of all-*trans*-retinoic acid on carcinogenesis indicate that the main mechanism is inhibition of promotion, which is related to the ability of retinoids to antagonize the activity of tumour promoters and affect the proliferation, differentiation and apoptosis of premalignant and malignant cells. The ability of all-*trans*-retinoic acid to alter intercellular adhesion and inhibit host responses such as angiogenesis may also play a role in its chemopreventive activity.

4.3.1 Antagonism of tumour promotion and activator protein 1 activity

all-*trans*-Retinoic acid inhibits the action of tumour promoters by antagonizing tumour promoter signalling. For example, it inhibited the induction of ornithine decarboxylase by TPA in cultured tracheal cells (Jetten & Shirley, 1985) and mouse skin (Connor *et al.*, 1983). The mechanism by which ornithine decarboxylase expression is controlled by all-*trans*-retinoic acid appears to be suppression of gene transcription and involves liganded nuclear RAR (Mao *et al.*, 1993). all-*trans*-

Retinoic acid can also affect other down-stream events of TPA signalling. TPA activates protein kinase C and eventually activates the transcription activator protein 1 (AP-1). all-*trans*-Retinoic acid can exert anti-AP-1 activity by *trans*-repressing the AP-1 function and thereby inhibiting TPA-induced transformation of mouse epidermal JB6 cells (Li *et al.*, 1996). Furthermore, in DMBA-initiated skin of transgenic mice carrying an AP-1-luciferase transgene, inhibition of papilloma formation by all-*trans*-retinoic acid and by retinoids with anti-AP-1 activity appeared to be mediated by suppression of AP-1 activation. Retinoids capable of RAR element *trans*-activation but devoid of anti-AP-1 activity failed to inhibit papilloma formation (Huang *et al.*, 1997).

4.3.2 Inhibition of cell proliferation

The formation of a premalignant lesion requires that initiated cells proliferate to expand the initiated clone. Clearly, inhibition of such proliferation would be an important mechanism for cancer prevention. There is no direct evidence that all-*trans*-retinoic acid can block the proliferation of initiated cells *in vivo* because they cannot be identified at an early stage as such, but there is ample evidence that all-*trans*-retinoic acid can inhibit cell proliferation in a number of settings. It inhibited cell proliferation by regulating cell cycle progression from G1 to S phase by altering the levels of cell cycle controlling proteins.

4.3.2.1 Cyclins and cyclin-dependent kinase inhibitors

The inhibition of DNA synthesis and the G1 arrest in SV-40-T-immortalized human bronchial epithelial BEAS-2B cells and their NNK-transformed derivative cell lines was found to occur as a result of suppression of the protein levels of cyclins D1 and E at a post-translational level. all-*trans*-Retinoic acid promoted the degradation of cyclin D1 by targeting it for proteolysis in proteasomes via increased ubiquitinylation which depended on the C-terminal PEST[proline (P), glutamate (E), serine (S) and threonine (T)] sequence (Langenfeld *et al.*, 1996, 1997; Boyle *et al.*, 1999). Specific nuclear RARs have been implicated in this effect because the receptor-selective retinoids that activated RARβ or RXR pathways caused a greater decrease in the amount of cyclin D1 protein and corresponding inhibition of DNA synthesis (Boyle *et al.*, 1999). Studies with lymphoblastoid B cell lines immortalized with Epstein-Barr virus have shown that all-*trans*-retinoic acid-induced accumulation in the G0/G1 phase is associated with multiple effects on G1 regulatory proteins, including p27Kip1 up-regulation, decreased levels of cyclins D2, D3 and A and inhibition of cyclin-dependent kinase (CDK)2, CDK4 and CDK6 activity, which ultimately resulted in reduced pRb phosphorylation and G0/G1 growth arrest (Zancai *et al.*, 1998). p21, which has been shown to induce G1 arrest by inhibiting CDK and proliferating cell nuclear antigen dependent DNA replication, was recently found to possess an RAR element in its promoter and to be regulated by retinoic acid. This could be another mechanism for cell cycle regulation (Liu *et al.*, 1996).

4.3.2.2 trans-Repression of activator protein 1
As activated AP-1 is the ultimate mediator of signalling by many mitogens, the antagonistic effects of all-*trans*-retinoic acid on AP-1 may suppress growth. This was found to occur in normal bronchial epithelial cells in which growth had been inhibited by all-*trans*-retinoic acid but not in the all-*trans*-retinoic acid-resistant, tumorigenic derivatives of SV-40-T-immortalized BEAS-2B cells (Lee *et al.*, 1997).

4.3.2.3 Suppression of the human papillomavirus oncogenes E6 and E7
HPV-16 immortalized keratinocytes were very sensitive to growth inhibition by all-*trans*-retinoic acid because the retinoid inhibited the expression of HPV-16 *E6* and *E7* oncogenes, which are required for maintenance of the continuous proliferation of these immortalized cells (Pirisi *et al.*, 1992).

4.3.2.4 Modulation of autocrine and paracrine loops
Premalignant cells often have a growth advantage over normal cells, as they overexpress growth factor receptors that can mediate paracrine or autocrine growth stimulation. One example of such a receptor is the epidermal growth factor receptor (EGFR) which is overexpressed in various premalignant lesions and can enhance cell growth by autocrine or paracrine routes in conjunction with epidermal growth factor (EGF) or transforming growth factor α (TGF-α). all-*trans*-Retinoic acid

suppressed the expression of TGF-α and EGFR mRNA in head-and-neck squamous-cell carcinoma cells by decreasing gene transcription (Grandis *et al.*, 1996).

HPV immortalization increased EGF receptor levels in ectocervical cells, increasing their sensitivity to growth stimulation by EGF. all-*trans*-Retinoic acid reduced both EGF binding and EGF receptor protein levels in immortalized cells but not in normal ectocervical cells. Thus, it can attenuate the increased responsiveness to EGF by decreasing the EGFR level (Sizemore & Rorke, 1993). all-*trans*-Retinoic acid inhibition of the growth of HPV-immortalized ectocervical cells and cervical carcinoma cell lines has been proposed to result from an increase in insulin-like growth factor binding protein 3 mRNA and protein levels and a reduced extracellular concentration of free insulin-like growth factor I (Andreatta-Van Leyen *et al.*, 1994).

Transforming growth factor-β (TGF-β) plays a complex role in the regulation of proliferation and differentiation of many cell types, including cells of epithelial origin, for which TGF-β is usually a growth inhibitory factor. In the immortal mouse epidermal cell line JB6, TPA caused progression to anchorage independence and tumorigenicity, partly by decreasing the level of TGF-β receptor expression. all-*trans*-Retinoic acid counteracted both the promoting effect of TPA and its suppression of TGF-β receptor (De Benedetti *et al.*, 1991).

4.3.3 Restoration of normal differentiation
Carcinogenesis is characterized by aberrant differentiation, which is manifested by either blockage of cells at an early stage of differentiation or redirection of differentiation towards an abnormal pathway. Several reports described in the General Remarks (section 4) have demonstrated the ability of all-*trans*-retinoic acid to suppress squamous-cell differentiation and enhance mucociliary differentiation in epithelial cells as well as stimulate differentiation of numerous tumour cell lines. It is thought that restoration by all-*trans*-retinoic acid of normal differentiation in premalignant cells might be accompanied by restoration of normal growth control mechanisms as well, but there is no clear experimental evidence that the effect of all-*trans*-retinoic acid on differentiation of premalignant cells is the cause of either cell growth inhibition or cell apoptosis.

The clear demonstration that all-*trans*-retinoic acid can induce terminal differentiation *in vivo* even in a fully malignant condition, acute promyelocytic leukaemia, lends strong support to this concept (Castaigne *et al.*, 1990; Warrel *et al.*, 1993).

4.3.4 Inhibition of prostaglandin production

An excessive production of prostaglandins has been correlated with tumour promotion. More recently, it was found that expression of the enzyme cyclooxygenase-2 (Cox-2), which catalyses the synthesis of prostaglandins, can be induced by growth factors and tumour promoters and is up-regulated in transformed cells and tumours. Therefore, it has become a target for chemoprevention. Treatment of oral epithelial cells with either EGF or TPA enhanced transcription of Cox-2 and increased production of prostaglandin-2. These effects were inhibited by all-*trans*-retinoic acid (Mestre *et al.*, 1997). [The Working Group noted that the molecular mechanism of this effect of all-*trans*-retinoic acid has not been elucidated.]

4.3.5 Induction of apoptosis

Several studies summarized in the General Remarks (section 4) demonstrated the ability of all-*trans*-retinoic acid to induce apoptosis in various tumour cell lines. The mechanism by which apoptosis is induced is not clear, but several studies have implicated nuclear RARs and RXRs in the process on the basis of the results of experiments with receptor-selective retinoids and transfection (Nagy *et al.*, 1995; Melino *et al.*, 1997; Monczak *et al.*, 1997). It is still not clear which target genes are induced that trigger apoptosis. It has been suggested that induction of tissue transglutaminase by all-*trans*-retinoic acid may be related to apoptosis induction (Melino *et al.*, 1997).

4.3.6 Increased gap-junctional communication

Most normal cells are directly coupled via intercellular gap junctions formed by the assembly of connexin proteins. Loss of gap-junctional communication is an early event in neoplasia both *in vitro* and *in vivo*. Restoration of this communication by transfection of connexin genes into tumour cells results in enhanced growth control and/or suppression of the neoplastic phenotype (Trosko & Ruch, 1998). all-*trans*-Retinoic acid has been shown to increase the expression of connexin 43

(Cx43) in C3H/10T1/2 cells at the levels of mRNA and protein (Rogers *et al.*, 1990); the resulting increase in gap-junctional communication is highly correlated with the ability of all-*trans*-retinoic acid to inhibit neoplastic transformation in these cells (Hossain *et al.*, 1989) and the suppression of proliferation in normal and transformed cells (Mehta *et al.*, 1989). Inhibition of proliferation by all-*trans*-retinoic acid was dependent on cell–cell contact and was not seen in sparsely seeded cells, again implicating gap-junctional communication in this response (Hossain & Bertram, 1994). The relevance of induced gap-junctional communication to the chemopreventive activity of all-*trans*-retinoic acid *in vivo* is suggested by the demonstration that the retinoid upregulates Cx43 expression in human skin after topical application (Guo *et al.*, 1992). The mechanism by which it increases Cx43 expression is not clear, as the promoter region does not contain a known RAR element. In one study, stabilization of Cx43 mRNA by all-*trans*-retinoic acid was suggested (Clairmont *et al.*, 1996).

4.3.7 Modulation of cell adhesion and motility

Cell invasion through the basement membrane is the ultimate step that distinguishes a carcinoma *in situ* from a malignant tumour. As this process requires changes in cell adhesion and detachment, local proteolysis and migration, inhibition of invasion may suppress malignant conversion. It is noteworthy that all-*trans*-retinoic acid can up-regulate the function of the invasion-suppressor complex E-cadherin/catenin (Vermeulen *et al.*, 1995) and inhibit the expression of various enzymes that degrade the basement membrane, such as collagenase and stromelysine, at the level of transcription by antagonizing AP-1 (Nicholson *et al.*, 1990; Schüle *et al.*, 1991). In addition, all-*trans*-retinoic acid suppressed the level of autocrine motility factor receptor and decreased cell motility (Lotan *et al.*, 1992). These findings suggest that if it can suppress the expression of the invasive phenotype in carcinoma *in situ*, it may prevent the progression of a premalignant lesion to a malignant one.

4.3.8 Inhibition of angiogenesis

The progressive growth of solid tumours depends on the development of new blood vessels, a process known as neovascularization or angiogenesis. Tumour cells secrete factors that induce the directed migration and proliferation of endothelial cells from capillaries in normal tissue, which eventually differentiate and form vessels around and within tumours. It is likely that some premalignant lesions also depend on angiogenesis for conversion into invasive cancer. all-*trans*-Retinoic acid has demonstrated antiangiogenic effects in several systems. In one study, it caused the endothelial cells of large and small vessels to become refractory to stimulation of migration by tumour-conditioned media or purified angiogenic factors (α-fibroblast growth factor, basic fibroblast growth factor, vascular endothelial growth factor, platelet-derived growth factor, TGFβ-1, and interleukin-8) without affecting cell proliferation (Lingen *et al.*, 1996). Rats given all-*trans*-retinoic acid were unable to mount a neovascular response to tumours implanted in their corneas. These results indicated that all-*trans*-retinoic acid can affect directly both tumour cells and endothelial cells and thereby suppress the formation of new blood vessels *in vivo*. Treatment of mice xenotransplanted with a human squamous-cell carcinoma reduced the level of a binding protein for fibroblast growth factor. This inhibited angiogenesis and led to a decrease in the tumour growth rate.

5. Other Beneficial Effects

all-*trans*-Retinoic acid is of benefit to patients suffering from a variety of dermatological disorders (see section 2.3).

6. Carcinogenicity

6.1 Humans
No data were available to the Working Group.

6.2 Experimental models
No studies of the carcinogenicity of all-*trans*-retinoic acid were available to the Working Group, but all-*trans*-retinoic acid can act as a tumour promoter in mouse skin and can enhance liver carcinogenesis induced by NDEA in mice (for details, see section 4.2.1).

7. Other Toxic Effects

7.1 Adverse effects
7.1.1 Humans
At the recommended oral dose of all-*trans*-retinoic acid, 45 mg/m^2 per day as two evenly divided doses, virtually all patients experience some drug-related toxicity. The most frequent adverse events are similar to those described in patients taking high doses of retinol and its esters (IARC, 1998), especially headache, fever, weakness and fatigue. Rare adverse events associated with use of all-*trans*-retinoic acid in patients with acute promyelocytic leukaemia include hypercalcaemia, bone-marrow necrosis, bone-marrow fibrosis, acute pancreatitis, thromboembolic events, acute neutrophilic dermatosis, erythema nodosum, basophilia, hyperhistaminaemia, granulomatous proliferation and necrotizing vasculitis (reviewed by Hatake *et al.*, 1997; Paydas *et al.*, 1998). The toxicity associated with topically applied all-*trans*-retinoic acid at 0.025% or 0.01% is generally localized, dermal and reversible after discontinuation of treament (Arky, 1998).

7.1.1.1 Retinoic acid syndrome
About 25% of patients with acute promyelocytic leukaemia who have been treated with the recommended oral dose of all-*trans*-retinoic acid have experienced 'retinoic acid syndrome', a life-threatening disorder reported to be related to leukocyte activation (Fenaux & De Botton, 1998). The syndrome usually occurs within the first month of treatment, sometimes after the first dose, and is characterized by fever, dyspnoea, weight gain, radiographic pulmonary infiltrates and pleural or pericardial effusion. The syndrome has occasionally been accompanied by impaired myocardial contractility, and episodic hypotension and has been observed with or without concomitant leukocytosis. Glucocorticoids given at high doses when symptoms of the syndrome appear may reduce the morbidity and mortality; in the absence of prevention by chemotherapy, 60% or more of patients taking oral all-*trans*-retinoic acid may require this treatment (Arky, 1998).

Retinoic acid syndrome has been ascribed to infiltration of leukaemic or maturing myeloid cells into the lung parenchyma. Diffuse alveolar haemorrhage with pulmonary capillaritis was reported in one woman who was treated with all-*trans*-retinoic acid for acute promyelocytic leukaemia (Nicolls *et al.*, 1998). Thromboembolic complications have also been reported, including acute renal failure due to occlusion of renal vessels (Pogliani *et al.*, 1997). A study of the development of retinoic acid syndrome showed that clinical signs generally develop within a median of seven days. Respiratory distress (89%), fever (81%), pulmonary infiltrates (81%), weight gain (50%), pleural effusion (47%), renal failure (39%), pericardial effusion (19%), cardiac failure (17%) and hypotension (12%) were the main clinical signs, and almost all subjects with the syndrome experienced at least three of these events. Nine of 64 cases of retinoic acid syndrome resulted in death. No significant predictive factors of the syndrome were found, but its occurrence was associated with shorter event-free survival and shorter overall survival (De Botton *et al.*, 1998).

7.1.1.2 Relapse of acute promyelocytic leukaemia at unusual sites

Although the combination of all-*trans*-retinoic acid and chemotherapy with daunorubicin and cytosine arabinoside has become the standard therapy for acute promyelocytic leukaemia, concern has been raised that all-*trans*-retinoic acid in combination with the other agents may increase the risk for relapse at unusual sites. Myelodysplastic syndrome and central nervous system relapse, although rare, have been seen after treatment of acute promyelocytic leukaemia with all-*trans*-retinoic acid. Whether the frequency of such events is truly increased among these patients is being addressed in clinical trials (Bseiso *et al.*, 1997; Evans *et al.*, 1997).

7.1.1.3 Metabolic, nutritional and haematological toxicity

Up to 60% of patients given the prescribed oral dose of all-*trans*-retinoic acid experience hypercholesterolaemia and/or hypertriglyceridaemia, and 50–60% show increased activity of liver enzymes. These abnormalities can sometimes lead to more severe complications such as acute pancreatitis, hepatotoxicity, hyperleukocytosis, worsening of coagulopathy, renal dysfunction, myocardial infarct and thrombocytosis (Cull *et al.*, 1997;

Kentos *et al.*, 1997; Yutsudo *et al.*, 1997; Arky, 1998). Hypercalcaemia has also been observed after oral administration of all-*trans*-retinoic acid; in one case, the hypercalcaemia was controlled and complete remission of acute promyelocytic leukaemia was achieved after the dose of all-*trans*-retinoic acid was reduced from 45 to 27 mg/m² per day (Lemez, 1995).

A phase-I trial of orally administered all-*trans*-retinoic acid was conducted to establish the maximum tolerated dose when given once daily to patients with solid tumours. In 49 patients who received doses ranging from 45 to 309 mg/m² per day, hypertriglyceridaemia was the dose-limiting effect at 269 mg/m² per day; grade 3 hypertriglyceridaemia developed in one patient each at 110, 138 and 269 mg/m² per day, and grade 4 hypertriglyceridaemia developed in one patient each at 88, 215 and 269 mg/m² per day. Grade 3 hypercholesterolaemia was seen in one patient at 269 mg/m² per day. Grade 3 transient elevations of transaminase activity were seen in four patients treated at doses ≥ 56 mg/m² per day. Toxic effects at grade 3 and 4 occurred sporadically and included thrombocytopenia, dehydration and transient renal failure, localized desquamous rash, staphylococcal bacteraemia, probable pseudotumour cerebri, shortness of breath, severe cough, myalgia, severe exacerbation of neck pain, headache, anorexia, fatigue, dysphagia, scleral haemorrhage, anaemia, nausea and vomiting. Severe toxicity tended to occur when the initial peak plasma concentration of all-*trans*-retinoic acid was 0.5 µg/ml, and the frequency of toxicity did not change as the plasma concentration decreased. The daily dose of all-*trans*-retinoic acid in patients with solid tumours recommended on the basis of these findings is 215 mg/m² (Conley *et al.*, 1997). [The Working Group noted that the symptoms were not necessarily related to treatment.]

In a clinical study of the treatment of chronic myeloid leukaemia, 18 patients were given 12 courses of 80 mg/m² per day, divided into two equal doses, each course consisting of one week of drug followed by one week's rest. Eleven patients left the study before the sixth course because of progressive hyperleukocytosis, thrombocytosis or refusal. Five additional subjects were withdrawn before the twelfth course because of elevated leukocyte counts, and one withdrew for other reasons. Hepatic toxicity of grades 1–2 was observed in 5% of participating subjects (Russo et al., 1998). Conversely, there were no documented instances of increased liver function or triglyceride concentration in 13 patients with chronic myeloid leukaemia who carried the Philadelphia chromosomal translocation and were treated for a median duration of 56 days with 175 mg/m² per day, divided into two equal daily doses (Cortes et al., 1997).

7.1.1.4 Mucocutaneous toxicity
(a) Topical application
The most frequent adverse effects of topically applied all-*trans*-retinoic acid are dermal. Local peeling, dry skin, burning, stinging, erythema and pruritus were reported by almost all of 179 patients who applied 0.05% all-*trans*-retinoic acid cream to their faces. The reactions were usually of mild to moderate severity, occurred early during therapy and recurred after an initial 24-week decline. Patients using topical all-*trans*-retinoic acid have a heightened sensitivity to sunlight and extreme wind or cold. Temporary hyper- or hypopigmentation has also been reported (Arky, 1998). Skin irritation caused by topically applied all-*trans*-retinoic acid does not appear to involve injury to the skin barrier but may be caused by dilatation of the cutaneous vasculature (Fullerton & Serup, 1997). Modified delivery systems such as polymer complexes and microsponge particles have been developed to reduce the irritating effects of topical all-*trans*-retinoic acid (Leyden, 1998).

The effectiveness of topical all-*trans*-retinoic acid (0.05.%) in reversing signs of photoageing was investigated under conditions of extended use (48 weeks). As expected, the adverse events were generally mild and were essentially dermal (dry skin, peeling, burning/stinging, erythema, irritation, pruritis and papules). The frequency of the adverse effects decreased with time (Olsen et al., 1997).

Topically applied all-*trans*-retinoic acid has been investigated as an intravaginal treatment for cervical intraepithelial neoplasia. In one study, doses of 0.05–0.2% applied to a sponge and inserted in a cervical cap for four days produced vaginal irritation, ulceration and discharge, with no evidence of systemic toxicity (Surwit et al., 1982). A study of doses increasing from 0.05% for four days showed that the maximum tolerated dose was 0.372% (Meyskens et al., 1983). In a subsequent study, 1 mL of 0.375% all-*trans*-retinoic acid induced only local, mild side-effects consisting primarily of increased vulvar burning, itching and irritation; again, no systemic side-effects were observed (Meyskens et al., 1994).

(b) Oral dosing
Mucocutaneous reactions are also common after treatment with oral all-*trans*-retinoic acid and include mucocutaneous dryness, xerostomia, dry skin, xerophthalmia, erythema and pruritis (Conley et al., 1997; Sutton et al., 1997; Budd et al., 1998; Russo et al., 1998). An oral dose of 230 mg/m² in combination with 20 mg/day tamoxifen resulted in unacceptable dermatological toxicity (moist desquamation) in patients with advanced breast cancer (Budd et al., 1998). Six of 13 patients with chronic myeloid leukaemia experienced dry skin or dry mucous membranes after administration of 175 mg/m² per day in two equal doses (Cortes et al., 1997).

7.1.1.5 Headache and general toxicity
Moderate to severe headaches are commonly experienced during oral therapy with all-*trans*-retinoic acid. Cases of pseudotumour cerebri with clinical signs of headache, nausea, double vision and bilateral papilloedema have been reported (Sano et al., 1998). General pain, bone pain, malaise and myalgia are also associated with such therapy (Conley et al., 1997; Budd et al., 1998; Russo et al., 1998).

Headache was the most common side-effect (54%) in a pilot study of orally administered all-*trans*-retinoic acid in patients with chronic myelogenous leukaemia who carried the Philadelphia chromosome and were given a dose of 175 mg/m² per day in two equal doses (Cortes et al., 1997). In a phase-II trial in patients with metastatic breast cancer, all-*trans*-retinoic acid was given orally at a dose of 50 mg/m² three times a day for 14 days of a 21-day cycle, which was repeated until progression of the disease, unacceptable toxicity or patient withdrawal. Of 17 subjects, 14 completed at least one course of therapy; the median time to progression for the remaining 14 subjects was six weeks. Two patients experienced grade 3 headache during the first cycle; the symptoms resolved after discontinuation of the drug, and returned after re-challenge. Six other subjects experienced grade 2 headache during treatment (Sutton et al., 1997).

The combination of all-*trans*-retinoic acid and interferon-α was investigated in a phase-I trial in children with refractory cancer. Pseudotumour cerebri or dose-limiting headache was observed in two of five patients over 12 years of age who had been treated at a dose of 120 mg/m^2 per day, and in one of six patients under 12 years who had been given 90 mg/m^2 per day (Adamson *et al.*, 1997).

A phase-I/II trial of all-*trans*-retinoic acid and tamoxifen was conducted in patients with potentially hormone-responsive advanced breast cancer. The patients received 20 mg/day tamoxifen and all-*trans*-retinoic acid on alternating weeks at doses of 70–230 mg/m^2 per day, divided into two equal doses per day. At all doses, headache, nausea, bone pain and skin changes were noted. The headaches were most severe during the first week of therapy and peaked at the end of the first week. The symptoms recurred in subsequent weeks of all-*trans*-retinoic acid therapy, although their severity tended to wane with each subsequent cycle. all-*trans*-Retinoic acid at a dose of 230 mg/m^2 produced unacceptable headache. Grade 3 headache, grade 2 nausea and vomiting and dermatological effects also occurred in some subjects given all-*trans*-retinoic acid at 190 mg/m^2. The maximum tolerated dose that could be given in alternating weeks with 20 mg/day tamoxifen was 190 mg/m^2 per day (Budd *et al.*, 1998).

7.1.1.6 Gastrointestinal toxicity

Gastrointestal toxicity ranging from constipation to severe nausea has been reported after oral administration of all-*trans*-retinoic acid. A dose of 80 mg/m^2 per day divided into two equal doses produced constipation (11%) and nausea (5%) in patients with chronic myeloid leukaemia (Russo *et al.*, 1998). When all-*trans*-retinoic acid at doses of 70–230 mg/m^2 per day was combined with 20 mg/day tamoxifen, grade 1 nausea and vomiting were observed in most subjects; grade 2 nausea and vomiting occurred in some subjects receiving doses ≥ 190 mg/m^2 per day (Budd *et al.*, 1998). Two of 17 patients with metastatic breast cancer experienced grade 3 nausea and vomiting at a dose of 50 mg/m^2 three times a day (Sutton *et al.*, 1997). Nausea was also experienced by four of 13 patients with chronic myelogenous leukaemia given 175 mg/m^2 per day in two equal doses; one of the cases was described as severe (Cortes *et al.*, 1997).

7.1.2 Experimental models

The LD$_{50}$ of orally administered all-*trans*-retinoic acid is approximately 2200 mg/kg bw in mice and 2000 mg/kg bw in rats (Kamm, 1982). The maximum tolerated dose in athymic nude mice was 20 mg/kg bw per day when given five times per week for four weeks. The dose was selected on the basis of acceptable weight loss and symptoms of hypervitaminosis A; a weight loss of 10–20% and mild to severe mucocutaneous reactions, such as dry or red skin, were seen at doses ≥ 30 mg/kg bw per day (Shalinsky *et al.*, 1995).

Rats given all-*trans*-retinoic acid orally at 5 or 50 mg/kg bw per day for 13 weeks showed hair loss, dermal and mucosal alterations, inhibition of spermatogenesis and weight loss at the low dose, and increased serum transaminase and alkaline phosphatase activities at the high dose. Similar signs were seen in dogs, but 50% of those at the high dose died. In mice, doses of 150–250 mg/kg bw per day caused alopecia, weight loss and skin and membrane changes after five days (Kamm *et al.*, 1984). In other studies in mice, the main dose-related findings included bone rarefaction, bone fracture, elevated serum alkaline phosphatase activity, testicular degeneration, dermal and epidermal inflammation and hyperkeratosis. In rats, decreases in plasma albumin and in haemoglobin concentration and an increase in serum alkaline phosphatase activity were seen. In a comparative study of all-*trans*-retinoic acid, etretinate and retinol palmitate/retinol acetate in rats, doses of 15, 7.5 and 40 mg/kg bw per day, respectively, had about the same negative effect on body weight. After four weeks of administration at these doses, bone fractures and increased serum alkaline phosphatase activity were observed with all agents, but all-*trans*-retinoic acid and retinol palmitate/retinol acetate were more lethal than etretinate. Retinol palmitate/retinol acetate resulted in the lowest frequency of bone fractures, and the increase in serum alkaline phosphatase activity was greatest with all-*trans*-retinoic acid, indicating that retinoids are not equipotent with respect to their short-term toxicity (reviewed by Kamm, 1982).

In male mice treated topically with 0.1% all-*trans*-retinoic acid in gel microspheres for 90 days at 2 or 5 mg/kg bw per day, testicular weight was reduced, with no pathological changes. This effect was not seen at 0.5 mg/kg bw per day. Females showed a reduction in ovarian weight at 5 mg/kg bw per day, with no pathological changes. A dose-related increase in the plasma concentration of all-*trans*-retinoic acid was seen 4 h after the first dose. Male and female dogs treated for 90 days with 0.1% all-*trans*-retinoic acid in gel microspheres at 0.2, 0.5 or 1 mg/kg bw per day showed no evidence of reduced testicular or ovarian weights or other pathological changes. The systemic exposure observed in preclinical studies of toxicity with topically applied all-*trans*-retinoic acid is probably the result of incidental ingestion (Arky, 1998). [The Working Group noted that topical administration of high doses of all-*trans*-retinoic acid gives rise to severe skin irritation, which is dose-limiting.]

7.2 Reproductive and developmental effects
7.2.1 Humans
7.2.1.1 Reproductive effects
Oral administration of all-*trans*-retinoic acid at 20–30 mg/day (~ 0.4 mg/kg bw per day) to 12 patients with acne for 90–300 days was associated with dry oral and nasal mucous membranes. The treatment had no measurable effect on sperm count, sperm density, total and progressive motility or morphology other than an increase in total ejaculate volume (Plewig *et al.*, 1979).

7.2.1.2 Developmental effects

(a)   Topical exposure
The available case reports and epidemiological studies do not provide evidence for developmental effects after administration of the standard dose of all-*trans*-retinoic acid (Rosa, 1992). In a retrospective study of 215 pregnant women with a history of dermal use of all-*trans*-retinoic acid, no evidence was found for an increased risk of major malformations (Jick *et al.*, 1993). In United States Medicaid data on 1120 cases of topical use of all-*trans*-retinoic acid during pregnancy, the frequency distribution of abnormal outcomes was no different from that expected for the country as a whole (Rosa, 1992).

Eighteen case reports of anomalies in children of mothers who had used all-*trans*-retinoic acid during pregnancy included four cases of holo-prosencephaly but which did not share all or most of the characteristic features of retinoid embryopathy, such as small or absent ears. The authors reviewed data to 1988 and concluded that any effect of topical all-*trans*-retinoic acid on human development would be weak (Rosa, 1992).

At least two other cases of congenital malformation have been associated with cosmetic or therapeutic topical application of all-*trans*-retinoic acid, which have features in common with retinoid embryopathy (Camera & Pregliasco, 1992; Lipson *et al.*, 1993).

(b)   Percutaneous absorption
The absence of teratogenic effects after topical application of all-*trans*-retinoic acid is compatible with its limited percutaneous absorption. Classical pharmacokinetics analyses were used to compare the circulating concentrations of all-*trans*-retinoic acid and its metabolites after topical application of 0.05% all-*trans*-retinoic acid cream. Topical application of all-*trans*-retinoic acid did not appreciably alter the endogenous plasma concentration of retinoids (Nau, 1993; Johnson, 1997). A physiologically based pharmacokinetics method for interspecies scaling of internal dose showed that the effective concentration of parent all-*trans*-retinoic acid and its metabolites across species was of the same order of magnitude (Clewell *et al.*, 1997). After topical application of 0.05% all-*trans*-retinoic acid to the face, arms and chest, the circulating levels of the compound and its metabolites were unchanged (Clewell *et al.*, 1997; Willhite & Clewell, 1999). The low dose that was absorbed, metabolized and delivered after topical application to intact human skin is consistent with the findings *in vivo* in humans (Jensen *et al.*, 1991; Buchan *et al.*, 1994; Latriano *et al.*, 1997), rodents (Willhite *et al.*, 1990) and lagomorphs (Christian *et al.*, 1997).

(c)   Oral exposure
Although all-*trans*-retinoic acid is an isomer of 13-*cis*-retinoic acid, which is responsible for retinoid embryopathy (Creech-Kraft & Willhite, 1997), clinical experience with all-*trans*-retinoic acid at the customary dose of 45 mg/m^2 per day as treatment for acute promyelocytic leukaemia in early or in late gestation has shown no evidence of fetotoxicity.

Three case reports have been published of oral administration of all-*trans*-retinoic acid during early pregnancy. Treatment at 45 mg/m^2 per day with prednisone at 1 mg/kg bw per day from day 36 through week 30 did not induce terata, and the infant showed neither retinoid dermatitis nor cheilitis, although it developed jaundice and respiratory distress shortly after delivery. These conditions resolved without sequelae after supporting therapy, at 7 and 11 days, respectively, and were considered not to be treatment-related. At 15 months, the child's growth and development were normal (Simone *et al.*, 1995). Similar treatment beginning at week 13 had no adverse effect on delivery, survival or early neonatal development (Morton *et al.*, 1995), and no effects were seen of treatment beginning at 14 weeks of gestation and continued for 60 days (Lin *et al.*, 1996).

Exposure late in pregnancy (week 30 until parturition) was not associated with fetotoxicity in four case reports. Oral administration of all-*trans*-retinoic acid at 45 mg/m^2 per day to patients at 23–28 weeks' gestation and continued for 30 days (Harrison *et al.*, 1994; Watanabe *et al.*, 1995) or reduced after remission of the leukaemia had been achieved after 28 days to 22 mg/m^2 per day for 14 days (Stentoft *et al.*, 1994) produced treatment-related changes in the mothers (gingival hypertrophy and increased activity of circulating liver enzymes). Spontaneous delivery at weeks 30–32 in each case was uneventful; evaluation of the children at five to eight months gave no evidence of ophthalmological or neurological abnormalities; growth and development were considered normal (Harrison *et al.*, 1994; Stentoft *et al.*, 1994; Watanabe *et al.*, 1995). Treatment with all-*trans*-retinoic acid at 45 mg/m^2 per day from week 34 through week 38 increased the concentration of 13-*cis*-retinoic acid in cord blood to 0.44 ng/mL and that of its 4-oxo metabolite to 1.3 ng/mL, but neither all-*trans*-retinoic acid nor all-*trans*-4-oxo-retinoic acid was detected. Exposure to all-*trans*-retinoic acid did not induce fetotoxicity, and delivery was uneventful; follow-up at nine months showed no complications (Lipovsky *et al.*, 1996).

Physical and mental development were normal in eight infants born to mothers given all-*trans*-retinoic acid orally at 70 mg/kg bw from week 30 until birth for treatment of acute promyelocytic leukaemia (Maeda *et al.*, 1997).

7.2.2 Experimental models

7.2.2.1 Reproductive effects

In rats given all-*trans*-retinoic acid by dietary supplementation at 0.03–0.75 mg/kg bw per day or by oral intubation at 0.4, 5, 10 or 50 mg/kg bw per day for 12 or 13 weeks, decreased testicular weights were observed, and there was histological evidence of decreased spermatogenesis. Similar results were found in dogs fed all-*trans*-retinoic acid by capsule at a dose of 5 or 50 mg/kg bw per day for 13 weeks (Kamm, 1982).

7.2.2.2 Developmental effects

Numerous studies have shown that embryos of mammalian species are susceptible to the embryotoxic effects of excess all-*trans*-retinoic acid (Table 7) at doses that do not cause overt maternal toxicity (Geelen, 1979; Agnish & Kochhar, 1993). The embryotoxic effects of retinoids can also be induced in other vertebrate classes, such as birds (Tickle *et al.*, 1982), amphibians (Durston *et al.*, 1989) and fish (Holder & Hill, 1991).

Since the initial studies, more than 70 types of anomalies affecting almost every organ system related to excess intake of all-*trans*-retinoic acid have been described in more than 100 reports (Soprano & Soprano, 1995). The anomalies described in mammalian embryos (monkeys, rabbits, rats, mice and hamsters) are microcephaly, holoprosencephaly, spina bifida, encephalocele, exencephaly, hydrocephaly, facial nerve palsy, cranial abnormalities, maxillary hypoplasia, mandibular hypoplasia, cleft palate, cleft lip, micrognathia, absent or deformed ear, exophthalmus, microphthalmus, anophthalmus, coloboma, nasal defects, facial clefting, oesophageal atresia, cardiovascular malformations, hypoplastic aorta, rib fusions, vertebral transformations, omphalocoele, multiple limbs, shortened limbs, ectrodactyly, syndactyly, anal atresia, thymic hypoplasia, amastia and defects of the uterus, testis, kidney, thyroid and pituitary. The important features of the teratogenicity of all-*trans*-retinoic acid are the wide spectrum of its effects on virtually every organ system of the body and the impressive stage-specificity of the induced effects, as described classically by Shenefelt (1972). For example, treatment of mice embryos before implantation (days 4.5–5.5 of gestation) resulted in a bizarre multiple hindlimb phenotype in which the pelvic girdle is

Table 7. Teratogenic effects of all-*trans*-retinoic acid

Species	Dose (mg/kg bw)	Effects	Reference
Mouse	70; GD 12	100% cleft palate; alteration of mesenchyme	Degitz *et al.* (1998)
		Thymic defects, increased expression of *Hoxa 3*	Mulder *et al.* (1998)
Chick embryo	Soaked bead, stage 20	Face and wing patterning; Sonic hedgehog expression	Helms *et al.* (1997)
Cynomolgus monkey	5; GD 16–26 2 x 5; GD 26–31	No teratogenic effects	Tzimas *et al.* (1996)
Rat	20–30; GD 10	Cranial facial defects	Tembe *et al.* (1996)
Rabbit	5–25; GD 10	Cranial facial defects; deformed tail	
NMRI mouse	20 mmol/kg bw GD 11	all-*trans*-Retinyl-β-D-glucuronide more teratogenic than all-*trans*-retinoic acid	Nau *et al.* (1996)
C57BL mouse	7.5; GD 7 1.25; GD 7	Holoprosencephaly, anophthalmia, microphthalmia	Sulik *et al.* (1995)
CD1 mouse	2.5; GD 7	Exencephaly	Sulik *et al.* (1995)
CD1 mouse	20; GD 9	Fused ribs and vertebrae tail; spina bifida increased by stress	Rasco & Hood (1995a,b)
Rat	40; GD 13, 14	Cleft palate	Ikemi *et al.* (1995)
Rat, rabbit	6; GD 12 6; GD 7–12	Decreased concentrations and effects after multiple applications	Collins *et al.* (1995)
Rat	6; GD 6–15	Axial skeletal defects	Collins *et al.* (1994)
Rabbit	6; GD 6–18	Low teratogenic response	Tzimas *et al.* (1994a)
C57BL mouse	28; GD 8 (3 x)	Spina bifida aperta	Alles & Sulik (1990)
Cynomolgus monkey	10; GD 10–20 2 x 10; GD 21–24	Ear defects, mandibular cleft palate	Hendrickx & Hummler (1992)
Rat	10; GD 6–15	Not specified	Kamm (1982)
Rabbit	6; GD 6–18	Not specified	
Mouse	3; GD 6–15	Not specified	
NMRI mouse	10; GD 11	Cleft palate, limb defects	Creech Kraft *et al.* (1989)
C57BL mouse	0–200; GD 10, 12	Cleft palate, synergistically increased by TCDD	Birnbaum *et al.* (1989)
Xenopus embryo	Stage 10; 10^{-5} mol/L	Microcephaly	Durston *et al.* (1989)

GD, gestation day; TCDD, 2,3,7,8-tetrachlordibenzo-*para*-dioxin duplicated (Rutledge *et al.*, 1994; Niederreither *et al.*, 1996). Exposure of postimplantation embryos (days 7–9.5 of gestation) typically results in the craniofacial, central nervous system, ear, cardiovascular and thymus defects listed above; and exposure at later stages of development (days 9.5–12 of gestation) is associated with defects of the limbs, palate and genitourinary tract (Kalter & Warkany, 1961; Shenefelt, 1972; Kistler, 1981; Sulik *et al.*, 1995). Even during the later phase, forelimb defects appear at slightly earlier times of treatment than hindlimb defects.

Studies have also been conducted on the effects of all-*trans*-retinoic acid on the viability and behaviour of offspring. For example, after administration of all-*trans*-retinoic acid on days 8–10, 11–13 and 14–16 of gestation in rats, hyperactivity in the open field and in running wheels was observed at doses > 4 mg/kg bw. Performance in the Morris maze was poorer than in the controls after a dose of 2.5 mg/kg bw on days 11–13. The scores on active avoidance tests were lower after a dose of 6 mg/kg bw. It was concluded that all-*trans*-retinoic acid induced functional defects at doses that did not cause morphological defects (Nolen, 1986).

The pharmacokinetics of all-*trans*-retinoic acid in pregnant animals has been studied extensively, and the findings shed light on the concentrations of this retinoid and its metabolites at the target site that are necessary to induce effects, the critical pharmacokinetics and the reasons for the species similarity in teratogenic responses. all-*trans*-Retinoic acid is rapidly eliminated from the circulation of mice, rats, hamsters, rabbits, monkeys and humans, with apparent half-lives < 3 h (Siegenthaler & Saurat, 1989; Allenby *et al.*, 1993; Fiorella *et al.*, 1993). The authors suggested that the presence of CRABPs in tissues of all species examined to date and their capacity to facilitate the metabolism of all-*trans*-retinoic acid may explain why it is rapidly eliminated. Studies in mice, rats and rabbits revealed that the embryonic concentrations of all-*trans*-retinoic acid and all-*trans*-4-oxoretinoic acid were similarly high or higher than those in plasma after administration of all-*trans*-retinoic acid (Tzimas *et al*, 1994b; Kochhar *et al.*, 1995). Binding of all-*trans*-retinoic acid to embryonic CRABPs or other as yet unidentified retinoid binding proteins in the embryo is likely to contribute to the greater concentrations

in the serum of embryos than dams (Dencker *et al.*, 1987, 1990).

The duration of exposure to retinoids is another major determinant of teratogenic outcome. For example, when 5 mg/kg bw of all-*trans*-retinoic acid were administered orally to rats on gestation day 9, no specific embryotoxicity was seen, whereas subcutaneous treatment induced a high incidence of embryolethality and skeletal anomalies. The AUC but not the C_{max} in maternal plasma correlated with the embryonic outcome (Tzimas *et al.*, 1997). Importantly, teratogenic outcomes in mice are observed at doses (10 mg/kg bw) well below those at which metabolism is saturated (100 mg/kg bw) (Tzimas *et al.*, 1995).

A common characteristic of the pharmacokinetics of all-*trans*-retinoic acid in rats, rabbits and cynomolgus monkeys is a diminution of the plasma concentrations after repeated dosing, although the extent and the time course of this phenomenon vary among species. In pregnant rats given all-*trans*-retinoic acid at a single oral dose of 6 mg/kg bw on day 12 of gestation or the last of six daily doses of 6 mg/kg bw on days 7–12 of gestation, multiple dosing resulted in a pronounced reduction in the exposure to this compound and to all-*trans*-4-oxoretinoic acid, since the plasma AUC values were ninefold and fivefold higher for the two compounds, respectively, after the single than after multiple administrations. In rabbits treated in the same way, the effect on the plasma concentration of all-*trans*-retinoic acid after repeated dosing was also evident, although it was less marked than in rats (Collins *et al.*, 1994). Similar results were found after rats were given all-*trans*-retinoic acid at 17 mg/kg bw three times at 3-h intervals (Tembe *et al.*, 1996) and in rats and rabbits given either a single dose of all-*trans*-retinoic acid on day 12 of gestation or multiple daily doses on days 7–12 (Collins *et al.*, 1995), although the change was smaller in rabbits. The decrease in plasma concentrations after repeated dosing has been attributed to up-regulation of all-*trans*-retinoic acid metabolism and excretion (Adamson *et al.*, 1993).

7.3. Genetic and related effects
7.3.1 Humans
No data were available to the Working Group.

7.3.2 Experimental models

Most of the information on the mutagenicity of all-*trans*-retinoic acid in the *Salmonella*/microsome test was generated in studies of the ability of this compound to modulate the mutagenic activity of known carcinogens (Table 8). The number of tester strains, the range of doses and the use of S9 mix is therefore somewhat incomplete. When the compound was tested at 2 and 4 µmol/plate in *Salmonella* strains TA101 and TA100 without S9 and TA98 with S9, no effect was observed on mutation frequencies (De Flora *et al.*, 1994). Treatment of *S. typhimurium* at doses of 2.5–40 µg/plate had no toxic effect and did not increase the mutation frequencies in TA98, TA100, TA102 and TA1535, with or without the addition of S9; however, the actual data were not shown (Qin & Huang, 1985). All the other studies were restricted to single tester strains. No effect was reported on the spontaneous mutation frequencies of TA104 tested only in the absence of S9 (Han, 1992), and the mutation frequencies in TA100 (Bhattacharya *et al.*, 1987) and TA98 (Wilmer & Spit, 1986; Whong *et al.*, 1988) were unchanged, in all cases tested only in the presence of S9.

In cultured mammalian cells, all-*trans*-retinoic acid did not induce unscheduled DNA synthesis in rat primary hepatocytes (Bhattacharya *et al.*, 1987), It did not alter the spontaneous mutation frequency at the *Hprt* locus in Chinese hamster ovary cells (Budroe *et al.*, 1988) and did not change chromosomal aberration frequencies in Chinese hamster ovary or human embryonic palatal mesenchymal cells (Patel *et al.*, 1998; Watanabe & Pratt, 1991). Although no effect on spontaneous sister chromatid exchange frequency was reported in three studies (Sirianni *et al.*, 1981; Cozzi *et al.*, 1990; Watanabe & Pratt, 1991), two other studies showed an effect. Juhl *et al.* (1978) reported a dose-dependent increase in sister chromatid exchange frequency in human diploid fibroblasts exposed to this retinoid. More recently, Patel *et al.* (1998) reported a statistically significant increase in sister chromatid exchange frequency in Chinese hamster ovary cells, but only after continuous treatment for 20 h and not after exposure for 3 h and only at the highest dose tested (0.8 µg/ml). S9 was used in neither of the latter two studies.

No reports were found of studies of the genotoxicity of all-*trans*-retinoic acid *in vivo*.

8. Summary of Data

8.1 Chemistry, occurrence and human exposure

all-*trans*-Retinoic acid is derived from retinol by oxidation of the C-15 alcohol group to a carboxylic acid. Like all members of the vitamin A family, it is lipophilic, sensitive to light, heat and oxygen and readily isomerized to a mixture of *cis* and *trans* isomers. Because of its acidic nature, it is slightly more soluble in water than retinol or retinal but still poorly so. Because of its conjugated tatraene structure, all-*trans*-retinoic acid has characteristic absorption spectra in the ultraviolet and visible, infrared and resonance Raman portions of the elctromagnetic spectrum.

all-*trans*-Retinoic acid is normally present in blood and tissues of animal species in smaller amounts than retinol and retinyl ester and is essentially absent from plant tissues. Human exposure occurs during topical or oral treatment for medical or cosmetic purposes.

all-*trans*-Retinoic acid has been used to treat dermatological disorders and several forms of cancer. The efficacious doses are 0.5–2 mg/kg of body weight per day when given orally and 0.1% as a cream or gel when administered topically.

all-*trans*-Retinoic acid is usually separated by high-performance liquid chromatography and detected by its absorption at 350 nm. After chemical formation of a suitable ester, it can also be separated and detected by gas–liquid chromatography and can be quantified by mass spectrometry.

8.2 Metabolism and kinetics

The metabolism, kinetics and distribution of all-*trans*-retinoic acid are complex but relatively well understood. It is present in most tissues of healthy animals, albeit at low concentrations. Most of the all-*trans*-retinoic acid in tissues is synthesized *in situ* from all-*trans*-retinol through the actions of two oxidoreductases (dehydrogenases) that catalyse the sequential oxidation of all-*trans*-retinol to all-*trans*-retinal and of all-*trans*-retinal to all-*trans*-retinoic acid. The identities and characteristics of these enzymes have not been established unequivocally. The low concentrations of all-*trans*-retinoic acid present in plasma (4–14 nmol/L) may be taken up by tissues.

Table 8. Genetic and related effects of retinoids in short-term tests *in vitro* and *in vivo*

End-point	Code	Test system	Result[a] Without exogenous metabolic system	With exogenous metabolic system	LED/HID[b]	Reference
G	SA0	TA100, reverse mutation	–	–	40 µg/plate	Qin & Huang (1985)
G	SA0	TA100, reverse mutation	0	+	0.5 µmol/plate	Bhattacharya et al. (1987)
G	SA2	TA102, reverse mutation	–	–	40 µg/plate	Qin & Huang (1985)
G	SA4	TA104, reverse mutation	–	0	10 µmol/plate	Han (1992)
G	SA5	TA1535, reverse mutation	–	–	40 µg/plate	Qin & Huang (1985)
G	SA8	TA98, reverse mutation	–	–	40 µg/plate	Qin & Huang (1985)
G	SA9	TA98, reverse mutation	0	–	500 nmol/plate	Wilmer & Spit (1986
G	SA9	TA98, reverse mutation	0	–	2.6 µmol/plate	Whong et al. (1988)
D	URP	Unscheduled DNA synthesis, rat primary hepatocytes	0	–	50 mmol/L	Budroe et al. (1987)
G	GCO	Gene mutation, Chinese hamster ovary cells, *Hprt* locus	–	–	25 mmol/L (+S9) 100 mmol/L (-S9)	Budroe et al. (1988)
C	CIC	Chromosomal aberrations, Chinese hamster ovary cells *in vitro*	–	0	1.6 mg/ml	Patel et al. (1998)
C	CIH	Chromosomal aberrations, human embryonic palatal mesenchymal cells *in vitro*	–	–	68 mmol/L (-S9) 140 mmol/L (+S9)	Watanabe & Pratt (1991)
S	SIC	Sister chromatid exchange, Chinese hamster ovary cells *in vitro*	(+)	0	0.8 mg/ml	Patel et al. (1988)
S	SIC	[c] Sister chromatid exchange, Chinese hamster epithelial liver cells *in vitro*	–	0	50 µmol/L	Cozzi et al. (1990)
S	SIS	Sister chromatid exchange, Chinese hamster V79 cells *in vitro*	–	0	25 mg/ml	Sirianni et al. (1981)
S	SIH	Sister chromatid exchange, human embryonic palatal mesenchymal cells *in vitro*	–	–	68 µmol/L (–S9) 140 µmol/L (+S9)	Watanabe & Pratt (1991)
S	SHF	[d] Sister chromatid exchange, human fibroblasts *in vitro*	+	0	1 µg/ml	Juhl et al. (1978)

[a] Result: +, positive; (+) weak positive, only one dose showed significant increase; – considered to be negative; 0, not tested
[b] LED, lowest effective dose that inhibits or enhances the investigted effect; HID, highest ineffective dose
[c] Isomer type was all-*trans*-retinoic acid, personal communication from author
[d] Presumed to be all-*trans*-retinoic acid since, exception for Juhl et al., all sources listed as Sigma. 13-*cis*-Retinoic acid listed only in Sigma catalogue from 1988 and 9-*cis*-retinoic acid from 1996. Budroe et al. (1988) probably used the same retinoic acid source as in 1987. The early study by Juhl et al. (1978) probably also involved all-*trans*-retinoic acid.
[d] Type of retinoid used most likely all-*trans*-retinoic acid, but it may have been13-*cis*-retinoic acid since publication date was after 1987.

Pharmacokinetic studies indicate that all-*trans*-retinoic acid is rapidly taken up from the gastrointestinal tract and rapidly cleared from the circulation. Repeated doses of all-*trans*-retinoic acid markedly lower both its maximal concentrations in plasma and the effective concentration in plasma integrated over time, implying that it induces its own catabolism *in vivo*. The recent identification and cloning of an all-*trans*-retinoic acid-inducible cytochrome P450 (CYP26) that catalyses oxidation of this retinoid adds to biochemical understanding of the observation. Although the metabolism of all-*trans*-retinoic acid in human beings and animal models is probably similar biochemically, the metabolite profiles and concentrations differ markedly among species. Although no animal model can be considered truly to reflect the human situation, the metabolite profiles and concentrations in monkeys most closely resemble those seen in humans.

8.3   Cancer-preventive effects
8.3.1   Humans
No studies have been reported of the use of all-*trans*-retinoic acid for the prevention of invasive cancer in humans.

The results of one randomized, controlled trial indicate that topically applied all-*trans*-retinoic acid is effective in reversing moderate dysplasia of the uterine cervix (cervical intra-epithelial neoplasia-II) but not against more severe dysplastic lesions. It was reported to be efficacious against actinic keratosis of the skin in one randomized trial but not in another at a lower dose; the descriptions of the studies were insufficient for detailed evaluation. Two further trials suggest that topically applied all-*trans*-retinoic acid is effective against dysplastic naevi.

8.3.2   Experimental models
The preventive efficacy of all-*trans*-retinoic acid was evaluated in models of skin, liver and mammary gland carcinogenesis. The results of several experiments in mice indicated that all-*trans*-retinoic acid was effective against two-stage skin carcinogenesis when 7,12 dimethylbenz[*a*]-anthracene was used as the initiator, whereas it enhanced skin carcinogenesis induced by this carcinogen alone or with ultraviolet radiation. One study in mice indicated that all-*trans*-retinoic acid

enhanced N-nitrosodiethylamine-induced liver carcinogenesis, but in one study in rats it was ineffective against N-methyl-N-nitrosourea-induced mammary carcinogenesis.

In vitro, all-*trans*-retinoic acid inhibited the transformation of normal cells by carcinogens and of immortalized cells by viral oncogenes. all-*trans*-Retinoic acid inhibited cell proliferation in monolayer cultures and modulated the differentiation of a large number of immortalized, transformed and tumorigenic cell types derived from trachea, skin and cervical epithelia. all-*trans*-Retinoic acid also suppressed the anchorage-independent growth of a variety of tumour cell lines. It suppressed abnormal squamous differentiation in immortalized and transformed cells and re-regulated growth control mechanisms by blocking cells in the G_1 phase of the cell cycle.

The inhibitory effects of all-*trans*-retinoic acid against carcinogen-induced genotoxicity were most often associated with agents that require bioactivation. Studies in animals and humans given topical applications of all-*trans*-retinoic acid have demonstrated alterations in enzymes that mediate carcinogen metabolism. all-*trans*-Retinoic acid can also act as a radical scavenger, suggesting that it acts on initiation by carcinogens. Carcinogen-induced neoplastic transformation *in vitro* was inhibited when all-*trans*-retinoic acid was added after removal of the carcinogen, while most studies in experimental animals in which inhibition of carcinogenesis was demonstrated involved treatment with all-*trans*-retinoic acid after exposure to the carcinogen. Thus, it can act in both the initiation and post-initiation phases of carcinogenesis.

8.3.3   Mechanisms of cancer prevention
Most studies of the effects of all-*trans*-retinoic acid on carcinogenesis indicate that inhibition of the post-initiation stage is the main mechanism of its putative preventive effects. The mechanisms of action may be related to the ability of retinoids to antagonize tumour promotion by *trans*-repressing the activity of AP-1. The ability of all-*trans*-retinoic acid to inhibit cell proliferation is associated with multiple effects on G_1 regulatory proteins which ultimately result in growth arrest in G_0 and G_1. Another possible mechanism is modulation of the autocrine and paracrine loops that mediate

positive and negative growth signals. Restoration of normal differentiation or enhancement of differentiation in cells with aberrant differentiation may contribute to the putative cancer-preventive effects of all-*trans*-retinoic acid. Restoration of controls on growth can also be mediated by enhancement of intercellular gap-junctional communication and suppression of prostaglandin biosynthesis. Induction of apoptosis provides the ultimate means for eradicating abnormal clones of premalignant cells. Enhancement of cell adhesion and inhibition of cell motility affect the invasive step in which carcinoma *in situ* is converted into a malignant tumour. Lastly, inhibition of angiogenesis may block the growth of advanced premalignant lesions and locally invasive malignancies.

8.4 Other beneficial effects

all-*trans*-Retinoic acid has been shown to be of benefit to patients suffering from a variety of dermatological disorders.

8.5 Carcinogenicity

No data were available to the Working Group.

8.6 Other toxic effects

8.6.1 Humans

The toxic effects associated with topical application of all-*trans*-retinoic acid are generally localized, cutaneous and reversible after treatment is discontinued. The most frequent adverse effects include peeling, dry skin, burning, stinging, erythema and pruritus. The reactions are usually of mild to moderate severity, occur early during therapy and recur after an initial decline. Patients using topical all-*trans*-retinoic acid have heightened sensitivity to sunlight and weather extremes, and temporary hyper- or hypopigmentation has been reported. Concentrations of 0.05–0.2% applied on a sponge inserted vaginally in a cervical cap for four days commonly produced vaginal irritation, ulceration and discharge, with no evidence of systemic toxicity.

all-*trans*-Retinoic acid administered orally at 45 mg/m^2 per day (the recommended daily dose) results in drug-related toxicity in virtually all patients with acute promyelocytic leukaemia. The most frequent adverse events are similar to those described in patients taking high doses of vitamin A (headache, fever, skin and mucous membrane

disturbances, bone pain and inflammation, nausea and vomiting, mucositis, pruritus, increased sweating, visual disturbances and alopecia). Transient increases in the concentration of triglycerides and the activity of transaminases are common and can sometimes lead to severe complications such as pancreatitis and hepatotoxicity. Moderate to severe headaches are commonly experienced during oral therapy with all-*trans*-retinoic acid and may limit the dose that can be given. Cases of pseudotumour cerebri, with clinical signs of headache, nausea, double vision and bilateral papilloedema, have been reported. Concern has been raised that all-*trans*-retinoic acid may increase the risk for relapses at unusual sites in patients with acute promyelocytic leukaemia.

One of the most serious reactions to orally administered all-*trans*-retinoic acid is 'retinoic acid syndrome', an acute, life-threatening respiratory disorder experienced by about 25% of patients with acute promyelocytic leukaemia who are being treated with all-*trans*-retinoic acid. The syndrome is characterized by fever, dyspnoea, weight gain, radiographic pulmonary infiltrates and pleural or pericardial effusions and has been observed with and without concomitant leukocytosis. High doses of glucocorticoids given at the first sign of the syndrome appear to reduce the rates of morbidity and mortality, but as much as 60% of patients with acute promyelocytic leukaemia who are taking all-*trans*-retinoic acid orally require such treatment.

No signs of reproductive toxicity were seen in one study in which 12 fertile men were exposed to all-*trans*-retinoic acid for up to 300 days. There were no reports of adverse pregnancy outcomes after oral administration of all-*trans*-retinoic acid to one patient with acute promyelocytic leukaemia during early pregnancy, and no signs of retinoid embryopathy were seen in seven such patients treated with all-*trans*-retinoic acid later in pregnancy; however, there have been no retrospective or prospective follow-up studies of the children of such patients. The available data do not indicate an increased risk for teratogenic effects after dermal application of all-*trans*-retinoic acid.

8.6.2 Experimental models

In mice given all-*trans*-retinoic acid orally, the major dose-related findings included bone rarefaction, bone fracture, elevated serum alkaline phosphatase activity, testicular degeneration, dermal and epidermal inflammation and hyperkeratosis. In rats, decreased plasma albumin and haemoglobin concentrations and increased serum alkaline phosphatase activity were seen.

Few studies of genotoxicity with all-*trans*-retinoic acid *in vitro* are available, and the results of those that have been reported were largely negative. The frequency of sister chromatid exchange was increased in the presence of this retinoid in two studies but not in three others. No reports were available of the effects of all-*trans*-retinoic acid on mutation or chromosomal changes in animals *in vivo*.

all-*trans*-Retinoic acid applied topically at doses of 2–5 mg/kg of body weight per day for 90 days reduced testicular and ovarian weights in mice, with no pathological changes; no such effect was seen in dogs given doses up to 1 mg/kg of body weight per day for 13 weeks. all-*trans*-Retinoic acid was a potent teratogen in all experimental species examined; this finding is compatible with its extensive placental transfer, with consequent exposure of embryos, and its interaction with retinoic acid receptors. The extent of teratogenicity is similar in different mammalian species, reflecting its rate of elimination. The teratogenic effects, which involve nearly every fetal organ system, depend on the route and the time of administration during gestation. In general, administration during early organogenesis results in greater teratogenicity than administration during late organogenesis, partly because of decreasing placental transfer with advancing gestation. Behavioural defects have been observed in rodents exposed to all-*trans*-retinoic acid *in utero*. Topical application results in low bioavailability and little or no teratogenicity.

The extensive placental transfer of all-*trans*-retinoic acid is closely associated with its binding to the abundant embryonic cellular retinoic acid binding proteins. The effective concentration of all-*trans*-retinoic acid in plasma integrated over time that reaches the embryo during the sensitive stages of organogenesis defines the potency of the teratogenic effect. Multiple dosing results in a reduction in the concentration of the drug in maternal and fetal compartments, probably because induction of metabolic enzymes increases 4-oxidation and glucuronidation.

9. Recommendations for Research

9.1 General recommendations for research on all-trans-retinoic acid and other retinoids

The results of studies in which the protocols differed widely or in which proper controls and differences in the baseline conditions were neglected, omitted or inadequately described are difficult to evaluate and compare. Standard protocols are urgently needed to evaluate the cancer-preventive properties of retinoids. Such protocols should specify continuous quality control of supplements and the type of formulation to be used. Such a strategy should be developed for molecular, cellular, experimental animal and human studies, in order to:

• understand the role of nuclear retinoid receptors in cancer chemoprevention;

• develop more relevant models of chemoprevention with efficacious retinoids, including assays based on over-expression of oncogenes and ablation of tumour suppressor genes;

• identify suitable biomarkers that can serve as surrogate outcome measures of invasive cancer in assessing the efficacy of retinoids in chemoprevention trials;

• identify more precisely the structural properties of retinoids that affect their toxicity;

• identify the mechanisms of action by which retinoids effect their characteristic spectrum of toxicity;

• design and develop retinoids with improved therapeutic ratios for cancer chemoprevention;

• understand better the mechanisms by which retinoids target specific tissues;

• understand the factors that determine homeostatic mechanisms for retinoids in cells and whether these regulatory mechanisms are important in cancer chemoprevention;

• understand better the structural properties of retinoids that influence their pharmacokinetics;

- clarify the reasons underlying the loss of retinoid X receptors in the process of cellular transformation; and

- understand the interaction and potential chemopreventive efficacy of retinoids in combination with other drugs.

10. Evaluation

10.1 Cancer-preventive activity
10.1.1 Humans
There is *inadequate evidence* that all-*trans*-retinoic acid has cancer-preventive activity in humans.

10.1.2 Experimental animals
There is *inadequate evidence* that all-*trans*-retinoic acid has cancer-preventive activity in experimental animals.

10.2 Overall evaluation
all-*trans*-Retinoic acid has not been established to have cancer-preventive activity in humans. Therapy with this retinoid gives rise to significant toxic effects, and it is an established teratogen in experimental animals.

11. References

Acevedo, P. & Bertram, J.S. (1995) Liarozole potentiates the cancer chemopreventive activity of and the up-regulation of gap junctional communication and connexin43 expression by retinoic acid and beta-carotene in 10T1/2 cells. *Carcinogenesis*, **16**, 2215–2222

Adamson, P.C., Boylan, J.F., Balis, F.M., Murphy, R.F., Godwin, K.A., Gudas, L.J. & Poplack, D.G. (1993) Time course of induction of metabolism of all-*trans*-retinoic acid and the up-regulation of cellular retinoic acid-binding protein. *Cancer Res.*, **53**, 472–476

Adamson, P.C., Reaman, G., Finklestein, J.Z., Feusner, J., Berg, S.L., Blaney, S.M., O'Brien, M., Murphy, R.F. & Balis, F.M. (1997) Phase I trial and pharmacokinetic study of all-*trans*-retinoic acid administered on an intermittent schedule in combination with interferon-α2a in pediatric patients with refractory cancer. *J. Clin. Oncol.*, **15**, 3330–3337

Agarwal, C., Rorke, E.A., Irwin, J.C. & Eckert, R.L. (1991) Immortalization by human papillomavirus type 16 alters retinoid regulation of human ectocervical epithelial cell differentiation. *Cancer Res.*, **51**, 3982–3989

Agarwal, C., Chandraratna, R.A., Teng, M., Nagpal, S., Rorke, E.A. & Eckert, R.L. (1996) Differential regulation of human ectocervical epithelial cell line proliferation and differentiation by retinoid X receptor- and retinoic acid receptor-specific retinoids. *Cell Growth Differ.*, **7**, 521–530

Agnish, N.D. & Kochhar, D.M. (1993) Developmental toxicity of retinoids. In: Koren G., ed., *Retinoids in Clinical Practice. The Risk–Benefit Ratio*. New York, Marcel Dekker, pp. 47–76

Allenby, G., Bocquel, M.T., Saunders, M., Kazmer, S., Speck, J., Rosenberger, M., Lovey, A., Kastner, P., Grippo, J.F., Chambon, P. & Levin, A.A. (1993) Retinoic acid receptors and retinoid X receptors: Interactions with endogenous retinoic acids. *Proc. Natl Acad. Sci. USA*, **90**, 30–34

Alles, A.J. & Sulik, K.K. (1990) Retinoic acid-induced spina bifida: Evidence for a pathogenetic mechanism. *Development*, **108**, 73–81

Andreatta-Van Leyen, S., Hembree, J.R. & Eckert, R.L. (1994) Regulation of insulin-like growth factor 1 binding protein 3 levels by epidermal growth factor and retinoic acid in cervical epithelial cells. *J. Cell Physiol.*, **160**, 265–274

Anzano, M.A., Byers, S.W., Smith, J.M., Peer, C.W., Mullen, L.T., Brown, C.C., Roberts, A.B. & Sporn, M.B. (1994) Prevention of breast cancer in the rat with 9-*cis*-retinoic acid as a single agent and in combination with tamoxifen. *Cancer Res.*, **54**, 4614–4617

Arky, R. (1998) *Physicians' Desk Reference*. 52nd Ed. Montvale, NJ, Medical Economics Company, pp. 1986–1989, 2154–2155, 2518–2520

Armstrong, R.B., Ashenfelter, K.O., Eckhoff, C., Levin, A.A. & Shapiro, S.S. (1994) General and reproductive toxicology of retinoids. In: Sporn, M.B., Roberts, A.B. & Goodman, D.S., eds, *The Retinoids. Biology, Chemistry, and Medicine*. 2nd Ed. New York, Raven Press, pp. 545–572

Barua, A.B. & Furr, H.C. (1998) Properties of retinoids: Structure, handling, and preparation. In: Redfern, C.P.F., ed., *Retinoid Protocols*. Totowa, NJ, Humana Press, pp. 3–28

Barua, A.B., Furr, H.C., Olson, J.A. & van Breemen, R.B. (1999) Vitamin A and carotenoids. In: DeLeenheer, A., Lambert, W. & van Bocxlaer, J., eds, *Modern Chromatographic Analysis of the Vitamins*, 3rd Ed. New York, Marcel Dekker (in press)

Behbakht, K., DeGeest, K., Turyk, M.E. & Wilbanks, G.D. (1996) All-*trans*-retinoic acid inhibits the proliferation of cell lines derived from human cervical neoplasia. *Gynecol. Oncol.,* **61**, 31–39

Bertram, J.S. (1980) Structure–activity relationships among various retinoids and their ability to inhibit neoplastic transformation and to increase cell adhesion in the C3H/10T1/2 CL8 cell line. *Cancer Res.,* **40**, 3141–3146

Bhattacharya, R.K., Firozi, P.F. & Aboobaker, V.S. (1984) Factors modulating the formation of DNA adduct by aflatoxin B1 in vitro. *Carcinogenesis,* **5**, 1359–1362

Bhattacharya, R.K., Francis, A.R. & Shetty, T.K. (1987) Modifying role of dietary factors on the mutagenicity of aflatoxin B1: In vitro effect of vitamins. *Mutat. Res.,* **188**, 121–128

Birnbaum, L.S., Harris, M.W., Stocking, L.M., Clark, A.M. & Morrissey, R.E. (1989) Retinoic acid and 2,3,7,8-tetrachlorodibenzo-*p*-dioxin selectively enhance teratogenesis in C57BL/6N mice. *Toxicol. Appl. Pharmacol.,* **98**, 487–500

Blaner, W.S. & Olson, J.A. (1994) Retinol and retinoic acid metabolism. In: Sporn, M.B., Roberts, A.B. & Goodman, D.S., eds, *The Retinoids: Biology, Chemistry, and Medicine,* 2nd Ed. New York, Raven Press, pp. 229–255

Bodo, M., Todisco, T., Pezzetti, F., Dottorini, M., Moggi, L. & Becchetti, E. (1989) Ability of retinoic and ascorbic acid to interfere with the binding of benzo(a)pyrene to DNA in explants from donors with bronchial cancer. *Oncology,* **46**, 178–182

Bollag, W. (1974) Therapeutic effects of an aromatic retinoic acid analog on chemically induced skin papillomas and carcinomas of mice. *Eur. J. Cancer,* **10**, 731–737

Boyle, J.O., Langenfeld, J., Lonardo, F., Sekula, D., Reczek, P., Rusch, V., Dawson, M.I. & Dmitrovsky, E. (1999) Cyclin D1 proteolysis: A retinoid chemoprevention signal in normal, immortalized, and transformed human bronchial epithelial cells. *J. Natl Cancer Inst.,* **91**, 373–379

Breitkreutz, D., Stark, H.J., Plein, P., Baur, M. & Fusenig, N.E. (1993) Differential modulation of epidermal keratinization in immortalized (HaCaT) and tumorigenic human skin keratinocytes (HaCaT-ras) by retinoic acid and extracellular Ca²⁺. *Differentiation,* **54**, 201–217

Bseiso, A.W., Kantarjian, H. & Estey, E. (1997) Myelodysplastic syndrome following successful therapy of acute promyelocytic leukemia. *Leukemia,* **11**, 168–169

Buchan, P., Eckhoff, C., Caron, D., Nau, H., Shroot, B. & Schaefer, H. (1994) Repeated topical administration of all-*trans*-retinoic acid and plasma levels of retinoic acids in humans. *J. Am. Acad. Dermatol.,* **30**, 428–434

Budavari, S., O'Neil, M.J., Smith, A., Heckelman, P.E. & Kinneary, J.F. (1996) *The Merck Index. An Encyclopedia of Chemicals, Drugs, and Biologicals,* 12th Ed. Whitehouse Station, NJ, Merck & Co., p. 1404

Budd, G.T., Adamson, P.C., Gupta, M., Homayoun, P., Sandstrom, S.K., Murphy, R.F., McLain, D., Tuason, L., Peereboom, D., Bukowski, R.M. & Ganapathi, R. (1998) Phase I/II trial of all-*trans*-retinoic acid and tamoxifen in patients with advanced breast cancer. *Clin. Cancer Res.,* **4**, 635–642

Budroe, J.D., Shaddock, J.G. & Casciano, D.A. (1987) Modulation of ultraviolet light-, ethyl methanesulfonate-, and 7,12-dimethylbenz[a]anthracene-induced unscheduled DNA synthesis by retinol and retinoic acid in the primary rat hepatocyte. *Environ. Mol. Mutag.,* **10**, 129–139

Budroe, J.D., Schol, H.M., Shaddock, J.G. & Casciano, D.A. (1988) Inhibition of 7,12-dimethylbenz[a]-anthracene-induced genotoxicity in Chinese hamster ovary cells by retinol and retinoic acid. *Carcinogenesis,* **9**, 1307–1311

Caliaro, M.J., Vitaux, P., Lafon, C., Lochon, I., Nehme, A., Valette, A., Canal, P., Bugat, R. & Jozan, S. (1997) Multifactorial mechanism for the potentiation of cisplatin (CDDP) cytotoxicity by all-*trans*-retinoic acid (ATRA) in human ovarian carcinoma cell lines. *Br. J. Cancer,* **75**, 333–340

Camera, G. & Pregliasco, P. (1992) Ear malformation in baby born to mother using tretinoin cream. *Lancet,* **339**, 687–687

Camoirano, A., Balansky, R.M., Bennicelli, C., Izzotti, A., D'Agostini, F. & De Flora, S. (1994) Experimental databases on inhibition of the bacterial mutagenicity of 4-nitroquinoline 1-oxide and cigarette smoke. *Mutat. Res.,* **317**, 89–109

Castaigne, S., Chomienne, C., Daniel, M.T., Ballerini, P., Berger, R., Fenaux, P. & Degos, L. (1990) All-*trans* retinoic acid as a differentiation therapy for acute promyelocytic leukemia. I. Clinical results. *Blood,* **76**, 1704–1709

Chen, L.C., Sly, L. & De Luca, L.M. (1994) High dietary retinoic acid prevents malignant conversion of skin papillomas induced by a two-stage carcinogenesis protocol in female SENCAR mice. *Carcinogenesis,* **15**, 2383–2386

Choo, C.K., Rorke, E.A. & Eckert, R.L. (1995) Retinoid regulation of cell differentiation in a series of human papillomavirus type 16-immortalized human cervical epithelial cell lines. *Carcinogenesis*, **16**, 375–381

Christian, M.S., Mitala, J.J., Powers, W.J.J., McKenzie, B.E. & Latriano, L. (1997) A developmental toxicity study of tretinoin emollient cream (Renova) applied topically to New Zealand white rabbits. *J. Am. Acad. Dermatol.*, **36**, S67–S76

Clairmont, A., Tessmann, D. & Sies, H. (1996) Analysis of connexin43 gene expression induced by retinoic acid in F9 teratocarcinoma cells. *FEBS Lett.*, **397**, 22-24

Clewell, H.J., Andersen, M.E., Wills, R.J. & Latriano, L. (1997) A physiologically based pharmacokinetic model for retinoic acid and its metabolites. *J. Am. Acad. Dermatol.*, **36**, S77–S85

Collins, M.D., Tzimas, G., Hummler, H., Burgin, H. & Nau, H. (1994) Comparative teratology and transplacental pharmacokinetics of all-*trans*-retinoic acid, 13-*cis*-retinoic acid, and retinyl palmitate following daily administrations in rats. *Toxicol. Appl. Pharmacol.*, **127**, 132–144

Collins, M.D., Tzimas, G., Bürgin, H., Hummler, H. & Nau, H. (1995) Single versus multiple dose administration of all-*trans*-retinoic acid during organogenesis: Differential metabolism and transplacental kinetics in rat and rabbit. *Toxicol. Appl. Pharmacol.*, **130**, 9–18

Conley, B.A., Egorin, M.J., Sridhara, R., Finley, R., Hemady, R., Wu, S., Tait, N.S. & Van Echo, D.A. (1997) Phase I clinical trial of all-*trans*-retinoic acid with correlation of its pharmacokinetics and pharmacodynamics. *Cancer Chemother. Pharmacol.*, **39**, 291–299

Connor, M.J., Lowe, N.J., Breeding, J.H. & Chalet, M. (1983) Inhibition of ultraviolet-B skin carcinogenesis by all-*trans*-retinoic acid regimens that inhibit ornithine decarboxylase induction. *Cancer Res.*, **43**, 171–174

Cortes, J., Kantarjian, H., O'Brien, S., Beran, M., Estey, E., Keating, M. & Talpaz, M. (1997) A pilot study of all-*trans*-retinoic acid in patients with Philadelphia chromosome-positive chronic myelogenous leukemia. *Leukemia*, **11**, 929–932

Cozzi, R., Bona, R., Polani, S. & De Salvia, R. (1990) Retinoids as modulators of metabolism: Their inhibitory effect on cyclophosphamide and 7,12-dimethylbenz[*a*]anthracene induced sister chromatid exchanges in a metabolically competent cell line. *Mutagenesis*, **5**, 397–401

Creech Kraft, J. & Juchau, M.R. (1992) Conceptual biotransformation of 4-oxo-all-*trans*-retinoic acid, 4-oxo-13-*cis*-retinoic acid and all-*trans*-retinoyl-β-glucuronide in rat whole embryo culture. *Biochem. Pharmacol.*, **43**, 2289–2292

Creech Kraft, J. & Willhite, C.C. (1997) Retinoids in abnormal and normal embryonic development. In: Kacew, S. & Lambert, G.H., eds, *Environmental Toxicology and Pharmacology of Human Development*. Washington DC, Taylor & Francis, pp. 15–49

Creech Kraft, J., Kochhar, D.M., Scott, W.J. & Nau, H. (1987) Low teratogenicity of 13-*cis*-retinoic acid (isotretinoin) in the mouse corresponds to low embryo concentrations during organogenesis: Comparison to the all-*trans*-isomer. *Toxicol. Appl. Pharmacol.*, **87**, 474–482

Creech Kraft, J., Löfberg, B., Chahoud, I., Bochert, G. & Nau, H. (1989) Teratogenicity and placental transfer of all-*trans*-, 13-*cis*-, 4-oxo-all-*trans*-, and 4-oxo-13-*cis*-retinoic acid after administration of a low oral dose during organogenesis in mice. *Toxicol. Appl. Pharmacol.*, **100**, 162–176

Creech Kraft, J., Slikker, W., Bailey, J.R., Roberts, L.G., Fischer, B., Wittfoht, W. & Nau, H. (1991a) Plasma pharmacokinetics and metabolism of 13-*cis*- and all-*trans*-retinoic acid in the cynomolgus monkey and the identification of 13-*cis*- and all-*trans*-retinoyl-β-glucuronides. A comparison to one human case study with isotretinoin. *Drug Metab. Dispos.*, **19**, 317–324

Creech Kraft, J., Eckhoff, C., Kochhar, D.M., Bochert, G., Chahoud, I. & Nau, H. (1991b) Isotretinoin (13-*cis*-retinoic acid) metabolism, *cis*–*trans* isomerization, glucuronidation, and transfer to the mouse embryo: Consequences for teratogenicity. *Teratog. Carcinog. Mutag.*, **11**, 21–30

Creek, K.E., Geslani, G., Batova, A. & Pirisi, L. (1995) Progressive loss of sensitivity to growth control by retinoic acid and transforming growth factor-beta at late stages of human papillomavirus type 16-initiated transformation of human keratinocytes. *Adv. Exp. Med. Biol.*, **375**, 117–135

Cull, G.M., Eikelboom, J.W. & Cannell, P.K. (1997) Exacerbation of coagulopathy with concurrent bone marrow necrosis, hepatic and renal dysfunction secondary to all-*trans*-retinoic acid therapy for acute promyelocytic leukemia. *Hematol. Oncol.*, **15**, 13–17

Daoud, A.H. & Griffin, A.C. (1978) Effects of selenium and retinoic acid on the metabolism of N-acetylaminofluorene and N-hydroxyacetylaminofluorene. *Cancer Lett.*, **5**, 231–237

Dawson, M.I. & Hobbs, P.D. (1994) The synthetic chemistry of retinoids. In: Sporn, M.B., Roberts, A.B. & Goodman, D.S., eds., *The Retinoids: Biology, Chemistry, and Medicine,* 2nd Ed. New York, Raven Press, pp. 5–178

Dawson, M.I., Chao, W.R. & Helmes, C.T. (1987) Inhibition by retinoids of anthralin-induced mouse epidermal ornithine decarboxylase activity and anthralin-promoted skin tumor formation. *Cancer Res.,* **47,** 6210–6215

De Benedetti, F., Falk, L., Ruscetti, F.W., Colburn, N.H., Faltynek, C.R. & Oppenheim, J.J. (1991) Synergistic inhibition of phorbol ester-induced transformation of JB6 cells by transforming growth factor-β and retinoic acid. *Cancer Res.,* **51,** 1158–1164

De Botton, S., Dombret, H., Sanz, M., San Miguel, J., Caillot, D., Zittoun, R., Gardembas, M., Stamatoulas, A., Condé, E., Guerci, A., Gardin, C., Geiser, K., Cony Makhoul, D., Reman, O., de la Serna, J., Lefrere, F., Chomienne, C., Chastang, C., Degos, L. & Fenaux, P. (1998) Incidence, clinical features, and outcome of all-*trans*-retinoic acid syndrome in 413 cases of newly diagnosed acute promyelocytic leukemia. The European APL Group. *Blood,* **92,** 2712–2718

De Flora, S., Bennicelli, C., Rovida, A., Scatolini, L. & Camoirano, A. (1994) Inhibition of the 'spontaneous' mutagenicity in *Salmonella typhimurium* TA102 and TA104. *Mutat. Res.,* **307,** 157–167

Degitz, S.J., Francis, B.M. & Foley, G.L. (1998) Mesenchymal changes associated with retinoic acid induced cleft palate in CD-1 mice. *J. Craniofac. Genet. Dev. Biol.,* **18,** 88–99

Dencker, L., d'Argy, R., Danielsson, B.R., Ghantous, H. & Sperber, G.O. (1987) Saturable accumulation of retinoic acid in neural and neural crest derived cells in early embryonic development. *Dev. Pharmacol. Ther.,* **10,** 212–223

Dencker, L., Annerwall, E., Busch, C. & Eriksson, U. (1990) Localization of specific retinoid-binding sites and expression of cellular retinoic-acid-binding protein (CRABP) in the early mouse embryo. *Development,* **110,** 343–352

Denning, M.F. & Verma, A.K. (1994) The mechanism of the inhibition of squamous differentiation of rat tracheal 2C5 cells by retinoic acid. *Carcinogenesis,* **15,** 503–507

Duell, E.A., Aström, A., Griffiths, C.E., Chambon, P. & Voorhees, J.J. (1992) Human skin levels of retinoic acid and cytochrome P-450-derived 4-hydroxy-retinoic acid after topical application of retinoic acid

in vivo compared to concentrations required to stimulate retinoic acid receptor-mediated transcription *in vitro. J. Clin. Invest.,* **90,** 1269–1274

Durston, A.J., Timmermans, J.P., Hage, W.J., Hendriks, H.F., de Vries, N.J., Heideveld, M. & Nieuwkoop, P.D. (1989) Retinoic acid causes an antcroposterior transformation in the developing central nervous system. *Nature,* **340,** 140–144

Eckhoff, C. & Nau, H. (1990) Identification and quantitation of all-*trans*- and 13-*cis*-retinoic acid and 13-*cis*-4-oxo-retinoic acid in human plasma. *J. Lipid Res.,* **31,** 1445–1454

Eckhoff, C., Collins, M.D. & Nau, H. (1991) Human plasma all-*trans*-, 13-*cis*- and 13-*cis*-4-oxoretinoic acid profiles during subchronic vitamin A supplementation: Comparison to retinol and retinyl ester plasma levels. *J. Nutr.,* **121,** 1016–1025

Edwards, L. & Jaffe, P. (1990) The effect of topical tretinoin on dysplastic nevi. A preliminary trial. *Arch. Dermatol.,* **126,** 494–499

Englert, G. (1975) A ^{13}C-NMR. Study of *cis–trans* isomeric vitamins A, carotenoids and related compounds. *Helv. Chim. Acta,* **58,** 2367–2390

Evans, G., Grimwade, D., Prentice, H.G. & Simpson, N. (1997) Central nervous system relapse in acute promyelocytic leukaemia in patients treated with all-*trans*-retinoic acid. *Br. J. Haematol.,* **98,** 437–439

Fenaux, P. & De Botton, S. (1998) Retinoic acid syndrome. Recognition, prevention and management. *Drug Saf.,* **18,** 273–279

Fiorella, P.D., Giguère, V. & Napoli, J.L. (1993) Expression of cellular retinoic acid-binding protein (type II) in *Escherichia coli.* Characterization and comparison to cellular retinoic acid-binding protein (type I). *J. Biol. Chem.,* **268,** 21545–21552

Firozi, P.F., Aboobaker, V.S. & Bhattacharya, R.K. (1987) Action of vitamin A on DNA adduct formation by aflatoxin B_1 in a microsome catalyzed reaction. *Cancer Lett.,* **34,** 213–220

Fischer, S.M., Klein-Szanto, A.J., Adams, L.M. & Slaga, T.J. (1985) The first stage and complete promoting activity of retinoic acid but not the analog RO-10-9359. *Carcinogenesis,* **6,** 575–578

Fitzgerald, D.J., Barrett, J.C. & Nettesheim, P. (1986) Changing responsiveness to all-*trans*-retinoic acid of rat tracheal epithelial cells at different stages of neoplastic transformation. *Carcinogenesis,* **7,** 1715–1721

Forbes, P.D., Urbach, F. & Davies, R.E. (1979) Enhancement of experimental photocarcinogenesis by topical retinoic acid. *Cancer Lett.,* **7,** 85–90

Frickel, F. (1984) Chemistry and physical properties of retinoids. In: Sporn, M.B., Roberts, A.B. & Goodman, D.S., eds, *The Retinoids*. Orlando FL, Academic Press, pp. 7–145

Frolik, C.A. & Olson, J.A. (1984) Extraction, separation, and chemical analysis of retinoids. In: Sporn M.B., Roberts A.B. & Goodman, D.S., eds, *The Retinoids*. New York, Academic Press, pp. 181–233

Fullerton, A. & Serup, J. (1997) Characterization of irritant patch test reactions to topical D vitamins and all-*trans*-retinoic acid in comparison with sodium lauryl sulphate. Evaluation by clinical scoring and multiparametric non-invasive measuring techniques. *Br. J. Dermatol.*, **137**, 234–240

Furr, H.C., Barua, A.B. & Olson, J.A. (1992) Retinoids and carotenoids. In: De Leenheer A.P., Lambert W.E. & Nelis, H.J., Eds. *Modern Chromatographic Analysis of Vitamins*, 2nd Ed. New York, Marcel Dekker Inc., pp. 1–71

Furr, H.C., Barua, A.B. & Olson, J.A. (1994) Analytical methods. In: Sporn M.B., Roberts, A.B. & Goodman, D.S., eds, *The Retinoids: Biology, Chemistry, and Medicine*, 2nd ed. New York, Raven Press, pp. 179–209

Geelen, J.A. (1979) Hypervitaminosis A induced teratogenesis. *CRC Crit. Rev. Toxicol.*, **6**, 351–375

Graham, V., Surwit, E.S., Weiner, S. & Meyskens, F.L., Jr (1986) Phase II trial of β-all-*trans*-retinoic acid for cervical intraepithelial neoplasia delivered via a collagen sponge and cervical cap. *West.J. Med.*, **145**, 192–195

Grandis, J.R., Zeng, Q. & Tweardy, D.J. (1996) Retinoic acid normalizes the increased gene transcription rate of TGF-α and EGFR in head and neck cancer cell lines. *Nat. Med.*, **2**, 237–240

Gudas, L.J., Sporn, M.B. & Roberts, A.B. (1994) Cellular biology and biochemistry of the retinoids. In: Sporn M.B., Roberts, A.B. & Goodman, D.S., eds, *The Retinoids*. New York, Raven Press, pp. 443–520

Gunning, D.B., Barua, A.B. & Olson, J.A. (1993) Comparative teratogenicity and metabolism of all-*trans*-retinoic acid, all-*trans*-retinoyl β-glucose, and all-*trans*-retinoyl β-glucuronide in pregnant Sprague-Dawley rats. *Teratology*, **47**, 29–36

Guo, H., Acevedo, P., Parsa, F.D. & Bertram, J.S. (1992) Gap-junctional protein connexin 43 is expressed in dermis and epidermis of human skin: Differential modulation by retinoids. *J. Invest. Dermatol.*, **99**, 460–467

Guzman, K., Bader, T. & Nettesheim, P. (1996) Regulation of MUC5 and MUC1 gene expression: Correlation with airway mucous differentiation. *Am. J. Physiol.*, **270**, L846–L853

Halpern, A.C., Schuchter, L.M., Elder, D.E., Guerry, D., Elenitsas, R., Trock, B. & Matozzo, I. (1994) Effects of topical tretinoin on dysplastic nevi. *J. Clin. Oncol.*, **12**, 1028–1035

Han, J.S. (1992) Effects of various chemical compounds on spontaneous and hydrogen peroxide-induced reversion in strain TA104 of *Salmonella typhimurium*. *Mutat. Res.*, **266**, 77–84

Harrison, P., Chipping, P. & Fothergill, G.A. (1994) Successful use of all-*trans*-retinoic acid in acute promyelocytic leukaemia presenting during the second trimester of pregnancy. *Br. J. Haematol.*, **86**, 681–682

Hatake, K., Uwai, M., Ohtsuki, T., Tomizuka, H., Izumi, T., Yoshida, M. & Miura, Y. (1997) Rare but important adverse effects of all-*trans*-retinoic acid in acute promyelocytic leukemia and their management. *Int. J. Hematol.*, **66**, 13–19

Helms, J.A., Kim, C.H., Hu, D., Minkoff, R., Thaller, C. & Eichele, G. (1997) Sonic hedgehog participates in craniofacial morphogenesis and is down-regulated by teratogenic doses of retinoic acid. *Dev. Biol.*, **187**, 25–35

Hendrickx, A.G. & Hummler, H. (1992) Teratogenicity of all-*trans*-retinoic acid during early embryonic development in the cynomolgus monkey (*Macaca fascicularis*). *Teratology*, **45**, 65–74

Hennings, H., Robinson, V.A., Michael, D.M., Pettit, G.R., Jung, R. & Yuspa, S.H. (1990) Development of an *in vitro* analogue of initiated mouse epidermis to study tumor promoters and antipromoters. *Cancer Res.*, **50**, 4794–4800

Hill, E.M., Bader, T., Nettesheim, P. & Eling, T.E. (1996) Retinoid-induced differentiation regulates prostaglandin H synthase and cPLA2 expression in tracheal epithelium. *Am. J. Physiol.*, **270**, L854–L862

Holder, N. & Hill, J. (1991) Retinoic acid modifies development of the midbrain–hindbrain border and affects cranial ganglion formation in zebrafish embryos. *Development*, **113**, 1159–1170

Hong, W.K. & Itri, L.M. (1994) Retinoids and human cancer. In: Sporn, M.B., Roberts, A.B. & Goodman, D.S., eds, *The Retinoids: Biology, Chemistry, and Medicine*, 2nd Ed. New York, Raven Press, pp. 597–630

Hossain, M.Z. & Bertram, J.S. (1994) Retinoids suppress proliferation, induce cell spreading, and up-regulate connexin43 expression only in postconfluent 10T1/2 cells: Implications for the role of gap junctional communication. *Cell Growth Differ.*, **5**, 1253–1261

Hossain, M.Z., Wilkens, L.R., Mehta, P.P., Loewenstein, W. & Bertram, J.S. (1989) Enhancement of gap junctional communication by retinoids correlates with their ability to inhibit neoplastic transformation. *Carcinogenesis*, **10**, 1743–1748

Howell, S.R., Shirley, M.A. & Ulm, E.H. (1998) Effects of retinoid treatment of rats on hepatic microsomal metabolism and cytochromes P450. Correlation between retinoic acid receptor/retinoid X receptor selectivity and effects on metabolic enzymes. *Drug Metab. Dispos.*, **26**, 234–239

Huang, C., Ma, W.Y., Dawson, M.I., Rincon, M., Flavell, R.A. & Dong, Z. (1997) Blocking activator protein-1 activity, but not activating retinoic acid response element, is required for the antitumor promotion effect of retinoic acid. *Proc. Natl Acad. Sci. USA*, **94**, 5826–5830

IARC (1998) *IARC Handbooks of Cancer Prevention*, Vol. 3, *Vitamin A*, Lyon, International Agency for Research on Cancer, pp. 167–170

Ikemi, N., Kawata, M. & Yasuda, M. (1995) All-*trans*-retinoic acid-induced variant patterns of palatal rugae in Crj:SD rat fetuses and their potential as indicators for teratogenicity. *Reprod. Toxicol.*, **9**, 369–377

Jensen, B.K., McGann, L.A., Kachevsky, V. & Franz, T.J. (1991) The negligible systemic availability of retinoids with multiple and excessive topical application of isotretinoin 0.05% gel (Isotrex) in patients with acne vulgaris. *J. Am. Acad. Dermatol.*, **24**, 425–428

Jetten, A.M. & Shirley, J.E. (1985) Retinoids antagonize the induction of ornithine decarboxylase activity by phorbol esters and phospholipase C in rat tracheal epithelial cells. *J. Cell Physiol.*, **123**, 386–394

Jick, S.S., Terris, B.Z. & Jick, H. (1993) First trimester topical tretinoin and congenital disorders. *Lancet*, **341**, 1181–1182

Johnson, E.M. (1997) A risk assessment of topical tretinoin as a potential human developmental toxin based on animal and comparative human data. *J. Am. Acad. Dermatol.*, **36**, S86–S90

Joiakim, A.P. & Chopra, D.P. (1993) Retinoic acid and calcium regulation of p53, transforming growth factor-β1, and transforming growth factor-α gene expression and growth in adenovirus 12-SV40-transformed human tracheal gland epithelial cells. *Am. J. Respir. Cell. Mol. Biol.*, **8**, 408–416

Juhl, H.J., Schürer, C.C., Bartram, C.R., Kohl, F.V., Melderis, H., von-Wichert, P. & Rüdiger, H.W. (1978) Retinoids induce sister-chromatid exchanges in human diploid fibroblasts. *Mutat. Res.*, **58**, 317–320

Jurima-Romet, M., Neigh, S. & Casley, W.L. (1997) Induction of cytochrome P450 3A by retinoids in rat hepatocyte culture. *Hum. Exp. Toxicol.*, **16**, 198–203

Kaartinen, L., Nettesheim, P., Adler, K.B. & Randell, S.H. (1993) Rat tracheal epithelial cell differentiation in vitro. *In Vitro Cell Dev. Biol. Anim.*, **29A**, 481–492

Kalin, J.R., Wells, M.J. & Hill, D.L. (1984) Effects of phenobarbital, 3-methylcholanthrene, and retinoid pretreatment on disposition of orally administered retinoids in mice. *Drug Metab. Dispos.*, **12**, 63–67

Kalter, H. & Warkany, J. (1961) Experimental production of congenital anomalies in strains of inbred mice by maternal treatment with hypervitaminosis A. *Am. J. Pathol.*, **38**, 1–15

Kamm, J.J. (1982) Toxicology, carcinogenicity, and teratogenicity of some orally administered retinoids. *J. Am. Acad. Dermatol.*, **6**, 652–659

Kamm, J.J., Ashenfelter, K.O. & Ehmann, C.W. (1984) Preclinical and clinical toxicology of selected retinoids. In: Sporn, M.B., Roberts, A.B. & Goodman, D.S., eds, *The Retinoids*. Orlando, FL, Academic Press, Inc., pp. 287–326

Kentos, A., Le Moine, F., Crenier, L., Capel, P., Meyer, S., Muus, P., Mandelli, F. & Feremans, W. (1997) All-*trans*-retinoic acid induced thrombocytosis in a patient with acute promyelocytic leukaemia. *Br. J. Haematol.*, **97**, 685-685

Khan, M.A., Jenkins, G.R., Tolleson, W.H., Creek, K.E. & Pirisi, L. (1993) Retinoic acid inhibition of human papillomavirus type 16-mediated transformation of human keratinocytes. *Cancer Res.*, **53**, 905–909

Kim, Y.H., Dohi, D.F., Han, G.R., Zou, C.P., Oridate, N., Walsh, G.L., Nesbitt, J.C., Xu, X.C., Hong, W.K., Lotan, R. & Kurie, J.M. (1995) Retinoid refractoriness occurs during lung carcinogenesis despite functional retinoid receptors. *Cancer Res.*, **55**, 5603–5610

Kistler, A. (1981) Teratogenesis of retinoic acid in rats: Susceptible stages and suppression of retinoic acid-induced limb malformations by cycloheximide. *Teratology*, **23**, 25–31

Klein-Szanto, A.J., Iizasa, T., Momiki, S., Garcia, P., I, Caamano, J., Metcalf, R., Welsh, J. & Harris, C.C. (1992) A tobacco-specific N-nitrosamine or cigarette smoke condensate causes neoplastic transformation of xenotransplanted human bronchial epithelial cells. *Proc. Natl Acad. Sci. USA*, **89**, 6693-6697

Kligman, A.M. & Thorne, E.G. (1991) Topical therapy of actinic keratoses with tretinoin. In: Marks, R., ed., *Retinoids in Cutaneous Malignancy*. Oxford Blackwell Scientific, pp. 66–73

Kochhar, D.M., Jiang, H., Penner, J.D. & Heyman, R.A. (1995) Placental transfer and developmental effects of 9-*cis* retinoic acid in mice. *Teratology*, **51**, 257–265

Koo, J.S., Yoon, J.H., Gray, T., Norford, D., Jetten, A.M. & Nettesheim, P. (1999a) Restoration of the mucous phenotype by retinoic acid in retinoid-deficient human bronchial cell cultures: Changes in mucin gene expression. *Am. J. Respir. Cell. Mol. Biol.,* **20**, 43–52

Koo, J.S., Jetten, A.M., Belloni, P., Yoon, J.H., Kim, Y.D. & Nettesheim, P. (1999b) Role of retinoid receptors in the regulation of mucin gene expression by retinoic acid in human tracheobronchial epithelial cells. *Biochem. J.,* **338**, 351–357

Langenfeld, J., Lonardo, F., Kiyokawa, H., Passalaris, T., Ahn, M.J., Rusch, V. & Dmitrovsky, E. (1996) Inhibited transformation of immortalized human bronchial epithelial cells by retinoic acid is linked to cyclin E down-regulation. *Oncogene,* **13**, 1983–1990

Langenfeld, J., Kiyokawa, H., Sekula, D., Boyle, J. & Dmitrovsky, E. (1997) Posttranslational regulation of cyclin D1 by retinoic acid: A chemoprevention mechanism. *Proc. Natl Acad. Sci. USA,* **94**, 12070–12074

Latriano, L., Tzimas, G., Wong, F. & Wills, R.J. (1997) The percutaneous absorption of topically applied tretinoin and its effect on endogenous concentrations of tretinoin and its metabolites after single doses or long-term use. *J. Am. Acad. Dermatol.,* **36**, S37–S46

Lee, H.Y., Dawson, M.I., Claret, F.X., Chen, J.D., Walsh, G.L., Hong, W.K. & Kurie, J.M. (1997) Evidence of a retinoid signaling alteration involving the activator protein 1 complex in tumorigenic human bronchial epithelial cells and non-small cell lung cancer cells. *Cell Growth Differ.,* **8**, 283–291

Lemez, P. (1995) Hypercalcaemia caused by all-*trans*-retinoic acid (ATRA) treatment in a case of acute promyelocytic leukaemia was manageable after decreasing the ATRA dose to 27 mg/m²/day. *Eur. J. Haematol.,* **55**, 275–276

Leyden, J.J. (1998) Topical treatment of acne vulgaris: Retinoids and cutaneous irritation. *J. Am. Acad. Dermatol.,* **38**, S1–S4

Li, X.Y., Aström, A., Duell, E.A., Qin, L., Griffiths, C.E. & Voorhees, J.J. (1995) Retinoic acid antagonizes basal as well as coal tar and glucocorticoid-induced cytochrome P4501A1 expression in human skin. *Carcinogenesis,* **16**, 519–524

Li, J.J., Dong, Z., Dawson, M.I. & Colburn, N.H. (1996) Inhibition of tumor promoter-induced transformation by retinoids that transrepress AP-1 without transactivating retinoic acid response element. *Cancer Res.,* **56**, 483–489

Lin, C.P., Huang, M.J., Liu, H.J., Chang, I.Y. & Tsai, C.H. (1996) Successful treatment of acute promyelocytic leukemia in a pregnant Jehovah's Witness with all-*trans*-retinoic acid, rhG-CSF, and erythropoietin. *Am. J. Hematol.,* **51**, 251–252

Lingen, M.W., Polverini, P.J. & Bouck, N.P. (1996) Retinoic acid induces cells cultured from oral squamous cell carcinomas to become anti-angiogenic. *Am. J. Pathol.,* **149**, 247–258

Lipovsky, M.M., Biesma, D.H., Christiaens, G.C. & Petersen, E.J. (1996) Successful treatment of acute promyelocytic leukaemia with all-*trans*-retinoic-acid during late pregnancy. *Br. J. Haematol.,* **94**, 699–701

Lipson, A.H., Collins, F. & Webster, W.S. (1993) Multiple congenital defects associated with maternal use of topical tretinoin. *Lancet,* **341**, 1352–1353

Liu, M., Iavarone, A. & Freedman, L.P. (1996) Transcriptional activation of the human p21[WAF1/CIP1] gene by retinoic acid receptor. Correlation with retinoid induction of U937 cell differentiation. *J. Biol. Chem.,* **271**, 31723–31728

Lotan, R. (1993) Retinoids and squamous cell differentiation. In: Hong, W.K. & Lotan, R., eds, *Retinoids in Oncology.* New York, Marcel Dekker Inc., pp. 43–72

Lotan, R. (1995) Cellular biology of the retinoids. In: Degos, L. & Parkinson, D.R., eds, *Retinoids in Oncology.* Berlin, Springer Verlag, pp. 27–42

Lotan, R., Amos, B., Watanabe, H. & Raz, A. (1992) Suppression of melanoma cell motility factor receptor expression by retinoic acid. *Cancer Res.,* **52**, 4878–4884

Maeda, M., Tyugu, H., Okubo, T., Yamamoto, M., Nakamura, K. & Dan, K. (1997) A neonate born to a mother with acute promyelocytic leukemia treated by all-*trans*-retinoic acid. *Jpn. J. Clin. Hematol.,* **38**, 770–775

Mao, Y., Gurr, J.A. & Hickok, N.J. (1993) Retinoic acid regulates ornithine decarboxylase gene expression at the transcriptional level. *Biochem. J.,* **295**, 641–644

Marnett, L.J. & Ji, C. (1994) Modulation of oxidant formation in mouse skin *in vivo* by tumor-promoting phorbol esters. *Cancer Res.,* **54**, 1886s–1889s

Maron, D.M. & Ames, B.N. (1983) Revised methods for the *Salmonella* mutagenicity test. *Mutat. Res.,* **113**, 173–215

Massaro, G.D. & Massaro, D. (1997) Retinoic acid treatment abrogates elastase-induced pulmonary emphysema in rats. *Nat. Med.,* **3**, 675–677

McCormick, D.L., Bagg, B.J. & Hultin, T.A. (1987) Comparative activity of dietary or topical exposure to three retinoids in the promotion of skin tumor induction in mice. *Cancer Res.*, **47**, 5989–5993

McCormick, D.L., Hollister, J.L., Bagg, B.J. & Long, R.E. (1990) Enhancement of murine hepatocarcinogenesis by all-*trans*-retinoic acid and two synthetic retinamides. *Carcinogenesis*, **11**, 1605–1609

McPhillips, D.M., Kalin, J.R. & Hill, D.L. (1987) The pharmacokinetics of all-*trans*-retinoic acid and *N*-(2-hydroxyethyl)retinamide in mice as determined with a sensitive and convenient procedure. Solid-phase extraction and reverse-phase high performance liquid chromatography. *Drug Metab. Dispos.*, **15**, 207–211

Mehta, P.P., Bertram, J.S. & Loewenstein, W.R. (1989) The actions of retinoids on cellular growth correlate with their actions on gap junctional communication. *J. Cell. Biol.*, **108**, 1053–1065

Melino, G., Draoui, M., Bellincampi, L., Bernassola, F., Bernardini, S., Piacentini, M., Reichert, U. & Cohen, P. (1997) Retinoic acid receptors alpha and gamma mediate the induction of 'tissue' transglutaminase activity and apoptosis in human neuroblastoma cells. *Exp. Cell Res.*, **235**, 55-61

Merrick, D.T., Gown, A.M., Halbert, C.L., Blanton, R.A. & McDougall, J.K. (1993) Human papillomavirus-immortalized keratinocytes are resistant to the effects of retinoic acid on terminal differentiation. *Cell Growth Differ.*, **4**, 831–840

Mestre, J.R., Subbaramaiah, K., Sacks, P.G., Schantz, S.P., Tanabe, T., Inoue, H. & Dannenberg, A.J. (1997) Retinoids suppress phorbol ester-mediated induction of cyclooxygenase-2. *Cancer Res.*, **57**, 1081–1085

Meyskens, F.L., Jr, Graham, V., Chvapil, M., Dorr, R.T., Alberts, D.S. & Surwit, E.A. (1983) A phase I trial of β-all-*trans*-retinoic acid delivered via a collagen sponge and a cervical cap for mild or moderate intraepithelial cervical neoplasia. *J. Natl Cancer Inst.*, **71**, 921–925

Meyskens, F.L., Jr, Surwit, E., Moon, T.E., Childers, J.M., Davis, J.R., Dorr, R.T., Johnson, C.S. & Alberts, D.S. (1994) Enhancement of regression of cervical intraepithelial neoplasia II (moderate dysplasia) with topically applied all-*trans*-retinoic acid: A randomized trial. *J. Natl Cancer Inst.*, **86**, 539–543

Moghal, N. & Neel, B.G. (1998) Integration of growth factor, extracellular matrix, and retinoid signals during bronchial epithelial cell differentiation. *Mol. Cell. Biol.*, **18**, 6666–6678

Monczak, Y., Trudel, M., Lamph, W.W. & Miller, W.H.J. (1997) Induction of apoptosis without differentiation by retinoic acid in PLB-985 cells requires the activation of both RAR and RXR. *Blood*, **90**, 3345–3355

Morton, J., Taylor, K., Wright, S., Pitcher, L., Wilson, E., Tudehope, D., Savage, J., Williams, B., Taylor, D., Wiley, J., Tsoris, D. & O'Donnell, A. (1995) Successful maternal and fetal outcome following the use of ATRA for the induction of APML late in the first trimester. *Blood*, **86** (Suppl. 1), 772a–772a

Muindi, J.R., Frankel, S.R., Huselton, C., DeGrazia, F., Garland, W.A., Young, C.W. & Warrell, R.P, Jr (1992) Clinical pharmacology of oral all-*trans*-retinoic acid in patients with acute promyelocytic leukemia. *Cancer Res.*, **52**, 2138–2142

Mulder, G.B., Manley, N. & Maggio-Price, L. (1998) Retinoic acid-induced thymic abnormalities in the mouse are associated with altered pharyngeal morphology, thymocyte maturation defects, and altered expression of Hoxa3 and Pax1. *Teratology*, **58**, 263–275

Nagy, L., Thomazy, V.A., Shipley, G.L., Fesus, L., Lamph, W., Heyman, R.A., Chandraratna, R.A. & Davies, P.J. (1995) Activation of retinoid X receptors induces apoptosis in HL-60 cell lines. *Mol. Cell. Biol.*, **15**, 3540–3551

Napoli, J.L. (1994) Retinoic acid homeostatis. Prospective roles of β-carotene, retinol, CRBP and CRABP. In: Blomhoff, R., ed., *Vitamin A in Health and Disease*. New York, Marcel Dekker, pp. 135–188

Nau, H. (1993) Embryotoxicity and teratogenicity of topical retinoic acid. *Skin Pharmacol.*, **6** (Suppl. 1), 35–44

Nau, H., Elmazar, M.M., Ruhl, R., Thiel, R. & Sass, J.O. (1996) All-*trans*-retinoyl-β-glucuronide is a potent teratogen in the mouse because of extensive metabolism to all-*trans*-retinoic acid. *Teratology*, **54**, 150–156

Nettesheim, P., Fitzgerald, D.J., Kitamura, H., Walker, C.L., Gilmer, T.M., Barrett, J.C. & Gray, T.E. (1987) *In vitro* analysis of multistage carcinogenesis. *Environ. Health Perspect.*, **75**, 71–79

Newton, D.L., Henderson, W.R. & Sporn, M.B. (1980) Structure–activity relationships of retinoids in hamster tracheal organ culture. *Cancer Res.*, **40**, 3413–3425

Nicholson, R.C., Mader, S., Nagpal, S., Leid, M., Rochette-Egly, C. & Chambon, P. (1990) Negative regulation of the rat stromelysin gene promoter by retinoic acid is mediated by an AP1 binding site. *EMBO J.*, **9**, 4443–4454

Nicolls, M.R., Terada, L.S., Tuder, R.M., Prindiville, S.A. & Schwarz, M.I. (1998) Diffuse alveolar hemorrhage with underlying pulmonary capillaritis in the retinoic acid syndrome. *Am. J. Respir. Crit. Care Med.*, **158**, 1302–1305

Niederreither, K., Ward, S.J., Dolle, P. & Chambon, P. (1996) Morphological and molecular characterization of retinoic acid-induced limb duplications in mice. *Dev. Biol.*, **176**, 185–198

Nolen, G.A. (1986) The effects of prenatal retinoic acid on the viability and behavior of the offspring. *Neurobehav. Toxicol. Teratol.,* **8**, 643–654

Okai, Y., Higashi-Okai, K., Nakamura, S., Yano, Y. & Otani, S. (1996) Suppressive effects of retinoids, carotenoids and antioxidant vitamins on heterocyclic amine-induced *umu* C gene expression in *Salmonella typhimurium* (TA 1535/pSK 1002). *Mutat. Res.,* **368**, 133–140

Olsen, E.A., Katz, H.I., Levine, N., Nigra, T.P., Pochi, P.E., Savin, R.C., Shupack, J., Weinstein, G.D., Lufrano, L. & Perry, B.H. (1997) Tretinoin emollient cream for photodamaged skin: Results of 48-week, multicenter, double-blind studies. *J. Am. Acad. Dermatol.,* **37**, 217–226

Patel, I.H., Khoo, K.C. & Colburn, W.A. (1982) Pharmacokinetics of tretinoin and its in vivo isomeric conversion to isotretinoin in the dog. *Drug Metab. Dispos.,* **10**, 387–390

Patel, R.K., Trivedi, A.H., Jaju, R.J., Kukreti, M.S., Bhatavdekar, J.M., Shah, P.M. & Patel, D.D. (1998) Protection from pan masala induced genomic damage by beta-carotene and retinoic acid—An in vitro experience. *Neoplasma,* **45**, 169–175

Paydas, S., Sahin, B., Zorludemir, S. & Hazar, B. (1998) All *trans*-retinoic acid as the possible cause of necrotizing vasculitis. *Leuk. Res.,* **22**, 655–657

Peck, G.L. & DiGiovanna, J.J. (1994) Synthetic retinoids in dermatology. In: Sporn, M.B., Roberts, A.B. & Goodman, D.S., eds, *The Retinoids: Biology, Chemistry, and Medicine,* 2nd Ed. New York, Raven Press, pp. 631–658

Pirisi, L., Batova, A., Jenkins, G.R., Hodam, J.R. & Creek, K.E. (1992) Increased sensitivity of human keratinocytes immortalized by human papillomavirus type 16 DNA to growth control by retinoids. *Cancer Res.,* **52**, 187–193

Plewig, G., Schill, W.B. & Hofmann, C. (1979) Oral treatment with tretinoin: Andrological, trichological, ophthalmological findings and effects on acne. *Arch. Dermatol. Res.,* **265**, 37–47

Pogliani, E.M., Rossini, F., Casaroli, I., Maffe, P. & Corneo, G. (1997) Thrombotic complications in acute promyelocytic leukemia during all-*trans*-retinoic acid therapy. *Acta Haematol.,* **97**, 228–230

Qin, S. & Huang, C.C. (1985) Effect of retinoids on carcinogen-induced mutagenesis in Salmonella tester strains. *Mutat. Res.,* **142**, 115–120

Raina, V. & Gurtoo, H.L. (1985) Effects of vitamins A, C, and E on aflatoxin B1-induced mutagenesis in *Salmonella typhimurium* TA-98 and TA-100. *Teratog. Carcinog. Mutag.,* **5**, 29–40

Rasco, J.F. & Hood, R.D. (1995a) Maternal restraint stress-enhanced teratogenicity of all-*trans*-retinoic acid in CD-1 mice. *Teratology,* **51**, 57–62

Rasco, J.F. & Hood, R.D. (1995b) Enhancement of the teratogenicity of all-*trans*-retinoic acid by maternal restraint stress in mice as a function of treatment timing. *Teratology,* **51**, 63–70

Reddel, R.R., Ke, Y., Gerwin, B.I., McMenamin, M.G., Lechner, J.F., Su, R.T., Brash, D.E., Park, J.B., Rhim, J.S. & Harris, C.C. (1988) Transformation of human bronchial epithelial cells by infection with SV40 or adenovirus-12 SV40 hybrid virus, or transfection via strontium phosphate coprecipitation with a plasmid containing SV40 early region genes. *Cancer Res.,* **48**, 1904–1909

Rigas, J.R., Miller, V.A., Zhang, Z.F., Klimstra, D.S., Tong, W.P., Kris, M.G. & Warrell, R.P. (1996) Metabolic phenotypes of retinoic acid and the risk of lung cancer. *Cancer Res.,* **56**, 2692-2696

Rogers, M., Berestecky, J.M., Hossain, M.Z., Guo, H.M., Kadle, R., Nicholson, B.J. & Bertram, J.S. (1990) Retinoid-enhanced gap junctional communication is achieved by increased levels of connexin 43 mRNA and protein. *Mol. Carcinog.,* **3**, 335–343

Rook, A.H., Jaworsky, C., Nguyen, T., Grossman, R.A., Wolfe, J.T., Witmer, W.K. & Kligman, A.M. (1995) Beneficial effect of low-dose systemic retinoid in combination with topical tretinoin for the treatment and prophylaxis of premalignant and malignant skin lesions in renal transplant recipients. *Transplantation,* **59**, 714–719

Rosa, F.W. (1992) Retinoid embryopathy in humans. In: Koren, G., ed., *Retinoids in Clinical Practice. The Risk–Benefit Ratio.* New York, Marcel Dekker, pp. 77–109

Russo, D., Regazzi, M., Sacchi, S., Visani, G., Lazzarino, M., Avvisati, G., Pelicci, P.G., Dastoli, G., Grandi, C., Iacona, I., Candoni, A., Grattoni, R., Galieni, P., Rupoli, S., Liberati, A.M. & Maiolo, A.T. (1998) All-*trans*-retinoic acid (ATRA) in patients with chronic myeloid leukemia in the chronic phase. *Leukemia,* **12**, 449–454

Rutledge, J.C., Shourbaji, A.G., Hughes, L.A., Polifka, J.E., Cruz, Y.P., Bishop, J.B. & Generoso, W.M. (1994) Limb and lower-body duplications induced by retinoic acid in mice. *Proc. Natl Acad. Sci. USA,* **91**, 5436–5440

Sano, F., Tsuji, K., Kunika, N., Takeuchi, T., Oyama, K., Hasegawa, S., Koike, M., Takahashi, M. & Ishida, M. (1998) Pseudotumor cerebri in a patient with acute promyelocytic leukemia during treatment with all-*trans*-retinoic acid. *Intern. Med.,* **37**, 546–549

Sarma, D., Yang, X., Jin, G., Shindoh, M., Pater, M.M. & Pater, A. (1996) Resistance to retinoic acid and altered cytokeratin expression of human papillomavirus type 16-immortalized endocervical cells after tumorigenesis. *Int. J. Cancer*, **65**, 345–350

Schüle, R., Rangarajan, P., Yang, N., Kleiwer, S., Ransone, L.J., Bolado, J., Verma, I.M. & Evans, R.M. (1991) Retinoic acid is a negative regulator of AP-1-responsive genes. *Proc. Natl Acad. Sci. USA*, **88**, 6092–6096

Schweiter, U., Englert, G., Rigassi, N. & Vetter, W. (1969) Physical organic methods in carotenoid research. *Pure Appl. Chem.*, **20**, 365–420

Shah, G.M., Goswami, U.C. & Bhattacharya, R.K. (1992) Action of some retinol derivatives and their provitamins on microsome-catalyzed formation of benzo[a]-pyrene–DNA adduct. *J. Biochem. Toxicol.*, **7**, 177–181

Shalinsky, D.R., Bischoff, E.D., Gregory, M.L., Gottardis, M.M., Hayes, J.S., Lamph, W.W., Heyman, R.A., Shirley, M.A., Cooke, T.A., Davies, P.J. & Thomazy, V. (1995) Retinoid-induced suppression of squamous cell differentiation in human oral squamous cell carcinoma xenografts (line 1483) in athymic nude mice. *Cancer Res.*, **55**, 3183 3191

Shenefelt, R.E. (1972) Morphogenesis of malformations in hamsters caused by retinoic acid: Relation to dose and stage at treatment. *Teratology*, **5**, 103-118

Shetty, T.K., Francis, A.R. & Bhattacharya, R.K. (1988) Modifying role of vitamins on the mutagenic action of *N*-methyl-*N'*-nitro-*N*-nitrosoguanidine. *Carcinogenesis*, **9**, 1513–1515

Shindoh, M., Sun, Q., Pater, A. & Pater, M.M. (1995) Prevention of carcinoma in situ of human papillomavirus type 16-immortalized human endocervical cells by retinoic acid in organotypic raft culture. *Obstet. Gynecol.*, **85**, 721–728

Shoyab, M. (1981) Inhibition of the binding of 7,12-dimethylbenz[a]anthracene to DNA of murine epidermal cells in culture by vitamin A and vitamin C. *Oncology*, **38**, 187–192

Siegenthaler, G. & Saurat, J.H. (1989) Binding of isotretinoin to cellular retinoic acid binding protein: A reappraisal. In: Marks, R. & Plewig, G., eds, *Acne and Related Disorders*. London, Martin Dunitz, pp. 169–174

Simone, M.D., Stasi, R., Venditti, A., Del Poeta, G., Aronica, G., Bruno, A., Masi, M., Tribalto, M., Papa, G. & Amadori, S. (1995) All-*trans*-retinoic acid (ATRA) administration during pregnancy in relapsed acute promyelocytic leukemia. *Leukemia*, **9**, 1412–1413

Sirianni, S.R., Chen, H.H. & Huang, C.C. (1981) Effects of retinoids on plating efficiency, sister-chromatid exchange (SCE) and mitomycin-C-induced SCE in cultured Chinese hamster cells. *Mutat. Res.*, **90**, 175–182

Sizemore, N. & Rorke, E.A. (1993) Human papillomavirus 16 immortalization of normal human ectocervical epithelial cells alters retinoic acid regulation of cell growth and epidermal growth factor receptor expression. *Cancer Res.*, **53**, 4511–4517

Slaga, T.J., Klein-Szanto, A.J., Fischer, S.M., Weeks, C.E., Nelson, K. & Major, S. (1980) Studies on mechanism of action of anti-tumor-promoting agents: their specificity in two-stage promotion. *Proc. Natl Acad. Sci. USA*, **77**, 2251–2254

Soprano, D.R. & Soprano, K.J. (1995) Retinoids as teratogens. *Annu. Rev. Nutr.*, **15**, 111–132

Stam, C.H. & MacGillavry, C.H. (1963) The crystal structure of the triclinic modification of vitamin-A acid. *Acta Crystallogr.*, **16**, 62–68

Steele, V.E., Kelloff, G.J., Wilkinson, B.P. & Arnold, J.T. (1990) Inhibition of transformation in cultured rat tracheal epithelial cells by potential chemopreventive agents. *Cancer Res.*, **50**, 2068–2074

Stentoft, J., Nielscn, J.L. & Hvidman, L.E. (1994) All-*trans*- retinoic acid in acute promyelocytic leukemia in late pregnancy. *Leukemia*, **8**, 1585–1588

Stich, H.F., Tsang, S.S. & Palcic, B. (1990) The effect of retinoids, carotenoids and phenolics on chromosomal instability of bovine papillomavirus DNA-carrying cells. *Mutat. Res.*, **241**, 387–393

Sulik, K.K., Dehart, D.B., Rogers, J.M. & Chernoff, N. (1995) Teratogenicity of low doses of all-*trans*-retinoic acid in presomite mouse embryos. *Teratology*, **51**, 398–403

Surwit, E.A., Graham, V., Droegemueller, W., Alberts, D., Chvapil, M., Dorr, R.T., Davis, J.R. & Meyskens, F.L.J. (1982) Evaluation of topically applied *trans*-retinoic acid in the treatment of cervical intraepithelial lesions. *Am. J. Obstet. Gynecol.*, **143**, 821–823

Sutton, L.M., Warmuth, M.A., Petros, W.P. & Winer, E.P. (1997) Pharmacokinetics and clinical impact of all-*trans*-retinoic acid in metastatic breast cancer: A phase II trial. *Cancer Chemother. Pharmacol.*, **40**, 335–341

Szuts, E.Z. & Harosi, F.I. (1991) Solubility of retinoids in water. *Arch. Biochem. Biophys.*, **287**, 297–304

Takitani, K., Tamai, H., Morinobu, T., Kawamura, N., Miyake, M., Fujimoto, T. & Mino, M. (1995a) Pharmacokinetics of all-*trans*-retinoic acid in pediatric patients with leukemia. *Jpn. J. Cancer Res.*, **86**, 400–405

Takitani, K., Tamai, H., Morinobu, T., Kawamura, N., Miyake, M., Fujimoto, T. & Mino, M. (1995b) 4-Oxo retinoic acid for refractory acute promyelocytic leukemia in children with all-*trans*-retinoic therapy. *J. Nutr. Sci. Vitaminol. Tokyo*, **41**, 493–498

Tang, X. & Edenharder, R. (1997) Inhibition of the mutagenicity of 2-nitrofluorene, 3-nitrofluoranthene and 1-nitropyrene by vitamins, porphyrins and related compounds, and vegetable and fruit juices and solvent extracts. *Food Chem. Toxicol.*, **35**, 373–378

Tembe, E.A., Honeywell, R., Buss, N.E. & Renwick, A.G. (1996) All-*trans*-retinoic acid in maternal plasma and teratogenicity in rats and rabbits. *Toxicol. Appl. Pharmacol.*, **141**, 456–472

Tickle, C., Alberts, B., Wolpert, L. & Lee, J. (1982) Local application of retinoic acid to the limb bud mimics the action of the polarizing region. *Nature*, **296**, 564–566

Trosko, J.E. & Ruch, R.J. (1998) Cell–cell communication in carcinogenesis. *Front. Biosci.*, **3**, D208–D236

Tzimas, G., Bürgin, H., Collins, M.D., Hummler, H. & Nau, H. (1994a) The high sensitivity of the rabbit to the teratogenic effects of 13-*cis*-retinoic acid (isotretinoin) is a consequence of prolonged exposure of the embryo to 13-*cis*-retinoic acid and 13-*cis*-4-oxo-retinoic acid, and not of isomerization to all-*trans*-retinoic acid. *Arch. Toxicol.*, **68**, 119–128

Tzimas, G., Sass, J.O., Wittfoht, W., Elmazar, M.M., Ehlers, K. & Nau, H. (1994b) Identification of 9,13-di-*cis*-retinoic acid as a major plasma metabolite of 9-*cis*-retinoic acid and limited transfer of 9-*cis*-retinoic acid and 9,13-di-*cis*-retinoic acid to the mouse and rat embryos. *Drug Metab. Dispos.*, **22**, 928–936

Tzimas, G., Collins, M.D. & Nau, H. (1995) Developmental stage-associated differences in the transplacental distribution of 13-*cis*- and all-*trans*-retinoic acid as well as their glucuronides in rats and mice. *Toxicol. Appl. Pharmacol.*, **133**, 91–101

Tzimas, G., Nau, H., Hendrickx, A.G., Peterson, P.E. & Hummler, H. (1996) Retinoid metabolism and transplacental pharmacokinetics in the cynomolgus monkey following a nonteratogenic dosing regimen with all-*trans*-retinoic acid. *Teratology*, **54**, 255–265

Tzimas, G., Thiel, R., Chahoud, I. & Nau, H. (1997) The area under the concentration–time curve of all-*trans*-retinoic acid is the most suitable pharmacokinetic correlate to the embryotoxicity of this retinoid in the rat. *Toxicol. Appl. Pharmacol.*, **143**, 436–444

Vahlquist, A. (1994) Role of retinoids in normal and diseased skin. In: Blomhoff, R., ed., *Vitamin A in Health and Disease*. New York, Marcel Dekker, pp. 365–424

Vecchini, F., Lenoir, V.M., Cathelineau, C., Magdalou, J., Bernard, B.A. & Shroot, B. (1994) Presence of a retinoid responsive element in the promoter region of the human cytochrome P4501A1 gene. *Biochem. Biophys. Res. Commun.*, **201**, 1205–1212

Verma, A.K. (1988) Inhibition of tumor promoter 12-*O*-tetradecanoylphorbol-13-acetate-induced synthesis of epidermal ornithine decarboxylase messenger RNA and diacylglycerol-promoted mouse skin tumor formation by retinoic acid. *Cancer Res.*, **48**, 2168–2173

Verma, A.K., Shapas, B.G., Rice, H.M. & Boutwell, R.K. (1979) Correlation of the inhibition by retinoids of tumor promoter-induced mouse epidermal ornithine decarboxylase activity and of skin tumor promotion. *Cancer Res.*, **39**, 419–425

Vermeulen, S.J., Bruyneel, E.A., van Roy, F.M., Mareel, M.M. & Bracke, M.E. (1995) Activation of the E-cadherin/-catenin complex in human MCF-7 breast cancer cells by all-*trans*-retinoic acid. *Br. J. Cancer*, **72**, 1447–1453

Vetter, W., Englert, G., Rigassi, N. & Schwieter, U. (1971) Spectroscopic methods. In: Isler, O., Gutmann, H. & Solms, U., eds, *Carotenoids*. Basel, Birkhauser Verlag, pp. 189–266

Wang, C.C., Campbell, S., Furner, R.L. & Hill, D.L. (1980) Disposition of all-*trans*- and 13-*cis*-retinoic acids and *N*-hydroxyethylretinamide in mice after intravenous administration. *Drug Metab. Dispos.*, **8**, 8–11

Warrell, R.P., Jr, de Thé, H., Wang, Z.Y. & Degos, L. (1993) Acute promyelocytic leukemia. *N. Engl. J. Med.*, **329**, 177–189

Watanabe, T. & Pratt, R.M. (1991) Influence of retinoids on sister chromatid exchanges and chromosomes in cultured human embryonic palatal mesenchymal cells. *Teratog. Carcinog. Mutag.*, **11**, 297–304

Watanabe, R., Okamoto, S., Moriki, T., Kizaki, M., Kawai, Y. & Ikeda, Y. (1995) Treatment of acute promyelocytic leukemia with all-*trans*-retinoic acid during the third trimester of pregnancy. *Am. J. Hematol.*, **48**, 210–211

Westin, S., Mode, A., Murray, M., Chen, R. & Gustafsson, J.A. (1993) Growth hormone and vitamin A induce P4502C7 mRNA expression in primary rat hepatocytes. *Mol. Pharmacol.*, **44**, 997–1002

Whong, W.Z., Stewart, J., Brockman, H.E. & Ong, T.M. (1988) Comparative antimutagenicity of chlorophyllin and five other agents against aflatoxin B1-induced reversion in *Salmonella typhimurium* strain TA98. *Teratog. Carcinog. Mutag.*, **8**, 215–224

Willhite, C.C. & Clewell, H.J. (1999) Physiologically-based pharmacokinetic scaling in retinoid developmental toxicity. In: Livrea, M., ed., *Vitamin A and Retinoids: An Update of Biological Aspects and Clinical Applications*. Basel, Birkhäuser Verlag, pp. 121–128

Willhite, C.C., Sharma, R.P., Allen, P.V. & Berry, D.L. (1990) Percutaneous retinoid absorption and embryotoxicity. *J. Invest. Dermatol.,* **95**, 523–529

Wilmer, J.W. & Spit, B.J. (1986) Influence of retinoids on the mutagenicity of cigarette-smoke condensate in *Salmonella typhimurium* TA98. *Mutat. Res.,* **173**, 9–11

Yoon, J.H., Gray, T., Guzman, K., Koo, J.S. & Nettesheim, P. (1997) Regulation of the secretory phenotype of human airway epithelium by retinoic acid, triiodothyronine, and extracellular matrix. *Am. J. Respir. Cell. Mol. Biol.,* **16**, 724–731

Yutsudo, Y., Imoto, S., Ozuru, R., Kajimoto, K., Itoi, H., Koizumi, T., Nishimura, R. & Nakagawa, T. (1997) Acute pancreatitis after all-*trans*-retinoic acid therapy. *Ann. Hematol.,* **74**, 295–296

Zancai, P., Cariati, R., Rizzo, S., Boiocchi, M. & Dolcetti, R. (1998) Retinoic acid-mediated growth arrest of EBV-immortalized B lymphocytes is associated with multiple changes in G_1 regulatory proteins: p27^{Kip1} up-regulation is a relevant early event. *Oncogene,* **17**, 1827–1836

Zhuang, Y.H., Sainio, E.L., Sainio, P., Vedeckis, W.V., Ylikomi, T. & Tuohimaa, P. (1995) Distribution of all-*trans*-retinoic acid in normal and vitamin A deficient mice: Correlation to retinoic acid receptors in different tissues of normal mice. *Gen. Compar. Endocrinol.,* **100**, 170–178

Handbook 2

13-*cis*-Retinoic acid

1. Chemical and Physical Characteristics

1.1 Nomenclature
See General Remarks, section 1.4

1.2 Name: 13-*cis*-Retinoic acid

Chemical Abstracts Services Registry Number
4759-48-2

IUPAC Systematic name
(7*E*,9*E*,11*E*,13*Z*)-9,13-Dimethyl-7-(1,1,5-trimethyl-cyclohex-5-en-6-yl)-nona-7,9,11,13-tetraen-15-oic acid (see 1.3), or (2*Z*,4*E*,6*E*,8*E*)-3,7-dimethyl-9-(2,2,6-trimethylcyclohex-1-en-1-yl)nona-2,4,6,8-tetraen-1-oic acid

Synonyms
13*Z*-Retinoic acid, 13-*cis* vitamin A acid, 13-*cis* vitamin A_1 acid, Isotretinoin®, Accutane®, Isotrex®, Roaccutane

1.3 Structural formula

Composition: $C_{20}H_{28}O_2$
Relative molecular mass: 300.45

1.4 Physical and chemical properties
Description
Reddish-orange plates from isopropyl alcohol

Melting-point
174–175 °C (Budavari *et al.*, 1996).

Solubility
Soluble in most organic solvents, fats and oils; sparingly soluble in water

Spectroscopy
UV and visible: λ_{max} 354 (ethanol), $E^{1\%}_{1\ cm}$ 1325, E_M 39 750 (Frickel, 1984; Budavari *et al.*, 1996; Barua & Furr, 1998).

Nuclear magnetic resonance spectroscopy
^{1}H-NMR (CDCl$_3$, 220 MHz): δ 1.03 (1-CH$_3$), 1.46 (2-CH$_2$), 1.63 (3-CH$_2$), 1.72 (5-CH$_3$), 2.00 (9-CH$_3$, 4-CH$_2$), 2.10 (13-CH$_3$), 5.69 (14-H), 6.17 (8-H), 6.29 (7-H, 10-H), 7.03 (11-H), 7.77 (12-H); J$_{7,8}$ (16 Hz), J$_{10,11}$ (11.5 Hz), J$_{11,12}$ (15 Hz) (Schweiter *et al.*, 1969; Vetter *et al.*, 1971; Frickel, 1984; Barua & Furr, 1998).

^{13}C-NMR (CDCl$_3$, 68 MHz) δ 12.9 (9-CH$_3$), 19.4 (3-C), 21.1 (13-CH$_3$), 21.6 (5-CH$_3$), 29.0 (1,1-CH$_3$), 33.3 (4-C), 34.4 (1-C), 40.0 (2-C), 115.9 (14-C), 128.9 (7-C), 129.4 (12-C), 130.1 (5-C), 130.3 (10-C), 132.9 (11-C), 137.4 (8-C), 137.9 (6-C), 140.3 (9-C), 153.3 (13-C), 171.4 (15-C) (Englert, 1975; Frickel, 1984; Barua & Furr, 1998)

Resonance Raman, infrared and mass spectrometry
(Frickel, 1984; Barua & Furr, 1998)

X-Ray analysis
(Frickel, 1984).

Stability
Unstable to light, oxygen and heat. 13-*cis*-Retinoic acid in solution is protected by the presence of antioxidants, such as butylated hydroxytoluene and pyrogallol. A variety of factors influence the stability of 13-*cis*-retinoic acid in tissue culture media. Degradation and isomerization are minimized by storage under an inert gas such as argon, at ≤ –20 °C in the dark (Frickel, 1984; Barua & Furr, 1998).

2. Occurrence, Production, Use, Human Exposure and Analysis

2.1 Occurrence
The mean concentration of 13-*cis*-retinoic acid in the plasma of fasting individuals is 5.4 nmol/L (Eckhoff & Nau, 1990; Blaner & Olson, 1994). The

mean concentration of a major metabolite, 13-*cis*-4-oxoretinoic acid, is somewhat higher, i.e. 11.7 nmol/L (Eckhoff & Nau, 1990). Most other tissues of the body also contain 13-*cis*-retinoic acid, at concentrations 10 or more times higher than that of plasma (Napoli, 1994). The 13-*cis*-retinoic acid concentration is < 1% that of all-*trans* retinol in human plasma and < 5% that of total vitamin A in the tissues of healthy animals and humans. Since 13-*cis*-retinoic acid is present, if at all, in only traces in plants, it is a very minor constituent of the diet, and consequently contributes very little to the intake of dietary vitamin A. 13-*cis*-Retinoic acid, unlike vitamin A and carotenoids, is not available as a dietary supplement.

2.2   Production

The synthesis of 13-*cis*-retinoic acid is based on that of the all-*trans* isomer (see Handbook 1, p. 96), but with discrete modifications. Thus, condensation of a *trans*-β-C_{15}-aldehyde with ethyl senecioate in the presence of sodium or lithium amide in liquid ammonia gives 13-*cis*-retinoic acid, whereas use of potassium amide yields the all-*trans* isomer (Mayer & Isler, 1971). In several chemical syntheses, the final product is a mixture of the all-*trans* and 13-*cis* isomers of retinoic acid or its esters, which then can be separated (Frickel, 1984). Photoisomerization of all-*trans* retinoids in a nonpolar solvent like hexane yields significant mounts of the 13-*cis* isomer (Frickel, 1984). 13-*cis*-Retinal can also be converted to its acid by mild oxidants (Mayer & Isler, 1971; Frickel, 1984).

2.3   Use

13-*cis*-Retinoic acid is primarily used for treating dermatological disorders (Peck & DiGiovanna, 1994; Vahlquist, 1994) and has also been used to treat several types of human cancer (Hong & Itri, 1994). It was first marketed in the United States in 1982 and in Europe somewhat later, primarily for the treatment of severe nodulocystic acne (Nau *et al.*, 1994).

Skin disorders that have been treated with 13-*cis*-retinoic acid are summarized in Table 1. Although the usual oral doses are 1–2 mg/kg bw per day (Peck & DiGiovanna, 1994; Vahlquist, 1994), such doses often induce adverse side-effects, as discussed in section 7.1. Topical preparations of 13-*cis*-retinoic acid in creams or gels have sometimes been used to treat acne vulgaris, but few other skin disorders (Vahlquist, 1994).

Some precancerous conditions and cancers treated with 13-*cis*-retinoic acid are summarized in Table 2. Oral doses of 0.5–2 mg/kg bw per day have commonly been used, but lower oral doses (5–10 mg/day) have also been employed (Hong & Itri, 1994).

2.4   Human exposure

13-*cis*-Retinoic acid was first introduced into commerce in the United States in 1982, and over the next 60 months 800 000 patients received the drug (Orfanos, 1985; Stern, 1989). Approximately 40% of all 13-cis-retinoic acid prescriptions are written to women, and between 1990 and 1995, the number of prescriptions written to women doubled (Holmes *et al.*, 1998). As already indicated, the amount of retinoic acids in food is very small, probably in the range of 10–100 µg/day. Because 13-*cis*-retinoic acid is rapidly metabolized by the body and is not stored in the liver or other organs, it does not accumulate over time (Blaner & Olson, 1994). As a consequence, exposure to 13-*cis*-retinoic acid is limited, for all practical purposes, to the oral treatment of medical disorders.

Table 1. Some skin disorders treated with 13-*cis*-retinoic acid

Acne vulgaris	Lupus erythematosis
Darier's disease	Nodulocystic acne
Eruptive keratoacanthoma	Pityriasis rubra pilaris
Granuloma annulare	Psoriasis
Hydradenitis suppurativa	Rosacea
Ichthyosis congenita	Scleroderma
Lichen planus	Warts

Modified from Vahlquist (1994) and from Peck and DiGiovanna (1994)

Table 2.   Some precancerous conditions and cancers that have been treated with 13-*cis*-retinoic acid
Acute promyelocytic leukaemia
Chronic myelogenous leukaemia
Cutaneous T-cell lymphoma/mycosis fungoides
Skin cancer
Actinic keratosis
Bladder cancer
Cervix cancer
Breast cancer
Head and neck cancer
Oral leukoplakia
Laryngeal papillomatosis
Lung cancer
Myelodysplastic syndrome
Modified from Hong and Itri (1994)

2.5   Analysis

13-*cis*-Retinoic acid in plasma and tissues is commonly measured by high-performance liquid chromatography (HPLC) (Barua & Furr, 1998). Either plasma or a tissue homogenate is acidified to pH 3–4 and then extracted several times with a suitable volume of an organic solvent such as chloroform/methanol, diethyl ether, dichloromethane, acetonitrile, 2-propanol or ethyl acetate. After the combined extract with anhydrous sodium sulfate has been dried, the solvent is evaporated under yellow light (to avoid isomerization) in nitrogen or argon to dryness. The dried powder is immediately dissolved in the HPLC solvent and injected onto the HPLC column. In some cases, a solid-phase extraction or elution step is introduced to remove contaminants.

A reversed-phase C_{18} column is usually used for the separation. The compound is usually detected by measuring the absorption at 354 nm, and it is quantified by measuring the area of the absorption peak with an integrator. A known amount of a reference standard, usually all-*trans*-retinyl acetate, is added to the tissue, plasma or serum sample to correct for losses during extraction and analysis. An antioxidant, such as butylated hydroxytoluene, is also added at the outset to minimize oxidation of the retinoids present.

A large number of chromatographic systems have been devised for the separation and quantifi-

cation of retinoic acid (Frolik & Olson, 1984; Furr *et al.*, 1992, 1994; Barua & Furr, 1998; Barua *et al.*, 1999). In most reversed-phase HPLC systems, 13-*cis*-retinoic acid is eluted before all-*trans*-retinoic acid.

13-*cis*-Retinoic acid, as its methyl or pentafluorobenzyl ester, can also be separated by gas–liquid or liquid–liquid chromatography and quantified by mass spectrometry. New ionization methods and tandem mass spectrometry have further enhanced the sensitivity and selectivity with which 13-*cis*-retinoic acid can be measured (Barua *et al.*, 1999).

3.   Metabolism, Kinetics and Genetic Variation

It is well accepted that 13-*cis*-retinoic acid is a naturally occurring form of retinoic acid that is normally present in blood and tissues of humans and higher animals (Blaner & Olson, 1994). Since 13-*cis*-retinoic acid is not as active in *trans*-activation assays as the all-*trans*- and 9-*cis*-retinoic acid isomers (Mangelsdorf *et al.*, 1994), it is also generally believed not to be a key retinoic acid for regulating gene transcription. This isomer is, however, effective in inducing retinoid-responsiveness in cells in culture and in animal models when given in large pharmacological doses. 13-*cis*-Retinoic acid is effective in treating human disease, especially dermatological conditions, and it is proposed that many of its effects are mediated by all-*trans*-retinoic acid after isomerization of the 13-*cis* isomer.

Current understanding of the metabolism, plasma transport and tissue distribution of 13-*cis*-retinoic acid in humans and animal models after administration of large doses is reviewed below. More information about the endogenous (physiological) metabolism of 13-*cis*-retinoic acid is given in the General Remarks.

3.1 Humans
3.1.1 Metabolism

It is generally assumed that 13-*cis*-retinoic acid is formed by isomerization of all-*trans*-retinoic acid or possibly by isomerization of 9-*cis*-retinoic acid. As can be seen in Figure 1 of the General Remarks, however, it is theoretically possible that 13-*cis*-retinoic acid is formed in a manner analogous to all-*trans*-retinoic acid, through sequential oxidation of 13-*cis*-retinol and 13-*cis*-retinal. One enzyme that can catalyse the oxidation of 13-*cis*-

retinol to 13-*cis*-retinal has been described (Driessen *et al.*, 1998), but it has not been established that 13-*cis*-retinol or 13-*cis*-retinal is present in significant quantities in human tissues, and it is not presently clear whether 13-*cis*-retinoic acid can be formed through a biosynthetic pathway that does not involve all-*trans*- or 9-*cis*-retinoic acid as the immediate precursor.

13-*cis*-4-Oxoretinoic acid was identified by HPLC and gas chromatography–mass spectrometry as the major circulating metabolite of 13-*cis*-retinoic acid in pooled plasma from patients receiving 20–100 mg/day in the long-term treatment of dermatological disorders. The second most abundant metabolite was all-*trans*-4-oxoretinoic acid. Neither the concentrations of these metabolites nor their distribution relative to that of circulating 13-*cis*- or all-*trans*-retinoic acid was reported (Vane & Bugge, 1981).

The biliary metabolites of 13-*cis*-retinoic acid were investigated in two patients with biliary T-tube drainage after administration of a single oral 80-mg dose of 13-*cis*-[^{14}C]retinoic acid The two patients excreted 23 and 17% of the radiolabel in their bile within four days. HPLC measurements of the extracted bile samples indicated that the β-glucuronide metabolites of 13-*cis*-retinoic acid accounted for about 48% and 44% of the total radioactivity in the bile of the two patients. The two major glucuronide conjugates present were those of 13-*cis*-4-oxoretinoic acid and 13-*cis*-16-hydroxyretinoic acid, with relatively minor amounts of the glucuronide conjugates of 13-*cis*-retinoic acid and 13-*cis*-18-hydroxyretinoic acid (Vane *et al.*, 1990).

13-*cis*-Retinoic acid, 9-*cis*-retinoic acid and all-*trans*-retinol inhibited all-*trans*-retinoic acid 4-hydroxylation by human hepatic microsomes. 13-*cis*- and 9-*cis*-Retinoic acid were competitive inhibitors of all-*trans*-retinoic acid 4-hydroxylation, with $K_i:K_m$ ratios of 3.5 ± 0.8 and 6.3 ± 0.5, respectively. This may suggest that the two *cis*-retinoids are alternative but inferior substrates for the hepatic cytochrome P450 isoforms that mediate the 4-hydroxylation reaction of all-*trans*-retinoic acid (Nadin & Murray, 1996).

13-*cis*-Retinoic acid generated by photo-isomerization of topically administered all-*trans*-retinoic acid may be absorbed percutaneously. After application of a 0.1% cream of all-*trans*-retinoic acid to human cadaver skin *in vitro* with and without exposure to ambient light, 13-*cis*-retinoic acid was detected after 24 h in samples of skin exposed to light but was virtually absent from skin samples maintained in the dark. Since the concentration of 13-*cis*-retinoic acid in the exposed skin sample was similar to that of all-*trans*-retinoic acid, some 13-*cis*-retinoic acid may be absorbed through the skin after photo-isomerization of topically applied all-*trans*-retinoic acid (Lehman & Malany, 1989).

The β-glucuronides of all-*trans*- and 13-*cis*-retinoic acid were found in the circulation of a healthy female volunteer after repeated administration of 13-*cis*-retinoic acid orally at 2.3 μmol/kg bw per day for 27 days. The maximal plasma concentrations of the two β-glucuronides reportedly reached 105 and 13 nmol/L, respectively. The maximal plasma concentration of 13-*cis*-retinoic acid after its oral administration on day 27 was reported to be 90 nmol/L, whereas that of all-*trans*-retinoic acid was about 5.5 nmol/L (Creech Kraft *et al.*, 1991a).

3.1.2 Kinetics

In early work on the pharmacokinetics of 13-*cis*-retinoic acid in humans, phase I and II trials were performed in patients with advanced cancer who received oral doses starting at 0.5 mg/kg bw per day and increasing over four weeks to a maximum of 8 mg/kg bw per day. Although large interindividual differences in peak plasma concentrations were noted, the plasma concentration of 13-*cis*-retinoic acid showed a linear correlation with increasing dose. At the maximal dose, the mean peak plasma concentration was 4 μmol/L. Even after repeated dosing, the drug was rapidly cleared from the plasma. The patients receiving 13-*cis*-retinoic acid had lower plasma retinol concentrations than those of the general population (Kerr *et al.*, 1982).

The pharmacokinetics, blood concentrations and urinary, biliary and faecal excretion of 13-*cis*-[^{14}C]retinoic acid were studied in four healthy male volunteers given a single 80-mg oral dose. About 80% of the dose was recovered as radiolabel in excreta during the study, with approximately equal fractions present in the urine and faeces. A second peak in the blood concentration of radiolabel was observed, suggesting possible enterohepatic circulation of 13-*cis*-retinoic acid. The mean half-life in the blood was 14 h, whereas the corresponding value for the radiolabel was 90 h (Colburn *et al.*, 1985).

Differences in the pharmacokinetics of 13-*cis*-retinoic acid between cancer patients and healthy volunteers have been reported. In these studies, 0.5

mg/kg bw was given orally to four healthy female and four healthy male volunteers and to five patients with cervical carcinoma and 14 male patients with squamous-cell carcinomas of the head and neck. The cancer patients also simultaneously received treatment with interferon-α_{2a} (3×10^6 IU three times per week subcutaneously). The mean integrated area under the curve for concentration–time (AUC) for 13-*cis*-retinoic acid was 1.7-fold higher in female patients than in the female volunteers and 1.3 times higher in male patients than in the male volunteers. The maximal blood concentrations of 13-*cis*-retinoic acid in male and female patients were approximately 20% higher than those observed in sex-matched healthy volunteers. Qualitatively similar observations were made for the concentrations of 13-*cis*-4-oxoretinoic acid in the patients with cervical and head-and-neck cancers. The maximal blood concentration of 13-*cis*-4-oxoretinoic acid in female patients was 3.3 times greater than that of the female volunteers and 1.8 times greater in male patients than in the male volunteers. The maximal blood concentrations of 13-*cis*-retinoic acid and 13-*cis*-4-oxoretinoic acid and the AUC values for these retinoids were greater for the healthy women than for the healthy men studied. The authors suggested that the higher AUC values of 13-*cis*-retinoic acid observed in the cancer patients may have been due to the treatment with interferon-α_{2a} (Waladkhani & Clemens, 1997).

Twelve patients with melanoma and regional node metastases after radical surgery were randomized for combined treatment for three months with recombinant interferon-α_{2a} and oral 13-*cis*-retinoic acid at a dose of 20 or 40 mg/day. The pharmacokinetics of 13-*cis*-retinoic acid and its effects on plasma retinol concentrations were investigated on the first and last days of the treatment schedule. The maximal plasma concentrations of 13-*cis*-retinoic acid were observed 4 h after dosing, with average values of 1.3 and 2.1 μmol/L after the two doses, respectively. The average half-life of 13-*cis*-retinoic acid in the circulation was approximately 30 h. The maximal plasma concentration, the half-life in the circulation and the AUC value over 0–48 h did not change after multiple dosing, whereas the AUC over 48 h for the major blood metabolite, 13-*cis*-4-oxoretinoic acid, increased. Immediately after receipt of the dose of 13-*cis*-retinoic acid, the plasma retinol concentrations began to decline, and they reached a minimum concentration

(a reduction of approximately 20%) shortly after the time of the maximal 13-*cis*-retinoic acid concentration, 4–12 h after treatment. After clearance of 13-*cis*-retinoic acid from the circulation, the plasma concentration of retinol returned to baseline (Formelli *et al.*, 1997).

A reduction in plasma retinol concentrations in patients receiving 13-*cis*-retinoic acid at 1 mg/kg bw per day for six months was reported in a further study. Although 13-*cis*-retinoic significantly reduced the plasma concentrations of all-*trans*-retinol in the 13 women enrolled in the study, from 1.9 ± 0.67 μmol/L at baseline to 1.5 ± 0.40 μmol/L after treatment ($p = 0.03$), the concentrations of the 22 men enrolled in the study did not significantly change ($p = 0.43$). The reason for this sex difference is unknown (Lippman *et al.*, 1998).

3.1.3. Tissue distribution

No information was available about the tissue distribution of 13-*cis*-retinoic acid in humans after its administration as a drug.

3.1.4 Variations within human populations

Very limited information was available about possible differences in the metabolism of 13-*cis*-retinoic acid in different human populations. As mentioned above, the maximal blood concentration of 13-*cis*-4-oxoretinoic acid in male and female cancer patients treated with interferon-α_{2a} was greater than that in healthy male and female volunteers after an oral dose of 13-*cis*-retinoic acid. The maximal blood concentrations of 13-*cis*-retinoic acid and 13-*cis*-4-oxoretinoic acid and the AUC values for these retinoids were also greater in the four healthy women than in the four healthy men studied. Thus disease state, treatment and sex may affect the way in which 13-*cis*-retinoic acid is taken up and metabolized in humans (Waladkhani & Clemens, 1997).

3.2 Experimental models

Most of the information available on the metabolism, plasma transport and tissue distribution of 13-*cis*-retinoic acid is derived from studies in rats and mice, although significant studies have been carried out in dogs and primates.

3.2.1 Metabolism

In rats, 13-*cis*-retinoyl-β-glucuronide is a major metabolite of 13-*cis*-retinoic acid after its administration at pharmacological doses. In bile duct-cannulated vitamin A-sufficient male rats given large intravenous doses of 4–20 mg/kg bw, analysis of the bile by reversed-phase HPLC showed that treatment was followed by rapid excretion of metabolites. The major biliary metabolite was 13-*cis*-retinoyl-β-glucuronide, and its rate of excretion increased rapidly after injection to reach a maximum 55 min later but then decreased exponentially. After 330 min of collection, biliary excretion of 13-*cis*-retinoyl-β-glucuronide accounted for 35–38% of the dose. The authors concluded that 13-*cis*-retinoyl-β-glucuronide is a major pathway for the metabolism of pharmacological doses of 13-*cis*-retinoic acid in rats and that neither the glucuronidation nor the biliary excretion pathway is saturated after administration of high pharmacological doses of 13-*cis*-retinoic acid (Meloche & Besner, 1986).

3.2.2 Kinetics

The serum concentrations of 13-*cis*-retinoic acid in male BDF_1 mice given 13-*cis*-retinoic acid orally at 10 mg/kg bw were maximal within 15–30 min and then declined in a monoexponential fashion with a half-life of 19 min. The concentrations in liver, lung, small intestine, fat, kidney, brain, heart, spleen, large intestine, muscle, testis and urinary bladder reached their maxima within 15–30 min, then declined exponentially with half-lives of 11–19 min. The liver showed the highest concentration at each time it was examined, followed by fat, lung and kidney. Only a small amount of unmetabolized 13-*cis*-retinoic acid was observed in bile and faeces, and none was found in urine (Kalin et al., 1982).

The pharmacokinetics of three parenteral 13-*cis*-retinoic acid formulations was studied after intraperitoneal administration to rats of 2.5 mg/360 g bw [6.9 mg/kg bw]; the drug was administered as an alkaline solution, suspended in corn oil or as a mixture with polysorbate 80. The alkaline solution was also given intravenously via the tail vein as a control. The mean elimination rate constant, calculated after the intravenous dose, was 0.72 ± 0.088 per h. The peak concentration in plasma and the time to reach this maximum were 14 mg/L and 0.5 h, 22 mg/L and 2 h and 10 mg/L and 1 h for the three formulations, respectively. The AUC values were 35 ± 8.8 mg·h/L for the intravenous dose and 34 ± 10, 62 ± 32 and 26 ± 12 mg·h/L for the intraperitoneal doses of alkaline solution, suspension in oil and mixture with polysorbate 80, respectively (Guchelaar et al., 1992).

The first-pass metabolism of 13-*cis*-retinoic acid in the gut contents, gut wall and liver of dogs was studied after simultaneous administration of 13-*cis*-[^{12}C]retinoic acid intravenously and 13-*cis*-[^{14}C]retinoic acid orally. Blood samples were obtained from the jugular and the portal veins at specified times to quantify the concentrations of the two labelled compounds. In addition, blood, bile, urine and the gastrointestinal contents were analysed for ^{14}C-containing material. The harmonic mean elimination half-life for the simultaneous intravenous and oral administration of 13-*cis*-retinoic acid was approximately 5.5 h. The mean blood clearance after intravenous administration was 5.2 ± 2.4 ml/min per kg bw, and the intrinsic clearance after oral administration was 6.6 ± 3.7 ml/min per kg bw. The average absolute bioavailability of 13-*cis*-retinoic acid in dogs was 21%, indicating an overall first-pass effect of approximately 80%. About 72% of the first-pass effect occurred in the gut lumen, the gut wall and liver making lesser contributions. These results indicate that the low bioavailability of 13-*cis*-retinoic acid in dogs is due mainly to loss of the drug before it reaches the portal circulation, probably because of biological or chemical degradation in the gut lumen before absorption (Cotler et al., 1983).

The effect of the route of administration of 13-*cis*-retinoic acid and its biliary excretion on its pharmacokinetics was examined in dogs given oral, intraportal and intravenous doses of 13-*cis*-retinoic acid at 2.2–5 mg/kg bw before and after bile-duct cannulation. Blood and bile samples were collected and analysed by HPLC. The concentrations of 13-*cis*-retinoic acid in blood were decreased after bile-duct cannulation, and the decreases in the AUC values were greatest after oral dosing, intermediate after intraportal dosing and least after intravenous dosing. 13-*cis*-Retinoic acid was excreted in the bile primarily as the glucuronide. The largest percentage of the dose (27%) was excreted in the bile after intraportal infusion, an intermediate percentage (8.5%) after intravenous dosing and the smallest percentage (3.3%) after oral dosing. These data indicate that biliary excretion affects the blood profile of 13-*cis*-retinoic acid as a function of route of administration and that the differences are probably the result of differences in first-pass clearance. In addition, the apparent bioavailability of 13-*cis*-retinoic acid was 14% in bile-cannulated dogs and

54% in the uncannulated animals, suggesting that enterohepatic recycling of 13-*cis*-retinoic acid may contribute to its oral bioavailability (Cotler *et al.*, 1984).

After a single dose of 13-*cis*-retinoic acid at 100 mg/kg was given to NMRI mice on day 11 of gestation or three doses of 100 mg/kg bw were given 4 h apart, the major plasma metabolite was 13-*cis*-retinoyl-β-glucuronide, followed by 4-oxo metabolites and all-*trans*-retinoic acid. all-*trans*-Retinoic acid was transferred very efficiently to the mouse embryo, whereas the transfer of 13-*cis*-retinoic acid was 10% and that of 13-*cis*-retinoyl-β-glucuronide was 1% that of all-*trans*-retinoic acid. Interestingly, no embryotoxicity was observed after the single oral dose, whereas the multiple doses enhanced the teratogenicity of 13-*cis*-retinoic acid markedly (Creech Kraft *et al.*, 1991b). In a study of the effects of development stage (gestational age) on the transplacental distribution of 13-*cis*- and all-*trans*-retinoic acid and their glucuronides in rats and mice, 13-*cis*-retinoic acid showed more efficient transplacental passage later in development in both rats and mice. The authors suggested that transplacental transfer of 13-*cis*-retinoic acid is enhanced during late organogenesis because of the time of development of the chorioallantoic placenta in these species (Tzimas *et al.*, 1995).

The maternal kinetics and metabolism of 13-*cis*-retinoic acid were examined in cynomolgus monkeys in two studies. all-*trans*-Retinoic acid was eliminated more rapidly than 13-*cis*-retinoic acid, and the elimination rate tended to increase with repeated dosing. Administration of 13-*cis*-retinoic acid resulted primarily in *cis* metabolites, whereas treatment with all-*trans*-retinoic acid resulted primarily in all-*trans* metabolites. The main metabolites observed after treatment with 13-*cis*-retinoic acid at 2 or 10 mg/kg bw per day were 13-*cis*-4-oxoretinoic acid and 13-*cis*-retinoyl-β-glucuronide. Elimination of 13-*cis*-retinoic acid was more rapid in the monkeys than in humans, and the dose of 13-*cis*-retinoic acid required to produce AUC values comparable to those of humans was approximately 10-fold greater (Creech Kraft *et al.* 1991a).

Pregnant cynomolgus monkeys received 13-*cis*-retinoic acid at 2.5 mg/kg bw by nasogastric intubation once a day on days 16–26 of gestation and twice a day on days 27–31. Maternal plasma kinetics was determined after dosing on days 26 and 31, and placental transfer was studied after the last dose on day 31. The plasma half-life was 13 h.

The major plasma metabolite was 13-*cis*-4-oxo-retinoic acid. The concentration of all-*trans*-retinoic acid in maternal plasma was 2% that of 13-*cis*-retinoic acid. β-Glucuronides of both all-*trans*- and 13-*cis*-retinoic acid were found at low concentrations. The authors provided extensive characterization of the kinetics of transfer of 13-*cis*-retinoic acid to and its accumulation in the embryos of treated mothers (Hummler *et al.*, 1994).

In detailed multicompartmental studies of pharmacokinetics in female cynomolgus monkeys, all-*trans*- and 13-*cis*-retinoic acid were injected intravenously at a dose of 0.25 or 0.0125 mg/kg bw and all-*trans*-4-oxo- and 13-*cis*-4-oxoretinoic acid at 0.25 mg/kg bw. The elimination half-life was observed to be longer for the *cis* retinoids and was not dose-dependent: 13-*cis*-4-oxoretinoic acid, 837 min > 13-*cis*-retinoic acid, 301 ± 204 min > all-*trans*-retinoic acid, 38 ± 3 min > all-*trans*-4-oxoretinoic acid, 11 ± 2 min. A second plasma peak attributed to enterohepatic circulation were seen only after administration of 13-*cis*-4-oxoretinoic acid. The volume of distribution was greater for 13-*cis*-retinoic acid than for all-*trans*-retinoic acid (Sandberg *et al.*, 1994).

3.2.3   *Tissue distribution*

The distribution of 13-*cis*-retinoic acid was studied after its intravenous administration at 10 mg/kg bw to male DBA mice by assessing the concentrations in liver, lung, kidney, brain, testis and small intestine at intervals ranging from 5 min to 6 h after administration. At all the intervals studied, the liver took up the greatest concentration of 13-*cis*-retinoic acid, followed by lung, kidney, brain, small intestine and testis. The concentration present in the liver 5 min after administration was the highest in any tissue at any time (13 ± 1.2 µg/g). The concentration present in lung at any time was approximately 50% of that present in liver. In all tissues examined, two phases of elimination were observed (Wang *et al.*, 1980).

The mean tissue concentrations of 13-*cis*-retinoic acid in small intestine, liver, lung, fat, kidney, brain, heart, spleen, large intestine, muscle, testis and urinary bladder were studied after oral administration of 10 mg/kg bw to male BDF$_1$ mice. In good agreement with the study of Wang *et al.* (1980), the highest concentrations were found in the small intestine and then in the liver, lung and fat, throughout the 120 min of the study. All the tissues examined took up some 13-*cis*-retinoic acid (Kalin *et al.*, 1982).

3.2.4   Inter-species variation

The studies summarized in sections 3.2.2 and 3.2.3 indicate that rats, mice, dogs, monkeys and humans have different patterns of distribution and metabolism of 13-*cis*-retinoic acid. This is most obvious from the patterns of metabolites that are observed when pharmacological doses of 13-*cis*-retinoic acid are administered to animals and humans. Thus, no animal model truly reflects the metabolism or pharmacokinetics in humans.

4.   Cancer-preventive Effects

4.1   Humans
4.1.1   Epidemiological studies
No data were available to the Working Group.

4.1.2   Intervention trials
4.1.2.1   Cancers of the head and neck
The results of a secondary analysis of a randomized clinical trial of 13-*cis*-retinoic acid for the prevention of progression of primary squamous-cell carcinoma of the larynx, pharynx or oral cavity after primary treatment was reported. Patients received either placebo (n = 51) or 13-*cis*-retinoic acid (n = 49). The initial dose of 13-*cis*-retinoic acid was 100 mg/day, but this was later reduced to 50 mg/day because of toxicity. After a median follow-up of 32 months, there was no difference between the two groups with regard to the recurrence of the primary cancer (15 treated patients and 17 placebo patients, p = 0.77); however, there was a statistically significant difference in the number of patients who developed a second primary cancer (two treated patients and 12 on placebo, p = 0.005). All but one of the second primary tumours was in the upper aerodigestive tract (Hong *et al.*, 1990). A further reanalysis (Benner *et al.*, 1994a) after a median follow-up of 4.5 years indicated that the treated patients continued to have significantly fewer second primary tumours: seven (14%) in the 13-*cis*-retinoic acid arm and 16 (31%) in the placebo arm (p = 0.042). When only the second primary tumours that developed in the area of the upper aerodigestive tract or lungs exposed to tobacco were considered, there were only three tumours in the 49 patients treated with 13-*cis*-retinoic acid, whereas there were 13 in 51 patients receiving placebo (p = 0.008). [The Working Group noted that the results of tests of statistical significance are difficult to interpret when the tests are applied to hypotheses that were not specified at the onset of

the trial. The Group also noted that these investigators are conducting a much larger multicentre study to test the hypothesis raised by the findings in their earlier report.]

4.1.2.2   Skin
Clinical experience with high doses of 13-*cis*-retinoic acid for the treatment of basal-ccll and squamous-cell cancers of the skin (Peck & DiGiovanna, 1994) led to studies of its possible chemopreventive effects.

In a study of five patients with xeroderma pigmentosum and a history of more than two skin cancers per year during the previous two years, the patients were treated with 13-*cis*-retinoic acid at approximately 2 mg/kg bw per day for two years and then followed for an additional year with no therapy. During treatment, 25 tumours were diagnosed (three to nine per patient), which represented an average reduction of 63% from the number before treatment (p = 0.02). After discontinuation of treatment, the tumour occurrence increased by roughly eightfold (Kraemer *et al.*, 1988). [The Working Group noted that the study did not include an untreated control group or a cross-over design. The patients underwent intense surveillance, and the removal of all suspect skin cancers during the month before beginning 13-*cis*-retinoic acid treatment may have increased the number of cancers diagnosed in the pretreatment phase.]

A randomized, placebo-controlled trial of 13-*cis*-retinoic acid was conducted which involved 981 patients who had a history of prior non-melanoma skin cancer but no known inherited predilection to these tumours, such as xeroderma pigmentosum or basal-cell naevus syndrome. The dose of 13-*cis*-retinoic acid, 10 mg/day (roughly 0.15 mg/kg bw per day) was chosen to minimize the toxic side-effects but was substantially lower than those used in other studies of the treatment or prevention of skin cancer. The three-year cumulative incidence of new skin cancers was virtually identical in the treated and placebo groups. There also was no evidence that treatment had an effect in subgroups of patients categorized by sex, age, solar damage and number of prior tumours. The lack of efficacy pertained to both basal-cell and squamous-cell carcinomas (Tangrea *et al.*, 1992a).

A study to evaluate the efficacy of 13-*cis*-retinoic acid and retinol on the incidence of non-melanoma skin cancer involved 525 subjects with a history of at least four basal-cell carcinomas and/or cutaneous squamous-cell carcinomas. Subjects were equally assigned at random to receive 13-*cis*-retinoic acid (5–10 mg/day orally), retinol (25 000 units/day orally) or placebo, in a double-blind study design. The time to first occurrence of a new basal-cell and/or cutaneous squamous-cell carcinoma after three years of exposure was the primary end-point used to evaluate efficacy. During the study, 319 basal-cell and 125 cutaneous squamous-cell carcinomas were diagnosed. There was no statistically significant difference in the time to a first new occurrence of either tumour between the group treated with retinoid and that given placebo (Levine *et al.*, 1997).

4.1.2.3 Urinary bladder
A trial was reported in which 13-*cis*-retinoic acid was initially administered at a dose of 0.5 mg/kg bw per day, which was increased to 1 mg/kg bw per day, for the prevention of recurrent early-stage bladder cancer in 20 eligible patients. No control group was included. 13-*cis*-Retinoic acid was toxic, resulting in the dropping out of eight patients from the study before three months and four before six months. Most of the patients had a relapse within one year. The study was terminated because of toxicity and the absence of positive results (Prout & Barton, 1992).

4.1.3 Intermediate end-points
4.1.3.1 Oral cavity
13-*cis*-Retinoic acid has been used in two randomized, placebo-controlled studies on patients with oral premalignant lesions. In an evaluation of treatment of oral leukoplakia with 13-*cis*-retinoic acid in 44 patients, 24 were assigned randomly to treatment at 1–2 mg/kg bw per day for three months, followed by no treatment for six months, and 20 were assigned to placebo. An objective evaluation of the leukoplakias was based on clinical inspection and a requirement for a minimum of four weeks' duration. The size of the lesions was decreased by 50% or more in 16 patients (67%) given 13-*cis*-retinoic acid and two patients (10%) given placebo (p = 0.0002). Histological reversal of the severity of disease was reported in 13 patients (54%) given the retinoid and in two patients (10%) given placebo (p = 0.01). The clinical response correlated with histological response in 56% (9/16) of the patients evaluated. Relapse of leukoplakia occurred in 9/16 patients two to three months after treatment was stopped.

The toxic effects of 13-*cis*-retinoic acid were reported to be acceptable in all but two patients and included common retinoid mucocutaneous adverse events and hypertriglyceridaemia. All of the adverse events were reversed by reducing the dose or temporarily discontinuing treatment (Hong *et al.*, 1986).

Four of nine patients treated with 13-*cis*-retinoic acid at 1 mg/kg bw per day for three months showed complete resolution of their oral leukoplakia (Beenken *et al.*, 1994).

When 70 patients were treated with 13-*cis*-retinoic acid at 1.5 mg/kg bw per day for three months, the clinical response rate was 55% (95% confidence interval, 42–67%). The patients were then randomized into two groups, one of which received 13-*cis*-retinoic acid at 0.5 mg/kg bw per day and the other received β-carotene at 64 mg/day, for nine months. The group given 13-*cis*-retinoic acid showed an 8% rate of progression (2/24), whereas those given β-carotene showed a rate of 55% (16/29; p < 0.001). The low dose of 13-*cis*-retinoic acid was well tolerated, and no patients dropped out of the trial because of toxic effects (Lippmann *et al.*, 1995a).

Biopsy specimens from patients in the trials described above were evaluated for expression of retinoic acid nuclear receptors and *p53* before and after treatment with 13-*cis*-retinoic acid and compared with those from normal control subjects. In one report (Lotan *et al.*, 1995), all of the normal specimens but only 21/52 (40%) of those from oral premalignant lesions had detectable *RAR-β* mRNA levels at baseline. After three months of treatment with 13-*cis*-retinoic acid, 35/39 (90%) of the oral lesions available for evaluation expressed RAR-β (p < 0.001). The authors noted that RAR-β is selectively down-regulated in oral premalignant lesions and that treatment with 13-*cis*-retinoic acid can up-regulate RAR-β in these lesions (Lotan *et al.*, 1995). In a separate report, an inverse relationship was seen between accumulation of *p53* and response to the retinoid (p = 0.006). *p53* accumulation was not modulated by 13-*cis*-retinoic acid (Lippman *et al.*, 1995b). A discrete increase in the micronucleus count in mucosal scrapings of lesions was found when compared with scrapings from mucosa that appeared to be normal at baseline in the 57 patients studied (p = 0.035). A reduction in the micronucleus count was seen after treatment (p = 0.02) (Benner *et al.*, 1994b).

4.1.3.2 Lung

A group of 26 patients with documented cytological abnormalities in sputum samples, ranging from moderate atypical metaplasia to overt carcinoma, were treated with 1–2.5 mg/kg bw per day of 13-*cis*-retinoic acid. No improvement in the degree of atypia was seen. The authors reported alterations in cellular morphology, including increased intracytoplasmic vacuolization, bizarre nuclear shapes, rupture of the nuclear membranes and pyknotic nuclei (Saccomanno *et al.*, 1982).

In a randomized, double-blind, placebo-controlled trial of 13-*cis*-retinoic acid in 86 long-term smokers who had either bronchial dysplasia or a metaplasia index (defined as the number of tissue samples with metaplasia divided by the number of tissue samples counted, multiplied by 100) greater than 15%, the patients initially underwent bronchoscopy, and endobronchial biopsy samples were taken from six sites within the proximate lung field. They were then treated with 13-*cis*-retinoic acid at 1 mg/kg bw per day or placebo for six months. Of the 86 randomized patients, 69 could be assessed after the completion of therapy. There was no evidence of an effect of treatment. The extent of metaplasia had decreased in 19/35 patients (54%) treated with 13-*cis*-retinoic acid and in 20/35 (59%) given placebo (Lee *et al.*, 1994).

4.2   Experimental models
4.2.1   Cancer and preneoplastic lesions
These studies are summarized in Table 3.

4.2.1.1   Skin
Mouse: Groups of 30 female CD-1 mice, eight weeks of age, received skin applications of 200 nmol/L (51.2 µg) of 7,12-dimethylbenz[*a*]-anthracene (DMBA) and were treated topically with 8 nmol of 12-*O*-tetradecanoylphorbol 13-acetate (TPA) 14 days after initiation twice weekly for 18 weeks. 13-*cis*-Retinoic acid was given topically at a dose of 34 nmol 1 h before the TPA application. The incidence of papillomas 18 weeks after DMBA initiation was approximately 90% in controls and approximately 50% in mice treated with 13-*cis*-retinoic acid. The multiplicity of tumours was reduced from approximately 10 tumours per mouse to about four by 13-*cis*-retinoic acid (Verma *et al.*, 1979). [The numbers were derived from graphs; no statistics were provided.]

Groups of 20 female Swiss mice, eight weeks of age, were treated topically with 0.8% methylcholanthrene twice weekly for five weeks and once a week for weeks 6–9. One group also received 3 mg/mouse 13-*cis*-retinoic acid topically twice weekly during weeks 3–5 and once a week for weeks 6–9. The animals were killed 23 weeks after the first application of methylcholanthrene. The incidences of papillomas were 89% in controls and 30% in the group given 13-*cis*-retinoic acid [statistics not given]. The incidence of carcinomas was reduced from 26% in controls to 10% in 13-*cis*-retinoic acid-treated mice [statistics not given] (Abdel-Galil *et al.*, 1984).

Female CD-1 mice, eight weeks of age, were initiated with 400 nmol of benzo[*a*]pyrene and one week later stage-I tumour promotion was begun, consisting of twice weekly applications of 3.2 nmol of TPA for two weeks. The animals were then randomized into groups of 20 and stage-II tumour promotion, consisting of twice weekly applications of 8 nmol of TPA for 23 weeks, was begun. Starting on day 1, week 8 or week 23 of stage-II promotion, groups of mice were treated topically with 13-*cis*-retinoic acid, 30 min before TPA application. The control groups were treated with acetone. The experiment was terminated 38 weeks after the start of stage-II promotion. The papilloma yields were four tumours per mouse in the control group and 2.1, 2.9 and 3.3 tumours/mouse in the groups treated from day 1 to week 38, week 8 to week 38 and week 23 to week 38, respectively, with 13-*cis*-retinoic acid during stage-II promotion. The difference in the median number of papillomas per mouse between the group treated from day 1 through week 38 and the control group was statistically significant ($p < 0.05$; one-sided Wilcoxon rank sum test) (Gensler *et al.*, 1986). [The Working Group noted that no data on tumour incidence were given].

Groups of 20 female CD-1 mice, eight weeks of age, received 200 nmol of benzo[*a*]pyrene or 5 µmol of *N*-methyl-*N*'-nitro-*N*-nitrosoguanidine (MNNG) as initiator and either 17 nmol of TPA or 100 µg of anthralene as promotors for 16 weeks. 13-*cis*-Retinoic acid was applied topically at 34 nmol. The retinoid had no effect on tumour initiation when it was given once 0.5 h before benzo[*a*]pyrene or MNNG and had no effect on tumour promotion when applied 0.5 h before each application of anthralin. The controls had a 70–100% incidence of papillomas, and incidences

Table 3. Effects of 13-*cis*-retinoic acid on carcinogenesis in animals

Cancer site	Species, sex, age at carcinogen treatment	No. of animals per group	Carcinogen dose and route	13-*cis*-Retinoic acid dose and route (basal diet)	Duration in relation to carcinogen	Incidence Control	Incidence Treated	Multiplicity Control	Multiplicity Treated	Efficacy	Reference
Skin	CD-1 mice, female, 8 wks	30	0.2 mmol DMBA 8 nmol TPA	34 nmol topical	0 to 18 wk	90	50	10	4	Effective	Verma et al. (1979)
Skin	CD-1 mice, female, 8 wks	20	400 nmol B[a]P 8 nmol TPA/2x/wk,	17 nmol topical[a]	+2 wk to end	NR	NR	4.0	2.1*	Effective	Gensler et al. (1986)
Skin	CD-1 mice, female, 8 wks	20	200 nmol B[a]P 17 nmol TPA	34 nmol topical	−0.5 h	80	100	17	21	Ineffective	Gensler & Bowden (1984)
			5 µmol MNNG 17 nmol TPA	34 nmol topical	−0.5 h	100	100	8	7	Ineffective	
			400 nmol B[a]P 100 µg anthralene/2x wk	17 nmol topical	+1 wk to end	70	80	1.5	1.8	Ineffective	
Skin	CD-1 mice, female, 5–7 wks	30	200 nmol DMBA 444 nmol anthralene daily/32 wks	1.7 nmol, topical 17 nmol, topical 170 nmol, topical	+2 wk to end	64	50 55 45	1.52	0.96 1.1 0.6*	Ineffective Ineffective Effective	Dawson et al. (1987)
Skin	CD-1 mice, female, 7–9 wks	24	200 nmol DMBA 10 nmol TPA	5 mg/kg diet 50 100 200	−1 to 32 wk	84	84 64 40 25	5.5	4.0[b] 2.7[b] 1.2[b] 0.4[b]	Effective* Effective* Effective* Effective*	Verma et al. (1986)
Skin	Swiss mice, female, 8 wks	20	0.8% MCA, 14 applications	3 mg/0.1 mL acetone, topical	+3 to +9 wk	89	30	NR	NR	Effective[c]	Abdel-Galil et al. (1984)
Skin	Sencar mice, female, 7–8 wks	25	5 µg DMBA	225 mg/kg diet 30 nmol, topical	+2 wk to end +2 wk to end	4 4	79* 24*	0.1 0.1	5.9 1.4	Tumour enhancing	McCormick et al. (1987)
Urinary bladder	C57BL/6 mice, male, 6–7 wks	20–25	NBHBA 90 mg total 140 mg total i.g., 2 ×/wk/6 wks	200 mg/kg diet	+1 wk to end	38 55	5* 32	NR NR	NR NR	Effective Effective	Becci et al. (1978)
	Wistar/Lewis rats, female, 7 wks	20–23	1.5 mg MNU, 3 biweekly	120 mg/kg diet 300 mg/kg diet	0 to end	43 43	34 28	NR NR	NR NR	Effective[d] Effective[a]	Squire et al. (1977)

Table 3 (Contd)

Cancer site	Species, sex, age at carcinogen treatment	No. of animals per group	Carcinogen dose and route	13-cis-Retinoic acid dose and route (basal diet)	Duration in relation to carcinogen	Incidence Control	Incidence Treated	Multiplicity Control	Multiplicity Treated	Efficacy	Reference
Urinary bladder (contd)	Fischer 344 rats, female, 21 days	100	2 g/kg diet FANFT (1–10 wks)	120 mg/kg diet / 240 mg/kg diet	+ 2 to 50 wk	36 / 36	42 / 47	NR / NR	NR / NR	Ineffective / Ineffective	Croft et al. (1981)
	Fischer 344 rats, male, 7 wks	30	NBHBA 1200 mg total / 1800 mg total / 2400 mg total	240 mg/kg diet	1-, 5- and 9 wk delay periods combined	36 / 82 / 94	17 / 65 / 74*	NR	NR	Effective / Effective / Effective	Becci et al. (1979)
Oeso-phagus	Sprague-Dawley rats, male, 21 days	40	2 mg/kg bw NMBA Zn-deficient diet	67 mg/kg diet purified diet	0 d to end	76	94	3.04	2.3	Ineffective	Gabrial et al. (1982)
Liver	Sprague-Dawley rats, male (110–140 g)	12–24	3'-Me DAB 0.05% in diet	200 mg/kg diet	0 d to 4 wk	90	8	NR	NR	Effective	Daoud & Griffin (1980)
Kidney	Wistar rats, female, 4 wks	40	40 mg/kg bw NDMA i.p.	240 mg/kg diet	2 d to 26 wk	100	100	NR	NR	Ineffective[e]	Hard & Ogiu (1984)
Trachea	Syrian golden hamster, female (152 g)	40–46	MNU, 0.8% for 12 wks, i.t.	120 mg/kg	+1 wk to 6 mth	10	30	NR	NR	Tumour enhancing*	Stinson et al. (1981)
Trachea	Syrian, golden hamsters, male, 15 wks	40	MNU (23 times) i.t.(2 x/wk)	172 mg/kg	+1 wk to end	40	55	NR	NR	Ineffective[e]	Yarita et al. (1980)
Lung	A/J mice, male, 10 wks	20–40	Urethane i.p. 0.5 mg/kg bw / 0.5 mg/kg bw / 1.0 mg/kg bw / 1.0 mg/kg bw	150 mg/kg diet / 150 mg/kg diet / 300 mg/kg diet / 300 mg/kg diet	+2 d to 20 wk / +2 d to 20 wk / +2 d to 20 wk / +2 d to 20 wk	NR / NR / NR / NR	NR / NR / NR / NR	12 / 12 / 32 / 32	16 / 16 / 31 / 32	Inefffective / Ineffective / Ineffective / Ineffective	Frasca & Garfinkel (1981)
Salivary glands	Sprague-Dawley rats, male 130–160 g	15	1 mg DMBA injection into gland	100 mg/kg / 20 mg/kg AIN76-A diet	0 d to 22 wk	35 / 35	37 / 33	NR / NR	NR / NR	Ineffective	Alam et al. (1984)

NR, not reported; DMBA, 7,12-dimethylbenz[a]anthracene; TPA, 12-O-tetradecanoylphorbol 13-acetate; B[a]P, benzo[a]pyrene; MNNG, N-methyl-N-nitro-N-nitrosoguanidine; MCA, 3-methylcholanthrene; NBHBA, N-nitroso-N-butyl-N-4-hydroxybutylamine; MNU, N-methyl-N-nitrosourea; FANFT, N-[4-(5-nitro-2-furyl)-2-thiazolyl]formamide; MBN, N-nitrosomethylbenzylamine; 3'-Me DAB, 3'-methyl-4-dimethylaminoazobenzene; NDMA, N-nitrosodimethylamine; i.g. intragastrically; i.p., intraperitoneally; i.t., intratracheally; wk, week; d, day

* Statistically significant (see text)

[a] Stage-II tumour promotion

[b] Papillomas ≤ 4 mm diameter

[c] Carcinoma incidence was reduced from 27% in controls to 10% in treated mice.

[d] Based on histological classification of lesions

[e] Kaplan–Meier statistics indicate no protection but an increased risk for dying from tumour.

of 80–100% was seen for all combinations of skin carcinogenesis protocols. Similarly, no effect on tumour multiplicity was found [no statistics given] (Gensler & Bowden, 1984).

Groups of 30 female CD-1 mice, five to seven weeks of age, were treated with 200 nmol of DMBA. Two weeks after initiation, 13-*cis*-retinoic acid was given topically at a dose of 1.7, 17 or 170 nmol twice weekly 1 h before treatment with 444 nmol of anthralene for 32 weeks. At the end of 13-*cis*-retinoic acid treatment, the incidences of skin papillomas were 64% in control mice and 50%, 55% and 45% in the groups at the low, intermediate and high doses of 13-*cis*-retinoic acid. Tumour multiplicity was reduced from 1.5 per mouse in controls to 0.96 at the low dose, 1.1 at the intermediate dose and 0.6 ($p < 0.005$, Student's t test) at the high dose (Dawson *et al.*, 1987).

Groups of 24 female CD-1 mice, seven to nine weeks of age, were treated with 200 nmol of DMBA and 10 nmol of TPA to induce skin papillomas. 13-*cis*-Retinoic acid was included in the basal diet at concentrations of 5–200 mg/kg diet one week before and throughout the 18 weeks of TPA treatment. There were no significant differences in the number of papillomas (all sizes) per group [statistical method not given] or in the percent of animals with tumours [no statistics given]. When only papillomas $\leq$ 4 mm in diameter were counted, the papilloma yields were 4, 2.7, 1.2 and 0.4 in the mice at 5, 50, 100 and 200 mg/kg 13-*cis*-retinoic acid and 5.5 in controls ; the papilloma incidence sin these groups were 84, 64, 40 and 25% respectively, and 84% in controls (p value for tumour multiplicity = 0.0002) [statistical methods and statistics for tumour incidence not given]. In a repeat of the experiment, with 24 female CD1 mice per group, the papilloma multiplicity ($\leq$ 2 mm diameter) was 2.9 in the group receiving 100 mg/kg diet of 13-*cis*-retinoic acid and 4.9 in the controls. In this experiment the mice were allowed to live until carcinomas developed. The carcinoma incidences were 25% in the group receiving 13-*cis*-retinoic acid and 52% in controls [no statistics given]. In another experiment, with 24 female Sencar mice per group, dietary administration of 13-*cis*-retinoic acid at 50 or 100 mg/kg diet had no effect on the incidence or yield of papillomas of all sizes, but when only papillomas $\leq$ 2 mm in diameter were counted, the papilloma yield was 7.2, 5.3 and 2.1 in the control group and the groups on diets containing the two doses of 13-*cis*-retinoic acid [no statistics given] (Verma *et al.*, 1986).

Groups of 25 female Sencar mice, seven to eight weeks of age, were initiated with a single application of 5.0 µg DMBA. Two weeks after initiation, mice received either basal diet or a diet supplemented with 225 mg/kg 13-*cis*-retinoic acid. At 30 weeks after initiation, the control groups had 0.1 papillomas per mouse and a 4% incidence of skin papillomas, whereas mice treated with 13-*cis*-retinoic acid had 5.9 papillomas per mouse and an incidence of 79% ($p < 0.01$, log rank analysis). In the same study, a group of 25 mice was treated with 30 nmol of 13-*cis*-retinoic acid topically twice a week for 28 weeks. The incidence of papillomas was enhanced from 0.1 papillomas per mouse and an incidence of 4% in the controls to 1.4 papillomas per mouse and an incidence of 24% ($p < 0.05$, log rank analysis) in 13-*cis*-retinoic acid-treated animals (McCormick *et al.*, 1987).

4.2.1.2   Urinary bladder

Mouse: Groups of 20–25 male C57BL/6 mice, six to seven weeks of age, were treated intragastrically twice weekly for six weeks with a total dose of 90 or 140 mg *N*-nitroso-*N*-butyl-*N*-4-hydroxybutylamine (NBHBA). One week after the last dose of carcinogen, the mice were given either basal diet or a diet supplemented with 200 mg/kg 13-*cis*-retinoic acid as gelatinized beadlets. All animals were killed six months after the first dose of carcinogen. The incidence of bladder carcinomas was 38% with the low dose of carcinogen and 55% at the high dose; the retinoid treatment reduced the carcinoma incidences to 5% and 32%, respectively. The effect of 13-*cis*-retinoic acid on the low dose of carcinogen was significant ($p < 0.01$; χ^2 analysis) (Becci *et al.*, 1978).

Rat: Groups of 30 male Fischer 344 rats received 100, 150 or 200 mg of NBHBA intragastrically twice a week for six weeks for total doses of 1200, 1800 and 2400 mg. At one, five or nine weeks after the last intubation of NBHBA, the rats were fed either control diet or a diet containing 240 mg/kg 13-*cis*-retinoic acid. The animals were killed one year after the first administration of carcinogen. The incidence and average number of transitional-cell carcinomas was dependent on the dose of carcinogen, and 13-*cis*-retinoic acid reduced the incidences of transitional-cell carcinomas with severe atypia in all groups ($p < 0.01$; Poisson probability distribution) (Becci *et al.*, 1979).

Groups of 20–23 female Wistar/Lewis rats, six to seven weeks of age, were given three doses of 1.5 mg *N*-methyl-*N*-nitrosourea (MNU) by instillation into the bladder twice a week. 13-*cis*-Retinoic acid was included in their diet as gelatinized beadlets at concentrations of 120 or 300 mg/kg diet either with the first instillation of MNU or one day after the last instillation. All animals were killed nine months after the first MNU treatment. The results for the two groups given 13-*cis*-retinoic acid were combined for statistical analysis. The incidence of bladder tumours was 43% in controls and 34% and 28% at the low and high doses of 13-*cis*-retinoic acid (not statistically significant). When a histological classification was made of the preneoplastic lesions and invasion of epithelial cells was scored, a comparison between the control and 13-*cis*-retinoic acid groups showed statistically significant inhibition of the development of preneoplastic lesions and of cell invasion ($p < 0.05 - < 0.01$, one-sided trend test) (Squire *et al.*, 1977).

Groups of 100 female Fischer 344 rats, 21 days of age, were given 2 g/kg of diet of N-[4-(5-nitro-2-furyl)-2-thiazolyl]formamide for 10 weeks to induce urinary bladder carcinomas, and were then given 0, 120 or 240 mg/kg of diet of 13-*cis*-retinoic acid or a diet with gelatinized beadlets (extra control group of 20 animals), beginning at week 12 and continuing to the end of the study at 50 weeks. The incidence of urinary bladder transitional-cell carcinomas was 36% in the rats given the gelatinized beadlets and 42% and 47% ($p < 0.05$; exact method for contingency tables) with the low and high doses of 13-*cis*-retinoic acid, whereas the incidence of urinary bladder carcinomas in the controls on the basal diet was 85% ($p < 0.001$ as compared with the controls fed gelatinized beadlets) (Croft *et al.*, 1981).

4.2.1.3   Oesophagus
Groups of 40 male weanling Sprague Dawley rats were given N-nitrosomethylbenzylamine intragastrically twice a week for four weeks at a dose of 2 mg/kg bw, in combination with a zinc-restricted diet (7 ppm zinc). 13-*cis*-Retinoic acid was added to the diet at a concentration of 67 mg/kg from the beginning until the end of the study at 29 weeks. The incidence of oesophageal cancers was 76% in control rats and 94% in the 13-*cis*-retinoic acid-treated group. The multiplicity of tumours was 3 in the controls and 2.3 in the 13-*cis*-retinoic acid-treated group [no statistics given] (Gabrial *et al.*, 1982).

4.2.1.4   Liver
Groups of 12–25 male Sprague-Dawley rats weighing 110–140 g bw were given a diet containing 0.05%

3'-methyl-4-dimethylaminoazobenzene for nine weeks. The diet of one group of rats also contained 200 mg/kg 13-*cis*-retinoic acid during the first four weeks of the experiment. The study was terminated at nine weeks. The incidence of liver tumours was 90% in controls and 8% in rats receiving 13-*cis*-retinoic acid (Daoud & Griffin, 1980). [The Working Group noted the short duration of the experiment and that no statistics were given.]

4.2.1.5   Kidney
Groups of 40 female Wistar rats, 21 days of age, received 40 mg/kg bw N-nitrosodimethylamine intraperitoneally as a single injection and 13-*cis*-retinoic acid at a concentration of 240 mg/kg diet for 26 weeks. Both the control group and that given 13-*cis*-retinoic acid had a 100% incidence of kidney tumours [no statistics given] (Hard & Ogiu, 1984).

4.2.1.6   Respiratory tract
Groups of 40 male Syrian golden hamsters, 15 weeks of age, received two intratracheal instillations of a 1% solution of MNU each week for 18 or 23 exposures. 13-*cis*-Retinoic acid was given in the diet just after the last injection of carcinogen and continued until the end of the study 56 weeks after the last injection, at a concentration of 128 mg/kg of diet for those animals receiving 18 exposures and 172 mg/kg of diet for those receiving 23 exposures. Neither dietary concentration affected the number of tumour-bearing animals. The incidence of invasive carcinomas was 55% in the controls and 40% in the hamsters that received the dose of 172 mg/kg but the relative risk for dying from tracheal tumours was 1.7 for those animals that received 128 mg/kg and 2 for those that received 172 mg/kg ($p = 0.223$ and 0.043, respectively; χ^2 test of log-likelihood ratio) (Yarita *et al.*, 1981).

Similar results were reported by Stinson *et al.* (1981; see Table 3).

4.2.1.7   Lung
A/J male mice, 10 weeks of age were given a single intraperitoneal injection of urethane at a dose of 0.5 or 1 mg/g bw [500 or 1000 mg/kg bw]. Two days later, groups of 20–40 mice were given a basal diet containing control gelatin beadlets or a diet containing 13-*cis*-retinoic acid at 150 or 300 mg/kg. All animals were killed 20 weeks after urethane injection. The number of pulmonary adenomas per mouse (surface tumours) was 12 and

32 in mice injected with 0.5 and 1 mg/g bw of ure-thane, respectively, and maintained on control diet and 16 and 16 in the groups injected with the low dose of urethane and maintained on 150 or 300 mg/kg of diet of 13-*cis*-retinoic acid, respectively. The tumour multiplicity was 31 and 33 in the groups injected with the high dose of urethane and maintained on 150 or 300 mg/kg of diet of 13-*cis*-retinoic acid (Frasca & Garfinkel, 1981). [The Working Group noted that the tumour incidence was not given, and no statistical analysis was reported.]

4.2.1.8 Salivary gland

Groups of 14–16 male Sprague-Dawley rats were anaesthetized and dissected to expose their submandibular salivary glands. DMBA (1 mg in 20 µL olive oil) was injected into the glands and the wound was closed. The animals then received either semi-purified AIN 76A diet alone or supplemented with 13-*cis*-retinoic acid at 20 or 100 mg/kg. The study was terminated 22 weeks after initiation. The incidence of malignant salivary gland tumours was 35% in control rats, 37% in rats given the diet containing 20 mg/kg 13-*cis*-retinoic acid and 33% in rats given the diet containing 100 mg/kg (Alam *et al.*, 1984).

4.2.2 Intermediate biomarkers

Mice were given 0.2 µmol of DMBA in 0.2 mL of acetone as an initiator followed by twice weekly applications of 8 nmol of TPA; 13-*cis*-retinoic acid was applied topically 1 h before the TPA application. The mice were killed 4.5 h after the last of seven TPA treatments, and ornithine decarboxylase, which is considered a useful biomarker for experimental skin carcinogenesis, was measured. 13-*cis*-Retinoic acid reduced the activity from 3.5 to 0.04 nmol (Verma *et al.*, 1979).

4.2.3 In-vitro models

The effects of 13-*cis*-retinoic acid were analysed primarily on established tumour cell lines in monolayer culture. A few studies were carried out with immortalized cells.

4.2.3.1 Inhibition of cell proliferation

The inhibitory effects of 13-*cis*-retinoic acid were studied in various cultured cell types. The effects were usually dose-dependent in the concentration range between 1 nmol/L and 1 µmol/L and were time-dependent, being detected within 24–48 h. When changes in the cell cycle were analysed, it was found that 13-*cis*-retinoic acid treatment resulted in cell accumulation in the G_1 phase of the cell cycle. The inhibitory effects were often reversible within a few days after the drug was discontinued.

In most cell lines, the response to 13-*cis*-retinoic acid was similar to the response to all-*trans*-retinoic acid, but in some cells (e.g. head-and-neck carcinoma cell lines) 13-*cis*-retinoic acid and 9-*cis*-retinoic acid were more potent than all-*trans*-retinoic acid in inhibiting cell proliferation (Giannini *et al.*, 1997). In contrast, in other cells (e.g. gastric carcinoma) all-*trans*-retinoic acid was more potent than 13-*cis*-retinoic acid in growth suppression *in vitro* (Jiang *et al.*, 1996).

(a) Immortalized cells

13-*cis*-Retinoic acid, like all-*trans*-retinoic acid, inhibited the growth, increased the adhesiveness and induced tissue transglutaminase in spontaneously immortalized NIH-3T3 mouse fibroblasts (Cai *et al.*, 1991). 13-*cis*-Retinoic acid suppressed the proliferation of HPV-16-immortalized ectocervical epithelial cells (Agarwal *et al.*, 1996) and Epstein-Barr virus-immortalized lymphoblastoid B-cell lines (Dolcetti *et al.*, 1998). In the latter cells, inhibition of proliferation was associated with an increase in P27Kip1 and inhibition of the transition from the G_1 to S phase and appeared to be independent of induction of differentiation or of down-regulation of viral latent antigens. Unexpectedly, retinoid-induced growth arrest appeared to be irreversible at a concentration (1 µmol/L) that might be reached in humans after oral systemic therapy (Dolcetti *et al.*, 1998).

(b) Malignant cells

13-*cis*-Retinoic acid inhibited the growth of head-and-neck cancer cells, and the sensitivity of the cells was associated with the expression of RARβ (Giannini *et al.*, 1997). A similar association was found in renal cancer cell lines (Hoffman *et al.*, 1996). Other cell types whose growth was inhibited by 13-*cis*-retinoic acid include cells from prostate cancer (Dahiya *et al.*, 1994), melanoma (Lotan & Lotan, 1980; Schaber *et al.*, 1994), pancreatic cancer (Jimi *et al.*, 1998), astrocytoma (Rutka *et al.*, 1988), ovarian teratocarcinoma (Taylor *et al.*, 1990), endometrial adenocarcinoma (Carter *et al.*, 1996) and breast carcinoma (Toma *et al.*, 1997). 13-*cis*-Retinoic acid decreased the saturation cell density and mitotic indices of the human teratocarcinoma-derived cell line PA-1 after it reached confluence (Taylor *et al.*, 1990).

Inhibition of anchorage-independent growth of a human lung tumour cell line, A427, in a 28-day assay is used to screen new chemopreventive agents. In this assay, 13-*cis*-retinoic acid caused a 66 ± 16% inhibition at a concentration of 33 µmol/L (Korytynski *et al.*, 1996).

The growth of prostate cancer cells and their potential to form colonies in soft agar was decreased after 13-*cis*-retinoic acid treatment when compared with controls. In nude mice, 13-*cis*-retinoic acid-treated cells produced significantly smaller tumours than untreated cells (Dahiya *et al.*, 1994).

4.2.3.2 Modulation of differentiation

13-*cis*-Retinoic acid was found to enhance cell differentiation in several cell types. It enhanced melanogenesis in melanoma cells (Lotan & Lotan, 1980; Meyskens & Fuller, 1980), regulated the expression of cytokeratin K5, increased *RARβ* mRNA levels in immortalized ectocervical cells (Agarwal *et al.*, 1996) and caused endodermal differentiation in embryonal carcinoma F9 cells (Williams *et al.*, 1987). It was less potent than all-*trans*-retinoic acid but more potent than retinol in inducing differentiation of F9 EC cells. In the human acute promyelocytic leukaemia cell line NB4, 13-*cis*-retinoic acid was less potent than all-*trans*-retinoic acid in inducing granulocytic differentiation (Zhu *et al.*, 1995). [The Working Group noted that this difference in potency *in vitro* may partly explain the low efficacy of 13-*cis*-retinoic acid in inducing complete remission in patients with acute promyelocytic leukaemia.]

13-*cis*-Retinoic acid at 0.01 µmol/L increased the expression of keratins K13, K15 and K19 in human epidermal keratinocytes cultured on a 3T3-feeder layer, which represents an embryonic type of differentiation. The treated cells had decreased expression of the proliferation-associated K16 but an increase in the expression of K6, the other proliferation-associated keratin (Korge *et al.*, 1990).

13-*cis*-Retinoic acid at 10 µmol/L directed a human follicular cell line towards a more normal state of proliferation and differentiation, as evidenced by increases in various parameters of differentiation such as uptake of [¹²⁵I] and binding of epidermal growth factor and thyroid-stimulating hormone (Van Herle *et al.*, 1990).

Treatment of pancreatic carcinoma cells grown on collagen gels with 13-*cis*-retinoic acid resulted in a change from a fibroblastoid to epithelioid morphology. The effect was inhibited by receptor antagonists (Jimi *et al.*, 1998).

4.2.3.3 Induction of apoptosis

13-*cis*-Retinoic acid induced apoptosis in MCF-7 (ER⁺) and MDA-MB-231 (ER⁻) cell lines but not in ZR-75.1 (ER⁺) cells. The apoptotic phenomenon was time-dependent and not related to arrest in a specific phase of the cell cycle. After treatment, the expression of *bcl-2* was reduced in MCF-7, while no treatment-related modifications were observed in ZR-75.1 or MDA-MB-231 (Toma *et al.*, 1997). Induction of apoptosis in the MCF-7 breast carcinoma cell line was observed even at 0.01 µmol/L 13-*cis*-retinoic acid but required six days of incubation (Toma *et al.*, 1998).

4.2.3.4 Antimutagenicity in short-term tests for mutagenicity

(a) Mammalian cells

Few studies have investigated the possibility that 13-*cis*-retinoic acid might play a role in reducing the genotoxic damage induced by mutagens or carcinogens. In three studies of chromosomal alterations in carcinogen-treated mammalian cells involving phytohaemagglutin-stimulated human lymphocytes or lymphoblastoid cultures, the effect of retinoids on the activity of directly acting mutagens was analysed. Mixed results were obtained.

In one study, 13-*cis*-retinoic acid increased the frequencies of sister chromatid exchange and chromosomal breakage induced by diepoxybutane, a DNA cross-linking agent, in lymphocyte cultures from two persons (Auerbach *et al.*, 1984). In another, an anticlastogenic effect of this retinoid was seen against the free radical-generating agent bleomycin in four human lymphoblastoid cell lines and in primary lymphocyte cultures derived from the peripheral blood of 11 subjects. The study design involved preincubation of the cells with a wide range of concentrations of the retinoid (10^{-8} to 10^{-5} mol/L) for 24 h before addition of bleomycin (Trizna *et al.*, 1992, 1993). Addition of 13-*cis*-retinoic acid to lymphocyte cultures from a single normal individual for 1 h before X-irradiation significantly reduced the amount of chromatid damage, but no protective effect was observed when exposure to the retinoid occurred after X-ray treatment. This study also included a group of five patients with xeroderma pigmentosum who were receiving 13-*cis*-retinoic acid. Lymphocyte cultures from the blood of the patients had fewer chromatid breaks and gaps after

X-irradiation than cells from the same patients when they were not receiving retinoids. This radio-protective effect could be transferred to lympho-cytes from a normal control by co-cultivating them with plasma from a patient with xeroderma pigmentosum who was receiving 13-*cis*-retinoic acid. The authors concluded that the presence of the retinoid in the plasma of these patients during treatment was responsible for the protection (Sanford *et al.*, 1992).

13-*cis*-Retinoic acid did not significantly modu-late the binding of [³H]dimethylbenz[*a*]anthracene to the DNA of primary murine epidermal cells in culture when it was present concurrently with the carcinogen. In contrast, treatment with all-*trans*-retinoic acid, retinol and retinol acetate at the same concentrations was protective against car-cinogen–DNA binding (Shoyab, 1981).

When microsomal preparations from unin-duced Fischer female rats were incubated with 13-*cis*-retinoic acid in the presence of retinol or benzo[*a*]pyrene, the retinoid produced a signifi-cant reduction in the rate of retinol esterification and benzo[*a*]pyrene hydroxylation (Ball & Olson, 1988). In another study, the effect of exposure of primary rat hepatocyte cultures to 13-*cis*-retinoic acid for 48 h was examined on the activities of three cytochrome P450 mRNAs. The levels of P4503A mRNA were increased approximately eightfold ($p < 0.05$), and those of CYP1A1 showed a less than threefold increase (not statistically significant). In contrast, the levels of CYP1A2 mRNA were not altered (Jurima-Romet *et al.*, 1997).

(b)   Animals in vivo

Several studies in rodents also considered the effect of treatment with this drug on the activity of enzymes involved in carcinogen metabolism (Table 4). In an early study, female adult Wistar rats were fed diets containing 13-*cis*-retinoic acid at 1 or 5 mg/kg bw per day for 3, 7, 14 or 28 days. Their livers were then removed and the activities of arylhydrocarbon hydroxylase (AHH), aminopy-rine-*N*-demethylase and 7-ethoxycoumarin deethy-lase were assayed. A transitory increase in the activ-ity of aminopyrine-*N*-demethylase occurred after three days, which was decreased to control levels at seven days, and inhibition of AHH activity was seen after 28 days of treatment (Goerz *et al.*, 1984). In a later study, 13-*cis*-retinoic acid was given at a concentration of 6 mg/kg bw per day for 10 or 60 days and the effect on mono-oxygenase enzymes was measured in the liver and skin. After 10 days, a

statistically significant induction of aminopyrine-*N*-demethylase was observed in microsomes from livers of retinoid-treated animals. The activities of the other two enzymes, 7-ethoxyresorufin-*O*-deethylase and erythromycin-*N*-demethylase, were significantly reduced in both the liver and skin. In contrast, after 60 days of treatment, there was no significant difference in enzyme activity in liver or skin microsomes. Furthermore, 13-*cis*-retinoic acid reduced the inductive effects of hexachloroben-zene on aminopyrine-*N*-demethylase. Hexachloro-benzene is a potent inducer of several P450 isozymes and has been shown to be carcinogenic in various animal species (Ertürk *et al.*, 1986 ; Goerz *et al.*, 1994).

The effect of 13-*cis*-retinoic acid on the activi-ties of the hepatic and cutaneous mono-oxygenase enzymes AHH, ethoxycoumarin dealkylase and ethoxyresorufin dealkylase was studied in adult male mice. The retinoid decreased the basal activities of all three enzymes in both liver and skin, the effect on ethoxyresorufin dealkylase activity being the most marked (70% inhibition). When the retinoid was given at the same time as the carcinogen 3-methylcholanthrene, the induc-tion of each of these enzymes was suppressed by the retinoid in both tissues (Finnen & Shuster, 1984).

In a large-scale study of the induction of hepatic enzymes by 13-*cis*-retinoic acid in Sprague-Dawley rats, both a dose-range and a time-course analysis were carried out. The hepatic concentra-tions of AHH were significantly suppressed in animals fed 13-*cis*-retinoic acid, but this treatment increased the cytosolic concentrations of quinone reductase and had no effect on glutathione *S*-transferase. In order to determine the effect of this enzyme alteration on binding of a carcinogen to liver DNA *in vivo*, animals were dosed for seven days with 13-*cis*-retinoic acid at 120 mg/kg bw per day, the dose that gave maximal induction of hepatic quinone reductase and near maximal suppression of AHH. On the eighth day, the animals received an intraperitoneal injection of [³H]benzo[*a*]pyrene. Binding to DNA was reduced to 38% in the liver, 29% in the stomach and 23% in the lung but remained unchanged in the kidney (McCarthy *et al.*, 1987).

The ability of 13-*cis*-retinoic acid to inhibit the induction of micronuclei in bone-marrow poly-chromatic erythrocytes by a carcinogen has been examined in one study (Table 4). Administration of the retinoid by gavage 2 h before an intraperitoneal

Table 4. Inhibition by 13-*cis*-retinoic acid of genetic and related effects in rodents and in humans *in vivo*

Retinoid tested (dose and administration route)[a]	Carcinogen (dose and administration route)[a]	Animal strain and species	Investigated effect	Result[b]	LED/HID[c]	Reference
13-*cis*-Retinoic acid (1 or 5 mg/kg/day for 3, 7, 14 or 28 days by gavage)	None	Female adult Wistar rats	Mono-oxygenase activities			Goerz *et al.* (1984)
			Hepatic aminopyrine-*N*-demethylase	(#)		
			Hepatic arylhydrocarbon hydroxylase	+		
			Hepatic 7-ethoxycoumarin deethylase	–		
13-*cis*-Retinoic acid (6 mg/kg day orally for 10 and 60 days)	None	Female Wistar rats	Mono-oxygenase enzyme activities		No statistical difference for any enzyme at 60 days	Goerz *et al.* (1994)
			Hepatic aminopyrine-*N*-demethylase	#		
			Hepatic 7-ethoxyresorufin *O*-deethylase	#		
			Hepatic erythromycin-*N*-demethylase	#		
			Cutaneous 7-ethoxy-resorufin-*O*-deethylase	#		
			Cutaneous erythromycin-*N*-demethylase	#		
13-*cis*-Retinoic acid (0.3 µmol/kg bw i.p.)	None	Adult hairless mice	Basal mono-oxygenase enzyme activities			Finnen & Shuster (1984)
			Hepatic arylhydrocarbon hydroxylase	+	By 20%	
			Hepatic ethoxycoumarin dealkylase	+	By 20%	
			Hepatic ethoxyresorufin dealkylase	+	By 70%	
			Cutaneous arylhydrocarbon hydroxylase	+	By 24%	
			Cutaneous ethoxycoumarin dealkylase	+	By 20%	
			Cutaneous ethoxyresorufin dealkylase	+	By 70%	
13-*cis*-Retinoic acid (0.3 µmol/kg bw i.p.)	3-Methyl-cholanthrene (route not given for hepatic assay but was topical for cutaneous; no dose given)	Adult hairless mice	Induced mono-oxygenase enzyme activities			Finnen & Shuster (1984)
			Hepatic arylhydrocarbon hydroxylase	+	By 25%	
			Hepatic ethoxycoumarin dealkylase	+	By 25%	
			Hepatic ethoxyresorufin dealkylase	+	By 75%	
			Cutaneous arylhydro-carbon hydroxylase	+	By 20%	
			Cutaneous ethoxycoumarin dealkylase	+	By 20%	
			Cutaneous ethoxyresorufin dealkylase	+	By 80%	

		Table 4. (contd)				
Retinoid tested (dose and administration route)[a]	Carcinogen (dose and administration route)[a]	Animal strain and species	Investigated effect	Result[b]	LED/HID[c]	Reference
13-*cis*-Retinoic acid (Dose study: 25–235 mg/kg bw per day for 4 days; time study: 1,2,4, 7 or 14 days at 235 and 600 mg/kg bw per day; both by gavage)	None	Male Sprague-Dawley rats	Hepatic activity Microsomal arylhydro-carbon hydroxylase	+	400 mg/kg bw per day	McCarthy *et al.* (1987)
			Cytosolic glutathione-*S*-transferase	–		
			Cytosolic quinone reductase	#		
13-*cis*-Retinoic acid (120 mg/kg bw per day by gavage for 7 days)	Benzo[*a*]pyrene (2 mg/kg bw i.p. on the 8th day)	Male Sprague-Dawley rats	Covalent binding to DNA	+	ID_{38} for liver, ID_{28} for stomach, ID_{23} for lung. No effect for kidney	McCarthy *et al.* (1987)
13-*cis*-Retinoic acid (20–150 mg/kg by single gavage administration 2 h before carcinogen)	Benzo[*a*]pyrene (185 mg/kg bw i.p.)	B6C3F$_1$ mice	Micronucleus test, bone marrow	+	40 mg/kg bw	Al Dosari *et al.* (1996)
13-*cis*-Retinoic acid (1.5 mg/kg for 3 months followed by either 0.5 mg/kg 13-*cis*-retinoic acid or 30 mg/day β-carotene)	Cigarette smoke (27 current smokers, 9 former smokers, 4 never smokers)	Humans	Micronucleus test, buccal mucosal cells	+		Benner *et al.* (1994b)

i.p., intraperitoneally; ID, dose that inhibited the investigated end-point by x%, as indicated by the authors or calculated from their data
[a] Doses of retinoids and carcinogens and routes of administration are given as reported by the authors.
[b]+, inhibition of the investigated end-point; –, no effect on the investigated end-point, #, enhancement of investigated end-point; (#), weak transient enhancement on end-point
[c] LED, lowest effective dose that inhibits or enhances the investigated effect; HID, highest ineffective dose

injection of benzo[*a*]pyrene significantly reduced the frequency of micronucleus formation in the carcinogen-treated animals (Al Dosari *et al.*, 1996).

4.3 Mechanisms of cancer prevention

The studies summarized in section 4.2.3 suggest that some of the chemopreventive effects of 13-*cis*-retinoic acid may be mediated by increases in the activities of cytochrome P450 enzymes, suppression of carcinogen-induced mono-oxyge-nases and reduction of genotoxic damage induced by mutagens or carcinogens. Most of the cancer preventive activity of 13-*cis*-retinoic acid appears to occur at the promotion stage.

13-*cis*-Retinoic acid itself does not bind to retinoid receptors, but it can be considered to be a pro-drug of all-*trans*-retinoic acid because it can be isomerized to the *trans* conformation in animal systems. Therefore, 13-*cis*-retinoic acid probably exerts its effects by regulating gene expression after being converted to all-*trans*-retinoic acid, a direct ligand of retinoic acid receptors. Indeed, there is no evidence that 13-*cis*-retinoic acid exerts its effects by a receptor-independent mechanism. The reader is referred to section 4.3 in Handbook 1 for details of the mechanism of action of all-*trans*-retinoic acid.

5. Other Beneficial Effects

13-*cis*-Retinoic Acid is regarded as an effective drug when given systemically in severe forms of acne (see section 2.3).

6. Carcinogenicity

6.1 Humans

No data were available to the Working Group.

6.2 Experimental models

No data on the carcinogenicity of 13-*cis*-retinoic acid were available to the Working Group. In one study in male Sencar mice, a tumour-enhancing effect of 13-*cis*-retinoic acid was observed (McCormick *et al.*, 1987 ; see section 4.2.1.1).

7. Other Toxic Effects

7.1 Adverse effects

7.1.1 Humans

At the recommended oral dose of 13-*cis*-retinoic acid, 0.5–20 mg/kg bw as two evenly divided doses, the toxicity experienced by patients is similar to that observed after treatment with other retinoids or high doses of retinol and its esters (IARC, 1998) on vitamin A). Mucocutaneous skin reactions are the most common. Concurrent administration of α-tocopherol (800 IU/day) and 13-*cis*-retinoic acid significantly reduced the mucocutaneous toxicity, liver function abnormalities and hypertriglyceridaemia and increased overall activity in a phase-I clinical trial (Dimery *et al.*, 1997).

7.1.1.1 Mucocutaneous toxicity

(a)   Topical administration

In a comparison of the effectiveness and toxicity of topically applied 0.05% 13-*cis*-retinoic acid gel and 0.05% all-*trans*-retinoic acid cream for the treatment of acne vulgaris, the two agents were found to have similar efficacy, but 13-*cis*-retinoic acid was less toxic: 10 of 15 subjects given all-*trans*-retinoic acid complained of stinging, erythema and desquamation during the 12-week treatment, but only 7 of 15 subjects given 13-*cis*-retinoic acid complained of mild skin irritation (Dominguez *et al.*, 1998).

(b)   Oral administration

The most frequent side-effects experienced with orally administered 13-*cis*-retinoic acid are mucocutaneous reactions, which are generally dose-dependent. Skin reactions can usually be tolerated without interruption of therapy with the use of emollients and other treatments, and the effects generally resolve upon discontinuation of

therapy. Drying of the mucosa of the mouth, nose and eyes is common, and cheilitis occurs in over 90% of patients. Facial dermatitis, rash, increased sensitivity to ultraviolet light, varicella zoster infection, erythema nodosum, erythema multiforme, urticaria, paronychia and median canaliform dystrophy have also been reported (Bigby & Stern, 1988; Dharmagunawardena & Charles-Holmes, 1997; Meigel, 1997). Pyoderma gangrenosum requiring hospitalization occurred

in a 17-year-old boy taking 13-*cis*-retinoic acid therapy for acne. Two weeks after beginning therapy at 0.5 mg/kg bw per day, he developed an erythematous papule over the mid-line chest, which became ulcerated and enlarged rapidly even when 13-*cis*-retinoic acid was discontinued. The ulcer healed, with scarring, after treatment with hydrocortisone and prednisolone (Gangaram *et al.*, 1997).

In a phase-III study of the efficacy of 13-*cis*-retinoic acid at 0.15 mg/kg bw per day for three years in the chemoprevention of new basal-cell carcinoma, the prevalence of mucocutaneous reactions was significantly higher in the treated group (70% versus 35%) (Tangrea *et al.*, 1992b, 1993). In a phase-I/II study of the use of 13-*cis*-retinoic acid to prevent acute leukaemia, the starting dose of 1 mg/kg bw twice daily for one month was escalated by 0.5 mg/kg bw per day at monthly intervals. The highest dose achieved was 2 mg/kg bw per day because of significant toxicity, including severely dry skin, cheilitis, conjunctivitis and epistaxis (Greenberg *et al.*, 1985). In a phase-II investigation of the use of 13-*cis*-retinoic acid for regression of aggressive laryngeal papillomatosis, a dose of 1–2 mg/kg bw per day was used for 5–20 months. The reported effects include cheilosis, dry skin, balanitis, conjunctivitis and epistaxis (Alberts *et al.*, 1986). A phase-II study of its use in mycosis fungoides began with a dose of 2 mg/kg bw per day; however, since most subjects developed dryness of the skin and mucous membranes, subsequent patients started at 1 mg/kg bw per day (Kessler *et al.*, 1987). A dose of 1 mg/kg bw per day for six months was used in a phase-II double-blinded study in chronic smokers found to have squamous metaplasia and/or dysplasia in bronchial biopsies. The symptoms that were more frequent in the treated group were cheilitis, skin dryness, conjunctivitis, hypertriglyceridaemia, arthralgia and rash (Lee *et al.*, 1994). In a phase-II trial in patients with oral leukoplakia, an initiation phase of 1.5 mg/kg bw per day for three months was followed by a maintenance phase of 0.5 mg/kg bw per day for nine months. Sixty-eight subjects completed one month of induction, most reporting at least low-grade toxicity; 23 subjects experienced grade 3 or 4 toxicity during the induction phase. The effects seen were typical of those associated with orally administered 13-*cis*-retinoic acid and included dry skin, cheilitis, conjunctivitis and triglyceridaemia. No effects on the liver were observed at either the induction or maintenance dose (Lippman *et al.*, 1993).

7.1.1.2 Ocular toxicity
Dry eyes and conjunctivitis are common side-effects of 13-*cis*-retinoic acid. Development of cataracts, keratoconus, keratitis and blepharitis have also been reported, and headaches, a common effect of retinoid therapy, are sometimes accompanied by visual disturbances (Bigby & Stern, 1988). Retinoic acid analogues may be incorporated into the rod photoreceptor elements during the continuous process of outer disc shedding and renewal, and this may contribute to reported disturbances of night vision (Lerman, 1992). Adverse ocular reactions do not usually require discontinuation of treatment since they are often reversible; however, persistent dry eye syndrome and evidence of unresolved lens abnormalities have been reported in some subjects even after cessation of therapy (Brown & Grattan, 1989; Lerman, 1992; Meigel, 1997).

The ocular effects of 13-*cis*-retinoic acid were examined in 55 patients undergoing treatment [dose not given] for severe nodular acne. The adverse effects were decreased tear-film break-up time, increased blepharitis and a large increase in colonization of *Staphylococcus aureus*. All of the ocular complications manifested within four weeks of initiation and were fully reversible upon discontinuation of treatment (Egger *et al.*, 1995).

7.1.1.3 Musculoskeletal toxicity
In children and adolescents given prolonged courses (16–87 months) of treatment at doses up to 4 mg/kg per day, musculoskeletal complaints (myalgia, arthralgia), vertebral hyperostoses with diffuse fractures and hyperostoses in the greater and lesser trochanters and at fascial insertions can develop (Pittsley & Yoder, 1983). Most of the changes are dose-dependent (Ellis *et al.*, 1985) and subtle, with small hyperostoses at insertions of the spinal ligaments, the plantar fascia, clavicle or Achilles tendon (Carey *et al.*, 1988). The toxicity

seen in adolescents (Erhardt & Harangi, 1997) is similar to that in adults (Kilcoyne *et al.*, 1986). The upper trunk, middle and lower part of the thoracic and lumbar spine, the appendicular skeleton and the muscles of the legs can be involved (Shalita *et al.*, 1988). In some of these patients, the consequences are more severe, beginning with accumulations of small osteophytes along the anterior cervical and thoracic vertebrae, followed by ossification of the anterior and posterior longitudinal ligaments, leading to spinal cord compression (Pittsley & Yoder, 1983; Pennes *et al.*, 1984, 1985; Kilcoyne *et al.*, 1986; Carey *et al.*, 1988; Pennes *et al.*, 1988; Scuderi *et al.*, 1993). Of even greater concern is the frank skeletal toxicity in the long bones, manifest by radiodense metaphyseal bands, growth arrest (Marini *et al.*, 1988), relative narrowing of the diaphyses in femora and tibiae and premature epiphyseal closure (Milstone *et al.*, 1982; Valentic & Barr, 1985; Lawson & McGuire, 1987). Patients as young as three years have developed signs of early osteoporosis (Lawson & McGuire, 1987), and skeletal toxicity can become evident in as little as five weeks (Novick *et al.*, 1984).

Rheumatological symptoms are common in adults treated with 13-*cis*-retinoic acid, although these effects are generally subclinical (reviewed by Kaplan & Haettich, 1991). The rheumatoid symptoms include hyperostosis of the spine and appendicular bone, abnormalities of calcium metabolism, arthritis and musculoskeletal pain. Of the rheumatoid symptoms, hyperostosis is the most common and occurs mainly with protracted treatment and high doses. The incidence may exceed 80% after a few years of administration (Kaplan & Haettich, 1991). Achilles tenosynovitis, myalgia and arthralgia are also associated with oral administration of 13-*cis*-retinoic acid (Bigby & Stern, 1988).

In order to evaluate the chronic effect of 13-*cis*-retinoic acid, 10 subjects were given 0.15 mg/kg bw per day for nine months. One subject discontinued because of joint pain, and myalgia and/or arthralgia occurred in 30% of the participants (Edwards *et al.*, 1986). In a phase-II pilot study of patients with leukoplakia, the subjects started at a dose of 1 mg/kg bw per day until a clinical response was observed and then received 0.25 mg/kg bw per day indefinitely. Of the 15 subjects enrolled in the study, two withdrew because of persistent bone pain and photosensitivity. Of the nine subjects who completed therapy, 22% experienced bone pain (Beenken *et al.*, 1994).

The influence of 13-*cis*-retinoic acid on bone density was investigated in 15 male patients receiving a six-month treatment with average initial dose of 0.9 mg/kg bw per day, reduced every four weeks to an average final dose of 0.4 mg/kg bw per day (Kocijancic, 1995). Short-term treatment with low doses of 13-*cis*-retinoic acid thus has no clinically important effects on bone density. A similar conclusion was reached in a study of nine subjects treated with a six-month course of 13-*cis*-retinoic acid (average initial dose, 0.7 mg/kg bw adjusted to a maintenance dose of 0.9 mg/kg bw per day after 1–3 months), although transient inhibitory effects on markers of bone turnover were observed (Kindmark et al., 1998).

7.1.1.4 Metabolic and haematological disorders

Approximately 25% of patients treated with 13-*cis*-retinoic acid for acne have disturbances of lipid metabolism, manifesting as hyperlipidaemia with or without hypercholesterolaemia. Rarely, acute complications develop secondary to hyperglyceridaemia, such as pancreatitis (Meigel, 1997). Haematopoietic and lymphatic complications have been reported, including leukopenia and anaemia (Bigby & Stern, 1988).

In a phase-I/II study of the use of 13-*cis*-retinoic acid in myelodysplastic syndrome, a starting dose of 1 mg/kg bw per day was escalated by 0.5 mg/kg bw per day at monthly intervals. The dose-limiting toxic effect in this study was thrombocytopenia, an unexpected observation (Greenberg et al., 1985). In another study, the same population was given 20–125 mg/m² per day for 21 days. Hepatotoxicity (hyperbilirubinaemia and elevated serum alanine transaminase activity) was dose-limiting. The most common adverse effects were hyperkeratosis, cheilosis and haematological responses, and the concentration of serum lipids was increased at 80 mg/m² per day (Gold et al., 1983). In a phase-III study of the efficacy of 13-*cis*-retinoic acid on the prevention of new basal-cell carcinoma, a dose of 0.15 mg/kg bw per day for three years increased serum triglycerides in 7% of subjects (2% with placebo) (Tangrea et al., 1992b, 1993). In studies of the efficacy of orally administered 13-*cis*-retinoic acid in the prevention of skin cancer, the doses ranged from 5–10 mg per day to 2 mg/kg bw per day. Two of seven subjects given the highest dose were able to complete two years of therapy. Increased liver function and triglycerides were observed in some subjects; the liver function returned to normal during therapy, although one subject was required to withdraw from treatment because of persistent abnormalities in tests for liver function. The toxicity and abnormal clinical chemistry parameters were less severe when a dose of 0.5 mg/kg bw per day was used (Kraemer et al., 1992). With 5–10 mg per day for three years, approximately 1% of subjects experienced clinical adverse reactions, consisting primarily of elevated serum cholesterol concentration or liver enzyme activity (Moon et al., 1997).

In a phase-II clinical trial of the use of interferon-α (5 x 10⁶ U/m³) in combination with 13-*cis*-retinoic acid (1 mg/kg bw per day) in 13 patients with metastatic melanoma, all patients experienced elevated serum cholesterol and tryglyceride concentrations, in addition to fatigue, myalgia, anorexia, stomatitis and cheilitis. Seven patients required 50% reductions in the 13-*cis*-retinoic acid dose because of hypertriglyceridaemia, fatigue, severe stomatitis with anorexia and weight loss (Rosenthal & Oratz, 1998). The same combination was investigated in a phase-II trial in patients with recurrent squamous-cell cervical carcinoma. The starting doses were 1 mg/kg bw per day 13-*cis*-retinoic acid and 6 x 10⁶ U/day recombinant interferon-α$_{2a}$. Thirty- four patients were evaluable for toxicity. Four patients developed grade 3 or higher anaemia, 13 developed grades 1–3 leukopenia (median nadir of leukocytes, 2800), three developed grade 3 neutropenia and two developed grade 3 thrombocytopenia. Other severe events included gastro-intestinal toxicity of grade 3 or higher and grade 3 neurological toxicity (Look et al., 1998). The combination of interferon-α, interleukin-2 and 13-*cis*-retinoic acid was studied in patients with metastatic renal-cell carcinoma. Severe hyperlipidaemia was observed in a small fraction of patients, which was attributed to the 13-*cis*-retinoic acid (1 mg/kg bw per day) and appeared to be cumulative with successive cycles (Stadler et al., 1998). Hypercalcaemia was the dose-limiting toxic effect of 13-*cis*-retinoic acid in 39 children who had received a bone-marrow transplant, 23% of whom developed grades 1–3 hypercalcaemia (Villablanca et al., 1993).

Mild increases in the activity of aminotransferases were reported in 5–35% of patients receiving 0.5–3 mg/kg bw per day for three months, but these were reversible on discontinuation of therapy. Pharmacokinetic and clinical data suggested that 13-*cis*-retinoic acid is not concentrated in the liver, and there is little evidence that it causes significant hepatotoxicity (Fallon &

Boyer, 1990). This conclusion may not apply to all patient populations, however; in a phase-II trial in which 13-*cis*-retinoic acid was given at 1 mg/kg bw per day to people with HIV-associated Kaposi sarcoma, hepatotoxicity was observed in 27% (Bower *et al.*, 1997).

7.1.1.5   *Effects on the central nervous system*
Headache, often described as severe and unrelenting, decreased hearing acuity, dizziness, oculogyric crisis and personality disorder have been associated with oral administration of 13-*cis*-retinoic acid for dermatological conditions. Fixation of the eyes in one direction, facial spasm and loss of speech developed in one patient after two weeks. Loss of libido, impotence and insomnia were reported by one subject. Evidence of pseudo-tumour cerebri has been found in subjects complaining of headaches (Bigby & Stern, 1988). Reports of severe depression, psychosis and suicides prompted the United States Food and Drug Administration to warn that oral use of 13-*cis*-retinoic acid for treatment of acne may cause uncommon psychotic disorders. It was noted that such problems might be more common among patients likely to take the drug (Josefson, 1998; Nightingale, 1998)

7.1.1.6   *Urogenital toxicity*
Renal impairment developed in one 34-year-old man after treatment for acne with 40 mg/day of 13-*cis*-retinoic acid for two months. He developed a moderate inflammatory syndrome, elevated creatinine concentration, proteinuria and haematuria with no indication of infection or abnormal immunological responses. With hydration and discontinuation of 13-*cis*-retinoic acid, the creatinine concentration returned to normal within seven days and the proteinuria, haematuria and inflammatory syndrome resolved within three days (Pavese *et al.*, 1997). Several cases of urethritis have been associated with temporary administration of 13-*cis*-retinoic acid (Edwards & Sonnex, 1997).

7.1.1.7   *Other toxicity*
In a phase-II trial of 13-*cis*-retinoic acid in combination with interleukin-2 and interferon-α in patients with metastatic renal carcinoma, 13-*cis*-retinoic acid was administered at 1 mg/kg bw per day. Eleven patients required 15 dose reductions because of toxicity attributed to 13-*cis*-retinoic acid. Flu-like symptoms (fever, chill, rigor, myalgia,

arthralgia) developed in all patients and were considered severe in 21% of the patients during the first cycle. These symptoms tended to abate over time and with additional cycles, with the exception of fatigue, which worsened with prolonged therapy (Stadler *et al.*, 1998).

7.1.2   **Experimental models**
7.1.2.1   *Acute and short-term toxicity*
The LD_{50} of 13-*cis*-retinoic acid in mice and rats treated orally was 3400 and 4000 mg/kg bw, respectively; the LD_{50} was approximately 2000 mg/kg bw in rabbits (Kamm, 1982). In studies to find the maximum tolerated dose of 13-*cis*-retinoic acid in athymic nude mice before conducting studies of tumour suppression, no symptoms of hypervitaminosis A were seen over the dose range of 10–100 mg/kg bw per day, although body weight decreased by about 7%. A dose of 120 mg/kg was chosen for further evaluation (Shalinsky *et al.*, 1995). During examination of the effect of 13-*cis*-retinoic acid on MNU-induced tumours in Sprague-Dawley rats, oral doses of 25–200 mg/kg bw per day were administered for four weeks. Body-weight loss, alopecia and eye crusting were found in all animals, and 50% of those at the high dose died (Hsu, 1998).

Rats received 10–50 mg/kg bw per day in the diet for 90 days and dogs received 120 mg/kg bw by capsule for seven weeks. The dose-related effects included decreased food consumption and body-weight gain, erythema, alopecia, mucosal changes, elevated serum alkaline phosphatase and transaminase activities, increased liver weight and decreased testicular weight. The effects seen only in rats included long bone fractures and elevated serum triglyceride concentrations; those seen only in dogs were apparent joint pain and decreased spermatogenesis (Kamm, 1982; Kamm *et al.*, 1984). In an independent study, 4–40 mg/kg bw per day given to rats orally for 12 weeks caused significant dose-related decreases in plasma albumin concentration and increased haemoglobin and alkaline phosphatase activity. The changes in albumin and haemoglobin were greater in female than in male animals. Only one bone fracture and no histological changes occurred (Hixson *et al.*, 1979). In mice given 60–400 mg/kg bw per day orally for 21 days, the main dose-related effects included bone fractures, dermal or epidermal inflammation and hyperkeratosis. Alkaline phosphatase activity was increased only at 80, 160 and 320 mg/kg bw per day. The bone fractures were not always accompanied by increases in alkaline phosphatase activity (Hixson & Denine, 1978).

7.1.2.2 Ocular toxicity

The effect of long-term systemic use of 13-cis-retinoic acid on the eyelids was investigated in female New Zealand rabbits treated orally for 60 days with 2 mg/kg bw per day 13-cis-retinoic acid. All 20 treated animals showed mild clinical signs of blepharoconjunctivitis, including hyperaemia of the eyelid margins and tearing. Histopathological examination revealed marked degenerative changes in the meibomian glands of both upper and lower eyelids. The acini of the meibomian glands showed a decreased number of basaloid epithelial cells, and remnants of degenerated and necrotic acinar cells, and secretory debris were noted in the lumina of the affected glands. There was no evidence of an inflammatory reaction in the affected glands or the eyelid tissue surrounding them, and there was no evidence of significant periacinar fibrosis (Kremer et al., 1994).

7.1.2.3 Long-term toxicity

13-cis-Retinoic acid was administered to rats at doses of 2, 18 or 32 mg/kg bw per day to rats in the diet for two years, after an initial 13-week period at 1 mg/kg bw per day to avoid fractures in young, growing animals. The dose-related effects included increased mortality rate and decreased food consumption and body-weight gain. Decreased haemoglobin and haematocrit and elevated serum triglyceride concentrations were observed at the two highest doses. Increased alkaline phosphatase activity and increased liver and kidney weights were observed in all treated groups. The non-neoplastic histological changes that occurred at increased incidences in animals at the two highest doses included fibrosis and inflammation of the myocardium, arterial calcification, focal tissue calcification and focal osteolysis of the bone (Kamm, 1982; Kamm et al., 1984).

In a 55-week study in dogs, the animals were started at 3, 20 or 120 mg/kg bw per day by capsule. Within four weeks, the dogs at the highest dose had severe weight loss and debilitation, and dosing was resumed only eight weeks later on a cycle of 60 mg/kg bw per day for six weeks and no treatment for two weeks. The clinical signs of toxicity observed during the treatment cycle included severe weight loss, skin changes, ophthalmic changes (e.g. corneal ulcers and corneal opacity), decreased haemoglobin and

haematocrit and increased serum alkaline phosphatase activity; most of the signs diminished during the rest periods. The ocular changes tended to revert to normal with discontinuation of treatment but did not completely clear during the observation periods. The microscopic changes included fibrosis and focal calcification in the myocardium and aorta, increased liver weight, testicular atrophy with spermatogenic arrest and lymph node oedema. Although increased liver weight and testicular atrophy with spermatogenic arrest were also observed at the intermediate dose, no clinical or histological signs of toxicity were found at the lowest dose (Arky, 1998).

7.2 Reproductive and developmental effects

7.2.1 Humans

7.2.1.1 Reproductive effects

No evidence was found of changes in serum testosterone, follicle-stimulating hormone or luteinizing hormone or in testicular size, sperm count or morphological apperance in patients receiving a therapeutic course of 13-cis-retinoic acid (Peck et al., 1979, 1982; Török & Kasa, 1985). In 20 men aged 15–42 years with acne, two of whom had normozoospermia and 18 had oligospermia or other abnormal sperm parameters, given 0.2–2 mg/kg bw per day for three months (followed by drug withdrawal or 0.5 mg/kg per day for the next three months), no statistically significant changes in total sperm output, motility or morphology were observed. In those patients with pre-existing sperm abnormalities, the motility and morphology improved but returned to pre-treatment levels three months after withdrawal of the drug. The authors attributed the improvements in semen quality to the anti-inflammatory properties of 13-cis-retinoic acid at therapeutic doses (Schill et al., 1981). Among the adverse events associated with therapeutic use of 13-cis-retinoic acid in men are isolated reports of impotence, gynaecomastia, ejaculatory failure and local inflammation. Case reports of male reproductive tract toxicity constitute no more than 1% of all drug side-effects (Coleman & MacDonald, 1994).

Abnormal or irregular menses (less frequent or lighter bleeding, 'skipped' or 'late' menstrual periods or menorrhagia) associated with use of 13-cis-retinoic acid have been reported only infrequently (Christmas, 1988; Cox, 1988) but can occur in 2–11% (Bruno et al., 1984) to, in one report, all of five healthy women given the drug (Edwards et al., 1986). These reports are inconsistent in that a greater incidence of such complaints occurred in patients given lower doses (0.1–0.22 or 0.11–0.14 mg/kg bw per day) (Bruno *et al.*, 1984; Edwards *et al.*, 1986) than in those given higher doses (0.75–1.21 mg/kg bw per day) (Bruno *et al.*, 1984).

In general, urinary and circulating steroids were not clinically altered in women given 13-*cis*-retinoic acid orally for up to 20 weeks (Lookingbill *et al.*, 1988; Matsuoka *et al.*, 1989; Rademaker *et al.*, 1991).

Among 10 women aged 19–29 who were maintained on 0.5 mg/kg bw per day, there was no evidence for systemic interference or interaction between 13-*cis*-retinoic acid and orally administered laevonorgestrel and ethinyloestradiol. The authors therefore considered that 13-*cis*-retinoic acid at 1 mg/kg bw per day would probably not interfere with the actions of oral contraceptive steroids (Orme *et al.*, 1984a,b).

7.2.1.2 Developmental effects

In June 1983, the first United Stated Food and Drug Administration alert on 13-*cis*-retinoic acid-induced teratogenicity was issued, after two spontaneous abortions occurred in a prospective cohort study. Within the next two weeks, the first three cases of 13-*cis*-retinoic acid embryopathy had been identified (Rosa, 1992). Between 1982 and 1984, 120 000 women of childbearing potential in the USA were treated. Thirty-five pregnancies associated with 13-*cis*-retinoic acid treatment were reported to the Administration, 29 of which resulted in spontaneous abortion or infants with birth defects, while six infants were normal (Stern *et al.*, 1984; Orfanos, 1985).

While seven adverse pregnancy outcomes in which the father had been exposed were reported up to 1992, the pattern of congenital malformation was diverse. These cases are considered chance associations, particularly since maternal use of the father's prescription was not always excluded (Rosa, 1992). Since 13-*cis*-retinoic acid is not genotoxic and since the preclinical studies showed no sign of developmental toxicity after paternal exposure alone (reviewed by Howard & Willhite, 1986), the human risk for teratogenic effects due to transmission of 13-*cis*-retinoic acid in semen or by other means is considered negligible.

The symptoms of 13-*cis*-retinoic acid embryopathy in humans and animals are remarkably consistent (Braun *et al.*, 1984; Howard & Willhite, 1986; Willhite *et al.*, 1986; Rosa, 1992; Newman *et al.*, 1993). The neuropsychological deficits induced by 13-*cis*-retinoic acid in rodents are also reflected in human experience (Adams, 1993). From a case series of 61 infants who had been exposed to 13-*cis*-retinoic acid, Lynberg *et al.* (1990) calculated a rate of 25% for major defects (excluding neuropsychological delay or deficit) and an overall relative risk of 7.1 (Khoury *et al.*, 1991). If the risk for spontaneous and elective abortion and for developmental delay and mental retardation is excluded, the mean prospective risk for major craniofacial, cardiac, thymic and central nervous system terata is 21–26% [95% confidence interval, 11–58] (Koebert *et al.*, 1993; Lammer *et al.*, 1985; Dai *et al.*, 1992). These estimates do not account for under-diagnosis and under-reporting of identified cases (Ayme *et al.*, 1988; Rosa, 1992). As of 1993, 94 abnormal pregnancy outcomes had been confirmed, which did not include embryos that were spontaneously aborted (absolute risk, 40%), delivered prematurely (absolute risk, 16%) (Lammer, 1988), terminated by elective abortion or were not reported to the Food and Drug Administration (Schardein, 1993). Of women exposed to 13-*cis*-retinoic acid, 64% elect to have an abortion (Anon., 1986). For all courses of treatment, Chan *et al.* (1995) estimated that one elective abortion occurred for every 319 prescriptions for 13-*cis*-retinoic acid that were filled.

The period of exposure considered to incur the highest risk is two to five weeks after conception (Rosa, 1992). Even brief exposure (three days) during the first month of gestation is sufficient to induce terata (Hersh *et al.*, 1985), but not all mothers who have taken the drug before and during the most sensitive stages of embryogenesis have given birth to affected infants (Kassis *et al.*, 1985). If exposure is stopped at least 2 to > 60 days before conception, the risks for malformation (5%) or spontaneous abortion (9.1%) are not significantly different from those for women of reproductive age in the general population (Dai *et al.*, 1989). At least two cases of functional neurological deficit have been reported, however, with limited exposure until after completion of the first trimester (Rosa, 1992). The guidelines recommend that contraception be continued for at least one month after drug withdrawal (Teratology Society, 1991).

The structural terata observed in infants born to mothers given 0.5–1.5 mg/kg bw per day arise primarily in those organs and tissues derived from the cranial neural crest and branchial apparatus (Benke, 1984; Fernhoff & Lammer, 1984; Rosa,

1984; Coberly et al., 1996). Rudimentary pinnae, microtia or anotia (Lott et al., 1984; Hill, 1984; Tremblay et al., 1985; Jahn & Ganti, 1987; Lynberg et al., 1990), congenital deafness (due to a vestigal tympanic membrane and/or malformation of the middle and inner ear), conotruncal cardiac defects (double outlet right ventricle, atrial and ventricular septal defects), tetralogy of Fallot (pulmonary stenosis, ventricular septal defect, overriding aorta, right ventricular hypertrophy), preductal aortic coarctation and related aorticopulmonary septation abnormalities (interrupted/hypoplastic ascending aorta, patent ductus arteriosus, aortic/pulmonary stenosis; dysplastic pulmonary arch), ectopic, hypoplastic or aplastic thymic defects, retinal and optic nerve anomalies (evident in strabismus, nystagmus or eyes that cannot follow; abnormal visual-evoked potential), cleft palate, micrognathia, mandibular asymmetry, Dandy–Walker malformation of the central nervous system (deficient or absent vermis, cerebellar agenesis or hypoplasia, absent aqueduct, dysplastic or malformed inferior medullary olive and/or pontine nuclei, dilated ventricle, focal cortical agenesis), skull malformations (hypertelorism, depressed nasal bridge, maxillary hypoplasia) and facial nerve paralysis constitute the constellation of terata (Lammer, 1988; Lynberg et al., 1990). Elevation of the tentorium cerebelli and the prominent occiput arise from cystic dilatation of the fourth ventricle (Lammer & Armstrong, 1992). Cleft palate, hydrocephalus (usually secondary to aqueductal stenosis), microcephaly, lissencephaly, holoprosencephaly, microphthalmia and malformations of the axial (occult spina bifida) and appendicular skeleton (absent clavicle, synostosis, oligodactyly, camptodactyly) are rather less common (de la Cruz et al., 1984; McBride, 1985; Robertson & MacLeod, 1985; Lammer, 1988; Rizzo et al., 1991; Rosa, 1992). Autopsy of four neonates who died at weeks 14–156 showed membranous atresia of the external auditory canals and Mondini–Alexander defect (flattened cochlea with fewer turns than normal, near complete absence of cochlear neurons, abnormally large utricle and saccule) and malformation of the external ear (Siebert & Lammer, 1990 ; Burk & Willhite, 1992; Coberly et al., 1996). An evaluation of 61 cases of 13-cis-retinoic acid-exposed infants with birth defects showed that 70% had some type of ear malformation and 50% had some kind of ear defect combined with cardiovascular and/or central

nervous system defect (Lynberg et al., 1990; Khoury et al., 1991). Those infants who survive can develop congestive heart failure, acute respiratory distress and seizures (Jahn & Ganti, 1987) and become cyanotic. They may have difficulty in feeding because of an impaired ability to suck (Hill, 1984; Westerman et al., 1994). Clinical signs of impaired or abnormal neurological development include hypotonia, hypertonia and cranial nerve pareses (Lammer & Armstrong, 1992).

Longitudinal follow-up of children at five years of age who had been exposed to 13-cis-retinoic acid in utero showed that at least 20% were mentally retarded and 43–47% were of substandard intelligence. All children with an intelligence quotient (IQ) < 71 had structural terata, and the majority had malformations of the central nervous system; structural terata were found in 40% of children with an IQ of 71–85 and 10% of those with an IQ of 86–115. None of the children with an IQ > 116 (the smallest percentage of the population) had malformations of the central nervous system. Many of these children had considerable motor deficits and were unable to walk or sit. Having one or more major congenital malformations of the brain was always associated with borderline to frank mental retardation in children who otherwise showed no structural terata or malformation. Among those with a normal IQ, 16% had an uncommon non-verbal learning disability manifest in difficulties with spatial cognition (e.g. inability to understand shapes and forms and trouble reading a map). These problems were often evidenced by an inability to form complete sentences or to articulate complete thoughts (Adams & Lammer, 1991, 1993).

Despite a vigorous education programme aimed at patients and their physicians (Marwick, 1984) and requiring informed consent before prescription of the drug to pregnant women (Zarowny, 1984; Stern, 1989), cases of 13-cis-retinoic acid embryopathy persist (Rappaport & Knapp, 1989; Pilorget et al., 1995; Holmes et al., 1998). Mothers as young as 15 to women in their early 40s (average age, 25 ± 6.7 years) were affected; 31% of the mothers were adolescents, 77% were aware that the drug was teratogenic and most (86%) were high-school graduates (Adams & Lammer, 1993; Pastuszak et al., 1994), yet 38% still used no means of contraception and 8% had ceased contraception while on the drug (Pastuszak et al., 1994). Some 87% of the affected pregnancies occurred after a prescription by a dermatologist.

Early reports showed that 50% of the female patients practised no contraception and 33% were pregnant at the initiation of therapy (Strauss *et al.*, 1988). Between 1989 and 1993, 3.4 pregnancies occurred for every 1000 courses of treatment in the USA, and the rate of elective abortion was 2.3 for every 1000 courses of treatment (Mitchell *et al.*, 1995). The fact that 33–35% of all female patients capable of bearing children did not use any contraceptive methods while on the drug is a consistent finding (Lammer *et al.*, 1985; Hogan *et al.*, 1988). Patient compliance with contraception during therapy with 13-*cis*-retinoic acid has thus been problematic, despite required routine labelling, printed patient brochures, patient checklists and pregnancy testing before, during and after treatment, signature of a consent form acknowledging their instructions, suggestions for two simultaneous forms of contraception and viewing an instructional videotape (Pastuszak *et al.*, 1994; Moskop *et al.*, 1997). Moskop *et al.* (1997) concluded:

"The opportunity for benefit and the responsibility to prevent harm are inseparably linked in the use of 13-*cis*-retinoic acid — if patients are to reap the benefits of this drug, they must also share with the drug's manufacturer and its physician-prescribers, in the responsibility to prevent its harms."

The developmental and clinical toxicology of oral 13-*cis*-retinoic acid in paediatric patients has been summarized (DiGiovanna & Peck, 1983).

7.2.2 Experimental models

7.2.2.1 Reproductive effects

Rats treated with 13-*cis*-retinoic acid at 30 mg/kg bw daily for eight weeks did not show effects on spermatogenesis (Kuhlwein & Schütte 1985). In rats fed 10, 25 or 50 mg/kg bw 13-*cis*-retinoic acid daily for 13 weeks, however, there was a dose-dependent reduction in testicular weight and histological evidence of decreased spermatogenesis. Similar effects were found in dogs given 120 mg/kg bw daily for seven weeks (Kamm, 1982).

7.2.2.2 Developmental effects

Numerous studies have shown that embryos of every animal species are susceptible to the embryotoxic effects of excess 13-*cis*-retinoic acid (Table 5). The types of terata resemble those seen with all-*trans*-retinoic acid (see Handbook 1, section 7.2.1).

The bioavailability and potential developmental toxicity of 13-*cis*-retinoic acid after topical application were evaluated. [The Working Group noted that experiments with animals are difficult to interpret because potentially teratogenic doses may ulcerate or otherwise damage their skin. Studies in humans and animals suggest low bioavailability and low teratogenicity of topical 13-*cis*-retinoic acid (Chen *et al.*, 1997).

The teratogenic potency of 13-*cis*-retinoic acid has marked interspecies variation: the lowest teratogenic doses of this retinoid in mice and rats are one order of magnitude higher than those in rabbits and cynomolgus monkeys (see Table 5) and > 100-fold higher than those in humans (see section 7.2.1). In mice and rats, the lowest teratogenic doses are much higher than the corresponding doses of the all-*trans*-isomer. In contrast, in rabbits and cynomolgus monkeys, the differences between the two retinoids are not as marked, and 13-*cis*-retinoic acid appears to be a more potent teratogen than all-*trans*-retinoic acid in monkeys (Hummler *et al.*, 1990; Korte *et al.*, 1993).

The plasma elimination rate of 13-*cis*-retinoic acid shows much more pronounced interspecies variation than that of all-*trans*-retinoic acid (Nau, 1990, 1995). The plasma half-life of 13-*cis*-retinoic acid was comparable to that of all-*trans*-retinoic acid only in mice and rats, whereas it was one order of magnitude higher in rabbits, monkeys and humans (reviewed by Nau, 1995).

Embryonic concentrations of 13-*cis*-retinoic acid and 13-*cis*-4-oxoretinoic acid were one order of magnitude lower than the plasma concentrations after dosing of the maternal animals with 13-*cis*-retinoic acid. The embryonic concentrations of 13-*cis*-retinoic acid were < 5% of the plasma concentrations after administration to mice, rats and rabbits at mid-gestation; higher embryo:maternal plasma concentration ratios for 13-*cis*-retinoic acid were observed at later gestational stages in rats and mice (Tzimas *et al.*, 1995). The hypothesis that the relatively extensive placental transfer of 13-*cis*-retinoic acid to the monkey embryo, as compared with the rodent embryo at mid-gestation, is related to the type of placenta (Hummler *et al.*, 1994) was addressed by comparing the placental transfer of 13-*cis*-retinoic acid in mice and rats at gestational ages at which the chorioallantoic placenta is either starting to differentiate (day 11 of gestation for mice and day 12 for rats) or is well established (day 14 for mice and day 16 for rats) (Tzimas *et al.*,

Table 5. Teratogenic effects of 13-*cis*-retinoic acid			
Species	Dose (mg/kg bw)	Effects	Reference
Hamster	37.5; GD 8–11	Cranio-facial effect	Eckhoff & Willhite (1997)
Rabbit	15; GD 8–11	Resorptions, teratogenicity	Tembe *et al.* (1996)
Rabbit	10; GD 6–18	Low teratogenic response	Tzimas *et al.* (1994)
CF-1 mouse	100–400; GD 11–13	Delayed ossification, cleft palate, reduced by phenobarbital pretreatment	Yuschak & Gautieri (1993)
Cynomolgus monkey	2.5; GD 10–25 2 x 2.5; GD 26, 27	Heart defects External ears, thymus aplasia	Hummler *et al.* (1990, 1994)
Rat	75; GD 8–10	Craniofacial defects; tail defects, spina bifida	Collins *et al.* (1994)
Cynomolgus monkey	2.5; DG 10–20 2 x 2.5; GD 21–24	Craniofacial defects; ear and heart defects	Korte *et al.* (1993)
NMRI mouse	10; GD 11	2% cleft palate	Creech Kraft *et al.* (1989)
ICR mouse	100, 150; GD 11	Cleft palate and limb defects, multiple dosing more effective; 4-oxo metabolite more teratogenic than parent drug	Kochhar & Penner (1987); Kochhar *et al.* (1996)
NMRI mouse	> 100	Cleft palate and limb defects	Creech Kraft *et al.* (1987)

GD, gestation day

1995). With advancing gestation, there was a twofold higher embryo:maternal plasma concentration ratio of 13-*cis*-retinoic acid in both rats and mice. The finding supports the hypothesis that the extensive placental transfer of 13-*cis*-retinoic acid and 13-*cis*-4-oxo-retinoic acid in cynomolgus monkeys can be accounted for by the presence of a functional chorioallantoic placenta on day 31 of gestation (Hummler *et al.*, 1994).

The teratogenicity induced by 13-*cis*-retinoic acid may be due at least in part to the action of the all-*trans*-isomer (Creech Kraft *et al.*, 1987, 1991b; Soprano *et al.*, 1994). The situation is, however, different in rats, rabbits and cynomolgus monkeys. In rats and rabbits, the embryonic concentrations of all-*trans*-retinoic acid after administration of teratogenic doses of 13-*cis*-retinoic acid were comparable to the endogenous concentrations. In monkeys, all-*trans*-retinoic acid may contribute to the teratogenicity of 13-*cis*-retinoic acid, because a significant increase in all-*trans*-retinoic acid over endogenous concentrations was observed after 13-*cis*-retinoic acid treatment (Tzimas *et al.*, 1996). Thus, embryonic exposure to all-*trans*-retinoic acid is not a prerequisite for 13-*cis*-retinoic acid-induced teratogenicity in all instances.

These data indicate that much higher doses of 13-*cis*-retinoic acid are required to elicit teratogenic effects in mice and rats ('insensitive' species) than in rabbits, monkeys and humans ('sensitive' species). This is partly due to the greater degree of detoxification of 13-*cis*-retinoic acid via β-glucuronidation and the more rapid elimination of the drug in mice and rats than in the other species. In addition, the placental transfer of 13-*cis*-retinoic acid and 13-*cis*-4-oxo-retinoic acid is more extensive in monkeys (Hummler *et al.*, 1994) than in mice, rats and rabbits (Tzimas *et al.*, 1995).

7.3 Genetic and related effects

7.3.1 Humans

During an intervention trial involving patients with oral premalignant lesions, the micronucleus frequencies in mucosal scrapings of the lesions and in normal-appearing mucosa were evaluated in patients receiving 13-*cis*-retinoic acid at 1.5 mg/kg bw. The treatment was continued for three months and followed by maintenance at 0.5 mg/kg bw or treatment with β-carotene at 30 mg/day. Most of these patients were cigarette smokers (27 of 40 were current smokers). The micronucleus frequencies were significantly reduced in both lesions and normal mucosa after the three-month treatment, and this effect was maintained during the following nine months by supplementation with either 13-*cis*-retinoic acid or β-carotene (Benner *et al.*, 1994b).

7.3.2 Experimental models

7.3.2.1 In vitro

The genotoxicity of 13-*cis*-retinoic acid in cultured cells has been examined in three studies, all on alterations of chromosomes. Mixed results were obtained (Table 6). 13-*cis*-Retinoic acid induced a dose-dependent increase in the frequency of sister chromatid exchange in human diploid fibroblasts, but it had no effect on V79 Chinese hamster cells. The authors attributed these findings to a lack of a measurable mono-oxygenase activity in the V79 cells. In support of this hypothesis, the retinoid-induced increase in sister chromatid exchange frequency was shown to be prevented by the addition of an inhibitor of P448-dependent mono-oxygenase, α-naphthoflavone, to the fibroblasts (Tetzner *et al.*, 1980). An increase in sister chromatid exchange frequency was also seen in human lymphocyte cultures treated with the retinoid, although the chromosomal aberration frequencies were unchanged (Auerbach *et al.*, 1984). The effect of this retinoid on sister chromatid exchange and chromosomal aberration frequencies in human embryonic palatal mesenchymal cells was examined in the presence and absence of a microsomal activation system. The authors suggested that there was a slight decrease in sister chromatid exchange frequency in the absence of exogenous metabolic activation, but this effect was not statistically significant. No change was observed in chromosomal aberration frequency (Watanabe & Pratt, 1991).

7.3.2.2. In vivo

No data were available to the Working Group.

8. Summary of Data

8.1 Chemistry, occurrence and human exposure

13-*cis*-Retinoic acid is derived from 13-*cis*-retinol by oxidation of the C-15 alcohol group to a carboxylic acid or by isomerization of all-*trans*-retinoic acid. Like all members of the vitamin A family, 13-*cis*-retinoic acid is lipophilic, sensitive to light, heat and oxygen and readily isomerized to a mixture of *cis* and *trans* isomers. Because of its acidic nature, it is slightly more soluble in water than retinol or retinal, but still poorly so. Because of its conjugated tetraene structure, 13-*cis*-retinoic acid has characteristic absorption spectra in the ultraviolet and visible, infrared and resonance Raman portions of the electromagnetic spectrum.

13-*cis*-Retinoic acid and its 4-oxo metabolite are present in blood and tissues of animal species in smaller amounts than retinol or retinyl ester and are essentially absent from plant tissues. Human exposure occurs during treatment with oral preparations and, to a much smaller extent, with topical ointments for medical or cosmetic purposes.

13-*cis*-Retinoic acid has been used to treat dermatological disorders and several forms of cancer. The efficacious oral doses are 0.5–2 mg/kg of body weight per day.

13-*cis*-Retinoic acid is usually separated by high-performance liquid chromatography and detected by its absorption at 354 nm. After chemical formation of a suitable ester, it can also be separated and detected by gas–liquid chromatography and can be quantified by mass spectrometry.

8.2 Metabolism and kinetics

13-*cis*-Retinoic acid is present normally in blood and is widely distributed in tissues at concentrations similar to those of all-*trans*-retinoic acid. Sulf-hydryl groups, both those present in small dialysable molecules like glutathione and those present as amino-acid residues in proteins, can catalyse interconversion of all-*trans*-retinoic acid and the 13-*cis*-isomer. Since 13-*cis*-retinoic acid does not bind to retinoic acid receptors, it is generally assumed that it acts as a precursor for all-*trans*-retinoic acid. Pharmacokinetic studies indicate that 13-*cis*-retinoic acid has a much longer elimination half-life in most species than all-*trans*-retinoic acid.

Table 6. Genetic and related effects of 13-*cis*-retinoic acid in short-term tests *in vitro*

Test system	Result[a]		LED/HID[b]	Reference
	Without exogenous metabolic system	With exogenous metabolic system		
Sister chromatid exchange, human diploid fibroblasts	+	0	0.5 µg/ml	Tetzner *et al.* (1980)
Sister chromatid exchange, V79 Chinese hamster fibroblasts	–	0	8 µg/ml	Tetzner *et al.* (1980)
Sister chromatid exchange, human lymphocytes	+	0	25 µmol/L	Auerbach *et al.* (1984)
Sister chromatid exchange, human embryonic palatal mesenchymal cells	–	–	100 µmol/L (–S9) 200 µmol/L (+S9)	Watanabe & Pratt (1991)
Chromosomal aberrations, human lymphocytes	–	0	50 µmol/L	Auerbach *et al.* (1984)
Chromosomal aberrations, human embryonic palatal mesenchymal cells	–	–	250 µmol/L (–S9) 200 µmol/L (+S9)	Watanabe & Pratt (1991)

[a] Result: +, positive; – considered to be negative; 0, not tested
[b] LED, lowest effective dose that inhibits or enhances the investigated effect; HID, highest ineffective dose

8.3 Cancer-preventive effects

8.3.1 Humans

Secondary analyses of the results of one randomized trial of use of 13-*cis*-retinoic acid as adjuvant therapy for cancers of the head and neck indicated a statistically significant reduction in the incidence of second primary tumours of the upper aerodigestive tract. A study of use of 13-*cis*-retinoic acid at high doses and in a group at inherited high risk, with no controls, suggested that this compound is effective in preventing basal- and squamous-cell cancers of the skin. Two randomized controlled trials among patients at lower risk and involving lower (and better tolerated) doses of 13-*cis*-retinoic acid have shown no evidence of preventive efficacy.

High doses of 13-*cis*-retinoic acid were shown to be effective against oral leukoplakia in two randomized trials, one with controls receiving placebo and the other with persons receiving β-carotene. One controlled trial showed no effect of 13-*cis*-retinoic acid in reducing cytological changes in the bronchi. Studies of molecular markers

suggested that 13-*cis*-retinoic acid increases expression of human retinoic acid receptor β, but the relevance of these findings to cancer-preventive activity is unclear.

A single intervention study showed a decrease in micronucleus formation in cells of the buccal cavity in patients, some of whom were smokers, who had been treated with 13-*cis*-retinoic acid for 12 months.

8.3.2 Experimental models

The preventive efficacy of 13-*cis*-retinoic acid has been evaluated in two-stage skin carcinogenesis models in mice and in urinary bladder carcinogenesis models in mice and rats. 13-*cis*-Retinoic acid was effective in most studies with both models. It was ineffective in models of tracheal, salivary gland, oesophageal and renal carcinogenesis.

In vitro, 13-*cis*-retinoic acid inhibited proliferation in numerous cell lines, few of which were immortalized and most of which were established tumour cell lines. 13-*cis*-Retinoic acid inhibited growth in both monolayers of adherent cell cultures and in semi-solid medium (anchorage-independent growth). 13-*cis*-Retinoic acid also induced differentiation in transformed cells and triggered apoptosis in a few cell lines. In most cell lines, the response to 13-*cis*-retinoic acid was similar to that to all-*trans*-retinoic acid.

The ability of 13-*cis*-retinoic acid to inhibit genetic and related effects in cell cultures has been evaluated in a limited number of studies, and these have yielded mixed results. In two studies, a reduction in the frequency of chromosomal damage was seen in human lymphocytes exposed to radical-generating agents (bleomycin and X-irradiation) when they were pretreated with 13-*cis*-retinoic acid; in contrast, a third study showed an increase in the frequency of diepoxybutane-induced sister chromatid exchange and chromosomal damage in human lymphocytes treated concurrently with the mutagen and the retinoid.

Orally administered 13-*cis*-retinoic acid inhibited the induction of micronucleated cells in the bone marrow of animals treated with benzo[*a*]pyrene and reduced the binding of this carcinogen to DNA in the liver, stomach and lung, but not the kidney. Although the mechanism of this protective effect is unknown, several studies showed a significant alteration in microsomal enzyme activity in both liver and skin of mammals treated with 13-*cis*-retinoic acid.

8.3.3   Mechanisms of cancer prevention

13-*cis*-Retinoic acid is readily isomerized to all-*trans*-retinoic acid which may explain most, if not all, of its actions.

8.4   Other beneficial effects

Treatment with 13-*cis*-retinoic acid is of benefit to patients suffering from a wide variety of dermatological disorders.

8.5   Carcinogenicity

No data were available to the Working Group.

8.6   Other toxic effects
8.6.1   Humans

The toxicity of 13-*cis*-retinoic acid is similar to that seen in hypervitaminosis A; most of the adverse reactions are dose-dependent and reversible, although some persist after discontinuation of therapy. The doses of 13-*cis*-retinoic acid used for chemoprevention are generally within the range of doses recommended for the treatment of acne;

therefore, the toxicity seen in chemoprevention trials is essentially the same as that seen with use of 13-*cis*-retinoic acid for dermatological indications. The symptoms affect the skin and mucous membranes and the musculoskeletal system, including dry skin, cheilitis, conjunctivitis and arthralgia. Skin reactions can usually be tolerated without interruption of therapy by the use of emollients and other treatments, and the effects generally resolve after therapy is discontinued. The most common abnormalities seen in laboratory examinations include hypertriglyceridaemia, hypercholesterolaemia, decreased serum concentrations of high-density lipoproteins and elevated activity of serum liver enzymes. Rarely, acute complications develop secondary to these abnormalities. Headache, often described as severe, impaired hearing, dizziness and psychological disorders have been associated with oral administration of 13-*cis*-retinoic acid.

13-*cis*-Retinoic acid is a confirmed human teratogen. The potential developmental toxicity associated with maternal therapy with this retinoid depends on the dose, the stage of gestation or the age of the patient, the duration of treatment and the route of administration. Dose-dependent desquamation of the testicular germinal epithelium to the point of necrosis has been observed in preclinical studies with 13-*cis*-retinoic acid, but such changes have not been observed in patients given the standard therapeutic dose.

There are no reports of genotoxic activity of 13-*cis*-retinoic acid in humans.

8.6.2   Experimental models

In short-term studies of toxicity in rats and dogs, dose-related effects were seen in both species, including decreased food consumption and body-weight gain, erythema, alopecia, mucosal changes, elevated serum alkaline phosphatase and transaminase activities and increased liver weight. Long-bone fractures and elevated serum triglyceride concentrations were seen in rats, while apparent joint pain was seen in dogs.

The dose-related effects seen in long-term studies of toxicity in rats included increased mortality rates and decreased food consumption and body-weight gain. Decreased haemoglobin concentration and haematocrit and elevated serum triglyceride concentrations were observed at higher doses, and increased alkaline phosphatase activity and increased liver and kidney weights were observed in all treated groups. Fibrosis and inflammation of the myocardium, arterial calcification, focal tissue calcification and focal osteolysis were seen at higher doses. In dogs, a dose of 120 mg/kg bw per day led to severe weight loss and debilitation within four weeks. With a dose cycle of 60 mg/kg bw per day for six weeks and no treatment for two weeks, toxic clinical effects observed during the treatment cycle included severe weight loss and skin changes, decreased haemoglobin concentration and haematocrit and increased serum alkaline phosphatase activity. Fibrosis and focal calcification in the myocardium and aorta and increased liver weight and lymph node oedema were observed at higher doses.

Long-term oral administration of 13-*cis*-retinoic acid can induce testicular toxicity in animals and interfere with spermatogenesis. 13-*cis*-Retinoic acid is an even more potent teratogen than all-*trans*-retinoic acid in monkeys, because of its relatively long half-life, metabolism to an active metabolite (13-*cis*-4-oxoretinoic acid) and efficient placental transfer.

The capacity of 13-*cis*-retinoic acid to induce chromosomal damage and sister chromatid exchange in cultured mammalian cells was examined in three studies. No change in the frequency of chromosomal aberrations was seen, but the results for sister chromatid exchange were contradictory, two showing an increase and the third showing no effect.

9. Recommendations for Research

9.1 General recommendations for 13-*cis*-retinoic acid and other retinoids

See section 9 of Handbook on all-*trans*-retinoic acid.

9.2 Recommendations specific to 13-*cis*-retinoic acid

None.

10. Evaluation

10.1 Cancer-preventive activity
10.1.1 Humans
There is *limited evidence* that 13-*cis*-retinoic acid has cancer-preventive activity in humans. This evaluation is based on its effectiveness against oral leukoplakia and preliminary evidence for prevention of second primary cancers of the aerodigestive tract.

10.1.2 Experimental animals
There is *limited evidence* that 13-*cis*-retinoic acid has cancer-preventive activity in experimental animals. This evaluation is based on the observation of inhibitory effects in most but not all studies with models of skin and urinary bladder carcinogenesis.

10.2 Overall evaluation
13-*cis*-Retinoic acid probably has cancer-preventive activity in humans, but it has a relatively low therapeutic ratio of efficacy to toxicity and is an established human teratogen. 13-*cis*-Retinoic acid is of value for treating a variety of dermatological disorders.

11. References

Abdel-Galil, A.M., Wrba, H. & El-Mofty, M.M. (1984) Prevention of 3-methylcholanthrene-induced skin tumors in mice by simultaneous application of 13-*cis*-retinoic acid and retinyl palmitate (vitamin A palmitate). *Exp. Pathol.*, **25**, 97–102

Adams, J. (1993) Structure–activity and dose–response relationships in the neural and behavioral teratogenesis of retinoids. *Neurotoxicol. Teratol.*, **15**, 193–202

Adams, J. & Lammer, E.J. (1991) Relationship between dysmorphology and neuro-psychological function in children exposed to isotretinoin 'in utero'. In: Fujii, T. & Boer, G.J., eds, *Functional Neuroteratology of Short-term Exposure to Drugs*, Teikyo, Teikyo University Press, pp. 159–170

Adams, J. & Lammer, E.J. (1993) Neurobehavioral teratology of isotretinoin. *Reprod. Toxicol.*, **7**, 175–177

Agarwal, C., Chandraratna, R.A., Teng, M., Nagpal, S., Rorke, E.A. & Eckert, R.L. (1996) Differential regulation of human ectocervical epithelial cell line proliferation and differentiation by retinoid X receptor- and retinoic acid receptor-specific retinoids. *Cell Growth Differ.*, **7**, 521–530

Alam, B.S., Alam, S.Q., Weir, J.C., Jr & Gibson, W.A. (1984) Chemopreventive effects of β-carotene and 13-*cis*-retinoic acid on salivary gland tumors. *Nutr. Cancer*, **6**, 4–12

Alberts, D.S., Coulthard, S.W. & Meyskens, F.L. (1986) Regression of aggressive laryngeal papillomatosis with 13-*cis*-retinoic acid (accutane). *J. Biol. Response Mod.*, **5**, 124–128

Al Dosari, A., McDonald, J., Olson, B., Noblitt, T., Li, Y. & Stookey, G. (1996) Influence of benzylisothiocyanate and 13-*cis*-retinoic acid on micronucleus formation induced by benzo[*a*]pyrene. *Mutat. Res.*, **352**, 1–7

Anonymous (1986) Isotretinoin and human teratogenicity. *Nutr.Rev.*, **44**, 297–299

Arky, R., ed. (1998) *Physicians' Desk Reference*, 52nd Ed. Montvale, NJ, Medical Economics Co., pp. 2433–2435

Armstrong, R.B., Ashenfelter, K.O., Eckhoff, C., Levin, A.A. & Shapiro, S.S. (1994) General and reproductive toxicology of retinoids. In: Sporn, M.B., Roberts, A.B. & Goodman, D.S., eds. *The Retinoids. Biology, Chemistry, and Medicine,* 2nd Ed. New York, Raven Press, pp. 545–572

Auerbach, A.D., Sagi, M. & Carter, D.M. (1984) Enhancement of carcinogen-induced chromosome breakage and sister chromatid exchange by 13-*cis*-retinoic acid. *Basic Life Sci.*, **29 Pt A**, 333–341

Ball, M.D. & Olson, J.A. (1988) 13-*cis*-Retinoic acid stimulates in vitro mannose 6-phosphate hydrolysis and inhibits retinol esterification and benzo[a]pyrene hydroxylation by rat-liver microsomes. *Biochim. Biophys. Acta,* **961**, 139–143

Barua, A.B. & Furr, H.C. (1998) Properties of retinoids: Structure, handling, and preparation. In: Redfern C.P.F., ed. *Retinoid Protocols.* Totowa, NJ, Humana Press, pp. 3–28

Barua, A.B., Furr, H.C., Olson, J.A. & van Breemen, R.B. (1999) Vitamin A and carotenoids. In: DeLeenheer A., Lambert W. & van Bocxlaer J., eds. *Modern Chromatographic Analysis of the Vitamins,* 3rd Ed. New York, Marcel Dekker (in press)

Becci, P.J., Thompson, H.J., Grubbs, C.J., Squire, R.A., Brown, C.C., Sporn, M.B. & Moon, R.C. (1978) Inhibitory effect of 13-*cis*-retinoic acid on urinary bladder carcinogenesis induced in C57BL/6 mice by N-butyl-N-(4-hydroxybutyl)nitrosamine. *Cancer Res.*, **38**, 4463–4466

Becci, P.J., Thompson, H.J., Grubbs, C.J., Brown, C.C. & Moon, R.C. (1979) Effect of delay in administration of 13-*cis*-retinoic acid on the inhibition of urinary bladder carcinogenesis in the rat. *Cancer Res.*, **39**, 3141–3144

Beenken, S.W., Huang, P., Sellers, M., Peters, G., Listinsky, C., Stockard, C., Hubbard, W., Wheeler, R. & Grizzle, W. (1994) Retinoid modulation of biomarkers in oral leukoplakia/dysplasia. *J. Cell Biochem.*, **19** (Suppl.), 270–277

Benke, P.J. (1984) The isotretinoin teratogen syndrome. *J. Am. Med. Asspc,* **251**, 3267–3269

Benner, S.E., Pajak, T.F., Lippman, S.M., Earley, C. & Hong, W.K. (1994a) Prevention of second primary tumors with isotretinoin in patients with squamous cell carcinoma of the head and neck: long-term follow-up. *J. Natl Cancer Inst.*, **86**, 140–141

Benner, S.E., Lippman, S.M., Wargovich, M.J., Lee, J.J., Velasco, M., Martin, J.W., Toth, B.B. & Hong, W.K. (1994b) Micronuclei, a biomarker for chemoprevention trials: Results of a randomized study in oral pre-malignancy. *Int. J. Cancer,* **59**, 457–459

Bigby, M. & Stern, R.S. (1988) Adverse reactions to isotretinoin. A report from the Adverse Drug Reaction Reporting System. *J. Am. Acad. Dermatol.,* **18**, 543–552

Blaner, W.S. & Olson, J.A. (1994) Retinol and retinoic acid metabolism. In: Sporn, M.B., Roberts, A.B. & Goodman, D.S., eds. *The Retinoids: Biology, Chemistry, and Medicine.* 2nd Ed. New York, Raven Press, pp. 229–255

Bower, M., Fife, K., Landau, D., Gracie, F., Phillips, R.H. & Gazzard, B.G. (1997) Phase II trial of 13-*cis*-retinoic acid for poor risk HIV-associated Kaposi's sarcoma. *Int. J. STD AIDS,* **8**, 518–521

Braun, J.T., Franciosi, R.A., Mastri, A.R., Drake, R.M. & O'Neil, B.L. (1984) Isotretinoin dysmorphic syndrome. *Lancet,* **i**, 506–507

Brown, R.D. & Grattan, C.E. (1989) Visual toxicity of synthetic retinoids. *Br. J. Ophthalmol.,* **73**, 286–288

Bruno, N.P., Beacham, B.E. & Burnett, J.W. (1984) Adverse effects of isotretinoin therapy. *Cutis,* **33**, 484–486

Budavari, S., O'Neil, M.J., Smith, A., Heckelman, P.E. & Kinneary, J.F. (1996) *The Merck Index. An Encyclopedia of Chemicals, Drugs, and Biologicals.* 12th Ed. Whitehouse Station, NJ, Merck & Co., p. 1404

Burk, D.T. & Willhite, C.C. (1992) Inner ear malformations induced by isotretinoin in hamster fetuses. *Teratology,* **46**, 147–157

Cai, D., Ben, T. & De Luca, L.M. (1991) Retinoids induce tissue transglutaminase in NIH-3T3 cells. *Biochem. Biophys. Res. Commun.,* **175**, 1119–1124

Carey, B.M., Parkin, G.J., Cunliffe, W.J. & Pritlove, J. (1988) Skeletal toxicity with isotretinoin therapy: A clinico-radiological evaluation. *Br. J. Dermatol.,* **119**, 609–614

Carter, C.A., Pogribny, M., Davidson, A., Jackson, C.D., McGarrity, L.J. & Morris, S.M. (1996) Effects of retinoic acid on cell differentiation and reversion toward normal in human endometrial adenocarcinoma (RL95-2) cells. *Anticancer Res.,* **16**, 17–24

Chan, A., Keane, R.J., Hanna, M. & Abbott, M. (1995) Terminations of pregnancy for exposure to oral retinoids in South Australia, 1985–1993. *Aust. N.Z. J. Obstet. Gynaecol.,* **35**, 422–426

Chen, C., Jensen, B.K., Mistry, G., Wyss, R., Zultak, M., Patel, I.H. & Rakhit, A.K. (1997) Negligible systemic absorption of topical isotretinoin cream: Implications for teratogenicity. *J. Clin. Pharmacol.,* **37**, 279–284

Christmas, T. (1988) Roaccutane and menorrhagia. *J. Am. Acad. Dermatol.,* **18**, 576–577

Coberly, S., Lammer, E. & Alashari, M. (1996) Retinoic acid embryopathy: Case report and review of literature. *Pediatr. Pathol. Lab. Med.,* **16**, 823–836

Colburn, W.A., Vane, F.M., Bugge, C.J., Carter, D.E., Bressler, R. & Ehmann, C.W. (1985) Pharmacokinetics of ^{14}C-isotretinoin in healthy volunteers and volunteers with biliary T-tube drainage. *Drug Metab. Dispos.*, **13**, 327–332

Coleman, R. & MacDonald, D. (1994) Effects of isotretinoin on male reproductive system. *Lancet*, **344**, 198–198

Collins, M.D., Tzimas, G., Hummler, H., Burgin, H. & Nau, H. (1994) Comparative teratology and transplacental pharmacokinetics of all-trans-retinoic acid, 13-cis-retinoic acid, and retinyl palmitate following daily administrations in rats. *Toxicol. Appl. Pharmacol.*, **127**, 132–144

Cotler, S., Bugge, C.J. & Colburn, W.A. (1983) Role of gut contents, intestinal wall, and liver on the first pass metabolism and absolute bioavailability of isotretinoin in the dog. *Drug Metab. Dispos.*, **11**, 458–462

Cotler, S., Chen, S., Macasieb, T. & Colburn, W.A. (1984) Effect of route of administration and biliary excretion on the pharmacokinetics of isotretinoin in the dog. *Drug Metab. Dispos.*, **12**, 143–147

Cox, N.H. (1988) Amenorrhoea during treatment with isotretinoin. *Br. J. Dermatol.*, **118**, 857–858

Creech Kraft, J., Kochhar, D.M., Scott, W.J. & Nau, H. (1987) Low teratogenicity of 13-*cis*-retinoic acid (isotretinoin) in the mouse corresponds to low embryo concentrations during organogenesis: comparison to the all-trans isomer. *Toxicol. Appl. Pharmacol.*, **87**, 474–482

Creech Kraft, J., Löfberg, B., Chahoud, I., Bochert, G. & Nau, H. (1989) Teratogenicity and placental transfer of all-trans-, 13-cis-, 4-oxo-all-trans-, and 4-oxo-13-cis-retinoic acid after administration of a low oral dose during organogenesis in mice. *Toxicol. Appl. Pharmacol.*, **100**, 162–176

Creech Kraft, J., Slikker, W., Bailey, J.R., Roberts, L.G., Fischer, B., Wittfoht, W. & Nau, H. (1991a) Plasma pharmacokinetics and metabolism of 13-*cis*- and all-*trans*-retinoic acid in the cynomolgus monkey and the identification of 13-*cis*- and all-*trans*-retinoyl-β-glucuronides. A comparison to one human case study with isotretinoin. *Drug Metab. Dispos.*, **19**, 317–324

Creech Kraft, J., Eckhoff, C., Kochhar, D.M., Bochert, G., Chahoud, I. & Nau, H. (1991b) Isotretinoin (13-*cis*-retinoic acid) metabolism, *cis-trans* isomerization, glucuronidation, and transfer to the mouse embryo: consequences for teratogenicity. *Teratog. Carcinog. Mutag.*, **11**, 21–30

Croft, W.A., Croft, M.A., Paulus, K.P., Williams, J.H., Wang, C.Y. & Lower, G.M., Jr (1981) Synthetic retinamides: Effect on urinary bladder carcinogenesis by

FANFT in Fischer rats. *Carcinogenesis*, **2**, 515–517

de la Cruz, E., Sun, S., Vangvanichyakorn, K. & Desposito, F. (1984) Multiple congenital malformations associated with maternal isotretinoin therapy. *Pediatrics*, **74**, 428–430

Dahiya, R., Boyle, B., Park, H.D., Kurhanewicz, J., Macdonald, J.M. & Narayan, P. (1994) 13-*cis*-Retinoic acid-mediated growth inhibition of DU-145 human prostate cancer cells. *Biochem. Mol. Biol. Int.*, **32**, 1–12

Dai, W.S., Hsu, M.A. & Itri, L.M. (1989) Safety of pregnancy after discontinuation of isotretinoin. *Arch. Dermatol.*, **125**, 362–365

Dai, W.S., LaBraico, J.M. & Stern, R.S. (1992) Epidemiology of isotretinoin exposure during pregnancy. *J. Am. Acad. Dermatol.*, **26**, 599–606

Daoud, A.H. & Griffin, A.C. (1980) Effect of retinoic acid, butylated hydroxytoluene, selenium and sorbic acid on azo-dye hepatocarcinogenesis. *Cancer Lett.*, **9**, 299–304

Dawson, M.I., Chao, W.R. & Helmes, C.T. (1987) Inhibition by retinoids of anthralin-induced mouse epidermal ornithine decarboxylase activity and anthralin-promoted skin tumor formation. *Cancer Res.*, **47**, 6210–6215

Dharmagunawardena, B. & Charles-Holmes, R. (1997) Median canaliform dystrophy following isotretinoin therapy. *Br. J. Dermatol.*, **137**, 658–659

Di Giovanna, J.J. & Peck, G.L. (1983) Oral synthetic retinoid treatment in children. *Pediatr. Dermatol.*, **1**, 77–88

Dimery, I.W., Hong, W.K., Lee, J.J., Guillory Perez, C., Pham, F., Fritsche, H.A.J. & Lippman, S.M. (1997) Phase I trial of alpha-tocopherol effects on 13-cis-retinoic acid toxicity. *Ann. Oncol.*, **8**, 85–89

Dolcetti, R., Zancai, P., Cariati, R. & Boiocchi, M. (1998) In vitro effects of retinoids on the proliferation and differentiation features of Epstein–Barr virus-immortalized B lymphocytes. *Leuk. Lymphoma*, **29**, 269–281

Dominguez, J., Hojyo, M.T., Celayo, J.L., Dominguez-Soto, L. & Teixeira, F. (1998) Topical isotretinoin vs. topical retinoic acid in the treatment of acne vulgaris. *Int. J. Dermatol.*, **37**, 54–55

Driessen, C.A., Winkens, H.J., Kuhlmann, E.D., Janssen, A.P., van-Vugt, A.H., Deutman, A.F. & Janssen, J.J. (1998) The visual cycle retinol dehydrogenase: Possible involvement in the 9-*cis* retinoic acid biosynthetic pathway. *FEBS Lett.*, **428**, 135–140

Eckhoff, C. & Nau, H. (1990) Identification and quantitation of all-*trans*- and 13-*cis*-retinoic acid and 13-*cis*-4-oxoretinoic acid in human plasma. *J. Lipid Res.*, **31**, 1445–1454

Eckhoff, C. & Willhite, C.C. (1997) Embryonic delivered dose of isotretinoin (13-*cis*-retinoic acid) and its metabolites in hamsters. *Toxicol. Appl. Pharmacol.*, **146**, 79–87

Edwards, S. & Sonnex, C. (1997) Urethritis associated with isotretinoin therapy. *Acta Derm. Venereol.*, **77**, 330–330

Edwards, L., Alberts, D.S. & Levine, N. (1986) Clinical toxicity of low-dose isotretinoin. *Cancer Treat. Rep.*, **70**, 663–664

Egger, S.F., Huber Spitzy, V., Bohler, K., Raff, M., Scholda, C., Barisani, T. & Vecsei, V.P. (1995) Ocular side effects associated with 13-cis-retinoic acid therapy for acne vulgaris: Clinical features, alterations of tearfilm and conjunctival flora. *Acta Ophthalmol. Scand.*, **73**, 355–357

Ellis, C.N., Pennes, D.R., Martel, W. & Voorhees, J.J. (1985) Radiographic bone surveys after isotretinoin therapy for cystic acne. *Acta Derm. Venereol.*, **65**, 83–85

Englert, G. (1975) A ^{13}C-NMR study of cis-trans isomeric vitamins A, carotenoids and related compounds. *Helv. Chim. Acta*, **58**, 2367–2390

Erhardt, E. & Harangi, F. (1997) Two cases of musculoskeletal syndrome associated with acne. *Pediatr. Dermatol.*, **14**, 456–459

Ertürk, E., Lambrecht, R.W., Peters, H.A., Cripps, D.J., Gocmen, A., Morris, C.R. & Bryan, G.T. (1986) Oncogenicity of hexachlorobenzene. *IARC Sci. Publ.*, **77**, 417–423

Fallon, M.B. & Boyer, J.L. (1990) Hepatic toxicity of vitamin A and synthetic retinoids. *J. Gastroenterol. Hepatol.*, **5**, 334–342

Fernhoff, P.M. & Lammer, E.J. (1984) Craniofacial features of isotretinoin embryopathy. *J. Pediatr.*, **105**, 595–597

Finnen, M.J. & Shuster, S. (1984) The effects of 13-*cis* retinoic acid on hepatic and cutaneous monoxygenase activities: possible cancer-protective mechanism. *Br. J. Dermatol.*, **111**, 704–704

Formelli, F., Cavadini, E., Mascheroni, L., Belli, F. & Cascinelli, N. (1997) Pharmacokinetics and effects on plasma retinol concentrations of 13-*cis*-retinoic acid in melanoma patients. *Br. J. Cancer*, **76**, 1655–1660

Frasca, J.M. & Garfinkel, L. (1981) 13-*cis* Retinoic acid and murine pulmonary adenomas: A preliminary report. *Nutr. Cancer*, **3**, 72–74

Frickel, F. (1984) Chemistry and physical properties of retinoids. In: Sporn, M.B., Roberts, A.B. & Goodman, D.S., eds. *The Retinoids*. Orlando, Academic Press, pp. 7–145

Frolik, C.A. & Olson, J.A. (1984) Extraction, separation, and chemical analysis of retinoids. In: Sporn, M.B., Roberts, A.B. & Goodman, D.S., eds. *The Retinoids*. Orlando, Academic Press, pp. 181–233

Furr, H.C., Barua, A.B. & Olson, J.A. (1992) Retinoids and carotenoids. In: De Leenheer A.P., Lambert W.E. & Nelis H.J., eds. *Modern Chromatographic Analysis of Vitamins*. 2nd Ed. New York, Marcel Dekker, pp. 1–71

Furr, H.C., Barua, A.B. & Olson, J.A. (1994) Analytical methods. In: Sporn, M.B., Roberts, A.B. & Goodman, D.S., eds. *The Retinoids: Biology, Chemistry, and Medicine*. 2nd Ed. New York, Raven Press, pp. 179–209

Gabrial, G.N., Schrager, T.F. & Newberne, P.M. (1982) Zinc deficiency, alcohol, and a retinoid: association with esophageal cancer in rats. *J. Natl Cancer Inst.*, **68**, 785–789

Gensler, H. & Bowden, G.T. (1984) Influence of 13-*cis*-retinoic acid on mouse skin tumor initiation and promotion. *Cancer Lett.*, **22**, 71–75

Gensler, H.L., Sim, D.A. & Bowden, G.T. (1986) Influence of the duration of topical 13-*cis*-retinoic acid treatment on inhibition of mouse skin tumor promotion. *Cancer Res.*, **46**, 2767–2770

Giannini, F., Maestro, R., Vukosavljevic, T., Pomponi, F. & Boiocchi, M. (1997) All-*trans*, 13-*cis* and 9-*cis* retinoic acids induce a fully reversible growth inhibition in HNSCC cell lines: Implications for *in vivo* retinoic acid use. *Int. J. Cancer*, **70**, 194–200

Goerz, G., Hamm, L., Bolsen, K. & Merk, H. (1984) Influence of 13-cis retinoic acid and of arotinoid on the cytochrome P-450 system in rat liver. *Dermatologica*, **168**, 117–121

Goerz, G., Bolsen, K., Kalofoutis, A. & Tsambaos, D. (1994) Influence of oral isotretinoin on hepatic and cutaneous P-450-dependent isozyme activities. *Arch. Dermatol. Res.*, **286**, 104–106

Gold, E.J., Mertelsmann, R.H., Itri, L.M., Gee, T., Arlin, Z., Kempin, S., Clarkson, B. & Moore, M.A. (1983) Phase I clinical trial of 13-*cis*-retinoic acid in myelodysplastic syndromes. *Cancer Treat. Rep.*, **67**, 981–986

Greenberg, B.R., Durie, B.G., Barnett, T.C. & Meyskens, F.L.J. (1985) Phase I–II study of 13-*cis*-retinoic acid in myelodysplastic syndrome. *Cancer Treat. Rep.*, **69**, 1369–1374

Guchelaar, H.J., Wouda, S., Beukeveld, G.J., Mulder, N.H. & Oosterhuis, J.W. (1992) Pharmacokinetics of parenteral 13-*cis*-retinoic acid formulations in rats. *J Pharm. Sci.*, **81**, 432–435

Hard, G.C. & Ogiu, T. (1984) Null effects of vitamin A analogs on the dimethylnitrosamine kidney tumor model. *Carcinogenesis*, **5**, 665–669

Hersh, J.H., Danhauer, D.E., Hand, M.E. & Weisskopf, B. (1985) Retinoic acid embryopathy: Timing of exposure and effects on fetal development. *J. Am. Med. Assoc.*, **254**, 909–910

Hill, R.M. (1984) Isotretinoin teratogenicity. *Lancet*, **i**, 1465–1465

Hixson, E.J. & Denine, E.P. (1978) Comparative subacute toxicity of all-*trans*- and 13-*cis*-retinoic acid in Swiss mice. *Toxicol. Appl. Pharmacol.*, **44**, 29–40

Hixson, E.J., Burdeshaw, J.A., Denine, E.P. & Harrison, S.D.J. (1979) Comparative subchronic toxicity of all-*trans*- and 13-*cis*-retinoic acid in Sprague-Dawley rats. *Toxicol. Appl. Pharmacol.*, **47**, 359–365

Hoffman, A.D., Engelstein, D., Bogenrieder, T., Papandreou, C.N., Steckelman, E., Dave, A., Motzer, R.J., Dmitrovsky, E., Albino, A.P. & Nanus, D.M. (1996) Expression of retinoic acid receptor β in human renal cell carcinomas correlates with sensitivity to the antiproliferative effects of 13-*cis*-retinoic acid. *Clin. Cancer Res.*, **2**, 1077–1082

Hogan, D.J., Strand, L.M. & Lane, P.R. (1988) Isotretinoin therapy for acne: A population-based study. *Can. Med. Assoc. J*, **138**, 47–50

Holmes, S.C., Bankowska, U. & Mackie, R.M. (1998) The prescription of isotretinoin to women: Is every precaution taken? *Br. J. Dermatol.*, **138**, 450–455

Hong, W.K. & Itri, L.M. (1994) Retinoids and human cancer. In: Sporn, M.B., Roberts, A.B. & Goodman, D.S., eds. *The Retinoids: Biology, Chemistry, and Medicine.* 2nd Ed. New York, Raven Press, pp. 597–630

Hong, W.K., Endicott, J., Itri, L.M., Doos, W., Batsakis, J.G., Bell, R., Fofonoff, S., Byers, R., Atkinson, E.N., Vaughan, C., Toth, B.B., Kramer, A., Dimery, I.W., Skipper, P. & Strong, S. (1986) 13-*cis* -Retinoic acid in the treatment of oral leukoplakia. *N. Engl. J. Med.*, **315**, 1501–1505

Hong, W.K., Lippman, S.M., Itri, L.M., Karp, D.D., Lee, J.S., Byers, R.M., Schantz, S.P., Kramer, A.M., Lotan, R., Peters, L.J., Dimery, I.W., Brown, B.W. & Goepfert, H. (1990) Prevention of second primary tumors with isotretinoin in squamous-cell carcinoma of the head and neck. *N. Engl. J. Med.*, **323**, 795–801

Howard, W.B. & Willhite, C.C. (1986) Toxicity of retinoids in humans and animals. *J. Toxicol. Toxin Rev.*, **5**, 55–94

Hsu, M.C. (1998) Systemic treatment of neoplastic conditions with retinoids. *J. Am. Acad. Dermatol.*, **39**, S108–S113

Hummler, H., Korte, R. & Hendrickx, A.G. (1990) Induction of malformations in the cynomolgus monkey with 13-*cis* retinoic acid. *Teratology,* **42**, 263–272

Hummler, H., Hendrickx, A.G. & Nau, H. (1994) Maternal toxicokinetics, metabolism, and embryo exposure following a teratogenic dosing regimen with 13-cis-retinoic acid (isotretinoin) in the cynomolgus monkey. *Teratology,* **50**, 184–193

IARC (1998) *IARC Handbooks of Cancer Prevention*, Vol. 3, *Vitamin A*, Lyon, International Agency for Research on Cancer, pp. 167–175

Jahn, A.F. & Ganti, K. (1987) Major auricular malformations due to Accutane® (isotretinoin). *Laryngoscope*, **97**, 832–835

Jiang, S.Y., Shyu, R.Y., Chen, H.Y., Lee, M.M., Wu, K.L. & Yeh, M.Y. (1996) In vitro and in vivo growth inhibition of SC-M1 gastric cancer cells by retinoic acid. *Oncology*, **53**, 334–340

Jimi, S., Shono, T., Tanaka, M., Kono, A., Yamada, Y., Shudo, K. & Kuwano, M. (1998) Effect of retinoic acid on morphological changes of human pancreatic cancer cells on collagen gels: A possible association with the metastatic potentials. *Oncol. Res.*, **10**, 7–14

Josefson, D. (1998) Acne drug is linked to severe depression. *BMJ*, **316**, 723–723

Jurima-Romet, M., Neigh, S. & Casley, W.L. (1997) Induction of cytochrome P450 3A by retinoids in rat hepatocyte culture. *Hum. Exp. Toxicol.*, **16**, 198–203

Kalin, J.R., Wells, M.J. & Hill, D.L. (1982) Disposition of 13-*cis*-retinoic acid and N-(2-hydroxyethyl)retinamide in mice after oral doses. *Drug Metab. Dispos.*, **10**, 391–398

Kamm, J.J. (1982) Toxicology, carcinogenicity, and teratogenicity of some orally administered retinoids. *J. Am. Acad. Dermatol.*, **6**, 652–659

Kamm, J.J., Ashenfelter, K.O. & Ehmann, C.W. (1984) Preclinical and clinical toxicology of selected retinoids. In: Sporn, M.B., Roberts, A.B. & Goodman, D.S., eds, *The Retinoids*. Orlando, Academic Press, Inc., pp. 287–326

Kaplan, G. & Haettich, B. (1991) Rheumatological symptoms due to retinoids. *Baillieres Clin. Rheumatol.*, **5**, 77–97

Kassis, I., Sunderji, S. & Abdul-Karim, R. (1985) Isotretinoin (Accutane®) and pregnancy. *Teratology*, **32**, 145–146

Kerr, I.G., Lippman, M.E., Jenkins, J. & Myers, C.E. (1982) Pharmacology of 13-cis-retinoic acid in humans. *Cancer Res.*, **42**, 2069–2073

Kessler, J.F., Jones, S.E., Levine, N., Lynch, P.J., Booth, A.R. & Meyskens, F.L.J. (1987) Isotretinoin and cutaneous helper T-cell lymphoma (mycosis fungoides). *Arch. Dermatol.*, **123**, 201–204

Khoury, M.J., James, L.M. & Lynberg, M.C. (1991) Quantitative analysis of associations between birth defects and suspected human teratogens. *Am. J. Med. Genet.*, **40**, 500–505

Kilcoyne, R.F., Cope, R., Cunningham, W., Nardella, F.A., Denman, S., Franz, T.J. & Hanifin, J. (1986) Minimal spinal hyperostosis with low-dose isotretinoin therapy. *Invest. Radiol.*, **21**, 41–44

Kindmark, A., Rollman, O., Mallmin, H., Petren-Mallmin, M., Ljunghall, S. & Melhus, H. (1998) Oral isotretinoin therapy in severe acne induces transient suppression of biochemical markers of bone turnover and calcium homeostasis. *Acta Derm. Venereol.*, **78**, 266–269

Kochhar, D.M. & Penner, J.D. (1987) Developmental effects of isotretinoin and 4-oxo-isotretinoin: The role of metabolism in teratogenicity. *Teratology*, **36**, 67–75

Kochhar, D.M., Jiang, H., Penner, J.D., Beard, R.L. & Chandraratna, R.A. (1996) Differential teratogenic response of mouse embryos to receptor selective analogs of retinoic acid. *Chem.–Biol. Interact.*, **100**, 1–12

Kocijancic, M. (1995) 13-cis-Retinoic acid and bone density. *Int. J. Dermatol.*, **34**, 733–734

Koebert, M.K., Haun, J.M. & Pauli, R.M. (1993) Temporal evolution of risk estimates for presumed human teratogens. *Reprod. Toxicol.*, **7**, 343–348

Korge, B., Stadler, R. & Mischke, D. (1990) Effect of retinoids on hyperproliferation-associated keratins K6 and K16 in cultured human keratinocytes: a quantitative analysis. *J. Invest. Dermatol.*, **95**, 450–455

Korte, R., Hummler, H. & Hendrickx, A.G. (1993) Importance of early exposure to 13-*cis* retinoic acid to induce teratogenicity in the cynomolgus monkey. *Teratology*, **47**, 37–45

Korytynski, E.A., Kelloff, G.J., Suk, W.A., Sharma, S. & Elmore, E. (1996) The development of an anchorage-independence assay using human lung tumor cells to screen potential chemopreventive agents. *Anticancer Res.*, **16**, 1091–1094

Kraemer, K.H., DiGiovanna, J.J., Moshell, A.N., Tarone, R.E. & Peck, G.L. (1988) Prevention of skin cancer in xeroderma pigmentosum with the use of oral isotretinoin. *N. Engl. J. Med.*, **318**, 1633–1637

Kraemer, K.H., DiGiovanna, J.J. & Peck, G.L. (1992) Chemoprevention of skin cancer in xeroderma pigmentosum. *J. Dermatol.*, **19**, 715–718

Kremer, I., Gaton, D.D., David, M., Gaton, E. & Shapiro, A. (1994) Toxic effects of systemic retinoids on meibomian glands. *Ophthalmic Res.*, **26**, 124–128

Kuhlwein, A. & Schütte, B. (1985) Light microscopic studies of spermatogenesis in rats following the administration of a high dose of 13-*cis*-retinoic acid. *Z. Hautkr.*, **60**, 245–248

Lammer, E.J. (1988) Developmental toxicity of synthetic retinoids in humans. *Prog. Clin. Biol. Res.*, **281**, 193–202

Lammer, E.J. & Armstrong, D.L. (1992) Malformations of hindbrain structures among humans exposed to isotretinoin (13-*cis*-retinoic acid) during early embryogenesis. In: Morriss-Kay, G., ed., *Retinoids in Normal Development and Teratogenesis*, Oxford, Oxford University Press, pp. 281–295

Lammer, E.J., Chen, D.T., Hoar, R.M., Agnish, N.D., Benke, P.J., Braun, J.T., Curry, C.J., Fernhoff, P.M., Grix, A.W., Jr, Lott, I.T., Richard, J.M. & Sun, S.C. (1985) Retinoic acid embryopathy. *N. Engl. J. Med.*, **313**, 837–841

Lawson, J.P. & McGuire, J. (1987) The spectrum of skeletal changes associated with long-term administration of 13-cis-retinoic acid. *Skeletal. Radiol.*, **16**, 91–97

Lee, J.S., Lippman, S.M., Benner, S.E., Lee, J.J., Ro, J.Y., Lukeman, J.M., Morice, R.C., Peters, E.J., Pang, A.C., Fritsche, H.A.J. & Hong, W.K. (1994) Randomized placebo-controlled trial of isotretinoin in chemoprevention of bronchial squamous metaplasia. *J. Clin. Oncol.*, **12**, 937–945

Lehman, P.A. & Malany, A.M. (1989) Evidence for percutaneous absorption of isotretinoin from the photoisomerization of topical tretinoin. *J. Invest. Dermatol.*, **93**, 595–599

Lerman, S. (1992) Ocular side effects of accutane therapy. *Lens Eye Toxicol. Res.*, **9**, 429–438

Levine, N., Moon, T.E., Cartmel, B., Bangert, J.L., Rodney, S., Dong, Q., Peng, Y.M. & Alberts, D.S. (1997) Trial of retinol and isotretinoin in skin cancer prevention: A randomized, double-blind, controlled trial. Southwest Skin Cancer Prevention Study Group. *Cancer Epidemiol. Biomarkers Prev.*, **6**, 957–961

Lippman, S.M., Batsakis, J.G., Toth, B.B., Weber, R.S., Lee, J.J., Martin, J.W., Hays, G.L., Goepfert, H. & Hong, W.K. (1993) Comparison of low-dose isotretinoin with beta carotene to prevent oral carcinogenesis. *N. Engl. J. Med.*, **328**, 15–20

Lippman, S.M., Hong, W.K. & Benner, S.E. (1995a) The chemoprevention of cancer. In: Greenwald P., Kramer B.S. & Weed D.L.., eds. *Cancer Prevention and Control.* New York, Marcel Dekker, pp. 329–352

Lippman, S.M., Shin, D.M., Lee, J.J., Batsakis, J.G., Lotan, R., Tainsky, M.A., Hittelman, W.N. & Hong, W.K. (1995b) p53 and retinoid chemoprevention of oral carcinogenesis. *Cancer Res.*, **55**, 16–19

Lippman, S.M., Benner, S.E., Fritsche, H.A.J., Lee, J.S. & Hong, W.K. (1998) The effect of 13-*cis*-retinoic acid chemoprevention on human serum retinol levels. *Cancer Detect. Prev.*, **22**, 51–56

Look, K.Y., Blessing, J.A., Nelson, B.E., Johnson, G.A., Fowler, W.C.J. & Reid, G.C. (1998) A phase II trial of isotretinoin and alpha interferon in patients with recurrent squamous cell carcinoma of the cervix: A Gynecologic Oncology Group study. *Am. J. Clin. Oncol.*, **21**, 591–594

Lookingbill, D.P., Demers, L.M., Tigelaar, R.E. & Shalita, A.R. (1988) Effect of isotretinoin on serum levels of precursor and peripherally derived androgens in patients with acne. *Arch. Dermatol.*, **124**, 540–543

Lotan, R. & Lotan, D. (1980) Stimulation of melanogenesis in a human melanoma cell line by retinoids. *Cancer Res.*, **40**, 3345–3350

Lotan, R., Xu, X.C., Lippman, S.M., Ro, J.Y., Lee, J.S., Lee, J.J. & Hong, W.K. (1995) Suppression of retinoic acid receptor-β in premalignant oral lesions and its up-regulation by isotretinoin. *N. Engl. J. Med.*, **332**, 1405–1410

Lott, I.T., Bocian, M., Pribram, H.W. & Leitner, M. (1984) Fetal hydrocephalus and ear anomalies associated with maternal use of isotretinoin. *J. Pediatr.*, **105**, 597–600

Lynberg, M.C., Khoury, M.J., Lammer, E.J., Waller, K.O., Cordero, J.F. & Erickson, J.D. (1990) Sensitivity, specificity, and positive predictive value of multiple malformations in isotretinoin embryopathy surveillance. *Teratology*, **42**, 513–519

Mangelsdorf, D.J., Umesono, K. & Evans, R.M. (1994) The retinoid receptors. In: Sporn, M.B., Roberts, A.B. & Goodman, D.S., eds. *The Retinoids: Biology, Chemistry, and Medicine*. 2nd Ed. New York, Raven Press, pp. 319–350

Marini, J.C., Hill, S. & Zasloff, M.A. (1988) Dense metaphyseal bands and growth arrest associated with isotretinoin therapy. *Am. J. Dis. Child.*, **142**, 316–318

Marwick, C. (1984) More cautionary labeling appears on isotretinoin. *J. Am. Med. Assoc.*, **251**, 3208–3209

Matsuoka, L.Y., Wortsman, J., Lifrak, E.T., Parker, L.N. & Mehta, R.G. (1989) Effect of isotretinoin in acne is not mediated by adrenal androgens. *J. Am. Acad. Dermatol.*, **20**, 128–129

Mayer, H. & Isler, O. (1971) Total syntheses. In: Isler, O., ed. *Carotenoids*. Basel, Birkhauser Verlag, pp. 325–575

McBride, W.G. (1985) Limb reduction deformities in child exposed to isotretinoin in utero on gestation days 26–40 only. *Lancet*, **i**, 1276–1276

McCarthy, D.J., Lindamood, C, 3rd & Hill, D.L. (1987) Effects of retinoids on metabolizing enzymes and on binding of benzo(a)pyrene to rat tissue DNA. *Cancer Res.*, **47**, 5014–5020

McCormick, D.L., Bagg, B.J. & Hultin, T.A. (1987) Comparative activity of dietary or topical exposure to three retinoids in the promotion of skin tumor induction in mice. *Cancer Res.*, **47**, 5989–5993

Meigel, W.N. (1997) How safe is oral isotretinoin? *Dermatology*, **195** (Suppl 1), 22–28

Meloche, S. & Besner, J.G. (1986) Metabolism of isotretinoin. Biliary excretion of isotretinoin glucuronide in the rat. *Drug Metab. Dispos.*, **14**, 246–249

Meyskens, F.L.J. & Fuller, B.B. (1980) Characterization of the effects of different retinoids on the growth and differentiation of a human melanoma cell line and selected subclones. *Cancer Res.*, **40**, 2194–2196

Milstone, L.M., McGuire, J. & Ablow, R.C. (1982) Premature epiphyseal closure in a child receiving oral 13-*cis*-retinoic acid. *J. Am. Acad. Dermatol.*, **7**, 663–666

Mitchell, A.A., Van-Bennekom, C.M. & Louik, C. (1995) A pregnancy-prevention program in women of childbearing age receiving isotretinoin [see comments]. *N. Engl. J. Med.*, **333**, 101–106

Moon, T.E., Levine, N., Cartmel, B. & Bangert, J.L. (1997) Retinoids in prevention of skin cancer. *Cancer Lett.*, **114**, 203–205

Moskop, J.C., Smith, M.L. & De Ville, K. (1997) Ethical and legal aspects of teratogenic medications: The case of isotretinoin. *J. Clin. Ethics*, **8**, 264–278

Nadin, L. & Murray, M. (1996) All-*trans*-retinoic acid 4-hydroxylation in human liver microsomes: In vitro modulation by therapeutic retinoids. *Br. J. Clin. Pharmacol.*, **41**, 609–612

Napoli, J.L. (1994) Retinoic acid homeostatis. Prospective roles of β-carotene, retinol, CRBP and CRABP. In: Blomhoff, R., ed. *Vitamin A in Health and Disease*. New York, Marcel Dekker, pp. 135–188

Nau, H. (1990) Correlation of transplacental and maternal pharmacokinetics of retinoids during organogenesis with teratogenicity. *Methods Enzymol.*, **190**, 437–448

Nau, H. (1995) Chemical structure–teratogenicity relationships, toxicokinetics and metabolism in risk assessment of retinoids. *Toxicol. Lett.*, **82–83**, 975–979

Nau, H., Chahoud, I., Dencker, L., Lammer, E.J. & Scott, W.J. (1994) Teratogenicity of vitamin A and retinoids. In: Blomhoff, R., ed. *Vitamin A in Health and Disease*. New York, Marcel Dekker, pp. 615–663

Newman, L.M., Johnson, E.M. & Staples, R.E. (1993) Assessment of the effectiveness of animal developmental toxicity testing for human safety. *Reprod. Toxicol.*, **7**, 359–390

Nightingale, S.L. (1998) From the Food and Drug Administration. *JAMA*, **279**, 984–984

Novick, N.L., Lawson, W. & Schwartz, I.S. (1984) Bilateral nasal bone osteophytosis associated with short-term oral isotretinoin therapy for cystic acne vulgaris. *Am. J. Med.*, **77**, 736–739

Orfanos, C.E. (1985) Retinoids in clinical dermatology: An update. In: Saurat, J.H., ed., *Retinoids: New Trends in Research and Therapy*, Basel, Karger, pp. 314–334

Orme, M., Back, D.J., Shaw, M.A., Allen, W.L., Tjia, J., Cunliffe, W.J. & Jones, D.H. (1984a) Isotretinoin and contraception. *Lancet*, **ii**, 752–753

Orme, M., Back, D.J., Cunliffe, W.J., Jones, D.H., Allen, W.L. & Tjia, J. (1984b) Isotretinoin and oral contraceptive steroids. In: Cunliffe, W.J. & Miller, A.J., eds, *Retinoid Therapy*, Lancaster, MTP Press, pp. 277–283

Pastuszak, A., Koren, G. & Rieder, M.J. (1994) Use of the Retinoid Pregnancy Prevention Program in Canada: Patterns of contraception use in women treated with isotretinoin and etretinate. *Reprod. Toxicol.*, **8**, 63–68

Pavese, P., Kuentz, F., Belleville, C., Rougé, P.E. & Elsener, M. (1997) Renal impairment induced by isotretinoin. *Nephrol. Dial. Transplant.*, **12**, 1299–1299

Peck, G.L. & DiGiovanna, J.J. (1994) Synthetic retinoids in dermatology. In: Sporn,, M.B., Roberts, A.B. & Goodman, D.S., eds. *The Retinoids: Biology, Chemistry, and Medicine*. 2nd Ed. New York, Raven Press, pp. 631–658

Peck, G.L., Olsen, T.G., Yoder, F.W., Strauss, J.S., Downing, D.T., Pandya, M., Butkus, D. & Arnaud-Battandier, J. (1979) Prolonged remissions of cystic and conglobate acne with 13-*cis*-retinoic acid. *N. Engl. J. Med.*, **300**, 329–333

Peck, G.L., Olsen, T.G., Butkus, D., Pandya, M., Arnaud-Battandier, J., Gross, E.G., Windhorst, D.B. & Cheripko, J. (1982) Isotretinoin versus placebo in the treatment of cystic acne. A randomized double-blind study. *J. Am. Acad. Dermatol.*, **6**, 735–745

Pennes, D.R., Ellis, C.N., Madison, K.C., Voorhees, J.J. & Martel, W. (1984) Early skeletal hyperostoses secondary to 13-cis-retinoic acid. *Am. J. Roentgenol.*, **142**, 979–983

Pennes, D.R., Martel, W. & Ellis, C.N. (1985) Retinoid-induced ossification of the posterior longitudinal ligament. *Skeletal. Radiol.*, **14**, 191–193

Pennes, D.R., Martel, W., Ellis, C.N. & Voorhees, J.J. (1988) Evolution of skeletal hyperostoses caused by 13-*cis*-retinoic acid therapy. *Am. J. Roentgenol.*, **151**, 967–973

Pilorget, H., Alessandri, J.L., Montbrun, A., Ah-Hot, M., Orvain, E. & Tilmont, P. (1995) Isotretinoin (RoAccutane®) embryopathy. A case report. *J. Gynecol. Obstet. Biol. Reprod. Paris*, **24**, 511–515

Pittsley, R.A. & Yoder, F.W. (1983) Retinoid hyperostosis. Skeletal toxicity associated with long-term administration of 13-*cis*-retinoic acid for refractory ichthyosis. *N. Engl. J. Med.*, **308**, 1012–1014

Prout, G.R., Jr & Barton, B.A. (1992) 13-*cis*-Retinoic acid in chemoprevention of superficial bladder cancer. The National Bladder Cancer Group. *J. Cell Biochem. Suppl.*, **16I**, 148–152

Rademaker, M., Wallace, M., Cunliffe, W. & Simpson, N.B. (1991) Isotretinoin treatment alters steroid metabolism in women with acne. *Br. J. Dermatol.*, **124**, 361–364

Rappaport, E.B. & Knapp, M. (1989) Isotretinoin embryopathy—A continuing problem. *J. Clin. Pharmacol.*, **29**, 463–465

Rizzo, R., Lammer, E.J., Parano, E., Pavone, L. & Argyle, J.C. (1991) Limb reduction defects in humans associated with prenatal isotretinoin exposure. *Teratology*, **44**, 599–604

Robertson, R. & MacLeod, P.M. (1985) Accutane-induced teratogenesis. *Can. Med. Assoc. J.*, **133**, 1147–1148

Rosa, F.W. (1984) A syndrome of birth defects with maternal exposure to a vitamin A congener: isotretinoin. *J. Clin. Dysmorphol.*, **2**, 13–17

Rosa, F.W. (1992) Retinoid embryopathy in humans. In: Koren, G., ed., *Retinoids in Clinical Practice. The Risk–Benefit Ratio,* New York, Marcel Dekker, pp. 77–109

Rosenthal, M.A. & Oratz, R. (1998) Phase II clinical trial of recombinant alpha 2b interferon and 13-*cis* retinoic acid in patients with metastatic melanoma. *Am. J. Clin. Oncol.*, **21**, 352–354

Rutka, J.T., De Armond, S.J., Giblin, J., McCulloch, J.R., Wilson, C.B. & Rosenblum, M.L. (1988) Effect of retinoids on the proliferation, morphology and expression of glial fibrillary acidic protein of an anaplastic astrocytoma cell line. *Int. J. Cancer*, **42**, 419–427

Saccomanno, G., Moran, P.G., Schmidt, R., Hartshorn, D.F., Brian, D.A., Dreher, W.H. & Sowada, B.J. (1982) Effects of 13-cis retinoids on premalignant and malignant cells of lung origin. *Acta Cytol.*, **26**, 78–85

Sandberg, J.A., Eckhoff, C., Nau, H. & Slikker, W. (1994) Pharmacokinetics of 13-*cis*-, all-*trans*-, 13-*cis*-4-oxo-, and all-*trans*-4-oxo retinoic acid after intravenous administration in the cynomolgus monkey. *Drug Metab. Dispos.*, **22**, 154–160

Sanford, K.K., Parshad, R., Price, F.M., Tarone, R.E. & Kraemer, K.H. (1992) Retinoid protection against X-ray-induced chromatid damage in human peripheral blood lymphocytes. *J. Clin. Invest.*, **90**, 2069–2074

Schaber, B., Mayer, P., Schreiner, T., Rassner, G. & Fierlbeck, G. (1994) Anti-proliferative activity of natural interferon-alpha, isotretinoin and their combination varies in different human melanoma cell lines. *Melanoma Res.*, **4**, 319–326

Schardein, J.L. (1993) Human studies: retinoic acid embryopathy. In: Schardein, J.L., ed., *Chemically Induced Birth Defects,* New York, Marcel Dekker, pp. 558–567

Schill, W.B., Wagner, A., Nikolowski, J. & Plewig, G. (1981) Aromatic retinoid and 13-*cis*-retinoic acid: spermatological investigations. In: Orfanos, C.E., Braun-Falco, O., Farber, E.M., Grupper, C., Polano, M.K., & Schuppli, R., eds, *Retinoids. Advances in Basic Research and Therapy,* Berlin, Springer Verlag, pp. 389–395

Schweiter, U., Englert, G., Rigassi, N. & Vetter, W. (1969) Physical organic methods in carotenoid research. *Pure Appl. Chem.*, **20**, 365–420

Scuderi, A.J., Datz, F.L., Valdivia, S. & Morton, K.A. (1993) Enthesopathy of the patellar tendon insertion associated with isotretinoin therapy. *J. Nucl. Med.*, **34**, 455–457

Shalinsky, D.R., Bischoff, E.D., Gregory, M.L., Gottardis, M.M., Hayes, J.S., Lamph, W.W., Heyman, R.A., Shirley, M.A., Cooke, T.A., Davies, P.J. & Thomazy, V. (1995) Retinoid-induced suppression of squamous cell differentiation in human oral squamous cell carcinoma xenografts (line 1483) in athymic nude mice. *Cancer Res.*, **55**, 3183–3191

Shalita, A.R., Armstrong, R.B., Leyden, J.J., Pochi, P.E. & Strauss, J.S. (1988) Isotretinoin revisited. *Cutis*, **42**, 1–19

Shoyab, M. (1981) Inhibition of the binding of 7,12-dimethylbenz[a]anthracene to DNA of murine epidermal cells in culture by vitamin A and vitamin C. *Oncology*, **38**, 187–192

Siebert, J.R. & Lammer, E.J. (1990) Craniofacial anatomy of retinoic acid embryopathy. *Teratology*, **41**, 592–592

Soprano, D.R., Gyda, M., 3rd, Jiang, H., Harnish, D.C., Ugen, K., Satre, M., Chen, L., Soprano, K.J. & Kochhar, D.M. (1994) A sustained elevation in retinoic acid receptor-β2 mRNA and protein occurs during retinoic acid-induced fetal dysmorphogenesis. *Mech. Dev.*, **45**, 243–253

Squire, R.A., Sporn, M.B., Brown, C.C., Smith, J.M., Wenk, M.L. & Springer, S. (1977) Histopathological evaluation of the inhibition of rat bladder carcinogenesis by 13-*cis*-retinoic acid. *Cancer Res.*, **37**, 2930–2936

Stadler, W.M., Kuzel, T., Dumas, M. & Vogelzang, N.J. (1998) Multicenter phase II trial of interleukin-2, interferon-α, and 13-*cis*-retinoic acid in patients with metastatic renal-cell carcinoma. *J. Clin. Oncol.*, **16**, 1820–1825

Stern, R.S. (1989) When a uniquely effective drug is teratogenic. The case of isotretinoin. *N. Engl. J. Med.*, **320**, 1007–1009

Stern, R.S., Rosa, F. & Baum, C. (1984) Isotretinoin and pregnancy. *J. Am. Acad. Dermatol.*, **10**, 851–854

Stinson, S.F., Reznik, G. & Donahoe, R. (1981) Effect of three retinoids on tracheal carcinogenesis with *N*-methyl-*N*-nitrosourea in hamsters. *J. Natl Cancer Inst.*, **66**, 947–951

Strauss, J.S., Cunningham, W.J., Leyden, J.J., Pochi, P.E. & Shalita, A.R. (1988) Isotretinoin and teratogenicity. *J. Am. Acad. Dermatol.*, **19**, 353–354

Tangrea, J.A., Edwards, B.K., Taylor, P.R., Hartman, A.M., Peck, G.L., Salasche, S.J., Menon, P.A., Benson, P.M., Mellette, J.R., Guill, M.A., Robinson, J.K., Guin, J.D., Stoll, H.L., Grabski, W.J. & Winton, G.B. (1992a) Long-term therapy with low-dose isotretinoin for prevention of basal cell carcinoma: A multicenter clinical trial. Isotretinoin–Basal Cell Carcinoma Study Group. *J. Natl Cancer Inst.*, **84**, 328–332

Tangrea, J.A., Kilcoyne, R.F., Taylor, P.R., Helsel, W.E., Adrianza, M.E., Hartman, A.M., Edwards, B.K. & Peck, G.L. (1992b) Skeletal hyperostosis in patients receiving chronic, very-low-dose isotretinoin. *Arch. Dermatol.*, **128**, 921–925

Tangrea, J.A., Adrianza, E., Helsel, W.E., Taylor, P.R., Hartman, A.M., Peck, G.L. & Edwards, B.K. (1993) Clinical and laboratory adverse effects associated with long-term, low-dose isotretinoin: Incidence and risk factors. The Isotretinoin–Basal Cell Carcinoma Study Group. *Cancer Epidemiol. Biomarkers. Prev.*, **2**, 375–380

Taylor, D.D., Taylor, C.G., Black, P.H., Jiang, C.G. & Chou, I.N. (1990) Alterations of cellular characteristics of a human ovarian teratocarcinoma cell line after in vitro treatment with retinoids. *Differentiation*, **43**, 123–130

Tembe, E.A., Honeywell, R., Buss, N.E. & Renwick, A.G. (1996) All-*trans*-retinoic acid in maternal plasma and teratogenicity in rats and rabbits. *Toxicol. Appl. Pharmacol.*, **141**, 456–472

Teratology Society (1991) Recommendations for isotretinoin use in women of childbearing potential. *Teratology*, **44**, 1–6

Tetzner, C., Juhl, H.J. & Rüdiger, H.W. (1980) Sister-chromatid exchange induction by metabolically activated retinoids in human diploid fibroblast cultures. *Mutat. Res.*, **79**, 163–167

Toma, S., Isnardi, L., Raffo, P., Dastoli, G., De Francisci, E., Riccardi, L., Palumbo, R. & Bollag, W. (1997) Effects of all-*trans*-retinoic acid and 13-*cis*-retinoic acid on breast-cancer cell lines: Growth inhibition and apoptosis induction. *Int. J. Cancer*, **70**, 619–627

Toma, S., Isnardi, L., Riccardi, L. & Bollag, W. (1998) Induction of apoptosis in MCF-7 breast carcinoma cell line by RAR and RXR selective retinoids. *Anticancer Res.*, **18**, 935–942

Török, L. & Kasa, M. (1985) Spermatological and endocrinological examinations connected with isotretinoin treatment. In: Saurat, J.H., ed., *Retinoids. New Trends in Research and Therapy*, New York, Karger, pp. 407–410

Tremblay, M., Voyer, P. & Aubin, G. (1985) Congenital malformations due to accutane. *Can. Med. Assoc. J.*, **133**, 208–208

Trizna, Z., Hsu, T.C., Schantz, S.P., Lee, J.J. & Hong, W.K. (1992) Anticlastogenic effects of 13-*cis*-retinoic acid *in vitro*. *Eur. J. Cancer*, **29A**, 137–140

Trizna, Z., Schantz, S.P., Lee, J.J., Spitz, M.R., Goepfert, H., Hsu, T.C. & Hong, W.K. (1993) *In vitro* protective effects of chemopreventive agents against bleomycin-induced genotoxicity in lymphoblastoid cell lines and peripheral blood lymphocytes of head and neck cancer patients. *Cancer Detect. Prev.*, **17**, 575–583

Tzimas, G., Bürgin, H., Collins, M.D., Hummler, H. & Nau, H. (1994) The high sensitivity of the rabbit to the teratogenic effects of 13-*cis*-retinoic acid (isotretinoin) is a consequence of prolonged exposure of the embryo to 13-*cis*-retinoic acid and 13-*cis*-4-oxo-retinoic acid, and not of isomerization to all-*trans*-retinoic acid. *Arch. Toxicol.*, **68**, 119–128

Tzimas, G., Collins, M.D. & Nau, H. (1995) Developmental stage-associated differences in the transplacental distribution of 13-*cis*- and all-*trans*-retinoic acid as well as their glucuronides in rats and mice. *Toxicol. Appl. Pharmacol.*, **133**, 91–101

Tzimas, G., Nau, H., Hendrickx, A.G., Peterson, P.E. & Hummler, H. (1996) Retinoid metabolism and transplacental pharmacokinetics in the cynomolgus monkey following a nonteratogenic dosing regimen with all-trans-retinoic acid. *Teratology,* **54**, 255–265

Vahlquist, A. (1994) Role of retinoids in normal and diseased skin. In: Blomhoff, R., ed. *Vitamin A in Health and Disease.* New York, Marcel Dekker, pp. 365–424

Valentic, J. & Barr, R.J. (1985) Isotretinoin therapy and premature epiphyseal closure. *J. Am. Med. Assoc.,* **253**, 841–842

Vane, F.M. & Bugge, C.J. (1981) Identification of 4-oxo-13-cis-retinoic acid as the major metabolite of 13-cis-retinoic acid in human blood. *Drug Metab. Dispos.,* **9**, 515–520

Vane, F.M., Bugge, C.J., Rodriguez, L.C., Rosenberger, M. & Doran, T.I. (1990) Human biliary metabolites of isotretinoin: Identification, quantification, synthesis, and biological activity. *Xenobiotica,* **20**, 193–207

Van Herle, A.J., Agatep, M.L., Padua, D.N., Totanes, T.L., Canlapan, D.V., Van Herle, H.M. & Juillard, G.J. (1990) Effects of 13-*cis*-retinoic acid on growth and differentiation of human follicular carcinoma cells (UCLA R0 82 W-1) in vitro. *J. Clin. Endocrinol. Metab.,* **71**, 755–763

Verma, A.K., Shapas, B.G., Rice, H.M. & Boutwell, R.K. (1979) Correlation of the inhibition by retinoids of tumor promoter-induced mouse epidermal ornithine decarboxylase activity and of skin tumor promotion. *Cancer Res.,* **39**, 419–425

Verma, A.K., Duvick, L. & Ali, M. (1986) Modulation of mouse skin tumor promotion by dietary 13-*cis*-retinoic acid and α-difluoromethylornithine. *Carcinogenesis,* **7**, 1019–1023

Vetter, W., Englert, G., Rigassi, N. & Schwieter, U. (1971) Spectroscopic methods. In: Isler, O., Gutmann, H. & Solms, U., eds. *Carotenoids.* Basel, Birkhauser Verlag, pp. 189–266

Villablanca, J.G., Khan, A.A., Avramis, V.I. & Reynolds, C.P. (1993) Hypercalcemia: A dose-limiting toxicity associated with 13-cis-retinoic acid. *Am. J. Pediatr. Hematol. Oncol.,* **15**, 410–415

Waladkhani, A.R. & Clemens, M.R. (1997) Differences in the pharmacokinetics of 13-cis retinoic acid in cancer patients. *Int. J. Cancer,* **70**, 494–495

Wang, C.C., Campbell, S., Furner, R.L. & Hill, D.L. (1980) Disposition of all-*trans*- and 13-*cis*-retinoic acids and N-hydroxyethylretinamide in mice after intravenous administration. *Drug Metab. Dispos.,* **8**, 8–11

Watanabe, T. & Pratt, R.M. (1991) Influence of retinoids on sister chromatid exchanges and chromosomes in cultured human embryonic palatal mesenchymal cells. *Teratog. Carcinog. Mutag.,* **11**, 297–304

Westerman, S.T., Gilbert, L.M. & Schondel, L. (1994) Vestibular dysfunction in a child with embryonic exposure to accutane. *Am. J. Otolaryngol.,* **15**, 400–403

Willhite, C.C., Hill, R.M. & Irving, D.W. (1986) Isotretinoin-induced craniofacial malformations in humans and hamsters. *J. Craniofac. Genet. Dev. Biol.,* **2** (Suppl.), 193–209

Williams, J.B., Shields, C.O., Brettel, L.M. & Napoli, J.L. (1987) Assessment of retinoid-induced differentiation of F9 embryonal carcinoma cells with an enzyme-linked immunoadsorbent assay for laminin: Statistical comparison of dose–response curves. *Anal. Biochem.,* **160**, 267–274

Yarita, T., Nettesheim, P. & Mitchell, T.J. (1980) Failure of two retinoids to inhibit tracheal carcinogenesis in hamsters. *Carcinogenesis,* **1**, 255–262

Yuschak, M.M. & Gautieri, R.F. (1993) Teratogenicity of 13-cis retinoic acid and phenobarbital sodium in CF-1 mice. *Res. Commun. Chem. Pathol. Pharmacol.,* **82**, 259–278

Zarowny, D.P. (1984) Accutane™ Roche®: Risk of teratogenic effects. *Can. Med. Assoc. J.,* **131**, 273–273

Zhu, J., Shi, X.G., Chu, H.Y., Tong, J.H., Wang, Z.Y., Naoe, T., Waxman, S., Chen, S.J. & Chen, Z. (1995) Effect of retinoic acid isomers on proliferation, differentiation and PML relocalization in the APL cell line NB4. *Leukemia,* **9**, 302–309

9-*cis*-Retinoic acid

1. Chemical and Physical Characteristics

1.1 Nomenclature
See General Remarks Section 1.4.

1.2 Name: 9-*cis*-Retinoic acid

Chemical Abstracts Services Registry Number
5300-03-8

IUPAC systematic name
(7*E*,9*Z*,11*E*,13*E*)-9,13-dimethyl-7-(1,1,5-tri-methylcyclohex-5-en-6-yl)nona-7,9,11,13-tetraen-15-oic acid (see 1.3), or (2*E*,4*E*,6*Z*,8,*E*)-3,7-dimethyl-9-(2,2,6-trimethylcyclohex-1-en-1-yl)nona-2,4,6,8-tetraen-1-oic acid

Synonyms
9-*cis*-RA, 9-*cis*-vitamin A acid, 9-*cis*-vitamin A_1 acid, Panretin ®, LGD 1057

1.3 Structural formula

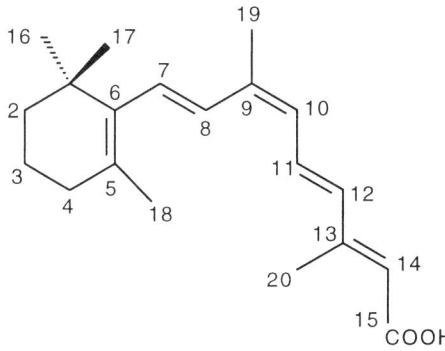

Composition: $C_{20}H_{28}O_2$
Relative molecular mass: 300.45

1.4 Physical and chemical properties
Description
Yellow crystals from ethanol

Melting-point
189–191 °C (Robeson *et al.*, 1955).

Solubility
Soluble in most organic solvents, fats, and oils; sparingly soluble in water.

Spectroscopy
UV and visible: λ_{max} 345 (ethanol), $E_{1\,cm}^{1\%}$ 1230, E_M 36 900 (Robeson *et al.*, 1955; Frickel, 1984; Barua & Furr, 1998)

Nuclear magnetic resonance
^{1}H-NMR (CDCl$_3$, 220 MHz): δ 1.04 (1-CH$_3$), 1.48 (2-CH$_2$), 1.64 (3-CH$_2$), 1.75 (5-CH$_3$), 2.01 (9-CH$_3$), 2.04 (4-CH$_2$), 2.37 (13-CH$_3$), 5.82 (14-H), 6.09 (10-H), 6.27 (12-H), 6.31 (7-H), 6.67 (8-H), 7.15 (11-H); J$_{7,8}$ (15.7 Hz), J$_{10,11}$ (11.3 Hz), J$_{11,12}$ (14.7 Hz) (Schweiter *et al.*, 1969; Vetter *et al.*, 1971; Frickel, 1984; Barua & Furr, 1998).

^{13}C-NMR (CDCl$_3$ 68 MHz); δ 13.4 (13-CH$_3$), 18.9 (3-C), 20.5 (9-CH$_3$), 21.6 (5-CH$_3$), 28.8 (1,1-CH$_3$), 32.7 (4-C), 33.9 (1-C), 39.3 (2-C), 119.6 (14-C), 128.1 (10-C), 129.0 (8-C), 129.4 (5-C), 129.6 (7-C, 11-C), 134.7 (12-C), 137.3 (6-C), 137.6 (9-C), 151.2 (13-C), 167.8 (15-C) (Englert, 1975; Frickel, 1984; Barua & Furr, 1998)

Resonance Raman, infrared and mass spectrometry
(Frickel, 1984; Barua & Furr, 1998).

X-Ray analysis
(Frickel, 1984).

Stability
Unstable to light, oxygen and heat. In solution is protected by the presence of antioxidants, such as butylated hydroxytoluene and pyrogallol. A variety of factors influence its stability in tissue culture media. Degradation and isomerization are minimized by storing under an inert gas such as argon, at –20 °C or lower in the dark (Frickel, 1984; Barua & Furr, 1998)

2. Occurrence, Production, Use, Human Exposure and Analysis

2.1 Occurrence

The concentration of 9-*cis*-retinoic acid in the plasma of fasting individuals is < 1 nmol/L. When a 70-kg man ate 140 g of turkey liver containing 0.25 mmol of vitamin A, however, the concentration of 9-*cis*-retinoic acid rose to 9 nmol/L and that of its 9,13-*cis* metabolite to 57 nmol/L within 4 h (Arnhold *et al.*, 1996). The concentrations were 100 pmol/g in mouse kidney and 13 pmol/g in liver, and may well be similar in human tissues (Blaner & Olson, 1994). Thus, the concentration of 9-*cis*-retinoic acid is < 0.1% that of all-*trans*-retinol in human plasma and < 2% that of total vitamin A in the tissues of healthy animals and humans. 9-*cis*-Retinoic acid is present only in traces in plants, if at all. It is therefore a very minor constituent of the diet, and, unlike vitamin A and carotenoids, is not available as a dietary supplement. The one notable exception is the concentration found in human plasma after consumption of liver (Arnhold *et al.*, 1996), possibly via formation from 9-*cis*-retinol, which is known to be present in that organ.

2.2 Production

The synthesis of 9-*cis*-retinoic acid is based on that of the all-*trans* isomer (see Handbook 1, **p.** 96), with several modifications. Thus, condensation of a 9-*cis*-β-C_{15}-aldehyde with ethyl senecioate in the presence of potassium amide in liquid ammonia gives 9-*cis*-retinoic acid (Mayer & Isler, 1971; Frickel, 1984). Use of a *trans* C_{14} aldehyde in Isler's industrial synthesis of retinol also yields predominantly the 9-*cis* isomer. Photoisomerization of all-*trans*-retinoids in a polar solvent such as acetonitrile yields a mixture of *cis* isomers, in which the 9-*cis* isomer predominates (Frickel, 1984). 9-*cis*-Retinal can also be converted to its acid by mild oxidants (Mayer & Isler, 1971; Frickel, 1984). Newer methods of synthesis for a large number of retinoids have been reviewed (Dawson & Hobbs, 1994).

2.3 Use

Although 9-*cis*-retinoic acid was identified, synthesized and characterized in the 1950s, it received attention as a potential therapeutic agent only after its identification in 1992 as an agonist for the retinoic acid receptor (RAR) and as the putative physiological ligand for the retinoid X receptor (RXR) (Heyman *et al.*, 1992 ; Levin *et al.*, 1992). The use of 9-*cis*-retinoic acid in the treatment of clinical disorders is therefore still in its infancy. The types of cancer that might be affected by treatment with 9-*cis*-retinoic acid are listed in Table 1 (Hong & Itri, 1994; Kelloff *et al.*, 1996; Makishima *et al.*, 1998; Soignet *et al.*, 1998).

Table 1. Types of cancer being considered for treatment with 9-*cis*-retinoic acid in planned or on-going clinical studies
Acute promyelocytic leukaemia
Breast carcinoma
Cervical carcinoma
Colon carcinoma
Kaposi sarcoma
Lung carcinoma
Neuroblastoma
Prostate carcinoma

[a] Modified from Hong & Itri (1994); Kelloff *et al.* (1996); Makishima *et al.* (1998); Soignet *et al.* (1998)

In clinical trials in which the dose was escalated gradually, the maximum tolerated oral dose of 9-*cis*-retinoic acid was found to be approximately 80 mg/m² per day (Rizvi *et al.*, 1998). A topical 0.1% formulation of 9-*cis*-retinoic acid (Panretin®) has been approved for the treatment of Kaposi sarcoma in the United States.

2.4 Human exposure

As indicated above, the total amount of 9-*cis*-retinoic acid in food is very small, probably 10–100 μg/day. 9-*cis*-Retinoic acid is one of the least prevalent of the retinoic acid isomers. Because it is rapidly metabolized in the body and is not stored in the liver or other organs, it does not accumulate over time (Blaner & Olson, 1994). The amount of 9-*cis*-retinoic acid ingested in the diet therefore poses neither benefit nor risk. Exposure to 9-*cis*-retinoic acid is limited, for all practical purposes, to topical and oral treatment of medical disorders. Although the various isomers of retinoic acid, including 9-*cis*-retinoic acid, are therapeutically effective, many adverse side-effects of therapeutic doses have been reported (Kamm *et al.*, 1984; Armstrong *et al.*, 1994; Nau *et al.*, 1994; Kelloff *et al.*, 1996; see section 7.1).

2.5 Analysis

9-*cis*-Retinoic acid is commonly measured in plasma and tissues by high-performance liquid chromatography (HPLC; Barua & Furr, 1998). Either plasma or a tissue homogenate is acidified to pH 3–4 and then extracted several times with a suitable volume of an organic solvent such as chloroform and methanol, diethyl ether, dichloromethane, acetonitrile, 2-propanol or ethyl acetate. After the combined extract has been dried with anhydrous sodium sulfate, the solvent is evaporated to dryness under yellow light (to avoid isomerization) in nitrogen or argon. The dried powder is immediately dissolved in the HPLC solvent and injected onto the HPLC column. In some cases, a solid-phase extraction or elution step is introduced to remove contaminants.

A reversed-phase C_{18} column is usually used for the separation. It is usually detected by measuring the absorption at 345 nm and quantified by measuring the area under the absorption peak with an integrator. A known amount of a reference standard, usually all-*trans*-retinyl acetate, is added to the tissue, plasma or serum sample to correct for losses during extraction and analysis. An antioxidant such as butylated hydroxytoluene is also added at the outset to minimize oxidation of any retinoids present.

A large number of chromatographic systems has been devised for the separation and quantification of 9-*cis*-retinoic acid (Frolik & Olson, 1984; Furr *et al.*, 1992, 1994; Barua & Furr, 1998; Barua *et al.*, in press). In most reversed-phase HPLC systems, 9-*cis*-retinoic acid is eluted between 13-*cis*-retinoic acid and all-*trans*-retinoic acid.

9-*cis*-Retinoic acid, as its methyl or pentafluorobenzyl ester, can also be separated by gas–liquid or liquid–liquid chromatography and quantified by mass spectrometry. New ionization methods and tandem mass spectrometry have further enhanced the sensitivity and selectivity with which various isomers of retinoic acid can be measured (Barua *et al.*, in press).

3. Metabolism, Kinetics and Genetic Variation

[The Working Group was concerned that there is insufficient experimental evidence to establish whether 9-*cis*-retinoic acid is 'the' or 'a' physiological ligand for the RXR family of receptors. Although there is a considerable body of literature on the formation of 9-*cis*-retinoic acid within cells, tissues and organisms and on its actions in living systems, decisive, unequivocal proof that 9-*cis*-retinoic acid is a physiological form of retinoic acid is lacking. In spite of this uncertainty, the literature on the metabolism, kinetics and tissue distribution of 9-*cis*-retinoic acid is reviewed below without bias, nevertheless referring to it as a 'putative' physiological ligand.]

3.1 Humans

3.1.1 Metabolism

9-*cis*-Retinoic acid was given to healthy men at 20 mg/day for 28 days, and plasma, urine and faeces were collected before treatment and after treatment on days 14 and 28. The major urinary metabolites were 9-*cis*-retinoyl-β-glucuronide and 9-*cis*-4-oxoretinoyl-β-glucuronide. High concentrations of unchanged 9-*cis*-retinoic acid were observed in the faeces. The authors consequently suggested that the substance is poorly absorbed in the gastrointestinal tract. The major metabolites in plasma 2 h after the last dose of 9-*cis*-retinoic acid on day 28 of the study were all-*trans*- and 13-*cis*-retinoic acid, 9,13-di-*cis*-retinoic acid and a mixture of 4-oxoretinoic acid isomers (Sass *et al.*, 1995).

A double-blind, placebo-controlled, randomized study was conducted in 40 healthy men given single increasing oral doses of 5, 15, 40, 80 and 150 mg of 9-*cis*-retinoic acid to assess the pharmacokinetics of single doses. The main metabolites in serum were all-*trans*- and 13-*cis*-retinoic acid and all-*trans*- and 9-*cis*-4-oxoretinoic acid. The main metabolite at all doses was 9-*cis*-4-oxoretinoic acid, which was present in blood at concentrations 41–83% of those observed for 9-*cis*-retinoic acid (Weber & Dumont, 1997).

9-*cis*-Retinoic acid was converted to more polar products very slowly by human endothelial cells in culture, whereas the same cells metabolized all-*trans*-retinoic acid rapidly. In contrast, cultured human hepatocytes metabolized 9-*cis*-retinoic acid faster than they did all-*trans*-retinoic acid (Lansink *et al.*, 1997).

3.1.2   Kinetics

9-*cis*-Retinoic acid was given orally twice daily at doses ranging from 20 to 150 mg/m^2 per day to 22 patients with carcinomas at various organ sites. On day 1 of the study, the time to the peak plasma concentration was 3–4 h at all doses of 9-*cis*-retinoic acid except the lowest and 6 h at the lowest dose. On day 22, the peak plasma concentrations were reached within 2–3.6 h at all doses. After 22 days of administration of 9-*cis*-retinoic acid, the peak concentrations and the values for the integrated area under the curve of plasma concentration–time (AUC) were markedly lower than those calculated for the same patients on day 1. The pharmacokinetics of 9-*cis*-retinoic acid was highly variable between patients, and the parameters overlapped widely between doses. The observed decrease in plasma concentration with increased length of administration also varied, but it was not possible to determine whether the reduction was dose-dependent because of the relatively small number of patients studied (Kurie *et al.*, 1996).

In the study of Weber and Dumont (1997) described above, the pharmacokinetics of 9-*cis*-retinoic acid were linear over the range of doses studied. The peak plasma concentrations were achieved on average within 3–4 h of dosing. The major pathway for elimination was reported to be by metabolism. The average AUC value for the 5-mg dose was 49 ng-h/mL, and that for the 150-mg dose was 1700 ng-h/mL. As has been reported after administration of all-*trans*- and 13-*cis*-retinoic acid to humans, 9-*cis*-retinoic acid induced a dose- or concentration-dependent reduction in plasma retinol concentration, by a maximum of 30% within 24 h after administration; however, the plasma concentration of retinol-binding protein remained unchanged.

3.1.3   Tissue distribution

The only systematic information about the concentrations of 9-*cis*-retinoic acid in human tissues is that reported by Arnhold *et al.* (1996; see Table 3 in General Remarks) and in the studies of pharmacokinetics discussed above. The limited information available suggests that the concentrations are

likely to be near the low limits of detection of modern analytical procedures based on HPLC.

3.1.4   Variation within human populations

No information was available about possible differences in the metabolism of 9-*cis*-retinoic acid within human populations.

3.2   Experimental models

3.2.1   Metabolism

9,13-Di-*cis*-retinoic acid was identified by HPLC–mass spectroscopy as a major metabolite of 9-*cis*-retinoic acid in the plasma of female mice given the compound orally at a dose of 50 mg/kg bw. A number of polar metabolites were found, including the β-glucuronides of 9-*cis*-retinoic acid and of 9-*cis*-4-oxoretinoic acid (Tzimas *et al.*, 1994a).

After radiolabelled 9-*cis*-retinoic acid was given orally at 10 or 100 mg/kg bw or intravenously at 10 mg/kg bw to male and female Sprague-Dawley rats, 9-*cis*-4-hydroxy- and 9-*cis*-4-oxoretinoic acid were the major metabolites. 9-*cis*-Retinoic acid also isomerized to 13-*cis*-retinoic acid, 9,13-di-*cis*-retinoic acid and all-*trans*-retinoic acid. The amount of volatile radiolabelled products increased with time after dosing, suggesting that β-oxidation of 9-*cis*-retinoic acid might occur. 9-*cis*-13,14 Dihydroretinoic acid was identified by nuclear magnetic resonance spectrometry as a metabolite, and the authors suggested that this represented an initial step in the β-oxidation of 9-*cis*-retinoic acid (Shirley *et al.*, 1996). The proposed oxidative and reductive metabolic pathways for 9-*cis*-retinoic acid in rats are shown in Figure 1.

In pregnant mice and rats given 9-*cis*-retinoic acid as a single oral dose of 100 mg/kg bw, 9-*cis*-retinoyl-β-glucuronide was the major metabolite in plasma and in all the tissues examined, but the concentrations were much larger in mouse than in rat plasma, suggesting species differences in the absorption and metabolism of this compound (Sass *et al.*, 1994).

Unanaesthetized and continuously anaesthetized male Wistar rats housed in metabolic cages were given 9-*cis*-retinoic acid at a single oral dose of 30 mg/kg bw and followed for 72 h. Urine and faeces collected at 24-, 48- and 72-h intervals. Most of the elimination occurred through the faeces, and about 75% was unchanged 9-*cis*-

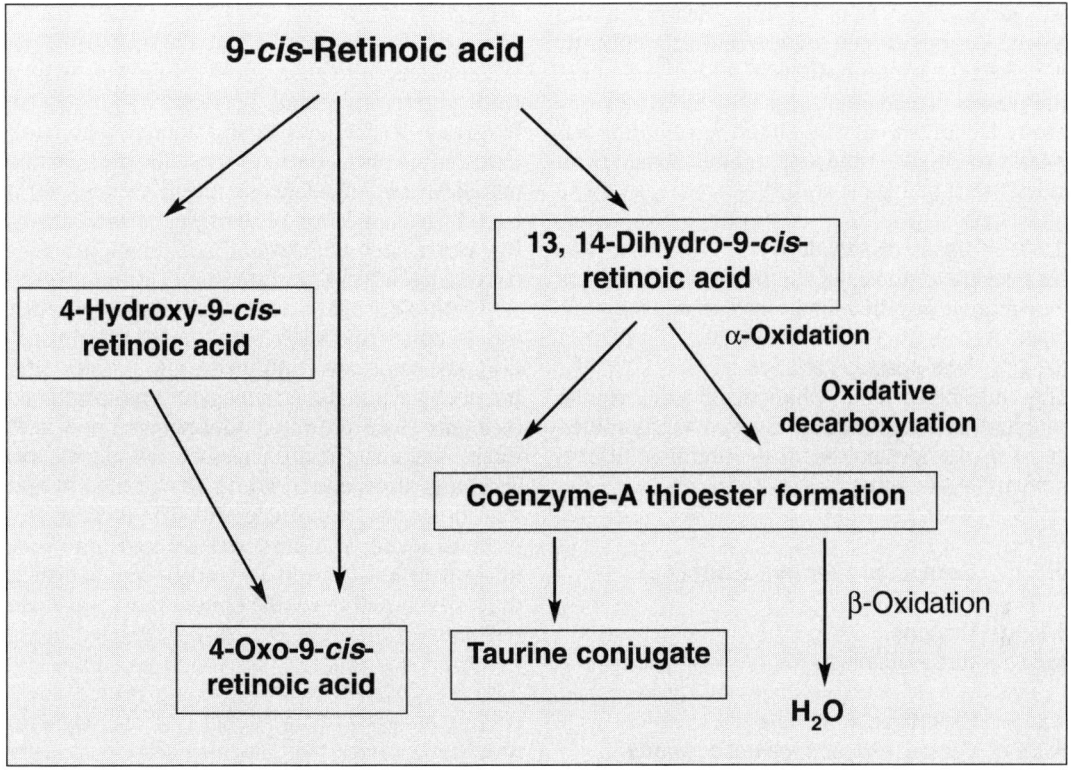

Figure 1. Proposed oxidative and reductive metabolic pathways for 9-*cis*-retinoic acid in rats

retinoic acid. The remainder of the excretion products were all-*trans*- and 13-*cis*-retinoic acid and 9-*cis*-, all-*trans*- and 13-*cis*-4-oxoretinoic acids (Disdier *et al.*, 1996). Unlike Sass *et al.* (1994, 1995), Disdier *et al.* (1996) found that very little 9-*cis*-retinoic acid is eliminated in either the urine or faeces of unanaesthetized rats as the glucuronide conjugate, and only small quantities of glucuronide conjugates were found in anesthetized rats. Disdier *et al.* (1996) suggested that the discrepancy was due to differences in experimental conditions and/or differences between species.

3.2.2   Kinetics

After female mice received 9-*cis*-retinoic acid at 50 mg/kg bw, the concentrations in plasma reached a maximum within 40–60 min and then declined in a mono-exponential manner with an apparent half-life of 64 ± 32 min. The plasma concentration of 9,13-di-*cis*-retinoic acid 90 min after treatment,

about 2 µmol/L, was nearly identical to that of 9-*cis*-retinoic acid (Tzimas *et al.*, 1994a). 9,13-Di-*cis*-retinoic acid was also identified as a major circulating metabolite after oral administration of 9-*cis*-retinal to rats and mice (Tzimas *et al.*, 1995).

In nude mice given all-*trans*- or 9-*cis*-retinoic acid at a single oral dose of 10 mg/kg bw, the peak concentration of 9-*cis*-retinoic acid in plasma occurred earlier (15–30 min) than that of all-*trans*-retinoic acid (60–180 min). Both the maximum plasma concentrations and the AUC values were lower for 9-*cis*-retinoic acid than all-*trans*-retinoic acid. In animals given a second dose of either compound two days after the first, the value for the AUC was decreased for all-*trans*-retinoic acid but increased for 9-*cis*-retinoic acid due apparently to the appearance of a second 9-*cis*-retinoic acid peak in the blood 180 min after dosing. The authors speculated that the increase was due to changes in the rate and/or site(s) of uptake or reabsorption of

9-*cis*-retinoic acid from the bile. Treatment with all-*trans*- and 9-*cis*-retinoic acid significantly decreased the concentrations of all-*trans*-retinol in the plasma of nude mice, by 50–60% within 4 h. The reduction was greater after a second dose was given two days after the first and was sustained for at least 48 h (Achkar *et al.*, 1994).

3.2.3 Tissue distribution
No systematic studies of the tissue distribution of 9-*cis*-retinoic acid in animals were available.

3.2.4 Inter-species variation
The metabolic and pharmacokinetic studies summarized above indicate marked species differences in the metabolism of 9-*cis*-retinoic acid in humans and rodents.

4. Cancer-preventive Effects

4.1 Humans
No data were available to the Working Group.

4.2 Experimental models
4.2.1 Cancer and preneoplastic lesions
These studies are summarized in Table 2.

4.2.1.1 Mammary gland
Groups of 24 (control) or 12 (treated) female Sprague-Dawley rats, 50 days of age, were injected intravenously with *N*-methyl-*N*-nitrosourea (MNU) at a dose of 50 mg/kg bw. One week later, the treated animals were given an experimental diet containing 60 or 120 mg/kg 9-*cis*-retinoic acid for 4.5 months. The incidence of mammary adenocarcinomas was 100% in controls and 58% and 25% at the low and high doses of 9-*cis*-retinoic acid ($p < 0.002$ and $p < 0.001$, respectively, Fisher's exact test). The tumour multiplicity was 3.6 for controls and 1.6 and 0.3 at the low and high dose, respectively ($p < 0.002$ in both cases; Mantel non-parametric test). The combination of 9-*cis*-retinoic acid with tamoxifen was more effective than either agent alone (Anzano *et al.*, 1994).

The experiment was repeated with similar results in a later study. 9-*cis*-Retinoic acid in combination with raloxifene was more effective than either agent alone (Anzano *et al.*, 1996).

4.2.1.2 Prostate
Groups of 30–40 male Wistar-Unilever (HsdCpb: WU) rats, seven to eight weeks of age, were treated with cyproterone acetate at a dose of 50 mg/kg bw by gavage for 21 days; then, one day later, with testosterone propionate at three daily doses of 100 mg/kg bw by subcutaneous injection; then, 60 h later, a single injection of 30 mg/kg bw MNU; then, two weeks later, with two Silastic tubing implants containing 40 mg testosterone. Treatment with 9-*cis*-retinoic acid at a dose of 50 or 100 mg/kg diet was initiated one week before MNU administration. The study was continued for 13 months after treatment with the carcinogen. The combined incidence of prostate adenocarcinomas and carcinosarcomas in all accessory sex glands was 79% in controls and 33% and 48% at the low and high doses of 9-*cis*-retinoic acid. The incidence of prostate adenocarcinomas was reduced from 65% in controls to 20% and 18% at the low and high doses of retinoid ($p < 0.01$; Fisher's exact two-sided test) (McCormick *et al.*, 1999).

4.2.1.3 Colon
Groups of 30–33 male Fischer 344 rats, eight to nine weeks of age, were injected intraperitoneally with azoxymethane at 15 mg/kg bw weekly for two weeks. The animals were maintained on a AIN76A diet alone or supplemented with 9-*cis*-retinoic acid at 0.1 mmol/kg of diet beginning one week before the first injection of carcinogen until the end of the study 36 weeks later. The incidence of colon adenocarcinomas was 33% in controls and 25% in rats given 9-*cis*-retinoic acid (not significant). 9-*cis*-Retinoic acid reduced the number of adenomas per rat from 3.2 to 2.2 ($p < 0.01$, ANOVA) and reduced the number of aberrant crypt foci per colon from 153 to 97 ($p < 0.01$, ANOVA) (Zheng *et al.*, 1997).

4.2.2 Intermediate biomarkers
9-*cis*-Retinoic acid at 0.1 mmol/kg of diet reduced the incidence of azoxymethane-induced aberrant crypt foci in the colon of rats (for details, see section 4.2.1.3; Zheng *et al.*, 1997).

4.2.3 In-vitro models
4.2.3.1 Cellular studies
The effects of 9-*cis*-retinoic acid have been analysed primarily in established tumour cell lines in monolayer culture, although a few studies were

Table 2. Effects of 9-cis-Retinoic acid (9-cis-RA) on carcinogenesis in rats

Cancer site	Strain, sex, age at carcinogen treatment	No. of animals per group	Carcinogen dose (mg/kg bw). route	9-cis-RA dose/route (basal diet)	Duration in relation to carcinogen	Incidence Control	Incidence 9-cis-RA	Multiplicity Control	Multiplicity 9-cis-RA	Efficacy	Reference
Mammary gland	Sprague-Dawley, female, 50 d	24	MNU 50 mg/kg bw, i.v.	60 mg/kg	+ 1 wk to end	100	58*	3.6	1.6*	Effective	Anzano et al. (1994)
		12		120 mg/kg		100	25*	3.6	0.3*	Effective	
Mammary gland	Sprague-Dawley, female, 50 d	24	MNU 50 mg/kg bw, i.v.	60 mg/kg	+ 1 wk to end	96	75	3.0	1.7	Effective	Anzano et al. (1996)
		12									
Colon	Fischer, 8–9 weeks	30–33	AOM, 15 mg/kg bw	0.1 mmol/kg diet	–1 wk to 36 wks	33	25	3.3	2.2*	Effective[a]	Zheng et al. (1997)
Prostate	Wistar, male, 7–8 weeks	30–40	50 mg/kg bw cyproterone acetate 21 d, 100 mg/kg bw testosterone proprionate s.c. 3 days, 30 mg/kg bw MNU i.v., 40 mg testosterone s.c.	50 mg/kg diet	–1 wk to end	65	20*	NR	NR	Effective	McCormick et al. (1999)
						65	18*	NR	NR	Effective	

MNU, N'-Methyl-N-nitrosourea; i.v., intravenously; AOM, azoxymethane; s.c., subcutaneously; NR, not reported

* Statistically significant (see text)

[a] Effective in reducing aberrant crypt foci and adenomas

carried out with immortalized cells. In general, the effects of 9-*cis*-retinoic acid were similar to those of all-*trans*-retinoic acid in that both inhibited cell proliferation and induced differentiation and apoptosis in some cell lines, perhaps because of their overlapping mechanisms of action. They were also found to have different effects on particular cell systems, perhaps because of their distinct mechanisms of action.

(a) Inhibition of cell proliferation

9-*cis*-Retinoic acid enhanced clonal growth of myeloid and erythroid cells from normal individuals and was more potent than all-*trans*-retinoic acid in stimulating the myeloid cells (Sakashita *et al.*, 1993).

9-*cis*-Retinoic acid, like all-*trans*-retinoic acid, inhibited the growth of the human HPV-16-immortalized ectocervical epithelial cells (Agarwal *et al.*, 1996) and inhibited the proliferation of a large panel of Epstein-Barr virus-immortalized lymphoblastoid cell lines with accumulation of cells in G_0/G_1 and no apparent direct cytotoxicity (Pomponi *et al.*, 1996).

9-*cis*-Retinoic acid inhibited the growth of gastric cancer cell lines without arresting them in G_0/G_1 (Naka *et al.*, 1997). Its inhibitory effects on DNA synthesis in cultured human breast cancer cell lines were equivalent to those of all-*trans*-retinoic acid (Anzano *et al.*, 1994). 9-*cis*-Retinoic acid also inhibited the growth of human breast cancer cells such as T47D under anchorage-dependent and anchorage-independent conditions (Darro *et al.*, 1998). Both 9-*cis*-retinoic acid and all-*trans*-retinoic acid at concentrations ranging from 10 nmol/L to 1 µmol/L inhibited the growth of all-*trans*-retinoic acid-sensitive NB4 cells and of fresh cells from 11 patients with acute promyelocytic leukaemia (Miller *et al.*, 1995). 9-*cis*-Retinoic acid was more potent than all-*trans*-retinoic acid in suppressing the clonal growth of two cell lines and samples from 13 patients with acute myelocytic leukaemia and samples from four patients with acute promyelocytic leukaemia (Sakashita *et al.*, 1993). Samples from three patients with acute myelocytic leukaemia responded to the growth inhibitory effects of 9-*cis*-retinoic acid but were refractory to all-*trans*-retinoic acid (Sakashita *et al.*, 1993). 9-*cis*-Retinoic acid, like all-*trans*-retinoic acid, inhibited the growth in monolayer culture of

several cells lines with oestrogen receptors (ERs) but not in those without. The inhibited cells accumulated in G_1. In addition, 9-*cis*-retinoic acid induced down-regulation of ER mRNA and protein and the expression of the oestrogen-responsive genes *PR* and *pS2* in MCF-7 cells (Rubin *et al.*, 1994). The growth of neuroblastoma cells was inhibited by 9-*cis*-retinoic acid in association with suppression of *myc* expression, and 9-*cis*-retinoic acid was 5–10 times more potent than all-*trans*-retinoic acid in this respect (Han *et al.*, 1995). The growth inhibitory effect of 9-*cis*-retinoic acid was reversible in studies in which this was examined, such as in human oral squamous-cell carcinoma cell lines (Giannini *et al.*, 1997).

(b) Modulation of differentiation

9-*cis*-Retinoic acid modulates differentiation in several types of cells. Treatment of human keratinocytes cultured in a submerged culture system with 9-*cis*-retinoic acid for up to five weeks induced a more proliferative phenotype with a longer lifespan than control cultures. The small proline-rich proteins, SPRR1 and SPRR2, were repressed weakly and strongly, respectively; the induction of involucrin was delayed, whereas expression of *Ki67* and of c-*jun* was maintained (Gibbs *et al.*, 1996). 9-*cis*-Retinoic acid induced differentiation in cells from patients with acute promyelocytic leukaemia and acute myeloid leukaemia (Sakashita *et al.*, 1993). Although similar effects on the induction of differentiation in NB4 acute promyelocytic leukaemia cells were observed after treatment with all-*trans*-retinoic acid or 9-*cis*-retinoic acid at 0.1 µmol/L, 9-*cis*-retinoic acid at 0.01 µmol/L was more active than all-*trans*-retinoic acid (Zhu *et al.*, 1995)

9-*cis*-Retinoic acid induced differentiation in cell lines from patients with acute promyelocytic and acute myelogenous leukaemia in primary culture and in HL60 and NB4 cells (Sakashita *et al.*, 1993; Zhu *et al.*, 1995). It is a more potent inducer of differentiation than all-*trans*-retinoic acid in HL60 cells but only at low concentrations in NB4 cells (Zhu *et al.*, 1995). 9-*cis*-Retinoic acid was 5–10 times more potent in inducing neuroblastoma cell differentiation (neurite outgrowth, increased acetylcholinesterase activity) than all-*trans*-retinoic acid (Han *et al.*, 1995). In human head-and-neck squamous carcinoma cells, 9-*cis*-retinoic acid, like all-*trans*-retinoic acid, suppressed squamous differentiation (decreased the level of keratin K1) and induced RARβ expression (Zou *et al.*, 1999).

(c)   Induction of apoptosis
9-*cis*-Retinoic acid induced apoptosis even in cells that did not undergo apoptosis after treatment with all-trans-retinoic acid. It induced apoptosis in some HL-60 sublines even without inducing differentiation, whereas all-trans-retinoic acid could not induce apoptosis unless the cells had first undergone differentiation to mature granulocytes. 9-*cis*-Retinoic acid also induced apoptosis in several human small-cell lung carcinoma cell lines (Güzey *et al.*, 1998), in adult T-cell leukaemia cell lines (Fujimura et al., 1998), in NB4 acute promyelocytic leukaemia cells (Bruel *et al.*, 1995) and in neuroblastoma cell lines (Lovat *et al.*, 1997a).

In one cellular system of apoptosis, in which activation of T-cell hybridomas induces a block at G_1/S in the cell cycle and apoptosis, 9-*cis*-retinoic acid inhibited apoptosis by suppressing the expression of Fas ligand (Yang *et al.*, 1995).

4.2.3.2   Antimutagenicity in short-term tests
No published reports were found of studies of the effect of 9-*cis*-retinoic acid on carcinogen- or mutagen-induced genotoxicity either *in vitro* or *in vivo*. The possible effect of this retinoid on cytochrome P450 (CYP) systems was examined in two studies (Table 3). The messenger RNA levels of three CYP isoenzymes were measured in primary rat hepatocytes cultured for 48 h in the presence of 9-*cis*-retinoic acid at 40 µmol/L. An eightfold increase was found for CYP3A ($p < 0.05$), a slight increase for CYPyp1A1 (not significant) and no change for CYPyp1A2 (Jurima-Romet *et al.*, 1997).

In male Sprague-Dawley rats treated with 9-*cis*-retinoic acid at a dose of 30 mg/kg bw per day by gavage for four days, the hepatic levels of CYP2B1/2 and CYP4A increased by over twofold ($p < 0.05$), while that of CYP2E was reduced by 33% ($p < 0.05$) and those of CYP1A2 by 27%, CYP2C11

Table 3. Effects of 9-*cis*-retinoic acid on metabolic activity *in vitro* and *in vivo*

Dose and route	Cells or animals	Investigated effect	Result[a]	LED/HID[b]	Reference
40 µmol/L	Rat hepatocytes	Cytochrome P450 (CYP) mRNA levels			Jurima-Romet et al. (1997)
		CYP1A1	–	40 µmol/L	
		CYP1A2	–	40 µmol/L	
		CYPCyp3a1/2	#	40 µmol/L	
30 mg/kg bw per day by gavage for 4 days	Male Sprague-Dawley rats	Liver CYP protein levels		30 mg/kg bw per day by gavage for 4 days	Howell et al. (1988)
		CYP2B1/2	#		
		CYP Cyp2C11	–		
		CYP2E	+		
		CYPCyp3A	–		
		CYP4A	#		
		Total CYP concentration	+		
		Effect on retinoid CYP metabolism (glucuronidation)	–		

[a] +, inhibition of the investigated end-point; –, no effect on the investigated end-point; #, enhancement of investigated end-point
[b] LED, lowest effective dose that inhibits or enhances the investigated effect; HID, highest ineffective dose

by 18% and CYP3A by 4% (all non-significant). When microsomal fractions from 9-*cis*-retinoic acid-treated animals were tested for the ability to metabolize this retinoid *in vitro*, PCYP-mediated metabolism was unchanged and a slight decrease was observed in glucuronidation, although the effect was not significant (Howell *et al.*, 1998).

4.3   Mechanisms of cancer prevention

Some reports and the more extensive information available on all-*trans*-retinoic acid suggest that 9-*cis*-retinoic acid exerts its effect on carcinogenesis at the promotion stage. The mechanisms that could account for the chemopreventive activities of 9-*cis*-retinoic acid are discussed below.

4.3.1   Antagonism of tumour promotion and AP-1 activity

In human bronchial epithelial cells, AP-1 transcriptional activity was reduced markedly by 9-*cis*-retinoic acid (Lee *et al.*, 1996). In a cell line of normal rabbit synovial fibroblasts, 9-*cis*-retinoic acid inhibited the induction of collagenase (metalloproteinase MMP-1) by antagonizing AP-1 at the transcriptional level (Pan *et al.*, 1995). These findings suggest that some of the chemopreventive effects of 9-*cis*-retinoic acid may derive from its antagonistic effects on AP-1.

4.3.2   Inhibition of cell proliferation

9-*cis*-Retinoic acid inhibited the proliferation of several cell lines *in vitro* (see section 4.2.3), including arrestation of some cells in the G_1 phase of the cell cycle (Fujimura *et al.*, 1998). *In vivo*, 9-*cis*-retinoic acid reduced mitotic activity and enhanced apoptosis in adenomas that develop *in vivo* in rats exposed to azoxymethane, and these effects were also considered to be the mechanism by which 9-*cis*-retinoic acid prevented aberrant crypt foci and colon tumours (Zheng *et al.*, 1999). The possible mechanisms of growth inhibition include changes in cell cycle regulatory proteins and modulation of autocrine loops.

4.3.2.1   Cyclins and cyclin D kinase inhibitors

Because lesions of human noninvasive breast carcinoma *in situ* overexpress cyclin D, agents that can reduce the level of this cyclin may be useful in chemoprevention. 9-*cis*-Retinoic acid inhibited the levels of expression of cyclins D1 and D3 in human

MCF-7, ZR-75 and T-47D breast carcinoma cells *in vitro*, and similar effects were observed in the immortalized HBL-100 and MCF-10A breast cell lines. 9-*cis*-Retinoic acid also suppressed the levels of Cdk2 and Cdk4. These data suggest that 9-*cis*-retinoic acid suppresses cell cycle progression from G_1 to S by reducing cyclin D expression in a variety of breast cell lines *in vitro* (Zhou *et al.*, 1997). In gastric cancer cell lines, 9-*cis*-retinoic acid inhibited growth after a transient increase in the amount of the cyclin-dependent kinase inhibitor, p21/Waf1/Cip1 protein, and also reduced the amount of cdk-7, epidermal growth factor receptor and cyclin D1 proteins. This was followed by a reduction in phosphorylation of the product of the retinoblastoma tumour suppressor gene in sensitive TMK-1 cells but not in resistant MKN-7 cells. These results suggest that the cytostatic effect of 9-*cis*-retinoic acid on gastric cancer cells is mediated through changes in the cell cycle regulatory machinery (Naka *et al.*, 1997).

4.3.2.2   Modulation of autocrine and paracrine loops

9-*cis*-Retinoic acid can interfere with autocrine loops, such as that associated with prolactin, which plays an important role in the induction and progression of mammary tumours. 9-*cis*-Retinoic acid down-regulated prolactin receptors in breast cancer cell lines within 1 h, and the maximal effect was achieved within 24 h. It was suggested that this effect on the prolactin signalling pathway is relevant for cancer prevention (Widschwendter *et al.*, 1999). Another growth stimulatory pathway affected by 9-*cis*-retinoic acid is that involving insulin-like growth factor. Treatment of Hs578T breast cancer cells with 9-*cis*-retinoic acid at 100 nmol/L increased the level of insulin-like growth factor binding protein 3 in the conditioned medium. It was suggested that this binding protein contributes to the growth inhibitory effect of 9-*cis*-retinoic acid by reducing the growth stimulatory effect of exogenous insulin-like growth factor-I (Colston *et al.*, 1998). The third example involves the estrogen and ER signalling pathway. 9-*cis*-Retinoic acid inhibited the growth in monolayer culture of several ER-positive, but not ER-negative, cell lines. MCF-7 cells exposed to 9-*cis*-retinoic acid showed a dose-dependent accumulation in G_1. 9-*cis*-Retinoic acid down-regulated ER mRNA and protein in MCF-7 cells, accompanied by decreased expression of the oestrogen-responsive genes *PR* and *pS2* in MCF-7 cells (Rubin *et al.*, 1994).

4.3.3   *Restoration of normal differentiation*
The ability of 9-*cis*-retinoic acid to modulate the differentiation of normal and malignant cells might be related to its chemopreventive effects. For example, normal human bronchial epithelial cells often undergo abnormal squamous differentiation in primary culture *in vitro* under certain conditions with exposure to certain growth factors. 9-*cis*-Retinoic acid could restore normal differentiation to such cells as it can inhibit the mRNA expression of the squamous differentiation markers transglutaminase type I, involucrin, keratin 5 and keratin 13 (Lee *et al.*, 1996). 9-*cis*-Retinoic acid also induced differentiation of neuroblastoma (Han *et al.*, 1995; Lovat *et al.*, 1997b) and acute promyelocytic cells (Elstner *et al.*, 1997).

4.3.3.1   *Induction of apoptosis*
The ability of 9-*cis*-retinoic acid to induce apoptosis in a variety of tumour cell lines even without inducing differentiation (Bruel *et al.*, 1995; Nagy *et al.*, 1995; Fujimura *et al.*, 1998) suggests that this effect may occur also in premalignant cells and thereby mediate some of its effects on carcinogenesis. Further support for this conclusion comes from the finding that 9-*cis*-retinoic acid enhanced the apoptotic index in non-involved crypts and in adenomas that developed in azoxymethane-treated rats (Zheng *et al.*, 1999).

4.3.3.2   *Increased cell adhesion*
9-*cis*-Retinoic acid induced E-cadherin in the human SK-BR-3 breast carcinoma cell line, and it was suggested that this could be a change towards a more normal phenotype (Anzano *et al.*, 1994). Because E-cadherin is not only an adhesion molecule but also functions as a tumour suppressor, its induction by 9-*cis*-retinoic acid could explain some of the chemopreventive effect of the latter.

4.3.3.3   *Mechanistic considerations*
9-*cis*-Retinoic acid is a pan-RAR, RXR agonist. As such, it can exert its action through RARs, as does all-*trans*-retinoic acid. There is considerable evidence both *in vitro* and in genetic studies that RAR and RXR ligands synergize within the RAR–RXR heterodimer, which is believed to be the major—albeit not the sole—molecular species that mediates retinoid action (Kastner *et al.*, 1995; Lotan *et al.*, 1995; Chambon, 1996). 9-*cis*-Retinoic acid is expected to be a more potent ligand of the RAR–RXR heterodimer and more potent *in vitro* than all-*trans*-retinoic acid owing to its ability to activate both subunits simultaneously. The affinity of 9-*cis*-retinoic acid for RARs is similar to that of all-*trans*-retinoic acid but about 20–50 times greater than the affinity of all-*trans*-retinoic acid for RXRs (Allenby *et al.*, 1993). Since in mammalian cell systems all-*trans*-retinoic acid and 9-*cis*-retinoic acid can be interconverted by unknown enzymatic systems, both isomers may contribute to the pharmacological response elicited when animals are exposed to either compound. In addition to acting through the RAR–RXR heterodimer, 9-*cis*-retinoic acid can act, at least in principle, through RXR homodimers and through a multitude of RXR heterodimers with other nuclear receptors, such as the thyroid hormone, vitamin D, peroxisome proliferator-activated (PPAR) and various so-called orphan receptors (see General Remarks, section 3). There is no firm evidence that a RXR homodimer signalling pathway exists, but the impact of RXR ligands on signalling pathways involving other RXR heterodimers such as, for example, PPAR–RXR (Mukherjee *et al.*, 1997) has to be taken into account when evaluating the biological action of an RXR ligand.

5.   Other Beneficial Effects
No reports of well-conducted studies with 9-*cis*-retinoic acid in humans on conditions other than cancer were available to the Working Group.

6.   Carcinogenicity

6.1   Humans
No data were available to the Working Group.

6.2   Experimental models
No data were available to the Working Group.

7. Other Toxic Effects

7.1 Adverse effects

7.1.1 Humans

The toxicity of 9-*cis*-retinoic acid is similar to that of other retinoids and mimics the symptoms of hypervitaminosis A. The most frequent effects include headache and adverse changes in the skin and mucous membranes. Commonly reported anomalies in clinical chemistry include hypercalcaemia and lipid abnormalities. Most of the adverse reactions are dose-dependent and reversible.

In a phase-I trial of 9-*cis*-retinoic acid in advanced cancer in which 34 patients received a single daily dose of 5–230 mg/m^2 per day for four weeks, the recommended single daily dose of 9-*cis*-retinoic acid was determined to be 140 mg/m^2 per day (Miller *et al.*, 1996). In another phase-I study, in 22 patients with solid tumours, the subjects received 20–150 mg/m^2 per day in two equal doses, and the recommended dose for continued evaluation was 100 mg/m^2 per day (Kurie *et al.*, 1996).

7.1.1.1 Retinoic acid syndrome

In a clinical study of 9-*cis*-retinoic acid in acute promyelocytic leukaemia, three of 12 patients receiving 30–230 mg/m^2 per day were treated with corticosteroids at high doses for signs suggestive of retinoic acid syndrome (Soignet *et al.*, 1998).

7.1.1.2 Toxicity in the central nervous system and general toxicity

One of the most commonly reported adverse effects of 9-*cis*-retinoic acid is headache, which can range from mild to severe. In 41 healthy men who received a single oral dose of 5–150 mg 9-*cis*-retinoic acid per day, the incidence but not the severity of headache increased with dose, affecting all subjects given doses ≥ 80 mg (Weber & Dumont, 1997). Headache occurred in all of seven subjects with acute promyelocytic leukaemia receiving 30–230 mg/m^2 per day (Miller *et al.*, 1995) and in 15 of 16 patients receiving 50–230 mg/m^2 per day (Soignet *et al.*, 1998). Headache was the most common and often the dose-limiting effect in three studies of 9-*cis*-retinoic acid in patients with cancer (Kurie *et al.*, 1996; Miller *et al.*, 1996; Rizvi *et al.*, 1998). Headaches associated with

administration of 9-*cis*-retinoic acid can often be controlled by medication, although unrelenting headache (Rizvi *et al.*, 1998) and migraine (Weber & Dumont, 1997) have been reported.

Other general signs associated with oral administration of 9-*cis*-retinoic acid include fatigue (Kurie *et al.*, 1996; Soignet *et al.*, 1998) and diffuse pain (Miller *et al.*, 1996).

Facial flushing is frequently observed after administration of 9-*cis*-retinoic acid, usually within a few hours, and is sometimes associated with headache (Miller *et al.*, 1995, 1996; Weber & Dumont, 1997; Rizvi *et al.*, 1998; Soignet *et al.*, 1998). Insomnia and changes in mental status have also been reported (Kurie *et al.*, 1996; Aboulafia *et al.*, 1998).

7.1.1.3 Mucocutaneous toxicity

In 41 healthy men given 9-*cis*-retinoic acid at a single oral dose of 5–150 mg, the most common adverse events were cutaneous and consisted primarily of mild xeroderma at doses > 80 mg/day, accompanied by pruritis in one participant (Weber & Dumont, 1997). No significant mucocutaneous reactions were reported in seven patients with acute promyelocytic leukaemia given 30–230 mg/m^2 per day for 3–62 days (Miller *et al.*, 1995). In another study in patients with this disease, dry skin was the second most common adverse effect at doses of 30–230 mg/m^2 per day (Soignet *et al.*, 1998). Cutaneous reactions were also the second most common adverse effects in patients with advanced cancer treated with 9-*cis*-retinoic acid once or twice daily at doses up to 140 mg/m^2 per day. The reactions consisted of grade-1 dry skin and erythema in 10 of 41 patients, and grade-2 peeling of the fingers in one subject (Rizvi *et al.*, 1998). Frequent mucocutaneous reactions of grades 1–2 were seen at doses of 15–230 mg/m^2 per day (Miller *et al.*, 1996), and frequent mucositis was seen at 20–150 mg/m^2 per day (Kurie *et al.*, 1996).

7.1.1.4 Metabolic, nutritional and haematological toxicity

The haematological effects seen after administration of 9-*cis*-retinoic acid appear to be dose-related. No significant change in haematological parameters was reported in five patients with acute promyelocytic leukaemia receiving doses ≤ 140 mg/m^2 per day (Miller *et al.*, 1995), and no relevant anomalies in serum chemistry were reported in a study of 34 healthy men receiving single doses of 5–150 mg (Weber & Dumont, 1997). Haematological effects occurred in a dose-dependent manner in a study of cancer patients receiving doses of 5–230 mg/m^2 per day and included grades 1–3 abnormalities in haemoglobin and leukocyte counts and grades 1–2 abnormalities in platelet count. No adverse effects were reported at 5 mg/m^2 per day, and most of the grades 2 and 3 events occurred at doses ≥ 180 mg/m^2 per day (Miller *et al.*, 1996).

Metabolic and nutritional events associated with use of 9-*cis*-retinoic acid include hypercalcaemia, hypercholesterolaemia, hypertriglyceridaemia, hyperbilirubinaemia, increased activities of alkaline phosphatase and aspartate aminotransferase, abnormal serum creatinine and glutamate oxaloacetate transferase activity, haematuria and proteinuria (Miller *et al.*, 1995; Kurie *et al.*, 1996; Miller *et al.*, 1996). In one study, the occurrence of hypertriglyceridaemia was related to dose and time, increasing with protracted use (Miller *et al.*, 1996). Elevated concentrations of triglycerides were present in 6 of 41 patients receiving 9-*cis*-retinoic acid at doses up to 140 mg/m^2 per day, but no symptomatic hypertriglyceridaemia was seen. The activity of transaminases was increased in 4 of 41 patients in this study and was dose limiting for one subject at 83 mg/m^2 per day and for another at 140 mg/m^2 per day. Dose-limiting hyperbilirubinaemia occurred in one subject receiving 70 mg/m^2 per day, and grade 4 hypercalcaemia was reported in two patients receiving 50 mg/m^2 per day; one of these subjects developed renal failure, seizures, sepsis and respiratory failure and ultimately died (Rizvi *et al.*, 1998). In a phase-II clinical trial of 9-*cis*-retinoic acid for AIDS-associated Kaposi sarcoma, the patients received 60 mg/m^2 per day for two weeks, followed by escalation to 100 mg/m^2 per day. After three weeks at the higher dose, a 46-year old man developed hypercalcaemia, changes in mental status and renal insufficiency; the symptoms improved within two days of cessation of use of 9-*cis*-retinoic acid (Aboulafia *et al.*, 1998).

Recently identified molecular interactions provide some insight into the mechanism of hyperlipoproteinaemia observed during clinical treatment with retinoids. The lipoprotein levels of 43 patients receiving 9-*cis*-retinoic acid or targretin were compared. Treatment with 9-*cis*-retinoic acid resulted in statistically significant dose- and time-dependent changes from baseline values for plasma triglycerides (increased by 59%), cholesterol (increased by 16%) and high-density lipoprotein cholesterol (decreased by 15%). Treatment with targretin had little effect on these parameters, but the level of apolipoprotein A-1 (apo A-I) tended to be substantially higher in patients taking targretin than in those given 9-*cis*-retinoic acid. In preclinical studies, transcription of the anti-atherogenic apo A-I of the high-density lipoprotein complex was found to be regulated by RXRs. These preliminary data suggested that RXR-selective ligands maintain high-density lipoprotein cholesterol and apo A-I and thus minimize the complications of chronic hyperlipidaemia seen with pan receptor agonists such as 9-*cis*-retinoic acid (Nervi *et al.*, 1997).

7.1.1.5 Musculoskeletal toxicity

Generalized bone pain with a slow onset of hypercalcaemia, eventually requiring medication, was reported in one patient with acute promyelocytic leukaemia receiving 9-*cis*-retinoic acid at 140 mg/m^2 per day (Miller *et al.*, 1995), and grades 1–3 bone pain occurred in 4 of 18 patients with this disease given 9-*cis*-retinoic acid at doses of 50–140 mg/m^2 per day (Soignet *et al.*, 1998). Arthralgia and myalgia have also been associated with administration of 9-*cis*-retinoic acid (Kurie *et al.*, 1996; Miller *et al.*, 1996).

7.1.1.6 Gastrointestinal effects

The gastrointestinal effects of 9-*cis*-retinoic acid appear to be dependent on the clinical state of the person taking the drug. Three of 41 healthy male subjects given a single oral dose of 5–150 mg experienced episodic vomiting; in one of these subjects, the vomiting was associated with a migraine headache (Weber & Dumont, 1997). No significant gastrointestinal effects were observed in one study of patients with acute promyelocytic leukaemia receiving 30–230 mg/m^2 per day (Miller *et al.*, 1995). In another study in this population, grade-1 nausea and vomiting were reported in one subject at 50 mg/m^2 per day (Soignet *et al.*, 1998). Nausea, vomiting, anorexia and diarrhoea have been reported in cancer patients participating in clinical trials with 9-*cis*-retinoic acid (Kurie *et al.*,

1996; Rizvi *et al.*, 1998). Diarrhoea was one of two dose-limiting effects of 9-*cis*-retinoic acid in one phase-I study, occurring in two patients with colorectal cancer taking 150 mg/m² per day.

7.1.1.7 Ocular disorders
As is commonly observed with retinoids, conjunctivitis and blurry vision have been reported during clinical evaluation of 9-*cis*-retinoic acid (Kurie *et al.*, 1996; Rizvi *et al.*, 1998). Ocular toxicity, characterized by detachments of the retinal pigment epithelium and retinal haemorrhage, was dose-limiting in one subject taking 9-*cis*-retinoic acid at 140 mg/m² per day (Rizvi *et al.*, 1998).

7.1.1.8 Respiratory effects
Six of 16 patients with lung cancer experienced dyspnoea when taking 9-*cis*-retinoic acid at doses of 50–230 mg/m² per day (Miller *et al.*, 1996). Dyspnoea was also reported in a phase-I trial of 9-*cis*-retinoic acid in patients with acute promyelocytic leukaemia given doses of 30–230 mg/m² per day (Soignet *et al.*, 1998).

7.1.2 Experimental models
The only toxic effect seen in a number of studies of chemoprevention with 9-*cis*-retinoic acid was weight loss. In athymic nude mice with xenografts of human oral squamous-cell carcinoma, the maximum tolerated oral dose of 9-*cis*-retinoic acid was 60 mg/kg bw, which produced a 4.2% decrease in body weight and mild mucocutaneous irritation after 24 days of treatment on five days per week. The weight loss and mucocutaneous reactions were dose-dependent: no adverse effects were seen at 10 or 30 mg/kg bw per day, while a 10% weight loss and mild-to-moderate mucocutaneous reactions were seen at 100 mg/kg bw per day (Shalinsky *et al.*, 1995). Five doses of 30 mg/kg bw per week were well tolerated in the same model (Shalinsky *et al.*, 1996).

In a model of mammary carcinogenesis induced by MNU, no signs of gross toxicity were observed in female rats fed 60 or 120 mg/kg of diet for 3 or 4.5 months, although some loss of body weight was observed (Anzano *et al.*, 1994). In another model of MNU-induced mammary tumours, rats were given 9-*cis*-retinoic acid intraperitoneally at 100 mg/kg bw per day on days 0, 1, 2, 3 and 9. Transient losses of body weight (up to

15%), alopecia and eye crusting were observed; daily dosing caused the death of some animals (Hsu, 1998). In a model of colon cancer induced by azoxymethane, 9-*cis*-retinoic acid was given to rats at a dose of 30 mg/kg of diet, since transient weight loss was observed after three weeks at 60 mg/kg, and the dose of 300 mg/kg was reported to be toxic [no details provided] (Zheng *et al.*, 1997).

Treatment of nude mice with 9-*cis*-retinoic acid at a single oral dose of 10 mg/kg bw decreased the plasma retinol concentration by 50–60% for at least 48 h; the decrease was greater after a second dose two days later (Achkar *et al.*, 1994).

7.2 Reproductive and developmental effects
7.2.1 Humans
No data were available to the Working Group.

7.2.2 Experimental models
7.2.2.1 Reproductive effects
In vitamin A-deficient mice, 9-*cis*-retinoic acid stimulated the differentiation and proliferation of growth-arrested spermatogonia in the testis (Gaemers *et al.*, 1998).

7.2.2.2 Developmental effects
The teratogenic effects of 9-*cis*-retinoic acid are summarized in Table 4. The teratogenic potency of this compound lies between that of the all-*trans* and 13-*cis* isomers. 9-*cis*-Retinoic acid induces cleft palate and limb defects in mice.

Studies with mice, rats and rabbits have shown a relationship between retinoid structure and the extent of placental transfer. Transfer of 9-*cis*-retinoic acid was intermediate between that of all-*trans*-retinoic acid and 13-*cis*-retinoic acid (Tzimas *et al.*, 1994b; Kochhar *et al.*, 1995), while the embryonic concentrations of 9-*cis*-retinoic acid β-glucuronide were < 5% of their plasma concentrations after administration of 9-*cis*-retinoic acid at mid-gestation (Tzimas *et al.*, 1995). [The Working Group noted that the poor transplacental passage of the β-glucuronide is in accordance with its hydrophilic character and high relative molecular mass.]

It is not clear how a small structural variation such as isomerization at C-13 and/or C-9 results in such drastic differences in the degree of placental transfer, because several physicochemical parameters of the retinoic acid isomers, such as relative

Table 4. Teratogenic effects of 9-*cis*-retinoic acid			
Species	Dose (mg/kg bw)	Effects	Reference
Mouse	25; GD 11	Cleft palate	Kochhar *et al.* (1995)
	100; GD 11	Limb defects	
Chick	Soaked bead implant, stage 20	Pattern duplication in wing	Thaller *et al.* (1993)
Xenopus embryo	Stages 8–18	Pattern formation in embryo	Creech Kraft *et al.* (1994)
Rat	Microinjection into cultured embryos on GD 10	Branchial arch and some somite defects	Creech Kraft & Juchau (1993)

GD, gestation day

molecular mass, pK_a and lipophilicity, are very similar or identical (Tzimas *et al.*, 1994b). In contrast, these retinoids display marked differences in their binding to embryonic cellular retinoic acid-binding proteins (CRABPs): whereas all-*trans*-retinoic acid is a high-affinity ligand of CRABP I and II, 13-*cis*-retinoic acid and 9-*cis*-retinoic acid bind to them with much lower affinity, if at all (Siegenthaler & Saurat, 1989; Allenby *et al.*, 1993; Fiorella *et al.*, 1993; Horst *et al.*, 1995).

7.3 Genetic and related effects
7.3.1 Humans
No data were available to the Working Group.

7.3.2 Experimental models
No data were available to the Working Group.

8. Summary of Data

8.1 Chemistry, occurrence and human exposure
9-*cis*-Retinoic acid is synthesized from 9-*cis*-retinol by oxidation of the C-15 alcohol group to a carboxylic acid. Like all members of the vitamin A family, 9-*cis*-retinoic acid is lipophilic, sensitive to light, heat and oxygen and readily isomerized to a mixture of *cis* and *trans* isomers. Because of its acidic nature, it is slightly more soluble in water than retinol or retinal, but still poorly so. 9-*cis*-

Retinoic acid has characteristic absorption spectra in the ultraviolet and visible, infrared and resonance Raman portions of the electromagnetic spectrum owing to its tetraene structure.

9-*cis*-Retinoic acid and its 4-oxo metabolite are present in blood and tissues of animal species in smaller amounts than retinol or retinyl ester and are not present in plant tissues. Human exposure occurs during treatment with topical or oral preparations for medical purposes.

9-*cis*-Retinoic acid has been used to treat acute promyelocytic leukaemia, and a topical formulation is approved for the treatment of Kaposi sarcoma. The maximal oral dose used in clinical studies of cancer is 100–150 mg/m² per day.

9-*cis*-Retinoic acid is usually separated by high-performance liquid chromatography and detected by its absorption at 345 nm. After chemical formation of a suitable ester, it can also be separated and detected by gas–liquid chromatography and can be quantified by mass spectrometry.

8.2 Metabolism and kinetics
Although 9-*cis*-retinoic acid is a potent ligand for retinoid X receptors, the mechanism for its endogenous presence in cells has not been established unequivocally. Three metabolic pathways have been proposed: (i) sulfhydryl groups in small molecules like glutathione and in proteins can catalyse the interconversion of 9-*cis*- and all-*trans*-retinoic acid; (ii) enzymes that can oxidize 9-*cis*-

retinol and 9-*cis*-retinal have been identified, suggesting that 9-*cis*-retinoic acid may be synthesized from 9-*cis*-retinol; and (iii) 9-*cis*-retinoic acid can be generated by cleavage of dietary 9-*cis*-β-carotene. Both 4-oxo- and glucuronide metabolites of 9-*cis*-retinoic acid have been identified in studies of pharmacokinetics in humans and animals.

8.3 Cancer-preventive effects
8.3.1 Humans
No data were available to the Working Group.

8.3.2 Experimental models
The preventive efficacy of 9-*cis*-retinoic acid was evaluated in two studies of carcinogen-induced mammary carcinogenesis, one on prostate carcinogenesis and one on colon carcinogenesis, in rats. 9-*cis*-Retinoic acid prevented mammary and prostate tumours but not colon tumours; however, it reduced the numbers of aberrant crypt foci and adenomas in the colon.

In general, the effects of 9-*cis*-retinoic acid *in vitro* were similar to those of all-*trans*-retinoic acid, in that both inhibited cell proliferation and induced differentiation and apoptosis in some cell lines; however, the 9-*cis* isomer was more potent than the all-*trans* isomer in several cell systems. 9-*cis*-Retinoic acid caused growth inhibition in normal, immortalized and malignant cell lines, often but not always in G_0 or G_1. Induction of differentiation and apoptosis were seen in several types of cells. The cells that were sensitive to 9-*cis*-retinoic acid responded to concentrations that are achieved in plasma with standard pharmacological doses *in vivo*.

The potential ability of 9-*cis*-retinoic acid to inhibit carcinogen-induced genotoxicity has not been studied *in vitro* or *in vivo*; however, two studies suggest that it could affect damage induced in DNA by a carcinogen by altering some cytochrome P450 isozymes both *in vitro* and *in vivo*.

8.3.3 Mechanisms of cancer prevention
9-*cis*-Retinoic acid appears to suppress cell proliferation and increase differentiation and apoptosis. The mechanisms by which proliferation can be inhibited involve antagonism of AP-1, decreased concentrations of cyclins and increased amounts of cyclin-dependent kinase inhibitor and interven-tion in growth-stimulating signalling pathways. Induction of apoptosis and differentiation also appear to contribute to the putative cancer-preventive effect of 9-*cis*-retinoic acid.

8.4 Other beneficial effects
No data were available to the Working Group.

8.5 Carcinogenicity
No data were available to the Working Group.

8.6 Other toxic effects
8.6.1 Humans
The toxicity of 9-*cis*-retinoic acid is similar to that of other retinoids and may result in symptoms similar to those of hypervitaminosis A. The most frequent signs and symptoms include headache and adverse skin and mucous membrane reactions. Most of the adverse reactions are dose-dependent and are reversible when therapy is discontinued. Symptoms of 'retinoic acid syndrome', a potentially life-threatening condition, have been observed during oral therapy with 9-*cis*-retinoic acid. The haematological effects that occur with administration of 9-*cis*-retinoic acid are reduced haemoglobin, leukocyte and platelet counts. The reported metabolic and nutritional effects include hypercalcaemia, hypercholesterolaemia, hyper-triglyceridaemia, hyperbilirubinaemia, elevated alkaline phosphatase and aspartate aminotransferase activity, abnormal serum creatinine and glutamate oxaloacetate transferase activity, haematuria and proteinuria. The gastrointestinal effects of 9-*cis*-retinoic acid appear to be dependent on the clinical state of the person taking the drug and can limit the dose that can be given in certain instances, such as in the treatment of patients with colorectal cancer. No studies were available on the reproductive or developmental effects of 9-*cis*-retinoic acid or on its genotoxicity in humans.

8.6.2 Experimental models
Administration of 9-*cis*-retinoic acid to athymic nude mice decreased body weight and caused mucocutaneous reactions, alopecia and eye crusting.

No data were available on the effects of 9-*cis*-retinoic acid on reproductive parameters in animals. Orally administered 9-*cis*-retinoic acid is teratogenic in mice.

9. Recommendations for research

9.1 General recommendations for 9-*cis*-retinoic acid and other retinoids

See section 9 of the Handbook on all-*trans*-retinoic acid.

9.2 Recommendations specific to 9-*cis*-retinoic acid

1. Clarify whether 9-*cis*-retinoic acid is a physiologically significant ligand in cell differentiation and its role in cancer chemoprevention.

2. Study in more detail the effects and mechanisms of action of 9-*cis*-retinoic acid in humans and in animal models.

10. Evaluation

10.1 Cancer-preventive activity
10.1.1 Humans
There is *inadequate evidence* that 9-*cis*-retinoic acid has cancer-preventive activity in humans.

10.1.2 Experimental animals
There is *limited evidence* that 9-*cis*-retinoic acid has cancer-preventive activity in experimental animals. This evaluation is based on the observation of inhibitory effects in two studies of mammary carcinogenesis and one of prostate carcinogenesis in rats.

10.2 Overall evaluation
There are no data on the cancer preventive activity of 9-*cis*-retinoic acid in humans. 9-*cis*-Retinoic acid is a known teratogen in mice.

11. References

Aboulafia, D.M., Bundow, D., Weaver, C. & Yokum, R.C. (1998) Retinoid-induced hypercalcemia in a patient with Kaposi sarcoma associated with acquired immunodeficiency syndrome. *Am. J. Clin. Oncol.*, **21**, 513–517

Achkar, C.C., Bentel, J.M., Boylan, J.F., Scher, H.I., Gudas, L.J. & Miller, W.H.J. (1994) Differences in the pharmacokinetic properties of orally administered all-*trans*-retinoic acid and 9-*cis*-retinoic acid in the plasma of nude mice. *Drug Metab. Dispos.*, **22**, 451–458

Agarwal, C., Chandraratna, R.A., Teng, M., Nagpal, S., Rorke, E.A. & Eckert, R.L. (1996) Differential regulation of human ectocervical epithelial cell line proliferation and differentiation by retinoid X receptor- and retinoic acid receptor-specific retinoids. *Cell Growth Differ.*, **7**, 521–530

Allenby, G., Bocquel, M.T., Saunders, M., Kazmer, S., Speck, J., Rosenberger, M., Lovey, A., Kastner, P., Grippo, J.F., Chambon, P. & Levin, A.A. (1993) Retinoic acid receptors and retinoid X receptors: Interactions with endogenous retinoic acids. *Proc. Natl Acad. Sci. USA*, **90**, 30–34

Anzano, M.A., Byers, S.W., Smith, J.M., Peer, C.W., Mullen, L.T., Brown, C.C., Roberts, A.B. & Sporn, M.B. (1994) Prevention of breast cancer in the rat with 9-*cis*-retinoic acid as a single agent and in combination with tamoxifen. *Cancer Res.*, **54**, 4614–4617

Anzano, M.A., Peer, C.W., Smith, J.M., Mullen, L.T., Shrader, M.W., Logsdon, D.L., Driver, C.L., Brown, C.C., Roberts, A.B. & Sporn, M.B. (1996) Chemoprevention of mammary carcinogenesis in the rat: Combined use of raloxifene and 9-*cis*-retinoic acid. *J. Natl Cancer Inst.*, **88**, 123–125

Armstrong, R.B., Ashenfelter, K.O., Eckhoff, C., Levin, A.A. & Shapiro, S.S. (1994) General and reproductive toxicology of retinoids. In: Sporn, M.B., Roberts, A.B. & Goodman, D.S., eds, *The Retinoids. Biology, Chemistry, and Medicine*, 2nd Ed. New York, Raven Press, pp. 545–572

Arnhold, T., Tzimas, G., Wittfoht, W., Plonait, S. & Nau, H. (1996) Identification of 9-*cis*-retinoic acid, 9,13-di-*cis*-retinoic acid, and 14-hydroxy-4,14-retro-retinol in human plasma after liver consumption. *Life Sci.*, **59**, L169–L177

Barua, A.B. & Furr, H.C. (1998) Properties of retinoids: Structure, handling, and preparation. In: Redfern, C.P.F., ed., *Retinoid Protocols*. Totowa, NJ, Humana Press, pp. 3–28

Barua, A.B., Furr, H.C., Olson, J.A. & van Breemen, R.B. (1999) Vitamin A and carotenoids. In: DeLeenheer, A., Lambert, W. & van Bocxlaer, J., eds, *Modern Chromatographic Analysis of the Vitamins*, 3rd Ed. New York, Marcel Dekker (in press)

Blaner, W.S. & Olson, J.A. (1994) Retinol and retinoic acid metabolism. In: Sporn, M.B., Roberts, A.B. & Goodman, D.S., eds, *The Retinoids. Biology, Chemistry, and Medicine*, 2nd Ed. New York, Raven Press, pp. 229–255

Bruel, A., Benoit, G., De-Nay, D., Brown, S. & Lanotte, M. (1995) Distinct apoptotic responses in maturation sensitive and resistant t(15;17) acute promyelocytic leukemia NB4 cells. 9-*cis* Retinoic acid induces apoptosis independent of maturation and Bcl-2 expression. *Leukemia*, **9**, 1173–1184

Chambon, P. (1996) A decade of molecular biology of retinoic acid receptors. *FASEB J.*, **10**, 940–954

Colston, K.W., Perks, C.M., Xie, S.P. & Holly, J.M. (1998) Growth inhibition of both MCF-7 and Hs578T human breast cancer cell lines by vitamin D analogues is associated with increased expression of insulin-like growth factor binding protein-3. *J. Mol. Endocrinol.*, **20**, 157–162

Creech Kraft, J. & Juchau, M.R. (1993) 9-*cis*-Retinoic acid: A direct-acting dysmorphogen. *Biochem. Pharmacol.*, **46**, 709–716

Creech Kraft, J., Willhite, C.C. & Juchau, M.R. (1994) Embryogenesis in cultured whole rat embryos after combined exposures to 3,3',5-triiodo-L-thyronine (T3) plus all-trans-retinoic acid and to T3 plus 9-*cis*-retinoic acid. *J. Craniofac. Genet. Dev. Biol.*, **14**, 75–86

Darro, F., Cahen, P., Vianna, A., Decaestecker, C., Nogaret, J.M., Leblond, B., Chaboteaux, C., Ramos, C., Petein, M., Budel, V., Schoofs, A., Pourrias, B. & Kiss, R. (1998) Growth inhibition of human *in vitro* and mouse *in vitro* and *in vivo* mammary tumor models by retinoids in comparison with tamoxifen and the RU-486 anti-progestagen. *Breast Cancer Res. Treat.*, **51**, 39–55

Dawson, M.I. & Hobbs, P.D. (1994) The synthetic chemistry of retinoids. In: Sporn, M.B., Roberts, A.B. & Goodman, D.S., eds, *The Retinoids. Biology, Chemistry, and Medicine*, 2nd Ed. New York, Raven Press, pp. 5–178

Disdier, B., Bun, H., Placidi, M. & Durand, A. (1996) Excretion of oral 9-*cis*-retinoic acid in the rat. *Drug Metab. Dispos.*, **24**, 1279–1281

Elstner, E., Linker Israeli, M., Le, J., Umiel, T., Michl, P., Said, J.W., Binderup, L., Reed, J.C. & Koeffler, H.P. (1997) Synergistic decrease of clonal proliferation, induction of differentiation, and apoptosis of acute promyelocytic leukemia cells after combined treatment with novel 20-epi vitamin D3 analogs and 9-*cis*-retinoic acid. *J. Clin. Invest.*, **99**, 349–360

Englert, G. (1975) A ^{13}C-NMR study of cis–*trans* isomeric vitamins A, carotenoids and related compounds. *Helv. Chim. Acta*, **58**, 2367–2390

Fiorella, P.D., Giguère, V. & Napoli, J.L. (1993) Expression of cellular retinoic acid-binding protein (type II) in *Escherichia coli*. Characterization and comparison to cellular retinoic acid-binding protein (type I). *J. Biol. Chem.*, **268**, 21545–21552

Frickel, F. (1984) Chemistry and physical properties of retinoids. In: Sporn, M.B., Roberts, A.B. & Goodman, D.S., eds, *The Retinoids*. Orlando, Academic Press, pp. 7–145

Frolik, C.A. & Olson, J.A. (1984) Extraction, separation, and chemical analysis of retinoids. In: Sporn, M.B., Roberts, A.B. & Goodman, D.S., eds, *The Retinoids*. New York, Academic Press, pp. 181–233

Fujimura, S., Suzumiya, J., Anzai, K., Ohkubo, K., Hata, T., Yamada, Y., Kamihira, S., Kikuchi, M. & Ono, J. (1998) Retinoic acids induce growth inhibition and apoptosis in adult T-cell leukemia (ATL) cell lines. *Leuk. Res.*, **22**, 611–618

Furr, H.C., Barua, A.B. & Olson, J.A. (1992) Retinoids and carotenoids. In: De Leenheer, A.P., Lambert, W.E. & Nelis, H.J., eds, *Modern Chromatographic Analysis of Vitamins*. New York, Marcel Dekker, pp. 1–71

Furr, H.C., Barua, A.B. & Olson, J.A. (1994) Analytical methods. In: Sporn, M.B., Roberts, A.B. & Goodman, D.S., eds, *The Retinoids. Biology, Chemistry, and Medicine*, 2nd Ed. New York, Raven Press, pp. 179–209

Gaemers, I.C., Sonneveld, E., Van Pelt, A.M., Schrans, B.H., Themmen, A.P., van der Saag, P.T. & De Rooij, D.G. (1998) The effect of 9-*cis*-retinoic acid on proliferation and differentiation of a spermatogonia and retinoid receptor gene expression in the vitamin A-deficient mouse testis. *Endocrinology*, **139**, 4269–4276

Giannini, F., Maestro, R., Vukosavljevic, T., Pomponi, F. & Boiocchi, M. (1997) All-*trans*, 13-*cis* and 9-*cis* retinoic acids induce a fully reversible growth inhibition in HNSCC cell lines: Implications for in vivo retinoic acid use. *Int. J. Cancer*, **70**, 194–200

Gibbs, S., Backendorf, C. & Ponec, M. (1996) Regulation of keratinocyte proliferation and differentiation by all-*trans*-retinoic acid, 9-*cis*-retinoic acid and 1,25-dihydroxy vitamin D3. *Arch. Dermatol. Res.*, **288**, 729–738

Güzey, M., Demirpence, E., Criss, W. & DeLuca, H.F. (1998) Effects of retinoic acid (all-*trans* and 9-*cis*) on tumor progression in small-cell lung carcinoma. *Biochem. Biophys. Res. Commun.*, **242**, 369–375

Han, G., Chang, B., Connor, M.J. & Sidell, N. (1995) Enhanced potency of 9-*cis* versus all-*trans*-retinoic acid to induce the differentiation of human neuroblastoma cells. *Differentiation*, **59**, 61–69

Heyman, R.A., Mangelsdorf, D.J., Dyck, J.A., Stein, R.B., Eichele, G., Evans, R.M. & Thaller, C. (1992) 9-*cis* Retinoic acid is a high affinity ligand for the retinoid X receptor. *Cell*, **68**, 397–406

Hong, W.K. & Itri, L.M. (1994) Retinoids and human cancer. In: Sporn, M.B., Roberts, A.B. & Goodman, D.S., eds, *The Retinoids. Biology, Chemistry, and Medicine*, 2nd Ed. New York, Raven Press, pp. 597–630

Horst, R.L., Reinhardt, T.A., Goff, J.P., Nonnecke, B.J., Gambhir, V.K., Fiorella, P.D. & Napoli, J.L. (1995) Identification of 9-*cis*,13-*cis*-retinoic acid as a major circulating retinoid in plasma. *Biochemistry*, **34**, 1203–1209

Howell, S.R., Shirley, M.A. & Ulm, E.H. (1998) Effects of retinoid treatment of rats on hepatic microsomal metabolism and cytochromes P450. Correlation between retinoic acid receptor/retinoid Xx receptor selectivity and effects on metabolic enzymes. *Drug Metab. Dispos.*, **26**, 234–239

Hsu, M.C. (1998) Systemic treatment of neoplastic conditions with retinoids. *J. Am. Acad. Dermatol.*, **39**, S108–S113

Jurima-Romet, M., Neigh, S. & Casley, W.L. (1997) Induction of cytochrome P450 3A by retinoids in rat hepatocyte culture. *Hum. Exp. Toxicol.*, **16**, 198–203

Kamm, J.J., Ashenfelter, K.O. & Ehmann, C.W. (1984) Preclinical and clinical toxicology of selected retinoids. In: Sporn, M.B., Roberts, A.B. & Goodman, D.S., eds, *The Retinoids*. Orlando, Academic Press, Inc., pp. 287–326

Kastner, P., Mark, M. & Chambon, P. (1995) Nonsteroid nuclear receptors: What are genetic studies telling us about their role in real life? *Cell*, **83**, 859–869

Kelloff, G.J., Crowell, J.A., Hawk, E.T., Steele, V.E., Lubet, R.A., Boone, C.W., Covey, J.M., Doody, L.A., Omenn, G.S., Greenwald, P., Hong, W.K., Parkinson, D.R., Bagheri, D., Baxter, G.T., Blunden, M., Doeltz, M.K., Eisenhauer, K.M., Johnson, K., Knapp, G.G., Longfellow, D.G., Malone, W.F., Nayfield, S.G., Seifried, H.E., Swall, L.M. & Sigman, C.C. (1996) Strategy and planning for chemopreventive drug development: clinical development plans. II. *J. Cell Biochem.*, **26** (Suppl.), 54–71

Kochhar, D.M., Jiang, H., Penner, J.D. & Heyman, R.A. (1995) Placental transfer and developmental effects of 9-*cis* retinoic acid in mice. *Teratology*, **51**, 257–265

Kurie, J.M., Lee, J.S., Griffin, T., Lippman, S.M., Drum, P., Thomas, M.P., Weber, C., Bader, M., Massimini, G. & Hong, W.K. (1996) Phase I trial of 9-*cis* retinoic acid in adults with solid tumors. *Clin. Cancer Res.*, **2**, 287–293

Lansink, M., Van Bennekum, A.M., Blaner, W.S. & Kooistra, T. (1997) Differences in metabolism and isomerization of all-*trans*-retinoic acid and 9-*cis*-retinoic acid between human endothelial cells and hepatocytes. *Eur. J. Biochem.*, **247**, 596–604

Lee, H.Y., Dawson, M.I., Walsh, G.L., Nesbitt, J.C., Eckert, R.L., Fuchs, E., Hong, W.K., Lotan, R. & Kurie, J.M. (1996) Retinoic acid receptor- and retinoid X receptor-selective retinoids activate signaling pathways that converge on AP-1 and inhibit squamous differentiation in human bronchial epithelial cells. *Cell Growth Differ.*, **7**, 997–1004

Levin, A.A., Sturzenbecker, L.J., Kazmer, S., Bosakowski, T., Huselton, C., Allenby, G., Speck, J., Kratzeisen, C., Rosenberger, M., Lovey, A. & Grippo, J.F. (1992) 9-*Cis* retinoic acid stereoisomer binds and activates the nuclear receptor RXRα. *Nature*, **355**, 359–361

Lotan, R., Dawson, M.I., Zou, C.C., Jong, L., Lotan, D. & Zou, C.P. (1995) Enhanced efficacy of combinations of retinoic acid- and retinoid X receptor-selective retinoids and α-interferon in inhibition of cervical carcinoma cell proliferation. *Cancer Res.*, **55**, 232–236

Lovat, P.E., Irving, H., Annicchiarico Petruzzelli, M., Bernassola, F., Malcolm, A.J., Pearson, A.D., Melino, G. & Redfern, C.P. (1997a) Apoptosis of N-type neuroblastoma cells after differentiation with 9-*cis*-retinoic acid and subsequent washout. *J. Natl Cancer Inst.*, **89**, 446–452

Lovat, P.E., Irving, H., Annicchiarico-Petruzzelli, M., Bernassola, F., Malcolm, A.J., Pearson, A.D., Melino, G. & Redfern, C.P. (1997b) Retinoids in neuroblastoma therapy: Distinct biological properties of 9-*cis*- and all-*trans*-retinoic acid. *Eur. J. Cancer*, **33**, 2075–2080

Makishima, M., Umesono, K., Shudo, K., Naoe, T., Kishi, K. & Honma, Y. (1998) Induction of differentiation in acute promyelocytic leukemia cells by 9-*cis* retinoic acid α-tocopherol ester (9-*cis* tretinoin tocoferil). *Blood*, **91**, 4715–4726

Mayer, H. & Isler, O. (1971) Total syntheses. In: Isler, O., ed., *Carotenoids*. Basel, Birkhauser Verlag, pp. 325–575

McCormick, D.L., Rao, K.V., Steele, V.E., Lubet, R.A., Kelloff, G.J. & Bosland, M.C. (1999) Chemoprevention of rat prostate carcinogenesis by 9-*cis*-retinoic acid. *Cancer Res.*, **59**, 521–524

Miller, W.H.J., Jakubowski, A., Tong, W.P., Miller, V.A., Rigas, J.R., Benedetti, F., Gill, G.M., Truglia, J.A., Ulm, E., Shirley, M. & Warrell, R.P.J. (1995) 9-*cis* Retinoic acid induces complete remission but does not reverse clinically acquired retinoid resistance in acute promyelocytic leukemia. *Blood*, **85**, 3021–3027

Miller, V.A., Rigas, J.R., Benedetti, F.M., Verret, A.L., Tong, W.P., Kris, M.G., Gill, G.M., Loewen, G.R., Truglia, J.A., Ulm, E.H. & Warrell, R.P.J. (1996) Initial clinical trial of the retinoid receptor pan agonist 9-*cis* retinoic acid. *Clin. Cancer Res.*, **2**, 471–475

Mukherjee, R., Jow, L., Croston, G.E. & Paterniti, J.R., Jr (1997) Identification, characterization, and tissue distribution of human peroxisome proliferator-activated receptor (PPAR) isoforms PPARγ2 versus PPARγ1 and activation with retinoid X receptor agonists and antagonists. *J. Biol. Chem.*, **272**, 8071–8076

Nagy, L., Thomazy, V.A., Shipley, G.L., Fesus, L., Lamph, W., Heyman, R.A., Chandraratna, R.A. & Davies, P.J. (1995) Activation of retinoid X receptors induces apoptosis in HL-60 cell lines. *Mol. Cell. Biol.*, **15**, 3540–3551

Naka, K., Yokozaki, H., Domen, T., Hayashi, K., Kuniyasu, H., Yasui, W., Lotan, R. & Tahara, E. (1997) Growth inhibition of cultured human gastric cancer cells by 9-*cis*-retinoic acid with induction of cdk inhibitor Waf1/Cip1/Sdi1/p21 protein. *Differentiation*, **61**, 313–320

Nau, H., Chahoud, I., Dencker, L., Lammer, E.J. & Scott, W.J. (1994) Teratogenicity of vitamin A and retinoids. In: Blomhoff, R., ed., *Vitamin A in Health and Disease*. New York, Marcel Dekker, pp. 615–663

Nervi, A.M., Rigas, J.R., Miller, V.A., Levine, D.M., Dain, B.J. & Warrell, R.P.J. (1997) Plasma lipoproteins associated with three novel retinoids: all-*trans* retinoic acid, 9-*cis* retinoic acid, and oral targretin™. *J. Invest. Med.*, **45**, 260A–260A

Pan, L., Eckhoff, C. & Brinckerhoff, C.E. (1995) Suppression of collagenase gene expression by all-*trans* and 9-*cis* retinoic acid is ligand dependent and requires both RARs and RXRs. *J. Cell Biochem.*, **57**, 575–589

Pomponi, F., Cariati, R., Zancai, P., De Paoli, P., Rizzo, S., Tedeschi, R.M., Pivetta, B., De Vita, S., Boiocchi, M. & Dolcetti, R. (1996) Retinoids irreversibly inhibit in vitro growth of Epstein–Barr virus-immortalized B lymphocytes. *Blood,* **88**, 3147–3159

Rizvi, N.A., Marshall, J.L., Ness, E., Yoe, J., Gill, G.M., Truglia, J.A., Loewen, G.R., Jaunakais, D., Ulm, E.H. & Hawkins, M.J. (1998) Phase I study of 9-*cis*-retinoic acid (ALRT1057 capsules) in adults with advanced cancer. *Clin. Cancer Res.*, **4**, 1437–1442

Robeson, C.D., Cawley, J.D., Weisler, L., Stern, M.H., Eddinger, C.C. & Chechak, A.J. (1955) Chemistry of vitamin A. XXIV. The synthesis of geometric isomers of vitamin A via methyl β-methylglutaconate. *J. Am. Chem. Soc.*, **77**, 4111–4119

Rubin, M., Fenig, E., Rosenauer, A., Menendez-Botet, C., Achkar, C., Bentel, J.M., Yahalom, J., Mendelsohn, J. & Miller, W.H.J. (1994) 9-*cis*-Retinoic acid inhibits growth of breast cancer cells and down-regulates estrogen receptor RNA and protein. *Cancer Res.*, **54**, 6549–6556

Sakashita, A., Kizaki, M., Pakkala, S., Schiller, G., Tsuruoka, N., Tomosaki, R., Cameron, J.F., Dawson, M.I. & Koeffler, H.P. (1993) 9-*cis*-Retinoic acid: Effects on normal and leukemic hematopoiesis in vitro. *Blood*, **81**, 1009–1016

Sass, J.O., Tzimas, G. & Nau, H. (1994) 9-*cis*-Retinoyl-beta-D-glucuronide is a major metabolite of 9-*cis*-retinoic acid. *Life Sci.*, **54**, L69–L74

Sass, J.O., Masgrau, E., Saurat, J.H. & Nau, H. (1995) Metabolism of oral 9-*cis*-retinoic acid in the human. Identification of 9-*cis*-retinoyl-β-glucuronide and 9-*cis*-4-oxo-retinoyl-β-glucuronide as urinary metabolites. *Drug Metab. Dispos.*, **23**, 887–891

Schweiter, U., Englert, G., Rigassi, N. & Vetter, W. (1969) Physical organic methods in carotenoid research. *Pure Appl. Chem.*, **20**, 365–420

Shalinsky, D.R., Bischoff, E.D., Gregory, M.L., Gottardis, M.M., Hayes, J.S., Lamph, W.W., Heyman, R.A., Shirley, M.A., Cooke, T.A., Davies, P.J. & Thomazy, V. (1995) Retinoid-induced suppression of squamous cell differentiation in human oral squamous cell carcinoma xenografts (line 1483) in athymic nude mice. *Cancer Res.*, **55**, 3183–3191

Shalinsky, D.R., Bischoff, E.D., Gregory, M.L., Lamph, W.W., Heyman, R.A., Hayes, J.S., Thomazy, V. & Davies, P.J. (1996) Enhanced antitumor efficacy of *cis*platin in combination with ALRT1057 (9-*cis* retinoic acid) in human oral squamous carcinoma xenografts in nude mice. *Clin. Cancer Res.*, **2**, 511–520

Shirley, M.A., Bennani, Y.L., Boehm, M.F., Breau, A.P., Pathirana, C. & Ulm, E.H. (1996) Oxidative and reductive metabolism of 9-*cis*-retinoic acid in the rat. Identification of 13,14-dihydro-9-*cis*-retinoic acid and its taurine conjugate. *Drug Metab. Dispos.*, **24**, 293–302

Siegenthaler, G. & Saurat, J.H. (1989) Binding of isotretinoin to cellular retinoic acid binding protein: A reappraisal. In: Marks, R. & Plewig, G., eds, *Acne and Related Disorders*, London, Martin Dunitz, pp. 169–174

Soignet, S.L., Benedetti, F., Fleischauer, A., Parker, B.A., Trugha, J.A., Crisp, M.R. & Warrell, R.P. (1998) Clinical study of 9-*cis* retinoic acid (LGD 1057) in acute promyelocytic leukemia. *Leukemia*, **12**, 1518–1521

Thaller, C., Hofmann, C. & Eichele, G. (1993) 9-*cis*-Retinoic acid, a potent inducer of digit pattern duplications in the chick wing bud. *Development,* **118**, 957–965

Tzimas, G., Sass, J.O., Wittfoht, W., Elmazar, M.M., Ehlers, K. & Nau, H. (1994a) Identification of 9,13-di*cis*-retinoic acid as a major plasma metabolite of

9-*cis*-retinoic acid and limited transfer of 9-*cis*-retinoic acid and 9,13-di-*cis*-retinoic acid to the mouse and rat embryos. *Drug Metab. Dispos.*, **22**, 928–936

Tzimas, G., Bürgin, H., Collins, M.D., Hummler, H. & Nau, H. (1994b) The high sensitivity of the rabbit to the teratogenic effects of 13-*cis*-retinoic acid (isotretinoin) is a consequence of prolonged exposure of the embryo to 13-*cis*-retinoic acid and 13-*cis*-4-oxo-retinoic acid, and not of isomerization to all-*trans*-retinoic acid. *Arch. Toxicol.*, **68**, 119–128

Tzimas, G., Collins, M.D. & Nau, H. (1995) Developmental stage-associated differences in the transplacental distribution of 13-*cis*- and all-*trans*-retinoic acid as well as their glucuronides in rats and mice. *Toxicol. Appl. Pharmacol.*, **133**, 91–101

Vetter, W., Englert, G., Rigassi, N. & Schwieter, U. (1971) Spectroscopic methods. In: Isler, O., Gutmann, H. & Solms, U., eds, *Carotenoids*. Basel, Birkhauser Verlag, pp. 189–266

Weber, C. & Dumont, E. (1997) Pharmacokinetics and pharmacodynamics of 9-*cis*-retinoic acid in healthy men. *J. Clin. Pharmacol.*, **37**, 566–574

Widschwendter, M., Widschwendter, A., Welte, T., Daxenbichler, G., Zeimet, A.G., Bergant, A., Berger, J., Peyrat, J.P., Michel, S., Doppler, W. & Marth, C. (1999) Retinoic acid modulates prolactin receptor expression and prolactin-induced STAT-5 activation in breast cancer cells *in vitro*. *Br. J. Cancer*, **79**, 204–210

Yang, Y., Mercep, M., Ware, C.F. & Ashwell, J.D. (1995) Fas and activation-induced Fas ligand mediate apop-tosis of T cell hybridomas: Inhibition of Fas ligand expression by retinoic acid and glucocorticoids. *J. Exp. Med.*, **181**, 1673–1682

Zheng, Y., Kramer, P.M., Olson, G., Lubet, R.A., Steele, V.E., Kelloff, G.J. & Pereira, M.A. (1997) Prevention by retinoids of azoxymethane-induced tumors and aber-rant crypt foci and their modulation of cell prolifera-tion in the colon of rats. *Carcinogenesis*, **18**, 2119–2125

Zheng, Y., Kramer, P.M., Lubet, R.A., Steele, V.E., Kelloff, G.J. & Pereira, M.A. (1999) Effect of retinoids on AOM-induced colon cancer in rats: Modulation of cell proliferation, apoptosis and aberrant crypt foci. *Carcinogenesis*, **20**, 255–260

Zhou, Q., Stetler-Stevenson, M. & Steeg, P.S. (1997) Inhibition of cyclin D expression in human breast carcinoma cells by retinoids *in vitro*. *Oncogene*, **15**, 107–115

Zhu, J., Shi, X.G., Chu, H.Y., Tong, J.H., Wang, Z.Y., Naoe, T., Waxman, S., Chen, S.J. & Chen, Z. (1995) Effect of retinoic acid isomers on proliferation, differentiation and PML relocalization in the APL cell line NB4. *Leukemia*, **9**, 302–309

Zou, C.P., Hong, W.K. & Lotan, R. (1999) Expression of retinoic acid receptor betaa is associated with inhibi-tion of keratinization in human head and neck squamous carcinoma cells. *Differentiation*, **64**, 123–132

Handbook 4

4-Hydroxyphenylretinamide

1. Chemical and Physical Characteristics

1.1. Nomenclature
See General Remarks, section 1.4.

1.2 Name
Chemical Abstracts Services Registry Number
65646-68-6

IUPAC systematic name
N-[4-(all-*E*)-9,13-Dimethyl-7-(1,1,5-trimethylcy-clohex-5-en-6-yl)nona-7,9,11,13-tetraen-15-oyl]aminophenol or N-[4-(all *E*)-3,7-dimethyl-9-(2,2,6-trimethylcyclohex-1-en-1-yl)nona-2,4,6,8-tetraen-1-oyl]aminophenol

Synonyms
Fenretinide, 4-HPR, N-(4-hydroxyphenyl)reti-namide, hydroxyphenyl-retinamide, N-(4-hydro-xyphenyl)retinamide, N-(4-hydroxyphenyl)-all-*trans*-retinamide

1.3 Structural formula

Composition: $C_{26}H_{33}NO_2$

Relative molecular mass: 391.55

1.4 Physical and chemical properties
Description
Yellow crystals from ethanol or water

Melting-point
173–175 °C (Shealy *et al.*, 1984; Budavari *et al.*, 1996)

Solubility
Soluble in most organic solvents, fats, oils and aqueous micellar solutions; sparingly soluble in water, e.g. 13 nmol/L at pH 6.5 (Li *et al.*, 1996).

Spectroscopy
UV and visible: λ_{max} 362 (methanol), $E_{1\,cm}^{1\%}$ 1225, E_M 47 900 (Budavari *et al.*, 1996; Barua & Furr, 1998). Higher E_M values, i.e. 57 100 and 56 400, have also been reported (Formelli *et al.*, 1996).

Nuclear magnetic resonance:
^{1}H-NMR [$(CD_3)SO_4$, 100 MHz]: δ 1.03 (1,1-CH_3), 1.3–1.8 (2-CH_2, 3-CH_3), 1.70 (5-CH_3), 1.8–2.2 (4-CH_2), 1.99 (9-CH_3), 2.36 (13-CH_3), 6.03 (14-H), 6.1–6.6 (7-H, 8-H, 10-H, 12-H), 6.99 (11-H), 6.6–6.8 and 7.3–7.6 (benzene ring -H), 9.15 (NH), 9.74 (OH) (Coburn *et al.*, 1983; Shealy *et al.*, 1984). Similar spectra with higher resolution were obtained by Barua and Olson (1985).

^{13}H-NMR [$(CD_3)SO_4$, 25.2 MHz]: δ 12.5 (9-CH_3), 13.2 (13-CH_3), 18.8 (3-C), 21.5 (5-CH_3), 28.9 (1,1-CH_3), 32.6 (4-C), 33.8 (1-C), 39.2 (2-C), 123.1 (14-C), 127.4-131.3 (5-C, 7-C, 10-C, 11-C), 136.2 (12-C), 137.1 (8-C), 137.3 (6-C), 137.9 (9-C), 147.4 (13-C), 164.2 (15-C); phenyl ring 115.1 (3′-C, 5′-C), 120.8 (2′-C, 6′-C), 153.3 (1′-C, 4′-C) (Coburn *et al*, 1983; Barua & Furr, 1998)

Resonance Raman
(Barua & Furr, 1998)

Infrared
(Coburn *et al.*, 1983; Shealy *et al.*, 1984; Barua & Furr, 1998)

Mass spectrometry
(Coburn *et al.*, 1983; Barua & Furr, 1998)

X-Ray analysis: (Chrzanowski *et al.*, 1984)

Stability
Unstable to light, oxygen and heat; protected in solution by the presence of antioxidants such as butylated hydroxytoluene and pyrogallol; degradation and isomerization are minimized by storage under an inert gas such as argon at –20 °C or less in the dark (Barua & Furr, 1998)

2. Occurrence, Production, Use, Human Exposure and Analysis

2.1 Occurrence
4-Hydroxyphenylretinamide is a synthetic compound and is available solely for testing in the treatment of some dermatological disorders and neoplasms.

2.2 Production
4-Hydroxyphenylretinamide is synthesized from all-*trans*-retinoic acid, which is converted to all-*trans*-retinoyl chloride by treatment with phosphorus trichloride in dry benzene under nitrogen. Retinoyl chloride in benzene is then added slowly to a cold, stirred solution of 4-aminophenol in dimethyl formamide. After the precipitate of 4-aminophenol hydrochloride has been filtered off, the filtrate is washed with water, concentrated and chilled to yield a crystalline product, which is recrystallized from methanol and water. Use of 13-*cis*-retinoic acid in the same procedure yields the 13-*cis* isomeric product (Shealy *et al.*, 1984). Other variations of this procedure have been used in producing a large number of related amide derivatives (Shealy *et al.*, 1984; Dawson & Hobbs, 1994).

2.3 Use
Clinical chemoprevention trials are under way with 4-hydroxyphenylretinamide as the primary therapeutic agent in tumours of the bladder, breast, cervix, lung, oral cavity, prostate and skin (Hong & Itri, 1994; Kelloff *et al.*, 1994; Formelli *et al.*, 1996). The most frequently used daily dose is 200 mg (Kelloff *et al.*, 1994; Formelli *et al.*, 1996).

2.4 Human exposure
Exposure to 4-hydroxyphenylretinamide is limited for all practical purposes to medical treatment for diseases and disorders. The intestinal absorption of this compound is markedly affected by the composition of the diet, as high-fat diets promote absorption whereas high-carbohydrate diets do not (Doose *et al.*, 1992). The major side-effects seen at the usual daily dose of 200 mg are cutaneous toxicity and occasional cases of night blindness due to a marked reduction in plasma retinol. A three-day drug 'holiday' per month during long-term treatment allows plasma retinol concentrations to recover and minimizes the visual toxicity (Kelloff *et al.*, 1994; Formelli *et al.*, 1996).

2.5 Analysis
4-Hydroxyphenylretinamide in plasma and tissues of treated patients is commonly measured by high-performance liquid chromatography (HPLC; Formelli *et al.*, 1989; Peng *et al.*, 1989; Doose *et al.*, 1992). Blood is collected in heparinized tubes and the plasma or a tissue homogenate is acidified to pH 3–4 and then extracted several times with a suitable volume of an organic solvent such as chloroform or methanol, diethyl ether, dichloromethane, acetonitrile, 2-propanol or ethyl acetate. A known amount of a reference standard, usually all-*trans*-retinyl acetate, is added to the sample to correct for losses during extraction and analysis. Furthermore, an antioxidant such as butylated hydroxytoluene is added at the outset to minimize oxidation of any retinoids present. After the combined extract has been dried with anhydrous sodium sulfate, the solvent is evaporated under yellow light (to avoid isomerization) in nitrogen or argon to dryness. The dried powder is immediately dissolved in the HPLC solvent and injected onto the HPLC column. In some cases, a solid-phase extraction or elution step is introduced to remove contaminants.

4-Hydroxyphenylretinamide is usually detected by measuring the absorption at 362 nm and is quantified by measuring the area of the absorption peak with an integrator. A reversed-phase C_{18} column is usually used for the separation.

A large number of chromatographic systems have been devised for the separation and quantification of retinoic acid and its derivatives (Frolik & Olson, 1984; Furr *et al.*, 1992, 1994; Barua & Furr,

1998; Barua *et al.,* 1999). Suitable procedures for 4-hydroxyphenylretinamide have been defined (Schrader & Sisco, 1987; Formelli *et al.,* 1989; Doose *et al.,* 1992).

3. Metabolism, Kinetics and Genetic Variation

3.1 Humans

3.1.1 Metabolism

The major metabolites of 4-hydroxyphenylretinamide include *N*-(4-methoxy-phenyl)retinamide, 4-hydroxyphenylretinamide-*O*-glucuronide and several other polar retinamides. 4-Hydroxyphenylretinamide is not detectably hydrolysed to all-*trans*-retinoic acid or to other retinoic acid isomers (Formelli *et al.,* 1996).

4-Hydroxyphenylretinamide and *N*-(4-methoxyphenyl)retinamide were found at high concentrations in plasma and breast tissue obtained at surgery from women participating in a trial of 4-hydroxyphenylretinamide for the prevention of contralateral breast cancer (Mehta *et al.,* 1991; see section 3.1.3.). In three human breast carcinoma cell lines and two melanoma cell lines *in vitro*, *N*-(4-methoxyphenyl)retinamide was the major metabolite of 4-hydroxyphenylretinamide, although other, unidentified polar and non-polar retinoids were also detected. The presence of serum in the medium did not affect the retention or metabolism of the compound by the cancer cells. Only cancer cell lines that metabolized 4-hydroxyphenylretinamide to *N*-(4-methoxyphenyl)retinamide were sensitive to the anti-proliferative effect of 4-hydroxyphenylretinamide, and *N*-(4-methoxyphenyl)retinamide did not block cell proliferation, indicating that it is not an active metabolite. The authors suggested that it could serve as an indirect biomarker of the response of cells to 4-hydroxyphenylretinamide (Mehta *et al.,* 1998).

A relevant metabolic effect of 4-hydroxyphenylretinamide is that on the normal transport and metabolism of retinol. In both cancer patients and healthy volunteers, it markedly lowered the plasma concentration of retinol (Formelli *et al.,* 1989; Peng *et al.,* 1989; Dimitrov *et al.,* 1990). This reduction accounts for the impaired night vision associated with administration of 4-hydroxyphenylretinamide. *In vitro* it also inhibited several rodent enzymes (acyl coenzyme A:retinol acyltransferase,

lecithin:retinol acyltransferase and retinal reductase) that are thought to be involved in normal retinol metabolism (Ball *et al.,* 1985; Dew *et al.,* 1993). [The Working Group noted that no inhibitory effects of 4-hydroxyphenylretinamide on the human homologues of these enzymes has been reported in the literature and it is unclear whether this observation *in vitro* is directly relevant to patients receiving 4-hydroxyphenylretinamide.]

3.1.2 Kinetics

In three cancer patients given 4-hydroxyphenylretinamide orally at a single dose of 300 mg/m^2, the average half-life in the circulation was 14 h with a mean value for the integrated area under the curve for plasma concentration–time (AUC) of 3.5 mg-h/mL. The half-life of *N*-(4-methoxyphenyl)retinamide is long but variable, ranging from 22 to 54 h, with a mean AUC value of 1.15 mg-h/mL. A rapid, significant reduction in plasma retinol concentration was seen within one to two weeks after treatment (Peng *et al.,* 1989).

Most of the studies of the pharmacokinetics of 4-hydroxyphenylretinamide have been conducted in women with breast cancer in trials of its use for preventing the recurrence of cancer in the contralateral breast (Formelli *et al.,* 1989). The plasma concentrations of both 4-hydroxyphenyretinamide and its methoxy metabolite are linearly related to the dose of 4-hydroxyphenylretinamide. Moreover, like all-*trans*-, 13-*cis*- and 9-*cis*-retinoic acid, 4-hydroxyphenylretinamide markedly reduces plasma retinol concentrations, which is thought to account for the impaired night vision observed in individuals receiving this compound (Formelli *et al.,* 1993). After a five-year treatment, 4-hydroxyphenylretinamide was cleared from the plasma with an average half-life of 27 h, while the rate of elimination of *N*-(4-methoxyphenyl)retinamide was lower. The half-life of 4-hydroxyphenylretinamide was slower after one oral dose (20 h) than after 28 consecutive days (27 h) (Formelli *et al.,* 1989).

3.1.3 Tissue distribution

In the study of Mehta *et al.* (1991), described above, of nine women who had been maintained on 4-hydroxyphenylretinamide at doses of 100, 200 or 300 mg for 15–639 days, the plasma concentrations of the drug were 0.077–1 mmol/L, while those of N-(4-methoxyphenyl)retinamide ranged from not detectable to 0.94 mmol/L, generally correlating well with those of the parent drug. The concentration of 4-hydroxyphenylretinamide in breast tissue was 0.08–6.7 nmol/mg of tissue while that of the methoxy metabolite was 2.6–34 nmol/mg. The breast therefore highly concentrates 4-hydroxyphenylretinamide, and N-(4-methoxyphenyl)retinamide even more so. Both compounds were also found at relatively high concentrations in mammary tumour tissue from these women. When the breast tissue from five women with breast cancer was resolved into fat and epithelial cells, 4-hydroxyphenylretinamide tended to be concentrated in the epithelial cells, and the methoxy metabolite tended to be associated with the fat (Mehta et al., 1991).

The concentrations of 4-hydroxyphenylretinamide and N-(4-methoxyphenyl)retinamide in plasma, breast tumour, normal breast tissue, breast muscle and breast fat from three patients who had received 4-hydroxyphenylretinamide for 5–252 days are shown in Table 1. The plasma concentrations of both retinoids were substantially lower than those in breast tissue. Their presence in plasma and in nipple discharge indicate that 4-hydroxyphenylretinamide enters breast epithelial cells (Formelli et al., 1993).

3.2 Experimental models
3.2.2 Metabolism

After female rats and mice had been given 4-hydroxyphenylretinamide at 5 mg/kg bw per day intraperitoneally for five days, the tissue concentrations of the drug and its metabolites were assessed in serum, liver, mammary gland and urinary bladder. Of the four metabolites detected, one co-eluted from the reversed-phase HPLC column with the cis isomer and a second with the same retention time as N-(4-methoxyphenyl)retinamide, a third was tentatively identified as a fatty acyl ester of the parent drug and the fourth remained unidentified. The amounts of each metabolite varied with tissue and species: for instance, the concentration of 4-hydroxyphenylretinamide was significantly lower and that of N-(4-methoxyphenyl)retinamide was higher in mouse tissues than in the corresponding tissues of rats, and the cis isomer and the putative acyl ester of 4-hydroxyphenylretinamide were detected in rat liver but not mouse liver. Thus, the drug and its metabolites are distributed to the liver, mammary gland and urinary bladder of rats and mice but the distribution is species dependent (Hultin et al., 1986).

Three metabolites of 4-hydroxyphenylretinamide were detected by reversed-phase HPLC in mammary gland extracts from BALB/c mice

Table 1. 4-Hydroxyphenylretinamide and N-(4-methoxyphenyl)retinamide concentrations (ng/ml or ng/g) in plasma and breast samples collected 12 h after the last dose, before surgery

	Patient 1: 4-hydroxyphenylretinamide, 200 mg for 7 days			Patient 2: 4-hydroxyphenylretinamide, 300 mg for 5 days			Patient 3: 4-hydroxyphenylretinamide, 100 mg for 168 days + 200 mg for 84 days		
Plasma	216		140	337		400	346		202
Breast tumour	499	2.3	1024	7.3	567	1.7	1291	3.2	ND	ND
Breast normal tissue	567	2.6	750	5.4	845	2.5	1024	2.6	473	1.4	6678	33.1
Breast muscle	311	1.4	1079	7.7	626	1.9	1076	2.7	299	0.9	2997	14.8
Breast fat	1776	8.2	1544	11.0	1871	5.5	1376	3.4	1096	3.2	7326	36.2

Reproduced from Formelli et al. (1993). ND, not detected

incubated in the presence of insulin, prolactin or steroid hormones (aldosterone, cortisol, progesterone and estradiol) for six days. Two were tentatively identified as 13-*cis*-4-hydroxyphenylretinamide and *N*-(4-methoxyphenyl)retinamide, while the third was not identified. The relative distribution of these metabolites in the organ culture was affected by the hormones added to the culture medium: addition of insulin at 5 mg/mL and prolactin at 5 mg/mL resulted in greater concentrations of *N*-(4-methoxyphenyl)retinamide than in mammary glands treated simultaneously with combinations of steroids. The concentrations of 13-*cis*-4-hydroxyphenylretinamide and of the unidentified metabolite were not markedly affected by inclusion of steroids in the culture medium (Mehta *et al.*, 1988).

3.2.3 Kinetics

After a single intravenous injection of 4-hydroxyphenylretinamide at 5 mg/kg bw to female rats, it was distributed to all the tissues examined (serum, liver, mammary gland and urinary bladder) with the highest concentration in the liver. The distribution continued for 4 h and was followed by first-order elimination kinetics. The half-life of elimination from the liver was 9.4 h, that from serum was 12 h (not significantly different from that in the liver), that from the mammary gland was 44 h and that from the urinary bladder was 9.3 h. In an experiment in which rats and mice were given 4-hydroxyphenylretinamide intraperitoneally at a dose of 5 mg/kg bw per day for five days, the compound was distributed to all tissues, the highest concentrations being reached in the urinary bladder followed by the liver and the mammary gland. The concentrations in the tissues were much greater than those in plasma, indicating that the tissues take up and concentrate 4-hydroxyphenyl-retinamide from the circulation (Hultin *et al.*, 1986).

Pretreatment of female BDF mice with 4-hydroxyphenylretinamide at 10 mg/kg bw for three days had no effect on its disposition in serum, liver, mammary gland or urinary bladder and had no effect on its pharmacokinetics or that of any of its four metabolites in liver. In contrast, pretreatment of the mice for three days with phenobarbital at 80 mg/kg bw per day had a significant effect on the disposition of 4-hydroxy-

phenylretinamide in all tissues examined, reduced the AUC values to half those of mice pretreated with the vehicle and significantly reduced the concentrations of the four metabolites in the liver. Thus, although pretreatment with 4-hydroxyphenylretinamide had no effect on its disposition or metabolism, pretreatment with the cytochrome P450 inducer phenobarbital significantly reduced the AUC for 4-hydroxyphenylretinamide in all tissues examined and consequently changed its disposition and metabolism (Hultin *et al.*, 1988).

The distribution of *N*-(4-methoxyphenyl)retinamide in serum, liver, mammary gland, urinary bladder and skin of female BDF mice was assessed after a single oral dose of 10 mg/kg bw. The highest concentrations were found in liver and mammary gland, and the largest AUC value was found for the mammary gland, followed by skin and liver. The elimination half-life of the metabolite was 5.1 h in liver, 5.6 h in serum, 19 h in urinary bladder, 23 h in skin and 27 h in mammary gland. Five metabolites of *N*-(4-methoxyphenyl)retinamide were detected but not identified, and their relative concentrations varied among the tissues. Thus, the metabolism of 4-hydroxyphenylretinamide to *N*-(4-methoxyphenyl)retinamide appears to be only the first of several metabolic steps that give rise to multiple other metabolites (Hultin *et al.*, 1990).

As reported in section 3.2.2, the tissues of female rats and mice receiving 4-hydroxyphenyl-retinamide intraperitoneally for five days show markedly different distributions and concentrations of metabolites, indicating a difference in the metabolism of this compound in the two species (Hultin *et al.*, 1986).

4. Cancer-preventive Effects

4.1 Humans
4.1.1 Epidemiological studies
No data were available to the Working Group.

4.1.2 Intervention trials
4.1.2.1 Breast
A large, multicentre, randomized, controlled trial of use of 4-hydroxyphenylretinamide for preventing breast cancer was begun in Milan, Italy, in 1987 (De Palo *et al.*, 1997). Patients aged 30–70 who had

been treated surgically for early breast cancer, without axillary lymph node involvement, were randomized to receive either no treatment or 4-hydroxyphenylretinamide at 200 mg/day for five years. The 1496 patients assigned to 4-hydroxyphenylretinamide treatment were instructed to take capsules containing the agent for all but the last three days of each month. Placebo capsules were not given to the 1476 women in the control group. The occurrence of a new, contralateral primary breast tumour was the primary end-point and was assessed by annual mammography and twice yearly clinical examinations. Other events, including new primary tumours in the ipsilateral breast, recurrence of the initial breast tumour or new primary cancers at other sites, were also recorded. Accrual to the study was closed prematurely in 1993, when opinion about use of adjuvant chemotherapy precluded accrual to the untreated control arm of the study. A preliminary report from this study (Decensi et al., 1997a) indicated that there was no difference overall in the incidence of contralateral breast cancer between treated and control women (53 and 54 cases, respectively). The authors noted, however, that there was a statistically significant interaction ($p = 0.018$) between menopausal status and the effect of treatment. The risk for contralateral cancer appeared to be reduced by treatment in premenopausal women (relative risk = 0.65) and increased in postmenopausal women (relative risk = 1.65). [The Working Group noted that the lack of blinding in the design of the study may complicate interpretation and that there was a significant imbalance in the assignment to study groups, with proportionally fewer premenopausal women assigned to the treatment arm. The Group also noted the difficulty of interpreting statistical analyses of data on subgroups and that the statistically significant interaction between menopausal status and treatment effect was not anticipated.]

4.1.2.2 Ovary

An incidental finding made during the trial described above of use of 4-hydroxyphenylretinamide for preventing breast cancer was the development of ovarian cancer in six women, none of whom were receiving 4-hydroxyphenylretinamide (De Palo et al., 1995a).

4.1.2.3 Prostate

Pienta et al. (1997) reported the results of a trial of 4-hydroxyphenylretinamide in 22 patients at risk for adenocarcinoma of the prostate who were given a dose of 100 mg/day for 12 scheduled 25-day cycles, with a three-day break between cycles. No untreated controls were included. Biopsies were performed 6 and 12 months after the start of therapy. Eight patients with no indication of adenocarcinoma in their biopsy samples before the study showed signs of this tumour before or at the time of their 12-month evaluation. This high frequency of cancer and the difficulty in accruing patients led to early closure of the study.

4.1.3 Intermediate end-points

4.1.3.1 Oral cavity

Tradati et al. (1994) studied eight patients with diffuse inoperable oral lichen planus or leukoplakia, who received topical applications of 4-hydroxyphenylretinamide twice daily. After one month of therapy, two patients had complete remission and the other six had a greater than 75% response. 4-Hydroxyphenylretinamide was well tolerated, and no local or distant side-effects were observed. [The Working Group noted that oral leukoplakia may regress spontaneously.]

A randomized study of patients with oral leukoplakia was begun in 1988 at the Milan Cancer Institute to evaluate the efficacy of 52 weeks of maintenance therapy with 4-hydroxyphenylretinamide administered systemically at a dose of 200 mg/day after complete laser resection of the lesions. A three-day period with no drug was prescribed at the end of each month to avoid the adverse effect on night blindness of lowering serum retinol concentrations. The most recent report (1993) gave the results for 153 patients, of whom 74 were randomized to 4-hydroxyphenylretinamide and 79 to no intervention (Chiesa et al., 1993; Costa et al., 1994). The proportion of patients with recurrence or new lesions during the trial was similar in the two treatment arms: 13/79 (10 recurrences and three new lesions) in the group receiving 4-hydroxyphenylretinamide and 21/79 (9 recurrences and 12 new lesions) among controls; however, the projected time to treatment failure was reported to be 6% with 4-hydroxyphenylretinamide and 30% for controls. [The Working Group observed differences between the rates of drop-out of patients in the two groups, which may partially explain the difference in rate of treatment failure, as determined by the crude proportions and the Kaplan-Meier method.]

4.1.3.2 Urinary bladder

Decensi *et al.* (1994a) reported the results of a trial in which 12 patients with superficial urinary bladder cancer were treated with 4-hydroxyphenylretinamide orally at a dose of 200 mg daily and compared with 12 non-randomized, untreated controls. The DNA content and the percent of cells in S or $G_2 + M$ phase were used as the end-points. A trend in recession from aneuploidy to a diploid state and a decrease in the number of cells in S or $G_2 + M$ phase were observed in the patients given 4-hydroxyphenylretinamide; however, few samples were studied (24 for ploidy and 8 for cell-cycle analysis). The proportion of patients with DNA aneuploidy in bladder-washed cells decreased from 8/12 to 6/12 in the group given 4-hydroxyphenylretinamide but increased from 8/12 to 10/12 in the control group. Positive or suspect results were found on cytological examination in 3/12 treated cases before administration of 4-hydroxyphenylretinamide, but all subsequently returned to normal. Two patients in the control group showed progression to invasive cancer. [The Working Group noted that some of these results were reported elsewhere (Costa *et al.*, 1995), with somewhat different data.]

4.1.3.3 Breast

A report from the trial for the prevention of breast cancer in Milan described above was based on data on 149 women who had been enrolled in the treatment arm of the study and had been assessed by mammography (Wolfe categories) before and after four years of treatment (Cassano *et al.*, 1993). No changes in mammographic pattern were observed. [The Working Group noted that no data on mammographic patterns after treatment were included in the report and that there were no data on control women.]

4.2 Experimental models
4.2.1 *Cancer and preneoplastic lesions*
These studies are summarized in Table 2.

4.2.1.1 Mammary gland

Mouse: Groups of 75–100 female C3H mice with mammary tumour virus were fed a diet supplemented with 4-hydroxyphenylretinamide at 1 mmol/kg of diet; nulliparous mice aged two months were fed the diet for 39 weeks and multiparous mice aged four to six months for up to 14 weeks. At the end of treatment, the animals were killed. The incidence of mammary adenocarcinomas was 85% in nulliparous mice maintained on the control diet, 71% in nulliparous mice fed the 4-hydroxyphenylretinamide-containing diet, 69% in multiparous mice on control diet and 80% in multiparous mice fed the treated diet. The numbers of tumours per animal were reduced from 2.4 in control nulliparous mice to 1.7 in those fed 4-hydroxyphenylretinamide ($p < 0.01$; χ^2 test), but no change in the number of tumours was found in multiparous mice (Welsch *et al.*, 1983).

Rat: Groups of 15–40 female Sprague-Dawley rats, 50 days of age, were given an intravenous injection of *N*-methyl-*N*-nitrosourea (MNU) at 15 or 50 mg/kg bw and a second injection on day 57. Three days later, the rats were fed either a basal diet or one supplemented with 391 mg/kg diet (1 mmol) or 782 mg/kg diet (2 mmol) of 4-hydroxyphenylretinamide until the end of the study 182 days after carcinogen treatment. The incidence of mammary adenocarcinomas was 100% in controls treated with the high dose of MNU, 65% in animals at the high dose of 4-hydroxyphenylretinamide ($p < 0.01$, Fisher's exact test) and 80% in animals at the low dose of 4-hydroxyphenylretinamide (not significant). At the low dose of MNU, the incidence of mammary adenocarcinomas was 30% in rats fed the control diet and 15% and 30% in the groups maintained on diets with the high and low doses of 4-hydroxyphenylretinamide, respectively (not significant). The tumour multiplicity of animals given the high dose of MNU was reduced from 5.2 in controls to 2.3 ($p < 0.01$, Mantel non-parametric test) in animals at the high dose of 4-hydroxyphenylretinamide and to 2.9 ($p < 0.05$) in rats fed the diet low in 4-hydroxyphenylretinamide. At the low dose of MNU, tumour multiplicity was not affected by 4-hydroxyphenylretinamide (Moon *et al.*, 1979). Several other experiments with similar concentrations of 4-hydroxyphenylretinamide and a single

Table 2. Effects of 4-hydroxyphenyl-retinamide on carcinogenesis in animals

Cancer site	Species, sex, age at carcinogen treatment	No. of animals per group	Carcinogen dose, route	4-Hydroxyphenyl-retinamide dose (mg/kg diet), route carcinogen (basal diet)	Duration in relation to carcinogen	Incidence Control	Incidence Treated	Multiplicity Control	Multiplicity Treated	Efficacy	Reference
Mammary gland	C3H mice Nulliparous Multiparous	75–100 75–100	Tumour virus	391 (Wayne Lab Chow)	0 d to end	85 69	71 80	2.4 1.5	1.7* 1.7	Effective Ineffective	Welsch et al. (1983)
Mammary gland	Sprague-Dawley rats, female, 50 d	15–17	MNU (50 mg/kg bw) twice, i.v.	782 391 (Wayne Lab Chow)	+3 d to end	100 100	65* 80	5.2 5.2	2.3* 2.9*	Effective Effective	Moon et al. (1979)
		40	MNU (15 mg/kg bw) twice, i.v.	782 391	+3 d to end	30 30	15 30	0.35 0.35	0.22 0.35	Ineffective Ineffective	
Mammary gland	Sprague-Dawley rats, female,120 d	40	MNU (50 mg/kg bw) single, i.v.	782 (AIN-76A)	−60 d to end	68	42*	1.7	1.3	Effective	Moon et al. (1992)
Mammary gland	Sprague Dawley rats, female, 50 d	30	MNU (50 mg/kg bw) single, i.v.	391 (Wayne Lab Chow)	−7 d to end	100	100	8.87	7.45*	Effective	McCormick & Moon (1986)
Mammary gland	Sprague-Dawley rats, female, 50 d	25	MNU (50 mg/kg) single i.v.	782 (Wayne Lab Chow)	+7 d to end	100	92	4.82	3.39*	Effective	McCormick et al. (1982a)
Mammary gland	Sprague-Dawley rat, female, 21 d	21–30	MNU (25 mg/kg bw) i.v.	782 (NIH-07)	−29 d to 12 wks	86	60	1.3	1.2	Ineffective	Silverman et al. (1983)
					−2 d to 12 wks +2 d to 17 wks	86 86	50* 60	1.3 1.3	0.7* 0.8	Effective	
		15	DMBA (10 mg/rat) i.g.	782 (NIH-07)	−21 d to 12 wks +10 d to 12 wks	53 53	60 47	0.9 0.9	0.9 0.8	Ineffective Ineffective	
Mammary gland	Fischer 344 rat, female, 50 d	25	MNU (45 mg/kg bw) i.v.	782 (AIN 76-A) 782 782 (Wayne Lab Chow) 782 (NIH-07)	−7 d to end +7 d to end −7 d to end +7 d to end −7 d to end	60 60 24 24 44	76 76 8 16 20*	1.04 1.04 0.48 0.48 0.64	1.52 1.92 0.20 0.32 0.20*	Ineffective Ineffective Ineffective Ineffective Effective	Cohen et al. (1994)

Table 2. (Contd)

Cancer site	Species, sex, age at carcinogen treatment	No. of animals per group	Carcinogen dose, route	4-Hydroxyphenyl-retinamide dose/route (mg/kg diet) route (basal diet)	Duration in relation to carcinogen	Incidence Control	Incidence Treated	Multiplicity Control	Multiplicity Treated	Efficacy	Reference
Mammary gland	Sprague-Dawley rats, female, 100 d	30	MNU (50 mg/kg bw) i.v.	782 (Wayne Lab Chow)	−60 d to 0 d −60 d to end	57 57	66 23*	1.4 1.4	2.7 0.3*	Ineffective Effective	Grubbs et al. (1990)
Mammary gland	Sprague-Dawley rats, female, 50 d	20	MNU (50 mg/kg bw) i.v.	391 (Wayne Lab Chow)	+7 d to −256 d	64	50	1.1	0.8*	Effective	McCormick et al. (1982b)
Mammary gland	Sprague-Dawley rats, female, 50 d	20	DMBA (75 mg/rat) i.g.	293 586	−14 d to 18 wks	70 70	65 30*	1 1	1.1 0.35*	Ineffective Effective	Abou-Issa et al. (1988)
Mammary gland	Sprague-Dawley rats, female, 50 d	30	DMBA (15 mg/rat)	90 mg/kg bw/d	0 d to end	84	89	3.65	2.45*	Effective	Bollag & Hartmann (1987)
Mammary gland	Sprague-Dawley rats, female, 50 d	22	DMBA (20 mg/rat) i.g.	782 (Wayne Lab Chow)	+7 d to end	91	85*	5.4	3.7*	Effective	McCormick et al. (1982a)
Mammary gland	Sprague-Dawley rats, female, 50 d	16	DMBA (15 mg/rat) i.g.	782 391 (AIN-76A)	−7 d to end	88 88	33* 73	2.1 2.1	0.6* 1.4	Effective Ineffective	Abou-Issa et al. (1993)
Skin	Sencar mice, female, 3–4 wks	25	DMBA (5 µg/mouse) topically	391 (Wayne Lab Chow) 30 nmol topically	+2 wks to end +2 wks to end	4 4	35 4	0.08 0.08	1.87 0.04	Ineffective Tumour enhancing Ineffective	McCormick et al. (1987)
Haematopoietic system (lymphoma)	PIM transgenic mice, 4 wks	30–40	50 mg/kg bw ENU i.p.	98 196 391	0 to 20 wks 0 to 35 wks 0 to 20 wks 0 to 35 wks 0 to 20 wks 0 to 35 wks	48 53 48 53 48 53	20* 43 37 52 20* 40	NR NR NR NR NR NR	NR NR NR NR NR NR	Effective Ineffective Ineffective Ineffective Effective Ineffective	McCormick et al. (1996)
Haematopoietic system (lymphoma)	AKR/J mice, female, 3–4 wks	10	MCF virus (50 ml)	391 782	−7 d to end	100 100	60* 50*	NR NR	NR NR	Effective Effective	Chan et al. (1997)

Table 2. (Contd)

Cancer site	Species, sex, age at carcinogen treatment	No. of animals per group	Carcinogen dose, route	4-hydroxyphenyl-retinamide dose/route (mg/kg diet) (basal diet)	Duration in relation to carcinogen	Incidence Control	Treated	Multiplicity Control	Treated	Efficacy	Reference
Prostate	Lobund-Wistar male rats, 3 months	20	MNU (30 mg/kg bw) i.v., after 1 wk TP (45 mg)	391 (L-485 (Tek-Lad))	+7 months to end (14 months)	88	21*	NR	NR	Effective	Pollard et al. (1991)
Prostate	WU, male rats, 7–8 wks	40	8 mg cyproterone acetate, daily/20 d i.p. 100 mg/kg TP, s.c. 50 mg MNU/kg i.v. s.c. implants of testosterone in silastic tubes	391 (Wayne Lab Chow)	+ 1 d to end (450 d)	45	59	NR	NR	Ineffective	McCormick et al. (1998)
Prostate	ACI rats, male, 21–25 months	44	None Spontaneous	78	NR	43.2	27.5	NR	NR	Ineffective	Ohshima et al. (1985)
Lung	A/J mice, female, 6 wks	30	NNK (2 mg per mouse), i.p	1556 783 (AIN-76-A1)	–7 d to 52 wks –7 d to 52 wks	73[b] 73[b]	50[b] 57[b]	16.4[a] 16.4[a]	15.4[a] 18.7[a]	Ineffective	Conaway et al. (1998)
Urinary bladder	BDF male mice, 4–56 wks	70	NBHBA (7.5 mg) i.g. 8 wkly	156 313 (AIN-76A)	–7 d to end	39 41	46 42	NR	NR	Ineffective Ineffective	Moon et al. (1994a)
Urinary bladder	BDF male mice, 4–5 wks	99	NBHBA (7.5 mg) i.g. 8 wkly	1.5 mmol/kg diet (Wayne Lab Chow)	0 to end	35	21*	NR	NR	Effective	Moon et al. (1982)
Colon	Fischer 344 male rats, 8 wks	25–33	AOM (15 mg/kg bw) Twice wkly, i.p.	391 782 (AIN-76A)	–1 to 36 wks	33	13* 12*	0.47 0.47	0.1* 0.08*	Effective Effective	Zheng et al. (1997)

MNU, N-methyl-N-nitrosourea; i.v., intravenously; d, days; DMBA, 7,12-dimethylbenz[a]anthracene; i.g., intragastrically; ENU, N-ethyl-N-nitrosourea; i.p., intraperitoneally; NR, not reported; TP, testosterone propionate; s.c., subcutaneously; NNK, 4-(N-nitrosomethylamino)-1-(3-pyridyl)-1-butanone; NBHBA, N-nitroso-N-butyl-N-4-hydroxybutylamine; AOM, azoxymethane

[a] Adenomas and adenocarcinomas combined

[b] Adenocarcinomas only

* Statistically significant (see text); effective, either incidence or multiplicity

intravenous dose of MNU at 50 mg/kg bw consistently showed the effectiveness of 4-hydroxyphenylretinamide at a concentration of 2 mmol/kg diet (McCormick *et al.*, 1982a; McCormick & Moon, 1986; Moon *et al.*, 1989; Ratko *et al.*, 1989; Moon & Mehta, 1990).

Groups of 40 female Sprague-Dawley rats, 60 days of age, received semipurified AIN-76A diet or the diet supplemented with 4-hydroxyphenylretinamide at 2 mmol/kg ; 60 days later, they were given a single intravenous injection of MNU at 50 mg/kg bw. The animals were killed 180 days after the carcinogen treatment. The incidence of mammary adenocarcinomas was 68% in controls and 42% in those given 4-hydroxyphenylretinamide ($p < 0.05$ χ^2 test). The multiplicity of tumours was unaffected (Moon *et al.*, 1992).

Groups of 21–30 female Sprague-Dawley rats received MNU at 25 mg/kg bw into the tail vein at 50 days of age and were given NIH-07 basal diet or NIH-07 diet containing 782 mg/kg diet 4-hydroxyphenylretinamide beginning at 21, 48 or 60 days of age. The diet was continued until 12 weeks after the carcinogen treatment in all groups except in a group that received 4-hydroxyphenylretinamide from 52 weeks of age until 17 weeks after exposure to the carcinogen. The incidence of mammary adenocarcinomas 28 weeks after exposure to the carcinogen was statistically significant inhibited only in the group that received 4-hydroxyphenylretinamide two days before the injection of MNU, the incidence being reduced to 50% as compared with 86% in controls ($p < 0.05$; Wilcoxon test). The tumour multiplicity was reduced from 1.3 to 0.7 tumours per rat. In a similar experiment within the same study with 7,12 dimethylbenz[*a*]anthracene (DMBA) as the carcinogen, groups of 15 rats were treated intragastrically with a single dose of 10 mg in sesame oil at 50 days of age, and dietary treatment with 4-hydroxyphenylretinamide was begun 21 or 60 days afterwards. 4-Hydroxyphenylretinamide showed no inhibitory effect in this study (Silverman *et al.*, 1983).

Groups of 25 female Fischer 344 rats were given MNU intravenously at a dose of 45 mg/kg bw at 50 days of age. The groups then received either Wayne lab chow or NIH-07 or AIN-76A semipurified diets containing 4-hydroxyphenylretinamide at 2 mmol/kg diet starting either seven days before or seven days after the carcinogen until the end of the study 25 weeks after administration of MNU. The mammary carcinoma incidence was 60% in control rats maintained on AIN-76A diet, 24% in those on Wayne lab chow and 44% in those on NIH-07 diet. Treatment with 4-hydroxyphenylretinamide had a significant effect only in animals on NIH-07 diet supplemented seven days before carcinogen treatment, the incidence being decreased from 44% to 20% and the tumour multiplicity from 0.64 to 0.20 ($p < 0.05$: Student's *t* test) (Cohen *et al.*, 1994).

Groups of 30 female Sprague-Dawley rats received an intravenous injection of MNU at 50 mg/kg bw at 100 days of age. The animals received Wayne lab chow alone or supplemented with 4-hydroxyphenylretinamide at 2 mmol/kg diet starting either 60 days before the carcinogen treatment or before, during and after the carcinogen treatment. The animals were killed 180 days after injection of the carcinogen. The incidence of mammary adenocarcinomas was increased from 57% in controls to 66% in the group given 4-hydroxyphenylretinamide before the carcinogen, and the tumour multiplicity was increased from 1.4 to 2.7 (not significant). In animals given 4-hydroxyphenylretinamide for the duration of the study, the adenocarcinoma incidence was reduced from 57% in controls to 23% in treated rats ($p < 0.05$; Fisher exact test) and the tumour multiplicity was reduced from 1.4 to 0.3 tumours per rat ($p < 0.05$; Wilcoxon rank test; Grubbs *et al.*, 1990).

Groups of 25 female Sprague-Dawley rats, 50 days of age, were treated by oral gavage with a single dose of 20 mg DMBA; seven days later, they received Wayne lab chow alone or supplemented with 4-hydroxyphenylretinamide at 2 mmol/kg for 180 days. Mammary tumours (fibroadenomas and carcinomas combined) developed in 91% of controls and 85% of the 4-hydroxyphenylretina-mide-treated rats ($p < 0.05$; log rank analysis), and the tumour multiplicity was reduced from 5.4 to 3.7 ($p < 0.05$; Student's *t* test; McCormick *et al.*, 1982a).

Groups of 20 female Sprague-Dawley rats received a semipurified AIN-76A diet alone or supplemented with 4-hydroxyphenylretinamide at 0.75 or 1.5 mmol/kg of diet and 14 days later, when they were 50 days of age, were given a single dose of 75 mg DMBA by gavage. The incidence of mammary adenocarcinomas 18 weeks later was 70% in controls, 65% in rats given the diet con-

taining the low dose of 4-hydroxyphenylreti-
namide and 30% in rats given the high dose
($p < 0.05$; Student's t test). The tumour multiplicity
was 1.0 in controls, 1.1 at the low dose of
4-hydroxy-phenylretinamide and 0.4 at the high
dose (Abou-Issa *et al.*, 1988). Similar results were
reported by Bollag and Hartman (1987),
McCormick *et al.* (1982a) and Abou-Issa *et al.*
(1993; see Table 2). [The Working Group noted
that the statistical test used is not appropriate for
the data analysed.]

4.2.1.2 Skin

Groups of 25 female Sencar mice, seven to eight
weeks of age, received topical applications of 5 µg
DMBA in acetone and, starting two weeks later,
4-hydroxyphenylretinamide either at 30 nmol in
acetone topically twice a week or at 1 mmol/kg of
diet for 30 weeks. DMBA by itself resulted in an
incidence of skin papillomas of only 4%. Topical
treatment of DMBA-initiated skin with 4-hydroxy-
phenylretinamide did not affect papilloma development, but dietary treatment increased the
incidence of skin papillomas to 35%. The tumour
multiplicity was increased from 0.1 per mouse in
controls to 1.9 with 4-hydroxyphenylretinamide
($p < 0.01$; log rank analyses ; McCormick *et al.*,
1987).

4.2.1.3 Lymphoma

Groups of 30–40 male PIM transgenic mice, which
are highly susceptible to the induction of T-cell
lymphomas owing to overexpression of the *pim-1*
oncogene, were given an intraperitoneal injection
of *N*-ethyl-*N*-nitrosourea (ENU) at 50 mg/kg bw
and immediately afterwards maintained on diets
containing 4-hydroxyphenylretinamide at a concentration of 98, 196 or 391 mg/kg of diet. The
lymphoma incidence was determined at 20 and at
35 weeks. The incidence 20 weeks after the
carcinogen injection was 48% in controls and 20%
at the low and high doses of 4-hydroxyphenyl-
retinamide ($p < 0.05$; Fisher's exact test). At 35
weeks, the incidence of lymphomas was 53% in
controls and 43, 52 and 40% at the low, intermediate
and high doses of 4-hydroxyphenylretinamide,
respectively (not significant). The rate of survival
at 35 weeks was 53% in control mice and 78% in
those at the high dose of 4-hydroxyphenylreti-
namide ($p < 0.01$; log rank analysis). The rate of

survival was also increased at the low and intermediate dietary concentrations, but not statistically
significantly so (McCormick *et al.*, 1996).

Groups of 10 female AKR/J mice, two to three
weeks of age, were maintained on lab chow diet
alone or supplemented with 4-hydroxyphenyl-
retinamide at 391 or 782 mg/kg of diet and one
week later received an injection of 50 µl of a solution containing 1 x 10^5 plaque-forming units per
ml of mink cell focus-forming virus into the thymus area. The animals were killed 20 weeks after
the virus injection. The incidence of lymphoma
was 100% in controls, 60% at the low dose of 4-
hydroxyphenylretinamide and 50% at the high
dose ($p < 0.01$; Student's t test; Chan *et al.*, 1997).
[The Working Group noted that the statistical
analysis and the presentation of the results were
difficult to interpret.]

4.2.1.4 Prostate

Groups of 20 male Lobund-Wistar rats, three
months of age, were given a single intravenous
injection of MNU at 30 mg/kg bw and then
received a Silastic tube implant containing 45 mg
of testosterone propionate, which was replaced
every two months. Seven months after the MNU
injection, 4-hydroxyphenylretinamide was added
to the basal diet at 1 mmol/kg. The animals were
killed 14 months after the carcinogen injection.
The incidence of prostate tumours was 88% in the
control rats and 21% in those given 4-hydrox-
yphenylretinamide ($p < 0.001$; statistical method
not given; Pollard *et al.*, 1991).

Groups of 40 male WU (HsdCpb:WU) rats,
seven to eight weeks of age, received intraperitoneal injections of 8 mg of cyproterone acetate
daily for 20 days; one day later, they received a single
subcutaneous injection of testosterone propionate
at 100 mg/kg bw, and 60 h after the testosterone
treatment, they were given an intravenous injection of MNU at 50 mg/kg bw. They then received
subcutaneous implants of Silastic tubes filled with
testosterone, which were replaced every 90 days.
One day after the injection of MNU, one group
received 4-hydroxyphenylretinamide at 1 mmol/kg
diet (391 mg/kg) for the duration of the experiment, which was terminated 450 days after the carcinogen treatment. The incidence of prostate adenocarcinomas was 45% in controls and 59% with
4-hydroxyphenylretinamide, and the incidence of

accessory gland tumours was 67% in controls and 62% with 4-hydroxyphenylretinamide (McCormick *et al.*, 1998).

Groups of 44 ACI/segHapBR retired breeder rats, 21–25 months of age, received either basal diet or diet supplemented with 4-hydroxyphenyl-retinamide at 783 mg/kg diet for 54 weeks. The incidence of prostate tumours was 43% in control rats and 28% in those given 4-hydroxyphenylreti-namide (not significant; Ohshima *et al.*, 1985).

4.2.1.5 Lung

Groups of 30 female A/J mice, five weeks old, were maintained on an AIN-76A diet alone or supple-mented with 4-hydroxyphenylretinamide at 2 or 4 mmol/kg diet and one week later were given an intraperitoneal injection of 4-(methylnitrosamino)-1-(3-pyridyl)-1-butanone (NNK) at 2 mg per mouse. At 52 weeks, when the animals were killed, the incidence of adenocarcinoma was 73% in con-trol mice, 50% in the group given the high dose of 4-hydroxyphenylretinamide and 57% in the group given the low dose (not significant); the incidence of adenoma was 27%, 43% and 43% and the tumour multiplicity was 17, 15 and 19 in the three groups, respectively (not significant). The body weights were reduced by > 30% in the group given 4-hydroxyphenylretinamide at 4 mmol/kg of diet (Conaway *et al.*, 1998). [The Working Group noted that the marked weight loss could have affected the tumour incidence.]

4.2.1.6 Urinary bladder

Groups of 99 male C57BL/6 x DBA/2F$_1$ (BDF) mice, five to six weeks of age, were given one intragastric instillation of 7.5 mg of *N*-nitroso-*N*-butyl-*N*-4-hydroxybutylamine (NBHBA) each week for eight weeks. The animals were fed either basal diet or diet supplemented with 4-hydroxyphenylreti-namide at 1.5 mmol/kg of diet for seven months after the first dose of NBHBA. The incidence of bladder carcinomas was 35% in control mice and 21% in those given 4-hydroxyphenylretinamide (*p* < 0.05; χ^2 test) (Moon *et al.*, 1982).

Groups of 70 male BDF mice, five to seven weeks of age, were maintained on an AIN-76A diet alone or supplemented with 4-hydroxyphenyl-retinamide at 156 or 313 mg/kg and one week later were given 7.5 mg of NBHBA by intragastric intu-bation each week for eight weeks. At 26 weeks,

when the animals were killed, the incidence of bladder carcinomas was 39% and 41% in the two control groups, 46% at the low dose of 4-hydrox-yphenylretinamide and 42% at the high dose (not significant; Moon *et al.*, 1994a).

4.2.1.7 Colon

Groups of 25–33 male Fischer 344 rats, seven to eight weeks of age, were maintained on a AIN-76A diet alone or supplemented with 4-hydroxy-phenylretinamide at 391 or 782 mg/kg diet and one week later received intraperitoneal injections of azoxymethane at 15 mg/kg bw weekly for two weeks. At 36 weeks after the carcinogen treatment, the incidence of colon adenocarcinoma was 33% in controls, 13% at the low dose of 4-hydroxy-phenylretinamide and 12% at the high dose (*p* < 0.05; ANOVA followed by Tukey test). The multi-plicity of adenocarcinomas was 0.47 in control rats and 0.1 at the low dose and 0.08 at the high dose of 4-hydroxyphenylretinamide (*p* < 0.01; ANOVA; Zheng *et al.*, 1997).

4.2.1.8 Combinations of 4-hydroxyphenylretinamide with other putative preventive agents

4-Hydroxyphenylretinamide has been evaluated for tumour-preventive activity in combination with other agents in models of experimental car-cinogenesis (Moon *et al.*, 1994b). For example, combinations with tamoxifen (Ratko *et al.*, 1989), ovariectomy (McCormick *et al.*, 1982a) or calcium glucarate (Abou-Issa *et al.*, 1993) were more effec-tive than the single agents alone.

4.2.2 Intermediate biomarkers

In two models of liver carcinogenesis in rats, with *N*-nitrosodiethylamine or a choline-deficient diet, 4-hydroxyphenylretinamide significantly decreased the size and number of glutathione *S*-transferase placental-form-positive foci, considered to be pre-neoplastic lesions, and the concentrations of 8-hydroxyguanine in the liver, an indicator of oxidative damage (Tamura *et al.*, 1997).

4.2.3 In-vitro models

4.2.3.1 Inhibition of cell transformation

Several studies have shown that 4-hydroxyphenyl-retinamide can act as a preventive agent at early stages of the carcinogenesis process. It was highly active in suppressing 3-methylcholanthrene-induced neoplastic transformation in the C3H/10T1/2 clone 8 mouse fibroblast line (Bertram, 1980), and it suppressed the transformation of rat tracheal epithelial cells induced by benzo[*a*]pyrene (Steele *et al.*, 1990). In a model of mammary carcinogenesis *in vitro* in cultures of the whole mammary organ from female BALB/c mice, N-nitrosodiethylamine induced transformation of mammary cells, resulting in nodule-like alveolar lesions, which are analogous to the precancerous hyperplastic alveolar nodules seen in mouse mammary gland *in vivo*. When 4-hydroxyphenylretinamide was added to the organ culture medium six days after the carcinogen, it suppressed the incidence of nodule-like alveolar lesions by 61%. The authors concluded that 4-hydroxyphenylretinamide can inhibit expression of the transformed phenotype at the promotional level (Chatterjee & Banerjee , 1982).

4.2.3.2 Inhibition of cell proliferation
4-Hydroxyphenylretinamide at concentrations below 1 µmol/L rarely affected the growth of cells of various types, whereas growth was inhibited at that dose. DNA synthesis was decreased by 51% in asynchronously growing PC3 prostate carcinoma cells or cells synchronized with serum deprivation when treated with 4-hydroxyphenylretinamide at 1 µmol/L. The reduction in proliferation rate was associated with accumulation of cells in the G_0/G_1 phase of the cell cycle (Igawa *et al.*, 1994; Roberson *et al.*, 1997). The inhibition is associated with suppression of c-*myc* gene expression (Igawa *et al.*, 1994). In other prostate carcinoma cells, however, 4-hydroxyphenylretinamide did not cause accumulation in G_1 (Sun *et al.*, 1999a). Similarly, 4-hydroxyphenylretinamide inhibited the growth of oesophageal squamous carcinoma cell lines without inducing arrest of cell growth in the G_1 phase nor apoptosis, but it caused down-regulation of epidermal growth factor receptors (Muller *et al.*, 1997).

4.2.3.3 Induction of cellular differentiation
Many retinoids are active in several models of cellular differentiation such as murine EC F9 cells, human HL-60 cells and neuroblastoma cells, but 4-hydroxyphenylretinamide was ineffective in most of these systems. No differentiation was induced in HL-60 cells (Delia *et al.*, 1993) or neuroblastoma cells (Ponzoni *et al.*, 1995), but 4-hydroxy-phenylretinamide induced primitive endodermal differentiation when added at a concentration of 1 µmol/L, a suboptimal concentration for induction of apoptosis (Clifford *et al.*, 1999).

4.2.3.4 Induction of apoptosis
Numerous studies over the past six years have highlighted induction of apoptosis as a major effect of 4-hydroxyphenylretinamide on tumour cells *in vitro*. This retinoid induced apoptosis in malignant haematopoietic (Delia *et al.*, 1993), neuroblastoma (Di Vinci, 1994; Mariotti *et al.*, 1994; Ponzoni *et al.*, 1995), cervical (Oridate *et al.*, 1995), breast (Swisshelm *et al.*, 1994; Sheikh *et al.*, 1994; Pellegrini *et al.*, 1995; Sheikh *et al.*, 1995), ovarian (Supino *et al.*, 1996; Sabichi *et al.*, 1998), head-and-neck (Oridate *et al.*, 1996; Sun *et al.*, 1999b), small-cell lung (Kalemkerian *et al.*, 1995), non-small-cell lung (Zou *et al.*, 1998; Sun *et al.*, 1999b) and prostate (Igawa *et al.*, 1994; Hsieh & Wu, 1997; Roberson *et al.*, 1997; Sun *et al.*, 1999a) cancer cell lines. It is noteworthy that many of the cell lines that are sensitive to 4-hydroxyphenylretinamide were resistant to doses of all-*trans*-retinoic acid or 9-*cis*-retinoic acid up to 10 µmol/L.

The induction of apoptosis often requires doses of 4-hydroxyphenylretinamide > 1 µmol/L and even as much as 10 µmol/L (Lotan, 1995; Supino *et al.*, 1996). [The Working Group noted that because the reported plasma concentration of 4-hydroxyphenylretinamide in patients treated with 200 mg/day is 1 µmol/L or less, the concentration in the target tissues may not be sufficient to induce apoptosis.]

4.2.3.5 Antimutagenicity in short-term tests
Little information is available on the effect of 4-hydroxyphenylretinamide on carcinogen-induced genotoxicity (Table 3). In a single study, it did not affect the ability of DMBA to induce sister chromatid exchange in mammary gland organ cultures during the 24-h exposure (Manoharan & Banerjee, 1985). [The Working Group noted that this study was limited to a single dose of both carcinogen and retinoid and the main focus of the study was on the effect of β-carotene and not 4-hydroxyphenylretinamide.] A second study showed a protective effect of 4-hydroxyphenylretinamide against the induction by bleomycin, which generates free radicals, of chromosomal breakage in two

Table 3. Effects of 4-hydroxyphenylretinamide on genetic and related effects *in vitro* and *in vivo*

Dose of retinoid	Genotoxic agent (dose)	Cells or animal	Investigated effect	Result[a]	LED/HID[b]	Reference
1 µmol/L	DMBA (7–8 µmol/L)	Mouse mammary cells	Sister chromatid exchange	–	1 µmol/L	Manorharan & Banerjee (1985)
1 pmol/L – 1 µmol/L (preincubation for 24 h)	Bleomycin (0.004 U/ml)	Two human lymphoblastoid cell lines	Chromosomal breakage	–	1 µmol/L	Trizna *et al.* (1993)
40 µmol/L	None	Rat hepatocytes	Cytochrome P450 (CYP) RNA levels			Jurima-Romet *et al.* (1997)
			CYP1A1	–	40 µmol/L	
			CYP1A2	–	40 µmol/L	
			CYP3a1/2	#	40 µmol/L	
800 mg/kg bw per day by gavage for 4 days	None	Male Sprague-Dawley rats	Hepatic levels of activity		800 mg/kg bw per day for 4 days	McCarthy *et al.* (1987)
			Arylhydrocarbon hydroxylase	+		
			Glutathione *S*-transferase	#		
			Quinone reductase	–		
600 mg/kg bw per day by gavage for 7 days	Benzo[a]pyrene (2 mg/kg bw i.p. on 8th day)	Male Sprague-Dawley rats	Covalent binding to DNA *in vivo*	+	600 mg/kg bw per day for 7 days (ID_{40} for liver, ID_{21} for stomach, ID_{11} for lung. No effect on kidney)	McCarthy *et al.* (1987)

DMBA, 7,12-dimethylbenz[a]anthracene; i.p., intaperitoneally; inhibitory dose
[a]+, inhibition of the investigated end-point; – no effect on investigated end-point; #, enhancement of investigated end-point
[b] LED, lowest effective dose that inhibits the investigated effect; HID, highest ineffective dose

human lymphoblastoid cell lines. In this study, the cells were preincubated with the retinoid for 24 h before addition of bleomycin (Trizna *et al.*, 1993).

Although there is no information on the effect of this retinoid on carcinogen metabolism *in vitro*, it may affect the activity of some metabolic enzymes. In primary rat hepatocyte cultures treated for 48 h with 4-hydroxyphenylretinamide, it affected the messenger RNA levels of cytochrome P450s (CYPs), the effects depending on the cytochrome being studied. The level of CYP3A RNA was increased approximately eightfold by the treatment ($p < 0.05$), whereas those of CYP1A1 and CYP1A2 were not affected (Jurima-Romet *et al.*, 1997). 4-Hydroxyphenylretinamide may also affect the enzyme activity *in vivo* (Table 3).

4.3   Mechanisms of cancer prevention
4.3.1   Inhibition of early stages
Several reports described above indicate that 4-hydroxyphenylretinamide can alter the activity of carcinogen-metabolizing enzymes, the level of expression of certain CYPs and the binding of benzo[a]pyrene to DNA in several tissues. Thus, it

may act at the very early stages of carcinogenesis. It inhibited transformation when added after a carcinogen at concentrations that did not inhibit proliferation, indicating activity after the initiation phase of carcinogenesis.

4.3.2 Inhibition of cell proliferation

4.3.2.1 Modulation of proteins regulating cell cycles
4-Hydroxyphenylretinamide down-regulates cyclin D1, p34^{cdc2} and cdk4 expression and Rb phosphorylation and increases ceramide synthesis in HL-60 cells (DiPietrantonio *et al.*, 1996, 1998). It also down-regulated proliferating cell nuclear antigen, cyclins D and E, p34^{cdc2}, p53 and Rb in the androgen-independent prostate cancer cell line JCA-1 (Hsieh *et al.*, 1995). Up-regulation of the Rb protein was observed in the breast cancer cell lines MCF-7 and T-47D (Kazmi *et al.*, 1996), and down-regulation of c-*myc* was demonstrated in PC3 prostate cancer cells (Igawa *et al.*, 1994). Increased expression of the cdk inhibitor p21/WAF1/Cip1 was observed in several prostate cancer cell lines (Sun *et al.*, 1999a).

4.3.2.2 Modulation of autocrine and paracrine loops
Several studies have shown that 4-hydroxyphenylretinamide can modulate components of growth factor and receptor signalling pathways that enhance or suppress growth stimulatory signals. Treatment of oesophageal carcinoma cells resulted in down-regulation of the c-erb-B1 epidermal growth factor receptor (Muller *et al.*, 1997), and similar results were obtained with breast cancer cells (Pellegrini *et al.*, 1995). Down-regulation of c-erb-B2 (*HER-2/neu*) mRNA and protein in breast carcinoma cells has also been described (Pellegrini *et al.*, 1995; Grunt *et al.*, 1998). Other families of factor and receptor systems were also modulated. Insulin-like growth factor (IGF) signalling was abrogated in several cancer cell types as a result of down-regulation of IGF-I-like protein in the medium, a reduction in IGF binding proteins 4 and 5, a decrease in type-I IGF receptor mRNA and IGF-I binding to breast cancer cells (Favoni *et al.*, 1998). Up-regulation of mac25, a putative member of the tumour suppressing IGF-BP family, in senescing mammary epithelial cells has also been reported (Swisshelm *et al.*, 1995). In contrast, 4-hydroxyphenylretinamide increased the activity of the negative growth regulator TGFβ1 and TGFβ receptor type II in prostate carcinoma cells (Roberson *et al.*, 1997).

4-Hydroxyphenylretinamide decreased the expression of androgen receptors in an androgen-dependent prostate carcinoma cell line, LNCaP (Hsieh & Wu, 1997).

4.3.3 Restoration of normal differentiation

4-Hydroxyphenylretinamide rarely induces differentiation of cancer cells, perhaps because it induces apoptosis within a relatively short time (see below). For example, in the neuroblastoma cell line (Ponzoni *et al.*, 1995) and in HL-60 cells, a classical retinoid-differentiated cell line, no differentiation was observed after treatment with 4-hydroxyphenylretinamide. This retinoid potentiated differentiation of HL-60 cells induced by all-*trans*-retinoic acid by suppressing the catabolism and enhancing retinoylation of the latter compound (Takahashi *et al.*, 1995; Taimi & Breitman, 1997).

The differentiation into primitive endoderm seen with all-*trans*-retinoic acid has, however, been detected in murine F9 EC cells treated with 4-hydroxyphenylretinamide at 1 µmol/L, a suboptimal concentration for induction of apoptosis (Clifford *et al.*, 1999). Therefore, some differentiation may occur *in vivo*, where the plasma concentration is at about this value.

4.3.4 Inhibition of prostaglandin production

4-Hydroxyphenylretinamide inhibited tumour promoter-induced cyclooxygenase-2 expression in human colon adenocarcinoma cells (Aliprandis *et al.*, 1997).

4.3.5 Induction of apoptosis

Since 4-hydroxyphenylretinamide induces apoptosis in a large number of tumour cell types, including those that are resistant to all-*trans*-retinoic acid (see above), it is reasonable to suggest that it acts through a mechanism that is either independent of retinoid receptors or includes, in addition to receptor activation, some other effects that trigger apoptosis.

4.3.6 Decreased cell adhesion

4-Hydroxyphenylretinamide abrogated neuroblastoma cell adhesion by down-modulation of integrin receptors such as integrin β 1, which may have resulted in detachment from the matrix and triggered programmed cell death (Rozzo *et al.*, 1997).

4.3.7 Molecular mechanisms
4.3.7.1 Retinoid receptor pathway
The biological activities of the natural retinoids are thought to be mediated by two classes of nuclear retinoid receptor: the RARs and the RXRs (see General remarks, section 3). There is no convincing evidence that 4-hydroxyphenylretinamide can bind to these receptors, but it was reported to compete with radiolabelled all-*trans*-retinoic acid for binding to a crude nuclear extract with 15% of the potency of unlabelled all-*trans*-retinoic acid (Sani *et al.*, 1995), and weak binding to retinoid receptors has been reported (Sheikh *et al.*, 1995). Doses of 4-hydroxyphenylretinamide > 1 mol/L were required for 50% inhibition of the binding of ^{3}H-4-(5,6,7,8-tetrahydro-5,5,8,8-tetramethyl-2-anthracenyl)benzoic acid to recombinant RARs (Sheikh *et al.*, 1995). Nonetheless, 4-hydroxyphenylretinamide activated the transcription of RARβ, which is a classical retinoid-regulated gene with a DR5 retinoic acid response element in its 5′ flanking region. 4-Hydroxyphenylretinamide activated the transcription of a reporter gene driven by RARβ RARE through co-transfected RARγ better than through RARβ and RARα (Fanjul *et al.*, 1996; Kazmi *et al.*, 1996). In addition, it activated a reporter gene via endogenous retinoid receptors (Sun *et al.*, 1999b) and induced the expression of RARβ in senescing mammary epithelial cells *in vitro* (Swisshelm *et al.*, 1995). These findings are a clear indication that, in some cells, 4-hydroxyphenylretinamide can activate RARs and some of their target genes. The status of RARβ may affect the response, as indicated by several reports of the greater sensitivity to 4-hydroxyphenylretinamideinduced apoptosis of ovarian cancer cells expressing transfected RARβ (Sabichi *et al.*, 1998; Pergolizzi *et al.*, 1999). In LNCaP prostate carcinoma cells, however, this retinoid suppressed RARβ mRNA levels yet induced apoptosis (Sun *et al.*, 1999a), and it does not induce apoptosis in some cells in which all-*trans*-retinoic acid induces RARβ (Zou *et al.*, 1998). Therefore, the presence of RARβ may not be necessary for induction of apoptosis by 4-hydroxyphenylretinamide.

4.3.7.2 Increased generation of reactive oxygen species
4-Hydroxyphenylretinamide can increase the generation of reactive oxygen species immediately after its addition to cultured leukaemic cells (Delia *et al.*, 1997) and cervical carcinoma cells (Oridate *et al.*, 1997). This increase is important for induction of apoptosis, since antioxidants can block apoptosis in these cell lines (Delia *et al.*, 1993, 1997; Oridate *et al.*, 1997; Sun *et al.*, 1999a). Since the concentrations of 4-hydroxyphenylretinamide that are required to induce apoptosis are rather high, it is difficult to block its effect with receptor antagonists at a high molar ratio. When such experiments were performed, however, no effective antagonism was observed (Sun *et al.*, 1999a). In five cell lines from head-and-neck tumours, five from lung cancers and three from prostate cancers, 4-hydroxyphenylretinamide induced generation of reactive oxygen species in only the three that were somewhat more sensitive (Sun *et al.*, 1999a,b). Thus, an additional, unknown mechanism besides RAR activation and induction of reactive oxygen species may mediate 4-hydroxyphenylretinamide-induced apoptosis.

5. Other Beneficial Effects

No data were available to the Working Group.

6. Carcinogenicity

6.1 Humans
No data were available to the Working Group.

6.2 Experimental models
No data were available to the Working Group. In a study of single-stage skin carcinogenesis, 4-hydroxyphenylretinamide enhanced development of DMBA-induced papillomas (see section 4.2.1).

7. Other Toxic Effects

7.1 Adverse effects
7.1.1 Humans
Unlike many other retinoids, 4-hydroxyphenylretinamide is usually well tolerated, and its clinical toxicity is considered to be 'mild and reversible' (Modiano *et al.*, 1990a). Intervention trials of 4-hydroxyphenylretinamide, including its clinical

toxicology, have been reviewed (Cobleigh, 1994; Costa *et al.*, 1994; De Palo *et al.*, 1995b; Veronesi *et al.*, 1996).

7.1.1.1 Ocular toxicity

In the earliest therapeutic trials, 4-hydroxyphenyl-retinamide was generally well tolerated, although some patients discontinued treatment with the drug due to night blindness and other side-effects, including increased concentrations of triglycerides and mucocutaneous complaints (Garewal *et al.*, 1989; Modiano *et al.*, 1989). The adverse events resolved upon cessation of treatment and were presumably related to the high doses administered (up to 800 mg/day) (Kaiser-Kupfer *et al.*, 1986). The frequent occurrence of visual abnormalities in these early trials led to the design of new dosing regimens and treatment intervals.

In 37 patients with advanced cancers who were treated with 300–400 mg/day of 4-hydroxyphenyl-retinamide for 13–300 days, 10% reported decreased night vision. One patient had electroretinogram changes, with a significant decrease in the amplitude for scotopic (dark-adapted or rod-mediated) vision after one month of treatment. All of the cases of night blindness resolved when treatment was discontinued (Modiano *et al.*, 1990b).

4-Hydroxyphenylretinamide was administered in a phase-I study to 100 surgically treated breast cancer patients at doses of 100, 200 and 300 mg/day for an initial six months and then at 200 mg per day for six months thereafter. One of the patients receiving 300 mg daily experienced impaired night vision after six months of treatment (Costa *et al.*, 1989).

Night blindness after administration of 4-hydroxyphenylretinamide is a consequence of interference with the formation of the retinol-binding protein and transthyretin complex (Berni & Formelli, 1992) and reductions in circulating retinol and retinol-binding protein. These effects can occur within hours after the first dose (Formelli *et al.*, 1989). The consequence is a reduction in retinal photoreceptor sensitivity (Decensi *et al.*, 1997b) and delay in rod–cone timing, which leads to an increased absolute luminance threshold (Caruso *et al.*, 1998). Of 14 men given 4-hydroxy-phenylretinamide at 100 mg/day for up to one year, 13 had normal age-matched electroretino-

graphic responses for the first six months; two subjects showed a gradual decline in rod-mediated a-wave amplitude, which returned to normal after treatment had ceased (Krzeminski *et al.*, 1996).

In order to overcome these effects, a three-day drug 'holiday' per month was instituted (Rotmensz *et al.*, 1991), to allow recovery of serum retinol concentrations and preservation of the ability to adapt to darkness (Formelli *et al.*, 1987). When this interrupted dosing regimen was used in an Italian phase-I trial extended to 30 months, the incidence of ophthalmic disturbances was 4% (Decensi *et al.*, 1997b). Although daily administration of 200 mg of 4-hydroxyphenylretinamide reduced the plasma concentrations of retinol and retinol-binding protein in all treated patients by an average of 71% 24 h after each dose, the plasma concentrations increased in all patients after the three-day interruption, some returning to baseline concentrations (Formelli *et al.*, 1993).

In a clinical trial for the prevention of bladder cancer, the main toxic effects were decreased dark adaptation and abnormal electroretinograms. The dose regimen used — 200 mg/day with a three-day holiday per month for two years — did produce night blindness but this was considered not to be severe enough to reduce or end treatment. Night blindness was reported in approximately 20% of the subjects assigned to 4-hydroxyphenylreti-namide and 2% of the untreated control group in both years of the study. After the end of treatment, all of the side-effects disappeared (Decensi *et al.*, 1997c).

In a phase-III clinical trial for the prevention of breast cancer, 1432 evaluable patients were treated daily with 200 mg of 4-hydroxyphenylretinamide with a three-day drug holiday each month. Mild and moderately diminished dark adaptation occurred at plasma retinol concentrations of 160 and 100 ng/ml, respectively, but only half of the subjects reported symptoms (Decensi *et al.*, 1993, 1994b). A constant 65% reduction in mean retinol concentration was seen during the five years of treatment (Formelli *et al.*, 1993; Veronesi *et al.*, 1996). In more complete reviews of the long-term effects of 4-hydroxyphenylretinamide on visual and retinal function (Mariani *et al.*, 1996; Decensi *et al.*, 1997b), the cumulative incidence of visual complaints, including loss of dark adaptation, was reported to have reached nearly 20% at five years, with more frequent occurrence at the start of treatment. Multivariate analysis of these data suggested an interaction between the age of the patients and the duration of treatment in predicting an impaired electroretinogram response resulting from treatment with 4-hydroxyphenylretinamide. The most recent review of ocular toxicity in another trial of breast cancer patients indicates that the incidence of complaints of night blindness in patients treated with 4-hydroxyphenylretinamide at 200 mg/day for four months is not cumulative, is proportional to dose and returns to normal after drug withdrawal (Caruso *et al.*, 1998).

The evaluation of 4-hydroxyphenylretinamide in the prevention of cancers at several other sites has also been associated with reduced retinol concentrations with and without ocular toxicity. In one study, 4-hydroxyphenylretinamide was applied topically at 100 mg twice daily for three months to patients with facial actinic keratoses. It was not absorbed into the circulation when given by this route (Moglia *et al.*, 1996). In another study, reported only as an abstract, oral treatment with 4-hydroxyphenylretinamide at 200, 300 or 400 mg/day was continued for three months in patients with more than 15 actinic keratoses, with either a two-day/week or a three-day/month drug holiday. Reversible symptomatic night blindness developed in two patients on 400 mg/day, and one patient at 200 mg/day had asymptomatic electroretinogram abnormalities (Sridhara *et al.*, 1997).

7.1.1.2 Other ophthalmic effects

Other ocular effects reported in chemoprevention trials with 4-hydroxyphenylretinamide are more reminiscent of the standard mucocutaneous toxicity seen with other synthetic retinoids. In one study, the incidence of visual disturbances was compared with that of other ophthalmic signs, which included ocular dryness, lachrymation, conjunctivitis and photophobia. The cumulative incidence of these complaints was 8% at five years, and they were not associated with a reduction in plasma retinol concentration as in the effect on dark adaptation but rather with the age of the patient. This suggests that the underlying mechanism is different for the direct effect on retinal function by retinol depletion and the effects on the conjunctival and lachrymal apparatus (Mariani *et al.*, 1996).

7.1.1.3 Dermatological effects

Cutaneous toxicity has been seen in clinical trials less frequently with 4-hydroxyphenylretinamide than with other synthetic retinoids, although patients in the early trials with high doses often discontinued the drug because of erythema and rash. A widespread, painful morbilliform skin eruption was reported in a patient with basal-cell carcinoma being treated with 800 mg/day of this retinoid (Gross *et al.*, 1991), and similar cutaneous side-effects were noted with 600 mg/day in the treatment of psoriasis (Kingston *et al.*, 1986).

In the Italian trial of 4-hydroxyphenylretinamide at 200 mg/day for breast cancer, dermatological complaints were the commonest symptoms reported and included pruritis, skin dryness and cheilitis. Two patients out of 53 experienced peeling of the palms and soles, and six patients reported alopecia, five had nail fragmentation, two had xerosis and one each had pruritis and urticaria (Rotmensz *et al.*, 1991).

4-Hydroxyphenylretinamide has been used in two trials for the treatment of oral leukoplakia. Topical application at 100 mg/day to patients with oral leukoplakia and lichen planus produced no local mucocutaneous side-effects (Tradati *et al.*, 1994). In 115 patients who had undergone laser resection of leukoplakic lesions and had been prescribed oral maintenance therapy with 4-hydroxyphenylretinamide at 200 mg/day or placebo for one year with a three-day drug holiday per month, the toxicity was mild with no evidence of night blindness. Twenty of the 39 patients taking the drug finished the year without interruption, four required dose reduction or interruption of treatment due to dermal toxicity including skin dryness and dermatitis, and one patient refused to continue the study because of dermatitis (Chiesa *et al.*, 1992).

7.1.1.4 Metabolic and biochemical effects

Clinical treatment with retinoids has been associated with hepatotoxicity and hyperlipoproteinaemia. Seven of 101 patients who had undergone surgery for breast cancer and were treated with 4-hydroxyphenylretinamide at 100–300 mg/day for six months had liver enzyme activities that were two to four times above baseline, but no serious permanent liver toxicity (Costa *et al.*, 1989).

In a phase-II trial for bladder cancer, not only ophthalmic disturbances but also increased plasma triglyceride concentrations and minor dermatological complaints were recorded. No significant difference in biochemical toxicity was observed between treated and untreated patients during the first two years of treatment, but a statistically significantly higher incidence of grade-1 hypertriglyceridaemia was observed in patients receiving 4-hydroxyphenylretinamide at completion of follow-up in the third year. This study suggests a possible relationship between treatment and delayed low-grade hypertriglyceridaemia (Decensi *et al.*, 1997c).

In an initial trial of 4-hydroxyphenylretinamide at 200 mg/day in the treatment of oral leukoplakia, three of 39 patients had to have dose reductions or interruption of treatment because of increased plasma concentrations of triglycerides or bilirubin, and two patients were dropped from the study because they had elevated concentrations of triglycerides or abnormal results in tests for liver function. The relationship of these abnormal findings in clinical chemistry to treatment was uncertain because several of these patients had other intercurrent diseases (Chiesa *et al.*, 1992).

7.1.1.5 Other toxic effects

In studies of short-term treatment with 4-hydroxyphenylretinamide in the interval between diagnosis and radical prostatectomy in patients with prostate carcinoma, the serum retinol concentrations were lower (1400 nmol/L) in the treated group than in those given placebo (2600 nmol/L), as in other clinical trials (Thaller *et al.*, 1996).

In eight patients with inoperable oral lichen planus or leukoplakia, topical application of 4-hydroxyphenylretinamide at 200 mg/day twice daily for one month did not elicit any sign of local or systemic toxicity (Tradati *et al.*, 1994). In 20 patients with actinic keratoses given 4-hydroxyphenylretinamide at 200 mg/day topically, twice daily for three months, no local or systemic toxicity was observed. Two of the 20 subjects refused to complete the study for cosmetic reasons, as 4-hydroxyphenylretinamide caused yellow blotches on their faces. After twice daily topical applications to the lesions on the face, the circulating concentrations of 4-hydroxyphenylretinamide were below the analytical limit of detection (Moglia *et al.*, 1996).

7.1.2 Experimental models

The Working Group was aware of studies of the short-term and long-term toxicity and carcinogenicity of 4-hydroxyphenylretinamide in rats, conducted by the pharmaceutical company that produces this drug. The results have not been published.

As part of a study of chemopreventive efficacy, 4-hydroxyphenylretinamide did not reduce body-weight gain in rats fed the compound at 2 mmol/kg of diet (0.1 mmol/kg bw per day) for six months. The livers of these rats were essentially normal, and there was no effect on total liver retinoid concentration. The oestrus cycles after four months were normal (Moon *et al.*, 1979). The lack of an effect of dietary 4-hydroxyphenylretinamide on final body weight was confirmed in another study, in which, however, the serum triglyceride and cholesterol concentrations were increased by 760% ($p < 0.01$) and 114% ($p < 0.01$), respectively, after 22 weeks. The liver weights were also significantly increased, although the concentrations of triglyceride and cholesterol in the liver were not affected (Radcliffe, 1983).

7.2 Reproductive and developmental effects

7.2.1 Humans

No reports of adverse effects on male or female reproductive function or of developmental toxicity were found in the open literature. The parent drug and its 4-methoxyphenyl metabolite cross the human placenta. After 20–27 months of treatment at 200 mg/day orally, 4-hydroxyphenylretinamide and *N*-(4-methoxyphenyl)retinamide were measured in the plasma, placenta and embryos of two women who conceived while receiving the drug and elected to abort. The plasma concentrations of 4-hydroxyphenylretinamide (5–26 ng/ml) and *N*-(4-methoxyphenyl)retinamide (49–87 ng/ml) reflected the 10–60-day interruptions of dosing in these two cases. In one patient who had had nearly two months' interruption, the concentrations of the two compounds in the placenta and embryo were at or near the limit of analytical detection (15 ng/g), whereas the concentrations in the placenta and embryo (25 and 75 ng/g, respectively)

Table 4. Teratogenic effects of 4-hydroxyphenylretinamide			
Species	Dose (mg/kg bw)	Effects	Reference
Rat	300 or 600	Resorptions; cardiac vessel defects	Turton *et al.* (1992)
Rat	125 or 800 GD 6–15	Hydrocephaly, microphthalmia	Kenel *et al.* (1988)
Rabbit	125 or 800 GD 6–18	Dome-shaped head, delay in skull bone ossification, microphthalmia	Kenel *et al.* (1988)

GD, gestation day

of the second case were nearly identical to those in maternal plasma. The embryos were not autopsied (Formelli *et al.*, 1998).

7.2.2 Experimental models

4-Hydroxyphenylretinamide has low teratogenic potency in rats and rabbits (Table 4), indicating that an acidic terminal group is necessary for the exertion of strong teratogenicity, probably via binding to retinoid receptors. In rats, 4-hydroxyphenylretinamide crosses the placenta readily, and the fetal concentrations are approximately one half of corresponding maternal values (Kenel *et al.*, 1988; Table 4).

7.3 Genetic and related effects
7.3.1 Humans

No data were available to the Working Group.

7.3.2 Experimental models

4-Hydroxyphenylretinamide was not mutagenic in *Salmonella typhimurium* strains TA100, TA1535, TA98, TA1537 or TA1538, either in the presence or absence of exogenous metabolic activation over a wide range of doses (0.5–400 mg/plate; Paulson *et al.*, 1985; Table 5), nor did it alter the mutation frequency at the *Tk* locus in L5178Y mouse lymphoma cells, either in the presence or absence of exogenous metabolic activation from rat liver (Paulson *et al.*, 1985). No increase in sister chromatid exchange frequency was found in mouse mammary cells in organ culture exposed to 4-hydroxyphenylretinamide, although the study was limited to a single dose of 1 mmol/L in the absence of exogenous activation (Manoharan & Banerjee, 1985).

4-Hydroxyphenylretinamide did not affect the chromosomal structure or number in bone-marrow cells of Crl:COBS(WI)BR rats receiving a single oral dose of 7000 mg/kg bw followed by sampling at 4, 16 and 24 h. Nor was any effect observed when rats were treated with 50, 200 or 800 mg/kg bw day for five days (Paulson *et al.*, 1985).

8. Summary of Data

8.1 Chemistry, occurrence and human exposure

4-Hydroxyphenylretinamide is a synthetic compound formed from all-*trans*-retinoic acid and 4-aminophenol. Because it contains retinoic acid, it is sensitive to light, heat and oxygen. As it is lipophilic, it is freely soluble in oils and non-polar solvents but poorly soluble in water. It has characteristic absorption spectra in the ultraviolet and visible, infrared and resonance Raman portions of the electromagnetic spectrum.

4-Hydroxyphenylretinamide and its methoxy metabolite are found in plasma after administration of the parent compound. 4-Hydroxyphenylretinamide is used mainly at a daily dose of 200 mg (0.51 mmol) in the treatment of several types of malignant and premalignant lesions.

4-Hydroxyphenylretinamide, like other retinoids, is analysed mainly by high-performance liquid chromatography and is quantified on the basis of its absorbance at 362 nm.

Table 5. Genetic and related effects of 4-hydroxyphenylretinamide in short-term tests *in vitro* and *in vivo*

Test system	Result[a] Without S9	With S9	HID[b]	Reference
Salmonella typhimurium TA100, reverse mutation	–	–	400 µg/plate	Paulson *et al.* (1985)
Salmonella typhimurium TA1535, reverse mutation	–	–	400 µg/plate	Paulson *et al.* (1985)
Salmonella typhimurium TA1537, reverse mutation	–	–	400 µg/plate	Paulson *et al.* (1985)
Salmonella typhimurium TA100, reverse mutation	–	–	400 µg/plate	Paulson *et al.* (1985)
Salmonella typhimurium TA98, reverse mutation	–	–	400 µg/plate	Paulson *et al.* (1985)
Mouse mammary organ cultures, sister chromatid exchange	–	–	1 µmol/L	Manoharan & Banerjee (1985)
Gene mutation, mouse lymphoma L5178Y cells, *Tk* locus	–	–	10 µg/ml (–S9) 150 µg/ml (+S9)	Paulson *et al.* (1985)
Chromosomal aberrations, rat bone-marrow cells *in vivo*	0 0	– –	7000 mg/kg bw by gavage Single dose of 800 mg/kg bw for 5 days	Paulson *et al.* (1985)

[a] –, No effect on the investigated end-point; 0, not tested; S9, exogenous metabolic system
[b] HID, highest ineffective dose

8.2 Metabolism and kinetics

The main metabolites of 4-hydroxyphenyl-retinamide include all-*trans*-N-(4-methoxy-phenyl)-retinamide, 4-hydroxyphenylretinamide-O-glucuronide and several other polar retinamides. 4-Hydroxyphenylretinamide given at clinically relevant doses is not detectably hydrolysed to all-*trans*-retinoic acid or other retinoic acid isomers. In women with breast cancer who have received 4-hydroxyphenyl-retinamide for five years, the drug is cleared from the plasma with a half-life of 24 h, which is much slower than the half-lives of all-*trans*- and 9-*cis*-retinoic acid. 4-Hydroxy-phenylretinamide accumulates in target tissues such as the breast. Studies in animal models suggests that it is both distributed and metabolized differently in mice and rats, and it is unclear whether either of these species can be used as a true model for humans.

8.3 Cancer-preventive effects
8.3.1 Humans

In a preliminary report of a large randomized trial of use of 4-hydroxyphenylretinamide, equivocal results were obtained with regard to the development of new contralateral tumours among women previously treated for early breast cancer. There were fewer new cancers among treated pre-menopausal women but more cancers among treated postmenopausal women. A decrease in the risk for ovarian cancer was reported among all treated women in this trial.

Two studies, only one of which was randomized, of intermediate end-points suggested an effect of 4-hydroxyphenylretinamide against oral leukoplakia. A possible effect on ploidy in urinary bladder cells has also been described.

8.3.2   Experimental models

The chemopreventive efficacy of 4-hydroxyphenylretinamide has been evaluated in animal models of mammary gland, prostate, lung, skin, urinary bladder and colon carcinogenesis and lymphomagenesis. It was effective in reducing the tumour incidence or multiplicity in 11 of 12 studies of mammary carcinogenesis in mice or rats. The results depended on the experimental conditions, including the strain and age of the animals, their diet and the dose of both carcinogen and retinoid. It was effective in one study in a model of urinary bladder carcinogenesis in mice and ineffective in another, and it was effective in one study of prostate carcinogenesis but not in two others. It was ineffective in one study of lung carcinogenesis in mice. It was effective in one study of carcinogenesis of the colon and in two studies of lymphomagenesis in mice. In one study in mice, 4-hydroxyphenylretinamide was ineffective or enhanced skin tumour development.

Studies *in vitro* suggest that 4-hydroxyphenylretinamide can affect carcinogenesis at several levels: it inhibited the transformation of cultured cells and of tissue in organ culture; it inhibited the proliferation of a variety of tumour cell lines and, rarely, induced apoptosis. It induced differentiation only rarely.

There are insufficient data to conclude whether 4-hydroxyphenylretinamide can reduce the genotoxic effects of carcinogens *in vitro* or *in vivo*. Indications that it alters the metabolism of carcinogens and thus affects DNA damage are provided by a study showing alterations to cytochrome P450 mRNA levels in cell cultures exposed to the retinoid, and a study in which phase I and phase II enzymes were shown to be altered in the livers of animals fed this compound. The altered metabolism was associated *in vivo* with a reduction in the binding to tissue DNA of a carcinogen known to be metabolized by these enzymes.

8.3.3   Mechanisms of cancer prevention

Few reports indicate any activity of 4-hydroxyphenylretinamide at the initiation stage of carcinogenesis, and most suggest it acts on promotion. The mechanisms that may account for the cancer-preventive effects of this retinoid appear to be associated with its ability to inhibit cell proliferation by increasing the amount of a cyclin-dependent kinase inhibitor and to down-regulate cyclin D1 and enhancing apoptosis. Its limited effects on differentiation raise doubts as to whether this is a mechanism for cancer prevention. The high doses required to affect apoptosis raise questions about the relevance *in vivo* of the effects on apoptosis seen *in vitro*.

8.4   Other beneficial effects

4-Hydroxyphenylretinamide was not effective in the treatment of several skin disorders or of rheumatoid arthritis.

8.5   Carcinogenicity
8.5.1   Humans
No data were available to the Working Group.

8.5.2   Experimental models
No data were available to the Working Group.

8.6   Other toxic effects
8.6.1   Humans
4-Hydroxyphenylretinamide has been safely administered in chemoprevention trials at 200 mg per day for prolonged periods with no significant toxicity. Night blindness and hypertriglyceridaemia are the most common side-effects of treatment and may necessitate discontinuation of treatment in some patients.

No reports were available on the reproductive, developmental or genotoxic effects of 4-hydroxyphenylretinamide in humans.

8.6.2   Experimental models
In rats, long term administration of 4-hydroxyphenylretinamide increased the serum concentrations of triglycerides and cholesterol.

4-Hydroxyphenylretinamide is transferred extensively to the rat conceptus, but its embryotoxicity and teratogenic potency are much lower that those of all-*trans*-retinoic acid, probably because it lacks a terminal acidic group. The few available studies show no genotoxic effects *in vitro* or *in vivo*.

9. Recommendations for Research

9.1 General recommendations for 4-hydroxyphenylretinamide and other retinoids
See section 9 of the Handbook on all-*trans*-retinoic acid.

9.2 Recommendations specific to 4-hydroxyphenylretinamide
1. Define the efficacy, extent and mechanism of action of 4-hydroxyphenylretinamide in the prevention of human breast and ovarian cancer.

2. Determine the mechanism of action of 4-hydroxyphenylretinamide in cancer chemoprevention.

10. Evaluation

10.1 Cancer-preventive activity
10.1.1 Humans
There is *inadequate evidence* that 4-hydroxyphenylretinamide has cancer-preventive activity in humans.

10.1.2 Experimental animals
There is *sufficient evidence* that 4-hydroxyphenylretinamide has cancer-preventive activity in experimental animals. This evaluation is based on the observation of inhibitory effects in models of mammary carcinogenesis in mice and rats and its effectiveness in a limited number of studies against prostate and colon carcinogenesis and lymphomagenesis.

10.2 Overall evaluation
There is inadequate evidence that 4-hydroxyphenylretinamide has cancer-preventive activity in humans, but there is sufficient evidence that 4-hydroxyphenylretinamide has cancer-preventive activity in experimental animals, supported by data from cellular systems *in vitro* and information on the mechanisms of the cancer-preventive

effects. 4-Hydroxyphenylretinamide does not have significant toxicity in humans treated at the usual dose. Therefore, 4-hydroxyphenylretinamide shows promise as a cancer-preventive agent in humans.

11. References

Abou-Issa, H.M., Duruibe, V.A., Minton, J.P., Larroya, S., Dwivedi, C. & Webb, T.E. (1988) Putative metabolites derived from dietary combinations of calcium glucarate and N-(4-hydroxyphenyl)retinamide act synergistically to inhibit the induction of rat mammary tumors by 7,12-dimethylbenz[*a*]anthracene. *Proc. Natl Acad. Sci. USA*, **85**, 4181–4184

Abou-Issa, H., Curley, R.W.J., Panigot, M.J., Wilcox, K.A. & Webb, T.E. (1993) *In vivo* use of N-(4-hydroxyphenyl retinamide)-O-glucuronide as a breast cancer chemopreventive agent. *Anticancer Res.*, **13**, 1431–1436

Aliprandis, E.T., Merritt, G., Prada, F., Rigas, B. & Kashfi, K. (1997) Fenretinide inhibits phorbol ester-induced cyclooxygenase-2 expression in human colon adenocarcinoma cells. *Biochem. Soc. Trans.*, **25**, 457S–457S

Ball, M.D., Furr, H.C. & Olson, J.A. (1985) Enhancement of acyl coenzyme A:Retinol acyltransferase in rat liver and mammary tumor tissue by retinyl acetate and its competitive inhibition by N-(4-hydroxyphenyl) retinamide. *Biochem. Biophys. Res. Commun.*, **128**, 7–11

Barua, A.B. & Furr, H.C. (1998) Properties of retinoids: Structure, handling, and preparation. In: Redfern, C.P.F., ed., *Retinoid Protocols*. Totowa, NJ, Humana Press, pp. 3–28

Barua, A.B. & Olson, J.A. (1985) Preparation of retinamides by use of retinoyl fluoride. *J. Lipid Res.*, **26**, 258–262

Barua, A.B., Furr, H.C., Olson, J.A. & van Breemen, R.B. (1999) Vitamin A and carotenoids. In: DeLeenheer, A., Lambert, W. & van Bocxlaer, J., eds, *Modern Chromatographic Analysis of the Vitamins*. 3rd Ed. *New York, Marcel Dekker* (in press)

Berni, R. & Formelli, F. (1992) In vitro interaction of fenretinide with plasma retinol-binding protein and its functional consequences. *FEBS Lett.*, **308**, 43–45

Bertram, J.S. (1980) Structure–activity relationships among various retinoids and their ability to inhibit neoplastic transformation and to increase cell adhesion in the C3H/10T1/2 CL8 cell line. *Cancer Res.*, **40**, 3141–3146

Bollag, W. & Hartmann, H.R. (1987) Inhibition of rat mammary carcinogenesis by an arotinoid without a polar end group (Ro 15-0778). *Eur. J. Cancer Clin. Oncol.*, **23**, 131–135

Budavari, S., O'Neil, M.J., Smith, A., Heckelman, P.E., & Kinneary, J.F., eds (1996) *The Merck Index. An Encyclopedia of Chemicals, Drugs, and Biologicals*, 12th Ed. Whitehouse Station, NJ, Merck & Co.

Caruso, R.C., Zujewski, J., Iwata, F., Podgor, M.J., Conley, B.A., Ayres, L.M. & Kaiser-Kupfer, M.I. (1998) Effects of fenretinide (4-HPR) on dark adaptation. *Arch. Ophthalmol.*, **116**, 759–763

Cassano, E., Coopmans de Yoldi, G., Ferranti, C., Costa, A., Mascotti, G., De Palo, G. & Veronesi, U. (1993) Mammographic patterns in breast cancer chemoprevention with fenretinide (4-HPR). *Eur. J. Cancer*, **29A**, 2161–2163

Chan, L.N., Zhang, S., Cloyd, M. & Chan, T.S. (1997) *N*-(4-Hydroxyphenyl)retinamide prevents development of T-lymphomas in AKR/J mice. *Anticancer Res.*, **17**, 499–503

Chatterjee, M. & Banerjee, M.R. (1982) *N*-Nitrosodiethylamine-induced nodule-like alveolar lesion and its prevention by a retinoid in BALB/c mouse mammary glands in the whole organ in culture. *Carcinogenesis*, **3**, 801–804

Chiesa, F., Tradati, N., Marazza, M., Rossi, N., Boracchi, P., Mariani, L., Clerici, M., Formelli, F., Barzan, L., Carrassi, A., Pastorini, A., Camerini, T., Giardini, R., Zurrida, S., Minn, F.L., Costa, A., De Palo, G. & Veronesi, U. (1992) Prevention of local relapses and new localisations of oral leukoplakias with the synthetic retinoid fenretinide (4-HPR). Preliminary results. *Eur. J. Cancer B. Oral Oncol.*, **28B**, 97–102

Chiesa, F., Tradati, N., Marazza, M., Rossi, N., Boracchi, P., Mariani, L., Formelli, F., Giardini, R., Costa, A., De Palo, G. & Veronesi, U. (1993) Fenretinide (4-HPR) in chemoprevention of oral leukoplakia. *J. Cell Biochem.*, **17F** (Suppl.), 255–261

Chrzanowski, F.A., Fegely, B.J., Sisco, W.R. & Newton, M.P. (1984) Analysis of *N*-(4-hydroxyphenyl)retinamide polymorphic forms by X-ray powder diffraction. *J. Pharm. Sci.*, **73**, 1448–1450

Clifford, J.L., Menter, D.G., Wang, M., Lotan, R. & Lippman, S.M. (1999) Retinoid receptor-dependent and -independent effects of *N*-(4-hydroxyphenyl)-retinamide in F9 embryonal carcinoma cells. *Cancer Res.*, **59**, 14–18

Cobleigh, M.A. (1994) Breast cancer and fenretinide, an analogue of vitamin A. *Leukemia*, **8** (Suppl. 3), S59–S63

Coburn, W.C., Jr, Thorpe, M.C., Shealy, Y.F., Kirk, M.C., Frye, J.L. & O'Dell, C.A. (1983) Spectroscopic charac-

terization of 13-*cis* and all-*trans*-retinamide. *J. Chem. Eng. Data*, **28**, 422–428

Cohen, L.A., Epstein, M., Saa-Pabon, V., Meschter, C. & Zang, E. (1994) Interactions between 4-HPR and diet in NMU-induced mammary tumorigenesis. *Nutr. Cancer*, **21**, 271–283

Conaway, C.C., Jiao, D., Kelloff, G.J., Steele, V.E., Rivenson, A. & Chung, F.L. (1998) Chemopreventive potential of fumaric acid, *N*-acetylcysteine, *N*-(4-hydroxyphenyl)retinamide and β-carotene for tobacco-nitrosamine-induced lung tumors in A/J mice. *Cancer Lett.*, **124**, 85–93

Costa, A., Malone, W., Perloff, M., Buranelli, F., Campa, T., Dossena, G., Magni, A., Pizzichetta, M., Andreoli, C., Del Vecchio, M., Formelli, F. & Barbieri, A. (1989) Tolerability of the synthetic retinoid Fenretinide® (HPR). *Eur. J. Cancer Clin. Oncol.*, **25**, 805–808

Costa, A., Formelli, F., Chiesa, F., Decensi, A., De Palo, G. & Veronesi, U. (1994) Prospects of chemoprevention of human cancers with the synthetic retinoid fenretinide. *Cancer Res.*, **54**, 2032s–2037s

Costa, A., De Palo, G., Decensi, A., Formelli, F., Chiesa, F., Nava, M., Camerini, T., Marubini, E. & Veronesi, U. (1995) Retinoids in cancer chemoprevention. Clinical trials with the synthetic analogue fenretinide. *Ann. N.Y. Acad. Sci.*, **768**, 148–162

Dawson, M.I. & Hobbs, P.D. (1994) The synthetic chemistry of retinoids. In: Sporn, M.B., Roberts, A.B. & Goodman, D.S., eds, *The Retinoids: Biology, Chemistry, and Medicine*, 2nd Ed. New York, Raven Press, pp. 5–178

Decensi, A., Formelli, F., Torrisi, R. & Costa, A. (1993) Breast cancer chemoprevention: Studies with 4-HPR alone and in combination with tamoxifen using circulating growth factors as potential surrogate endpoints. *J. Cell Biochem.*, **17G** (Suppl.), 226–233

Decensi, A., Bruno, S., Costantini, M., Torrisi, R., Curotto, A., Gatteschi, B., Nicolo, G., Polizzi, A., Perloff, M., Malone, W.F. & Bruzzi, P. (1994a) Phase IIa study of fenretinide in superficial bladder cancer, using DNA flow cytometry as an intermediate end point. *J. Natl Cancer Inst.*, **86**, 138–140

Decensi, A., Torrisi, R., Polizzi, A., Gesi, R., Brezzo, V., Rolando, M., Rondanina, G., Orengo, M.A., Formelli, F. & Costa, A. (1994b) Effect of the synthetic retinoid fenretinide on dark adaptation and the ocular surface. *J. Natl Cancer Inst.*, **86**, 105–110

Decensi, A., Costa, A., De Palo, G., Formelli, F., Marubini, E., Mariani, L., Fontana, V. & Veronesi, U. (1997a)

Retinoid–menopause interactions in a breast cancer prevention trial. *Proc. Am. Assoc. Cancer Res.,* **38,** 529–529

Decensi, A., Fontana, V., Fioretto, M., Rondanina, G., Torrisi, R., Orengo, M.A. & Costa, A. (1997b) Long-term effects of fenretinide on retinal function. *Eur. J. Cancer,* **33,** 80–84

Decensi, A., Torrisi, R., Bruno, S., Curotto, A., Malcangi, B., Nicolo, G., Bruttini, G.P., Costantini, M., Rondanina, G., Baglietto, L., Gatteschi, B., Varaldo, M. & Bruzzi, P. (1997c) Randomized trial of fenretinide in superficial bladder cancer using DNA flow cytometry as an intermediate endpoint. *Proc. Am. Soc. Clin. Oncol.,* **16,** 541A–541A

Delia, D., Aiello, A., Lombardi, L., Pelicci, P.G., Grignani, F., Formelli, F., Ménard, S., Costa, A., Veronesi, U. & Pierotti, M.A. (1993) N-(4-Hydroxyphenyl)retinamide induces apoptosis of malignant hemopoietic cell lines including those unresponsive to retinoic acid. *Cancer Res.,* **53,** 6036–6041

Delia, D., Aiello, A., Meroni, L., Nicolini, M., Reed, J.C. & Pierotti, M.A. (1997) Role of antioxidants and intra-cellular free radicals in retinamide-induced cell death. *Carcinogenesis,* **18,** 943–948

De Palo, G., Veronesi, U., Camerini, T., Formelli, F., Mascotti, G., Boni, C., Fosser, V., Del Vecchio, M., Campa, T., Costa, A. & Marubini, E. (1995a) Can fen-retinide protect women against ovarian cancer? *J. Natl Cancer Inst.,* **87,** 146–147

De Palo, G., Veronesi, U., Marubini, E., Camerini, T., Chiesa, F., Nava, M., Formelli, F., Del Vecchio, M., Costa, A., Boracchi, P. & Mariani, L. (1995b) Controlled clinical trials with fenretinide in breast cancer, basal cell carcinoma and oral leukoplakia. *J. Cell Biochem.,* **22** (Suppl.), 11–17

De Palo, G., Camerini, T., Marubini, E., Costa, A., Formelli, F., Del Vecchio, M., Mariani, L., Miceli, R., Mascotti, G., Magni, A., Campa, T., Di Mauro, M.G., Attili, A., Maltoni, C., Del Turco, M.R., Decensi, A., D'Aiuto, G. & Veronesi, U. (1997) Chemoprevention trial of contralateral breast cancer with fenretinide. Rationale, design, methodology, organization, data management, statistics and accrual. *Tumori,* **83,** 884–894

Dew, S.E., Wardlaw, S.A. & Ong, D.E. (1993) Effects of pharmacological retinoids on several vitamin A-metabolizing enzymes. *Cancer Res.,* **53,** 2965–2969

Dimitrov, N.V., Meyer, C.J., Perloff, M., Ruppenthal, M.M., Phillipich, M.J., Gilliland, D., Malone, W. & Minn, F.L. (1990) Alteration of retinol-binding-pro-tein concentrations by the synthetic retinoid fenre-tinide in healthy human subjects. *Am. J. Clin. Nutr.,* **51,** 1082–1087

DiPietrantonio, A., Hsich, T.C. & Wu, J.M. (1996) Differential effects of retinoic acid (RA) and N-(4-hydroxyphenyl)retinamide (4-HPR) on cell growth, induction of differentiation, and changes in p34^{cdc2}, Bcl-2, and actin expression in the human promyelo-cytic HL-60 leukemic cells. *Biochem. Biophys. Res. Commun.,* **224,** 837–842

DiPietrantonio, A.M., Hsieh, T.C., Olson, S.C. & Wu, J.M. (1998) Regulation of G1/S transition and induction of apoptosis in HL-60 leukemia cells by fenretinide (4HPR). *Int. J. Cancer,* **78,** 53–61

Di Vinci, A., Geido, E., Infusini, E. & Giaretti, W. (1994) Neuroblastoma cell apoptosis induced by the syn-thetic retinoid N-(4-hydroxyphenyl)retinamide. *Int. J. Cancer,* **59,** 422–426

Doose, D.R., Minn, F.L., Stellar, S. & Nayak, R.K. (1992) Effects of meals and meal composition on the bio-availability of fenretinide. *J. Clin. Pharmacol.,* **32,** 1089–1095

Fanjul, A.N., Delia, D., Pierotti, M.A., Rideout, D., Qiu, J. & Pfahl, M. (1996) 4-Hydroxyphenyl retinamide is a highly selective activator of retinoid receptors. *J. Biol. Chem.,* **271,** 22441–22446

Favoni, R.E., de Cupis, A., Bruno, S., Yee, D., Ferrera, A., Pirani, P., Costa, A. & Decensi, A. (1998) Modulation of the insulin-like growth factor-I system by N-(4-hydroxyphenyl)retinamide in human breast cancer cell lines. *Br. J. Cancer,* **77,** 2138–2147

Formelli, F., Carsana, R. & Costa, A. (1987) N-(4-Hydroxyphenyl)retinamide (4-HPR) lowers plasma retinol levels in rats. *Med. Sci. Res.,* **15,** 843–844

Formelli, F., Carsana, R., Costa, A., Buranelli, F., Campa, T., Dossena, G., Magni, A. & Pizzichetta, M. (1989) Plasma retinol level reduction by the syn-thetic retinoid fenretinide: A one year follow-up study of breast cancer patients. *Cancer Res.,* **49,** 6149–6152

Formelli, F., Clerici, M., Campa, T., Di Mauro, M.G., Magni, A., Mascotti, G., Moglia, D., De Palo, G., Costa, A. & Veronesi, U. (1993) Five-year administra-tion of fenretinide: Pharmacokinetics and effects on plasma retinol concentrations. *J. Clin. Oncol.,* **11,** 2036–2042

Formelli, F., Barua, A.B. & Olson, J.A. (1996) Bioactivities of N-(4-hydroxyphenyl)retinamide and retinoyl β-glucuronide. *FASEB J.,* **10,** 1014–1024

Formelli, F., De Palo, G., Costa, A. & Veronesi, U. (1998) Human transplacental passage of the retinoid fenre-tinide (4HPR). *Eur. J. Cancer,* **34,** 428–429

Frolik, C.A. & Olson, J.A. (1984) Extraction, separation, and chemical analysis of retinoids. In: Sporn, M.B., Roberts, A.B. & Goodman, D.S., eds, *The Retinoids.* New York, Academic Press, pp. 181–233

Furr, H.C., Barua, A.B. & Olson, J.A. (1992) Retinoids and carotenoids. In: De Leenheer, A.P., Lambert, W.E. & Nelis, H.J., eds, *Modern Chromatographic Analysis of Vitamins,* 2nd Ed. New York, Marcel Dekker Inc., pp. 1–71

Furr, H.C., Barua, A.B. & Olson, J.A. (1994) Analytical methods. In: Sporn, M.B., Roberts, A.B. & Goodman, D.S., eds, *The Retinoids: Biology, Chemistry, and Medicine,* 2nd Ed. New York, Raven Press, pp. 179–209

Garewal, H.S., List, A., Meyskens, F., Buzaid, A., Greenberg, B. & Katakkar, S. (1989) Phase II trial of fenretinide [*N*-(4-hydroxyphenyl) retinamide] in myelodysplasia: Possible retinoid-induced disease acceleration. *Leuk. Res., 13,* 339–343

Gross, E.G., Peck, G.L. & DiGiovanna, J.J. (1991) Adverse reaction to fenretinide, a synthetic retinoid. *Arch. Dermatol., 127,* 1849–1850

Grubbs, C.J., Eto, I., Juliana, M.M., Hardin, J.M. & Whitaker, L.M. (1990) Effect of retinyl acetate and 4-hydroxyphenylretinamide on initiation of chemically-induced mammary tumors. *Anticancer Res., 10,* 661–666

Grunt, T.W., Dittrich, E., Offterdinger, M., Schneider, S.M., Dittrich, C. & Huber, H. (1998) Effects of retinoic acid and fenretinide on the c-*erb*B-2 expression, growth and cisplatin sensitivity of breast cancer cells. *Br. J. Cancer, 78,* 79–87

Hong, W.K. & Itri, L.M. (1994) Retinoids and human cancer. In: Sporn, M.B., Roberts, A.B. & Goodman, D.S., eds, *The Retinoids: Biology, Chemistry, and Medicine,* 2nd Ed. New York, Raven Press, pp. 597–630

Hsieh, T.C. & Wu, J.M. (1997) Effects of fenretinide (4-HPR) on prostate LNCaP cell growth, apoptosis, and prostate-specific gene expression. *Prostate, 33,* 97–104

Hsieh, T.C., Ng, C. & Wu, J.M. (1995) The synthetic retinoid *N*-(4-hydroxyphenyl)retinamide (4-HPR) exerts antiproliferative and apoptosis-inducing effects in the androgen-independent human prostatic JCA-1 cells. *Biochem. Mol. Biol. Int., 37,* 499–506

Hultin, T.A., May, C.M. & Moon, R.C. (1986) *N*-(4-Hydroxyphenyl)-all-*trans*-retinamide pharmacokinetics in female rats and mice. *Drug Metab. Dispos., 14,* 714–717

Hultin, T.A., McCormick, D.L., May, C.M. & Moon, R.C. (1988) Effects of pretreatment with the retinoid *N*-(4-hydroxyphenyl)-all-*trans*-retinamide and phenobarbital on the disposition and metabolism of *N*-(4-hydroxyphenyl)-all-*trans*-retinamide in mice. *Drug Metab. Dispos., 16,* 783–788

Hultin, T.A., Filla, M.S. & McCormick, D.L. (1990) Distribution and metabolism of the retinoid, *N*-(4-methoxyphenyl)-all-*trans*-retinamide, the major meta-bolite of *N*-(4-hydroxyphenyl)-all-*trans*-retinamide, in female mice. *Drug Metab. Dispos., 18,* 175–179

Igawa, M., Tanabe, T., Chodak, G.W. & Rukstalis, D.B. (1994) *N*-(4-Hydroxyphenyl)retinamide induces cell cycle specific growth inhibition in PC3 cells. *Prostate, 24,* 299–305

Jurima-Romet, M., Neigh, S. & Casley, W.L. (1997) Induction of cytochrome P450 3A by retinoids in rat hepatocyte culture. *Hum. Exp. Toxicol., 16,* 198–203

Kaiser-Kupfer, M.I., Peck, G.L., Caruso, R.C., Jaffe, M.J., DiGiovanna, J.J. & Gross, E.G. (1986) Abnormal retinal function associated with fenretinide, a synthetic retinoid. *Arch. Ophthalmol., 104,* 69–70

Kalemkerian, G.P., Slusher, R., Ramalingam, S., Gadgeel, S. & Mabry, M. (1995) Growth inhibition and induction of apoptosis by fenretinide in small-cell lung cancer cell lines. *J. Natl Cancer Inst., 87,* 1674–1680

Kazmi, S.M., Plante, R.K., Visconti, V. & Lau, C.Y. (1996) Comparison of *N*-(4-hydroxyphenyl)retinamide and all-*trans*-retinoic acid in the regulation of retinoid receptor-mediated gene expression in human breast cancer cell lines. *Cancer Res., 56,* 1056–1062

Kelloff, G.J., Crowell, J.A., Boone, C.W., Steele, V.E., Lubet, R.A., Greenwald, P., Alberts, D.S., Covey, J.M., Doody, L.A., Knapp, G.G., Nayfield, S.G., Parkinson, D.R., Prasad, K., Prorok, P.C., Sausville, E.A. & Sigman, C.C. (1994) Clinical development plan: *N*-(4-Hydroxyphenyl)retinamide. *J. Cell Biochem., 20* (Suppl.), 176–196

Kenel, M.F., Krayer, J.H., Merz, E.A. & Pritchard, J.F. (1988) Teratogenicity of *N*-(4-hydroxyphenyl)-all-*trans*-retinamide in rats and rabbits. *Teratog. Carcinog. Mutag., 8,* 1–11

Kingston, T.P., Lowe, N.J., Winston, J. & Heckenlively, J. (1986) Visual and cutaneous toxicity which occurs during N-(4-hydroxyphenyl)retinamide therapy for psoriasis. *Clin. Exp. Dermatol., 11,* 624–627

Krzeminski, R., Zwas, F., Esper, P. & Pienta, K. (1996) Electroretinographic findings in subjects after administration of fenretinide. *Doc. Ophthalmol., 91,* 299–309

Li, C.Y., Zimmerman, C.L. & Wiedmann, T.S. (1996) Solubilization of retinoids by bile salt/phospholipid aggregates. *Pharm. Res.*, **13**, 907–913

Lotan, R. (1995) Retinoids and apoptosis: Implications for cancer chemoprevention and therapy. *J. Natl Cancer Inst.*, **87**, 1655–1657

Manoharan, K. & Banerjee, M.R. (1985) β-Carotene reduces sister chromatid exchanges induced by chemical carcinogens in mouse mammary cells in organ culture. *Cell Biol. Int. Rep.*, **9**, 783–789

Mariani, L., Formelli, F., De Palo, G., Manzari, A., Camerini, T., Campa, T., Di Mauro, M.G., Crippa, A., Delle Grottaglie, M., Del Vecchio, M., Marubini, E., Costa, A. & Veronesi, U. (1996) Chemoprevention of breast cancer with fenretinide (4-HPR): Study of long-term visual and ophthalmologic tolerability. *Tumori*, **82**, 444–449

Mariotti, A., Marcora, E., Bunone, G., Costa, A., Veronesi, U., Pierotti, M.A. & Della Valle, G. (1994) N-(4-Hydroxyphenyl)retinamide: A potent inducer of apoptosis in human neuroblastoma cells. *J. Natl Cancer Inst.*, **86**, 1245–1247

McCarthy, D.J., Lindamood, C., III & Hill, D.L. (1987) Effects of retinoids on metabolizing enzymes and on binding of benzo(a)pyrene to rat tissue DNA. *Cancer Res.*, **47**, 5014–5020

McCormick, D.L. & Moon, R.C. (1986) Retinoid–tamoxifen interaction in mammary cancer chemoprevention. *Carcinogenesis*, **7**, 193–196

McCormick, D.L., Mehta, R.G., Thompson, C.A., Dinger, N., Caldwell, J.A. & Moon, R.C. (1982a) Enhanced inhibition of mammary carcinogenesis by combined treatment with N-(4-hydroxyphenyl)retinamide and ovariectomy. *Cancer Res.*, **42**, 508–512

McCormick, D.L., Becci, P.J. & Moon, R.C. (1982b) Inhibition of mammary and urinary bladder carcinogenesis by a retinoid and a maleic anhydride–divinyl ether copolymer (MVE-2). *Carcinogenesis*, **3**, 1473–1476

McCormick, D.L., Bagg, B.J. & Hultin, T.A. (1987) Comparative activity of dietary or topical exposure to three retinoids in the promotion of skin tumor induction in mice. *Cancer Res.*, **47**, 5989–5993

McCormick, D.L., Johnson, W.D., Rao, K.V., Bowman-Gram, T., Steele, V.E., Lubet, R.A. & Kelloff, G.J. (1996) Comparative activity of N-(4-hydroxyphenyl)-all-*trans*-retinamide and α-difluoromethylornithine as inhibitors of lymphoma induction in PIM transgenic mice. *Carcinogenesis*, **17**, 2513–2517

McCormick, D.L., Rao, K.V., Dooley, L., Steele, V.E., Lubet, R.A., Kelloff, G.J. & Bosland, M.C. (1998) Influence of N-methyl-N-nitrosourea, testosterone, and N-(4-hydroxyphenyl)-all-*trans*-retinamide on prostate cancer induction in Wistar-Unilever rats. *Cancer Res.*, **58**, 3282–3288

Mehta, R.G., Hultin, T.A. & Moon, R.C. (1988) Metabolism of the chemopreventive retinoid N-(4-hydroxyphenyl)retinamide by mammary gland in organ culture. *Biochem. J.*, **256**, 579–584

Mehta, R.G., Moon, R.C., Hawthorne, M., Formelli, F. & Costa, A. (1991) Distribution of fenretinide in the mammary gland of breast cancer patients. *Eur. J. Cancer*, **27**, 138–141

Mehta, R.R., Hawthorne, M.E., Graves, J.M. & Mehta, R.G. (1998) Metabolism of N-[4-hydroxyphenyl]retinamide (4-HPR) to N-[4-methoxyphenyl]retinamide (4-MPR) may serve as a biomarker for its efficacy against human breast cancer and melanoma cells. *Eur. J. Cancer*, **34**, 902–907

Modiano, M., Pond, G., Holdsworth, M., Plezia, P. & Alberts, D. (1989) Phase I and pharmacokinetic (PK) study of selective intraarterial chemoembolization (CE) with angiostat collagen, CDDP, mitomycin, adriamycin for metastatic colorectal carcinoma to the liver. The University of Arizona experience. *Clin. Res.*, **37**, 143A–143A

Modiano, M.R., Dalton, W.S., Lippman, S.M., Joffe, L., Booth, A.R. & Meyskens, F.L.J. (1990a) Ocular toxic effects of fenretinide. *J. Natl Cancer Inst.*, **82**, 1063–1063

Modiano, M.R., Dalton, W.S., Lippman, S.M., Joffe, L., Booth, A.R. & Meyskens, F.L.J. (1990b) Phase II study of fenretinide (N-[4-hydroxyphenyl]retinamide) in advanced breast cancer and melanoma. *Invest. New Drugs*, **8**, 317–319

Moglia, D., Formelli, F., Baliva, G., Bono, A., Accetturi, M., Nava, M. & De Palo, G. (1996) Effects of topical treatment with fenretinide (4-HPR) and plasma vitamin A levels in patients with actinic keratoses. *Cancer Lett.*, **110**, 87–91

Moon, R.C. & Mehta, R.G. (1990) Cancer chemoprevention by retinoids: Animal models. *Methods Enzymol.*, **190**, 395–406

Moon, R.C., Thompson, H.J., Becci, P.J., Grubbs, C.J., Gander, R.J., Newton, D.L., Smith, J.M., Phillips, S.L., Henderson, W.R., Mullen, L.T., Brown, C.C. & Sporn, M.B. (1979) N-(4-Hydroxyphenyl)retinamide, a new retinoid for prevention of breast cancer in the rat. *Cancer Res.*, **39**, 1339–1346

Moon, R.C., McCormick, D.L., Becci, P.J., Shealy, Y.F., Frickel, F., Paust, J. & Sporn, M.B. (1982) Influence of 15 retinoic acid amides on urinary bladder carcinogenesis in the mouse. *Carcinogenesis*, **3**, 1469–1472

Moon, R.C., Pritchard, J.F., Mehta, R.G., Nomides, C.T., Thomas, C.F. & Dinger, N.M. (1989) Suppression of rat mammary cancer development by *N*-(4-hydroxyphenyl)retinamide (4-HPR) following surgical removal of first palpable tumor. *Carcinogenesis*, **10**, 1645–1649

Moon, R.C., Kelloff, G.J., Detrisac, C.J., Steele, V.E., Thomas, C.F. & Sigman, C.C. (1992) Chemoprevention of MNU-induced mammary tumors in the mature rat by 4-HPR and tamoxifen. *Anticancer Res.*, **12**, 1147–1153

Moon, R.C., Kelloff, G.J., Detrisac, C.J., Steele, V.E., Thomas, C.F. & Sigman, C.C. (1994a) Chemoprevention of OH-BBN-induced bladder cancer in mice by oltipraz, alone and in combination with 4-HPR and DFMO. *Anticancer Res.*, **14**, 5–11

Moon, R.C., Mehta, R.G. & Rao, K.V.N. (1994b) Retinoids and cancer in experimental animals. In: Sporn, M.B., Roberts, A.B. & Goodman, D.S., eds, *The Retinoids: Biology, Chemistry, and Medicine*, 2nd Ed. New York, Raven Press, pp. 573–595

Muller, A., Nakagawa, H. & Rustgi, A.K. (1997) Retinoic acid and N-(4-hydroxyphenyl)retinamide suppress growth of esophageal squamous carcinoma cell lines. *Cancer Lett.*, **113**, 95–101

Ohshima, M., Ward, J.M. & Wenk, M.L. (1985) Preventive and enhancing effects of retinoids on the development of naturally occurring tumors of skin, prostate gland, and endocrine pancreas in aged male ACI/segHapBR rats. *J. Natl Cancer Inst.*, **74**, 517–524

Oridate, N., Lotan, D., Mitchell, M.F., Hong, W.K. & Lotan, R. (1995) Induction of apoptosis by retinoids in human cervical carcinoma cell lines. *Int. J. Oncol.*, **7**, 433–441

Oridate, N., Lotan, D., Xu, X.C., Hong, W.K. & Lotan, R. (1996) Differential induction of apoptosis by all-*trans*-retinoic acid and *N*-(4-hydroxyphenyl)retinamide in human head and neck squamous cell carcinoma cell lines. *Clin. Cancer Res.*, **2**, 855–863

Oridate, N., Suzuki, S., Higuchi, M., Mitchell, M.F., Hong, W.K. & Lotan, R. (1997) Involvement of reactive oxygen species in *N*-(4-hydroxyphenyl)retinamide-induced apoptosis in cervical carcinoma cells. *J. Natl Cancer Inst.*, **89**, 1191–1198

Paulson, J.D., Oldham, J.W., Preston, R.F. & Newman, D. (1985) Lack of genotoxicity of the cancer chemopreventive agent *N*-(4-hydroxyphenyl)retinamide. *Fundam. Appl. Toxicol.*, **5**, 144–150

Pellegrini, R., Mariotti, A., Tagliabue, E., Bressan, R., Bunone, G., Coradini, D., Della Valle, G., Formelli, F., Cleris, L., Radice, P., Pierotti, M.A., Colnaghi, M.I. & Ménard, S. (1995) Modulation of markers associated with tumor aggressiveness in human breast cancer cell lines by *N*-(4-hydroxyphenyl)retinamide. *Cell Growth Differ.*, **6**, 863–869

Peng, Y.M., Dalton, W.S., Alberts, D.S., Xu, M.J., Lim, H. & Meyskens, F.L.J. (1989) Pharmacokinetics of *N*-4-hydroxyphenylretinamide and the effect of its oral administration on plasma retinol concentrations in cancer patients. *Int. J. Cancer*, **43**, 22–26

Pergolizzi, R., Appierto, V., Crosti, M., Cavadini, E., Cleris, L., Guffanti, A. & Formelli, F. (1999) Role of retinoic acid receptor overexpression in sensitivity to fenretinide and tumorigenicity of human ovarian carcinoma cells. *Int. J. Cancer*, **81**, 829–834

Pienta, K.J., Esper, P.S., Zwas, F., Krzeminski, R. & Flaherty, L.E. (1997) Phase II chemoprevention trial of oral fenretinide in patients at risk for adenocarcinoma of the prostate. *Am. J. Clin. Oncol.*, **20**, 36–39

Pollard, M., Luckert, P.H. & Sporn, M.B. (1991) Prevention of primary prostate cancer in Lobund-Wistar rats by *N*-(4-hydroxyphenyl)retinamide. *Cancer Res.*, **51**, 3610–3611

Ponzoni, M., Bocca, P., Chiesa, V., Decensi, A., Pistoia, V., Raffaghello, L., Rozzo, C. & Montaldo, P.G. (1995) Differential effects of *N*-(4-hydroxyphenyl)retinamide and retinoic acid on neuroblastoma cells: Apoptosis *versus* differentiation. *Cancer Res.*, **55**, 853–861

Radcliffe, J.D. (1983) Effect of N-4-hydroxyphenyl retinamide on lipid metabolism in rats. *Nutr. Rep. Int.*, **28**, 799–803

Ratko, T.A., Detrisac, C.J., Dinger, N.M., Thomas, C.F., Kelloff, G.J. & Moon, R.C. (1989) Chemopreventive efficacy of combined retinoid and tamoxifen treatment following surgical excision of a primary mammary cancer in female rats. *Cancer Res.*, **49**, 4472–4476

Roberson, K.M., Penland, S.N., Padilla, G.M., Selvan, R.S., Kim, C.S., Fine, R.L. & Robertson, C.N. (1997) Fenretinide: Induction of apoptosis and endogenous transforming growth factor β in PC-3 prostate cancer cells. *Cell Growth Differ.*, **8**, 101–111

Rotmensz, N., De Palo, G., Formelli, F., Costa, A., Marubini, E., Campa, T., Crippa, A., Danesini, G.M., Delle Grottaglie, M., Di Mauro, M.G., Filiberti, A., Gallazzi, M., Guzzon, A., Magni, A., Malone, W., Mariani, L., Palvarini, M., Perloff, M., Pizzichetta, M.

& Veronesi, U. (1991) Long-term tolerability of fenre-tinide (4-HPR) in breast cancer patients. *Eur. J. Cancer,* **27**, 1127–1131

Rozzo, C., Chiesa, V., Caridi, G., Pagnan, G. & Ponzoni, M. (1997) Induction of apoptosis in human neurob-lastoma cells by abrogation of integrin-mediated cell adhesion. *Int. J. Cancer,* **70**, 688–698

Sabichi, A.L., Hendricks, D.T., Bober, M.A. & Birrer, M.J. (1998) Retinoic acid receptor β expression and growth inhibition of gynecologic cancer cells by the syn-thetic retinoid *N*-(4-hydroxyphenyl)retinamide. *J. Natl Cancer Inst.,* **90**, 597–605

Sani, B.P., Shealy, Y.F. & Hill, D.L. (1995) *N*-(4-Hydroxyphenyl)retinamide: Interactions with retinoid-binding proteins/receptors. *Carcinogenesis,* **16**, 2531–2534

Schrader, P.A. & Sisco, W.R. (1987) High-performance liquid chromatographic analysis of fenretinide in rodent feed. *J. Chromatogr.,* **408**, 430–434

Shealy, Y.F., Frye, J.L., O'Dell, C.A., Thorpe, M.C., Kirk, M.C., Coburn, W.C., Jr & Sporn, M.B. (1984) Synthesis and properties of some 13-*cis*- and all-*trans*-retinamides. *J. Pharm. Sci.,* **73**, 745–751

Sheikh, M.S., Li, X.S., Chen, J.C., Shao, Z.M., Ordonez, J.V. & Fontana, J.A. (1994) Mechanisms of regulation of WAF1/Cip1 gene expression in human breast car-cinoma: Role of p53-dependent and independent signal transduction pathways. *Oncogene,* **9**, 3407–3415

Sheikh, M.S., Shao, Z.M., Li, X.S., Ordonez, J.V., Conley, B.A., Wu, S., Dawson, M.I., Han, Q.X., Chao, W.R., Quick, T., Niles, R.M. & Fontana, J.A. (1995) *N*-(4-Hydroxyphenyl)retinamide (4-HPR)-mediated biolog-ical actions involve retinoid receptor-independent pathways in human breast carcinoma. *Carcinogenesis,* **16**, 2477–2486

Silverman, J., Katayama, S., Radok, P., Levenstein, M.J. & Weisburger, J.H. (1983) Effect of short-term adminis-tration of *N*-(4-hydroxyphenyl)-all-*trans*-retinamide on chemically induced mammary tumors. *Nutr. Cancer,* **4**, 186–191

Sridhara, R., Peck, G., Wu, S., Edwards, P., Crowell, J., Fontana, J. & Conley, B. (1997) Pharmacokinetics (PK) and pharmacodynamics (PD) of fenretinide (4-HPR) in patients (pts) treated in a skin cancer preven-tion trial. *Proc. Am. Soc. Clin. Oncol.,* **16**, 540A–540A

Steele, V.E., Kelloff, G.J., Wilkinson, B.P. & Arnold, J.T. (1990) Inhibition of transformation in cultured rat tracheal epithelial cells by potential chemopreventive agents. *Cancer Res.,* **50**, 2068–2074

Sun, S.Y., Yue, P. & Lotan, R. (1999a) Induction of apop-tosis by *N*-(4-hydroxyphenyl)retinamide and its asso-ciation with reactive oxygen species, nuclear retinoic acid receptors, and apoptosis-related genes in human prostate carcinoma cells. *Mol. Pharmacol.,* **55**, 403–410

Sun, S.Y., Kurie, J.M., Yue, P., Dawson, M.I., Shroot, B., Chandraratna, R.A., Hong, W.K. & Lotan, R. (1999b) Differential responses of normal, premalignant, and malignant human bronchial epithelial cells to recep-tor-selective retinoids. *Clin. Cancer Res.,* **5**, 431–437

Supino, R., Crosti, M., Clerici, M., Warlters, A., Cleris, L., Zunino, F. & Formelli, F. (1996) Induction of apopto-sis by fenretinide (4HPR) in human ovarian carci-noma cells and its association with retinoic acid receptor expression. *Int. J. Cancer,* **65**, 491–497

Swisshelm, K., Ryan, K., Lee, X., Tsou, H.C., Peacocke, M. & Sager, R. (1994) Down-regulation of retinoic acid receptor beta in mammary carcinoma cell lines and its up-regulation in senescing normal mammary epithelial cells. *Cell Growth Differ.,* **5**, 133–141

Swisshelm, K., Ryan, K., Tsuchiya, K. & Sager, R. (1995) Enhanced expression of an insulin growth factor-like binding protein (mac25) in senescent human mam-mary epithelial cells and induced expression with retinoic acid. *Proc. Natl Acad. Sci. USA,* **92**, 4472–4476

Taimi, M. & Breitman, T.R. (1997) *N*-4-Hydroxyphenyl-retinamide enhances retinoic acid-induced differentia-tion and retinoylation of proteins in the human acute promyelocytic leukemia cell line, NB4, by a mechanism that may involve inhibition of retinoic acid catabolism. *Biochem. Biophys. Res. Commun.,* **232**, 432–436

Takahashi, N., Sausville, E.A. & Breitman, T.R. (1995) *N*-(4-Hydroxyphenyl)retinamide (Fenretinide) in com-bination with retinoic acid enhances differentiation and retinoylation of proteins. *Clin. Cancer Res.,* **1**, 637–642

Tamura, K., Nakae, D., Horiguchi, K., Akai, H., Kobayashi, Y., Andoh, N., Satoh, H., Denda, A., Tsujiuchi, T., Yoshiji, H. & Konishi, Y. (1997) Inhibition by *N*-(4-hydroxyphenyl)retinamide and all-*trans*-retinoic acid of exogenous and endoge-nous development of putative preneoplastic, glu-tathione *S*-transferase placental form-positive lesions in the livers of rats. *Carcinogenesis,* **18**, 2133–2141

Thaller, C., Eichele, G., Slawin, K., Thompson, T.C. & Kadmon, D. (1996) Retinoid alterations induced by fenretinide therapy in prostate cancer. *Proc. Am. Assoc. Cancer Res.,* **37**, 243–243

Tradati, N., Chiesa, F., Rossi, N., Grigolato, R., Formelli, F., Costa, A. & De Palo, G. (1994) Successful topical treatment of oral lichen planus and leukoplakias with fenretinide (4-HPR). *Cancer Lett.,* **76**, 109–111

Trizna, Z., Benner, S.E., Shirley, L., Furlong, C. & Hong, W.K. (1993) N-(4-Hydroxyphenyl)retinamide is anti-clastogenic in human lymphoblastoid cell lines. *Anticancer Res.*, **13**, 355–356

Turton, J.A., Willars, G.B., Haselden, J.N., Ward, S.J., Steele, C.E. & Hicks, R.M. (1992) Comparative terato-genicity of nine retinoids in the rat. *Int. J. Exp. Pathol.*, **73**, 551–563

Veronesi, U., De Palo, G., Costa, A., Formelli, F. & Decensi, A. (1996) Chemoprevention of breast cancer with fenretinide. In: Hakama, M., Beral, V., Buiatti, E., Faivre, J. & Parkin, D.M., eds, *Chemoprevention in Cancer Control* (IARC Scientific Publications No. 136). Lyon, International Agency for Research on Cancer, pp. 87–94

Welsch, C.W., DeHoog, J.V. & Moon, R.C. (1983) Inhibition of mammary tumorigenesis in nulliparous C3H mice by chronic feeding of the synthetic retinoid, N-(4-hydroxyphenyl)retinamide. *Carcino-genesis*, **4**, 1185–1187

Zheng, Y., Kramer, P.M., Olson, G., Lubet, R.A., Steele, V.E., Kelloff, G.J. & Pereira, M.A. (1997) Prevention by retinoids of azoxymethane-induced tumors and aber-rant crypt foci and their modulation of cell prolifera-tion in the colon of rats. *Carcinogenesis*, **18**, 2119–2125

Zou, C.P., Kurie, J.M., Lotan, D., Zou, C.C., Hong, W.K. & Lotan, R. (1998) Higher potency of N-(4-hydroxy-phenyl)retinamide than all-*trans*-retinoic acid in induction of apoptosis in non-small cell lung cancer cell lines. *Clin. Cancer Res.*, **4**, 1345–1355

Handbook 5

Etretinate

1. Chemical and Physical Characteristics

1.1 Nomenclature

Etretinate belongs to the class of synthetic aromatic retinoids in which the lipophilic trimethylcyclohexenyl group of retinoic acid has been replaced by an aromatic ring. In the case of etretinate, the cyclohexenyl group has been replaced by a 4-methoxy-2,3,6-trimethylphenyl group while the all-*trans*-tetraene structure of the retinoic acid side-chain has been retained. In a further departure from the retinoic acid structure, the terminal carboxyl group of etretinate has been derived as an ethyl ester. The free acid form of etretinate is acitretin (Figure 1).

When reference is made to 'etretinate' it is assumed to be the all-*trans* isomer, unlike the retinoic acids. In this nomenclature, the side-chain of etretinate is numbered starting from the carboxylate carbon; but since etretinate is a synthetic derivative of retinoic acid, the retinoid numbering system is often used for etretinate and its derivatives. Application of the numbering system commonly used for retinoic acid to the basic skeleton of etretinate is shown in Figure 2. For example, ethyl 2*Z*, 4*E*, 6*E*, 8*E*-3,7-dimethyl-9-(4-methoxy-2,3,6-trimethylphenyl)nona-2,4,6,8-tetraenoate, a geometric isomer of etretinate, is commonly referred to as 13-*cis*-etretinate (Figure 2). The methyl groups attached to the tetraene side-chain are often referred to as the C-9 and C-13 methyls, in keeping with retinoid nomenclature. The free-acid derivative of etretinate, which is a major metabolite and the biologically active form, is all-*trans*-3,7-dimethyl-9-(4-methoxy-2,3,6-trimethylphenyl)nona-2,4,6,8-tetraenoic acid, commonly known as acitretin or etretin (see Handbook on acitretin; Figure 1).

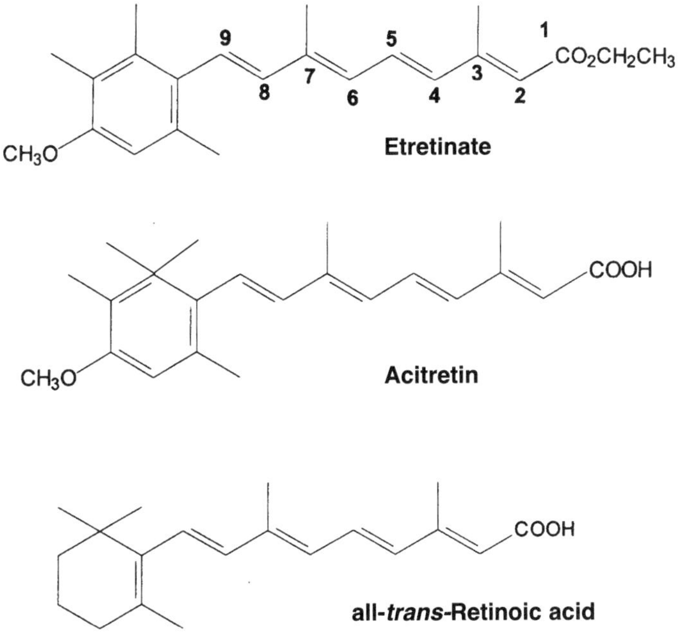

Figure 1. Structures of all-*trans*-retinoic acid, etretinate and acitretin

1.2 Name

Chemical Abstracts Services Registry Number
54350-48-0

IUPAC Systematic name
Ethyl all-*trans*-3,7-dimethyl-9-(4-methoxy-2,3,6-trimethylphenyl)nona-2,4,6,8-tetraenoate

Synonyms
Tetison® R010.98359; Tigason

1.3 Structural formula

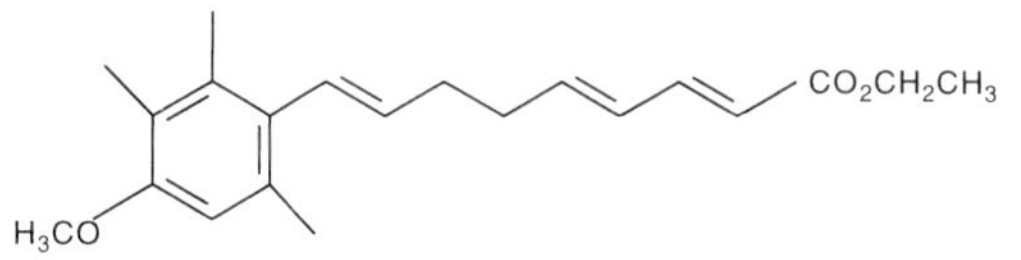

Composition: $C_{23}H_{30}O_3$
Relative molecular mass: 354

1.4 Physical and chemical properties

Melting-point

104–105 °C (Budavari *et al.*, 1989)

Spectroscopy
UV and visible spectrum: $\lambda_{max} = 351$ nm in 1.5% diisopropyl ether in hexane (Englert *et al.*, 1978)

Mass spectrum
(m/e, %): 354 (M⁺, 85), 339 (30), 293 (30), 281 (90), 191 (42), 203 (80),163 (86), 150 (100), 265 (38), 251 (53), 201 (55) (Hänni *et al.*, 1977)

^{1}H-NMR (CDCl$_3$, 270 MHz): δ 1.29 (3H, t, $J = 7.1$ Hz), 2.10 (3H, s), 2.15, 2.23 and 2.29 (9H, 3s), 2.36 (3H, s), 3.81 (3H,s), 4.17 (2H, q, $J = 7.1$ Hz), 5.78 (1H, s), 6.19 (1H, d, $J = 11.4$ Hz), 6.24 (1H, d, $J = 16.3$ Hz), 6.31 (1H, d, $J = 15.1$ Hz), 6.60 (1H, s), 6.68 (1H, d, $J = 16.3$ Hz), 7.02 (1H, dd, $J = 11.4, 15.11$ Hz) (Englert *et al.*, 1978).

^{13}C NMR (CDCl$_3$, 68 MHz): δ 11.82, 12.86, 13.84, 14.40, 17.36, 21.36, 55.41, 59.50, 110.24, 119.11, 122.84, 128.64, 130.02, 130.41, 130.53, 133.85, 135.82, 135.87, 138.18, 138.95, 152.28, 156.23, 166.85 (Englert *et al.*, 1978)

Geometric isomers
Sixteen possible isomers

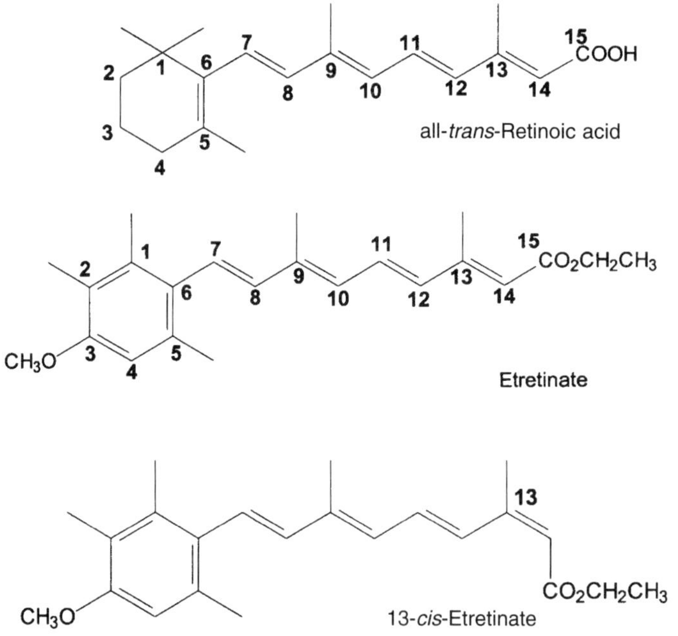

all-*trans*-Retinoic acid

Etretinate

13-*cis*-Etretinate

Figure 2. Common numbering scheme for retinoids

1.4.1 Photochemical properties

Etretinate is a yellow to greenish-yellow compound with an absorption maximum (λ_{max}) at 351 nm (1.5% diisopropylether in hexane) in the UV and visible spectrum. Because of its conjugated tetraene structure, etretinate can readily undergo photoisomerizaiton reactions when exposed to light, particularly in solution. Irradiation of dilute solutions of etretinate in hexane, benzene or ethanol under an inert atmosphere with a high-pressure xenon lamp gave complex mixtures of products which were shown by mass spectrometric analysis to consist entirely of geometric isomers. The equilibrium concentrations of the main isomers were obtained after 1 h of irradiation and consisted primarily of the 9,13-di-*cis*, 13-*cis*, 11-*cis*, 11,13 di-*cis*, all-*trans*, 9-*cis*, 7,13-di-*cis* and 7-*cis* isomers. Four other uncharacterized isomers were produced in minor amounts (Englert *et al.*, 1978).

1.4.2 Solubility and interactions in vivo

Etretinate is a very lipophilic molecule which readily partitions into hydrophobic environments. In humans, etretinate is stored in adipose tissue (Paravicini *et al.*, 1981). More than 99% of that which is found in the circulation is bound to plasma proteins, primarily lipoproteins. Acitretin, the free acid metabolite of etretinate, is bound predominantly to serum albumin in the circulation.

1.4.3 Relationships between chemical structure and biological activity

The pharmacological activity of etretinate is probably primarily due to activation of the retinoic acid receptors (RARs), which are ligand-inducible transcription factors belonging to the steroid-thyroid superfamily of nuclear receptors (Evans, 1988). The physiological hormone for the RARs is retinoic acid (Giguère *et al.*, 1987; Petkovich *et al.*, 1987), and extensive studies of structure–activity relationships with retinoid analogues have established that a terminal carboxylic acid group and a lipophilic head group are required for interaction with the RARs (Gale, 1993). Since etretinate is an ethyl ester derivative, it would not be expected to bend the RARs and it would require conversion to its free acid form, acitretin, to activate the RARs. The lipophilic group required for RAR activity is provided by 4-methoxy-2,3,6-trimethylphenyl on etretinate. The planar all-*trans* configuration of the

etretinate side-chain appears to be optimal for RAR activity, but 9-*cis*-retinoic acid, the putative physiological ligand for the retinoid X receptors (RXRs), also activates RARs (Heyman *et al.*, 1992). Thus, the 9-*cis* isomer of acitretin may activate RARs.

2. Occurrence, Production, Use, Human Exposure and Analysis

2.1 Occurrence

Etretinate is not a naturally occurring compound but can readily be synthesized by a variety of routes.

2.2 Production

The synthesis of etretinate starting from 2,3,5-trimethylphenol, **1**, is outlined in Scheme 1 (Soukup *et al.*, 1989). Compound **1** is first methylated to compound **2** and then subjected to Friedel-Crafts reaction conditions with the alcohol **3** to give a mixture of the terminal alkynes, **4**. Deprotonation of **4** followed by reaction with the aldehyde **5** gave the propargyl alcohol, **6**. Hydrogenation of **6** to give **7** followed by dehydration gave a mixture of geometric isomers, **8**. Isomerization of **8** gave the all-*trans* isomer, etretinate, as the major product with smaller amounts of the 9-*cis* and 13-*cis* isomers.

The chemistry described by Soukup *et al.* (1989) also provides alternative routes to etretinate, as outlined in Scheme 2. The anisole, **2**, can be formylated to give the aldehyde, **9**, which is formally equivalent to β-cyclocitral, the C_{10} unit employed in retinoic acid synthesis. Compound **9** can be used as the starting material in a variety of strategies for elaborating the tetraenoate side-chain of etretinate. Alternatively, the anisole, **2**, can be brominated to the aryl bromide, **10**, which can be reacted with the terminal alkyne, **11**, under Pd(0) catalysed conditions to give the alcohol, **12**, which is formally equivalent to the C_{15} unit used in retinoic acid synthesis. Conversion of **12** to the phosphonium salt, **13**, followed by hydrogenation gave **14**. Wittig reaction of **14** with the aldehyde, **5**, preceded or followed by isomerization, will yield etretinate.

An alternative synthesis of acitretin, the free acid form of etretinate, is outlined in Scheme 3 (Aurell *et al.*, 1995). The lithium trienediolate generated from the hexa-2,4-dienoic acid, **16**, when

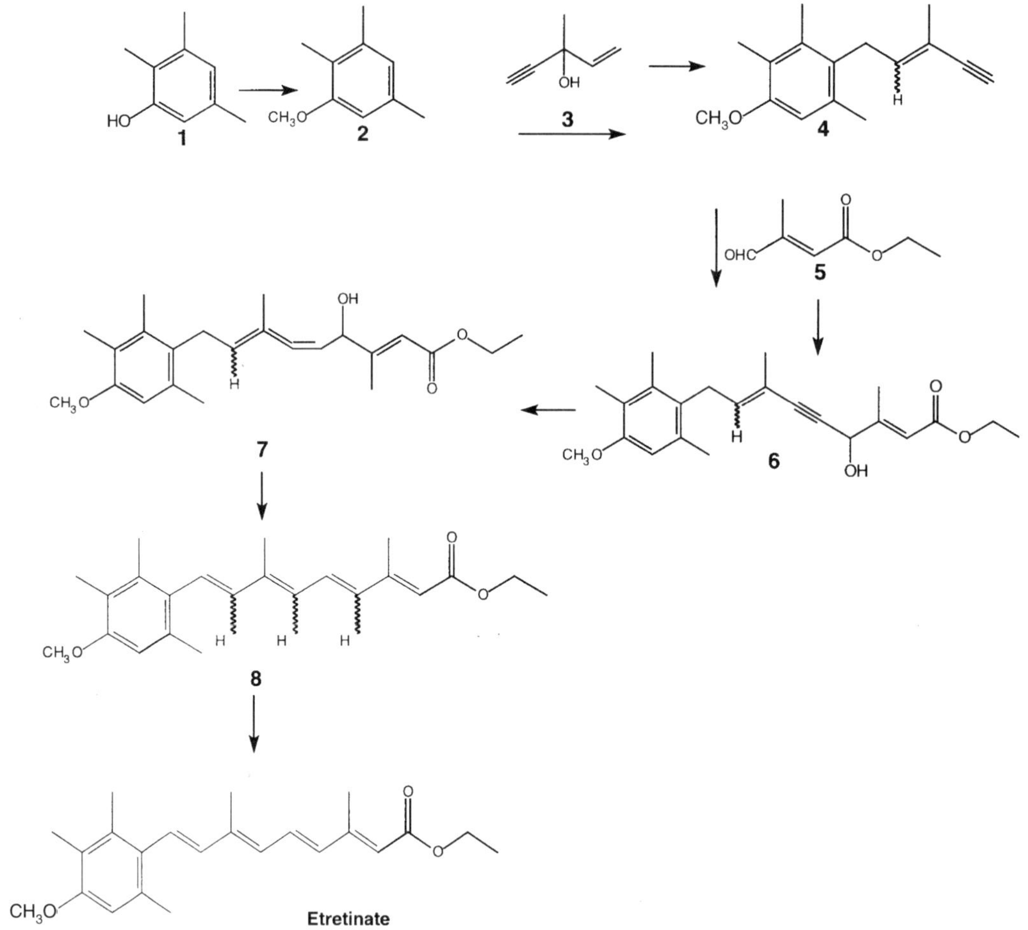

Scheme 1.
Geometric isomers are denoted by wavy lines.

reacted with the ketone, **17**, gave the alcohol, **18**. Dehydration of **18** followed by isomerization of the resultant mixture of geometric isomers gave acitretin, which can be esterified to etretinate. Synthesis of etretinate, derivatives of etretinate and geometric isomers of these compounds have also been described by Bestmann and Ermann (1984) and Makin *et al.* (1989). The large-scale synthesis of acitretin and various derivatives including etretinate was described by Bollag *et al.* (1978).

2.3   Use
Etretinate was approved by the appropriate regulatory agencies in most countries of the world for use in the treatment of severe recalcitrant psoriasis, including erythrodermic and generalized pustular psoriasis (Ellis & Voorhees, 1987). It is,

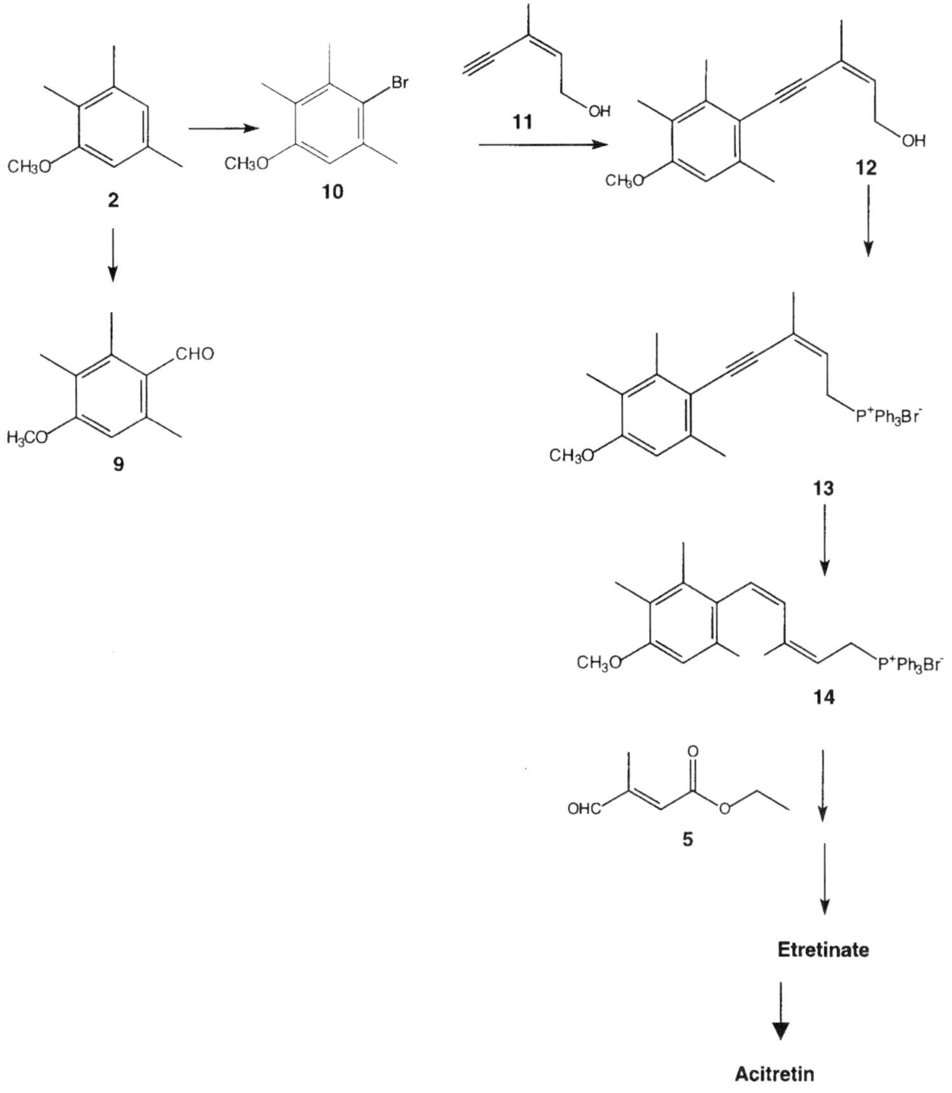

Scheme 2

however, no longer marketed and has been replaced by acitretin wherever the latter has been approved.

2.4   Human exposure

Etretinate has been shown to be effective in the treatment not only of severe recalcitrant psoriasis but also of a variety of other cutaneous disorders of keratinization including Darier disease, lamellar ichthyosis, nonbullous congenital ichthyosiform erythroderma, pityriasis rubra pilaris, epidermolytic hyperkeratosis, keratoderma palmaris et plantaris, X-linked ichthyosis, ichthyosis vulgaris, erythrokeratodermia variabilis and lichen planus (Peck, 1984). Etretinate has also been considered for treatment of certain skin cancers and premalignant conditions, including mycosis fungoides, basal-cell carcinoma, actinic keratoses, keratoacanthoma and epidermodysplasia verruciformis (see section 4.1.3). It has been recommended that

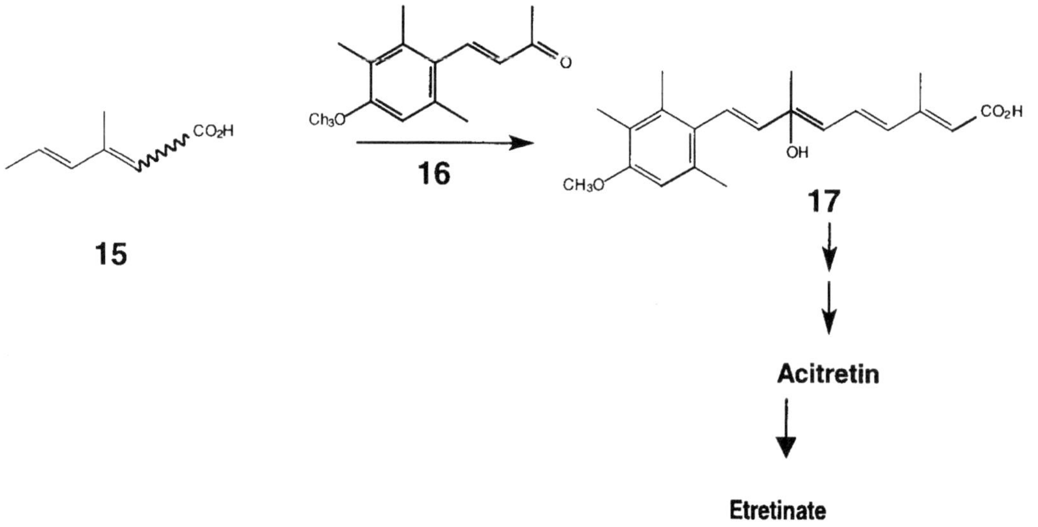

Scheme 3.

etretinate be taken with food to increase its absorption (DiGiovanna *et al.*, 1984).

Etretinate was marketed in 10-mg and 25-mg gelatin capsules for oral administration. Patients with psoriasis usually began with an initial daily dosage of 0.75–1 mg/kg bw given in divided doses (Goldfarb & Ellis, 1998; Paul & Dubertret, 1998). It was recommended that a maximum dose of 1.5 mg/kg bw per day not be exceeded. Maintenance doses of 0.5–0.75 mg/kg bw per day were recommended after an initial response was obtained. A dose of 0.25 mg/kg bw per day was recommended for the initial treatment of erythrodermic psoriasis. Initial responses were observed within 8–16 weeks, but patients were maintained on therapy for up to nine months. Similar doses of etretinate have been used for the treatment of cutaneous disorders of keratinization and cutaneous malignancies and premalignancies (Peck, 1984).

2.5   Analysis
Numerous methods based on high-performance liquid chromatography (HPLC) have been described for the quantitative analysis in plasma of etretinate, acitretin and their geometric isomers. The limit of detection of a reversed-phase HPLC method for analysis of etretinate and acitretin in

plasma was 10 ng/ml (Palmskog, 1980), while that of a normal-phase HPLC method for the same two compounds was 4 ng/ml (Paravicini & Busslinger, 1983). An alternative reversed-phase HPLC method for the simultaneous determination of etretinate and acitretin in rat blood required much smaller sample volumes and allowed for serial sampling (Thongnopnua & Zimmerman, 1988). Another normal-phase HPLC method which allowed for the determination of etretinate, acitretin and the 13-*cis* isomer of acitretin, with a detection limit of 3 ng/ml, was used to study the long-term pharmacokinetics of etretinate in patients with psoriasis who had been changed from etretinate to acitretin therapy (De Leenheer *et al.*, 1990). A reversed-phase HPLC method with shorter retention times was also used to detect these three compounds in human plasma (Jakobsen *et al.*, 1987). A programmed-gradient HPLC system for the analysis of etretinate, its metabolites and other retinoids in plasma allowed shortened analysis and better peak shapes (Annesley *et al.*, 1984). Problems of recovery arising from strong binding of retinoids to plasma proteins were addressed by column-switching techniques (Wyss & Bucheli, 1988; Wyss, 1990).

HPLC methods were used to isolate metabolites from the faeces and urine of persons treated with tritium-labelled etretinate. The structures of the metabolites were elucidated by mass spectrometry and ¹H-NMR spectroscopy (Hänni et al., 1977). Bile samples collected from patients treated with ¹⁴C-labelled etretinate were analysed by HPLC after β-glucuronidase treatment, and the structures of the metabolites were determined by mass spectrometry and ¹H-NMR spectroscopy (Vane et al., 1989a). Similarly, HPLC methods were used to isolate metabolites from the blood of persons with psoriasis treated with etretinate, and spectroscopic techniques were used to elucidate their structures (Vane et al., 1989b). Another reversed-phase HPLC method has been developed for the simultaneous assay of etretinate, acitretin and their metabolites in whole perfusate, perfusate plasma, bile and hepatic tissue obtained in a perfused rat liver model (Decker & Zimmerman, 1995).

3. Metabolism, Kinetics and Genetic Variation

Etretinate is a retinoid which requires metabolic conversion to its free acid form, acitretin, in order to exert its biological activity.

3.1 Humans

About 40% of an oral dose of etretinate is bioavailable. The pharmokinetics of etretinate after administration of single doses to healthy volunteers and patients with psoriasis has been studied extensively (Gollnick et al., 1990). The tabulated results of 10 such studies (Larsen, 1994) indicate that the vast majority were undertaken with a dose of 100 mg and the peak plasma concentration was 100–1400 ng/ml. The corresponding concentration of acitretin, recorded 3–6 h after administration of etretinate, was 100–600 ng/ml. The drug can be detected in plasma 30 min after oral intake. The pharmocokinetics of etretinate may be affected by intake of milk or food. No definitive correlation has been demonstrated between the plasma concentration and the therapeutic effects of etretinate.

The pharmocokinetics of etretinate after multiple oral doses has been the subject of at least eight studies, most of which involved patients with psoriasis (Lucek & Colburn, 1985; Larsen, 1994;

Orfanos et al., 1997). The mean terminal elimination half-life of etretinate ranged from 1 to 40 days, which was significantly longer than that determined after single doses (4–10 h). The mean terminal half-life was determined to be 25 days for etretinate, 6.5 days for the metabolite acitretin and 16 days for 13-cis-acitretin (Larsen, 1994).

Etretinate is an ethyl ester which undergoes extensive hydrolysis in the liver, gut and blood after oral absorption to yield the corresponding acid metabolite, acitretin. Hydrolysis initially takes place in the gut or gut wall. The methoxy group on the aromatic ring is subsequently demethylated, most probably in the liver. Other metabolic transformations include shortening of the side-chain, glucuronidation, hydroxylation of the methoxy group, isomerization to 13-cis-acitretin and reduction of one or two double-bonds in the side-chain (Hill & Sani, 1991; Larsen, 1994). In addition to the parent compound, 9-cis-acitretin, 13-cis-acitretin and three minor metabolites are found in plasma, and various metabolites are excreted in both the bile and the urine. The absorption and metabolism of etretinate have not been correlated with liver damage in patients with psoriasis. After administration of radiolabelled etretinate to healthy subjects, radiolabelled metabolites were detected in urine and faeces for as long as three weeks. The major reason for the observed decrease in the concentration of etretinate in blood after biliary cannulation was reduced absorption due to elimination of solubilizing bile salts in the duodenum (Lucek et al., 1988). In general, there is no correlation between drug dose and rate of elimination.

Etretinate is a highly lipophilic compound which is extensively bound in plasma to lipoproteins. The mean concentrations of serum lipids (triglyceride and cholesterol) increase after treatment with etretinate. The changes in very low-density and low-density lipoprotein suggest that the increase may be due to enhanced synthesis of lipoproteins (Marsden, 1986). Up to about 200 and 130 etretinate molecules can bind to one molecule of low-density lipoprotein and one molecule of high-density lipoprotein, respectively; human serum albumin binds about 10 etretinate molecules (Carrillet et al., 1990). After repetitive dosing, the compound accumulates in fat, liver and adrenals (Rollman et al., 1989).

3.2   Experimental models

After intravenous injection to rats, etretinate is distributed primarily in muscle, skin and particularly in adipose tissue. After 6 h, about 45% of a dose is metabolized to acitretin and about 40% to unidentified metabolites (Eisenhardt & Bickel, 1994). Body fat has a significant effect on etretinate disposition in rats, slowing the systemic clearance (Chien *et al.*, 1992).

In rats, 15% of an oral dose of etretinate is bioavailable. In the bile of rats given etretinate intravenously, the free acid (acitretin) and other conjugated metabolites are present in a conjugated form; one of these lacks the methyl of the methoxy group. Pregnant rats have a lower rate of clearance of etretinate because of a lower rate of formation of acitretin (Hill & Sani, 1991). Etretinate is transferred across the placenta and is secreted in milk (Reiners *et al.*, 1988; Gollnick *et al.*, 1990). In dogs dosed with etretinate, the oral bioavailability is 52%, and the terminal half-life for elimination from plasma is > 300 h (Gollnick *et al.*, 1990).

Etretinate accumulated in adipose tissue in a genetically obese rodent model. At doses up to 30 mg/kg bw, it did not change the mineral composition of bone, despite obvious macroscopic alterations (Krari *et al.*, 1989).

4.   Cancer-preventive Effects

4.1   Humans
4.1.1   Epidemiological studies
No data were available to the Working Group.

4.1.2   Intervention trials
4.1.2.1   Urinary bladder
Alfthan *et al.* (1983) studied the effect of etretinate in the prevention of recurrence of superficial bladder tumours in patients cleared of all visible tumours by electrocoagulation or trans-urethral resection. Fifteen patients were randomized to receive etretinate and 15 to placebo. One given the placebo died of a myocardial infarct within a month, and one receiving etretinate dropped out because of side-effects after four weeks. Etretinate was given to 15 patients at a dose of 50 mg/day for a month, which was reduced to 25 mg/day, and was given to the remaining patients at a dose of 25 mg/day for the duration of therapy. Therapy was continued for 10–26 (mean, 17.6) months. Of the

patients given etretinate, six had no recurrences, five had fewer recurrences than before treatment, four had no change, and none had progressive disease. Of those given placebo, two had no recurrences, two had fewer recurrences than before treatment, none had no change and two had progressive disease.

Charbit *et al.* (1983) undertook a double-blind study in a group of 20 patients of the possible effectiveness of etretinate in the prevention of recurrences of superficial tumours of the bladder. Etretinate was given at a dose of 30 mg/day; the 10 controls received a placebo. Treatment was given for an average of 16 months (range, 8–25 months for etretinate and 8–29 months for placebo). The rate of recurrence with etretinate (6/10) was not lower than that with placebo (3/10).

Pedersen *et al.* (1984) studied patients with non-invasive bladder tumours who had experienced at least two recurrences in the previous 18 months, which had been surgically removed. Forty-seven patients were randomized to receive etretinate at 50 mg/day and 49 to receive placebo. During the first four months, 11 patients given etretinate withdrew because of side-effects, and one died of intercurrent disease. Four patients given placebo also withdrew, and two died of intercurrent disease. At four months, cystoscopy was repeated, and recurrent tumours were resected. One patient with invasive cancer who had been given placebo was taken off the study. By eight months, six further patients given etretinate had stopped treatment because of toxic effects, but four could be evaluated and cystoscopy was repeated. There was no difference in the recurrence rate: nine of 33 evaluable patients given etretinate and 15 of 40 given placebo were free of tumour.

Studer *et al.* (1984) studied 86 patients with recurrent superficial bladder tumours treated by trans-urethral resection in a double-blind randomized trial. Etretinate was initially given at a dose of 50 mg/day, but this was reduced to 25 mg/day in 90% of the cases because of side-effects. At the time of the report, 25 patients had been followed for two or more years, 40 were still under observation and 21 had been withdrawn from the trial. Of the latter, three given etretinate had died of causes unrelated to treatment, and treatment of two patients given etretinate and nine on placebo had been stopped because of progression of the disease.

There were fewer recurrences at 3, 12 and 24 months in the group given etretinate than in the group given placebo, but the differences were not statistically significant. There was, however, a statistically significantly lower frequency of multi-focal recurrences in patients given etretinate. [The Working Group noted that the design of the study and the methods of statistical analysis were not clearly described.]

A subsequent report on this study (Studer *et al.*, 1995) provided additional information on outcomes. Data on 42 patients given placebo and 37 treated with etretinate showed no difference in the proportions who had a recurrence after randomization (74 and 70%, respectively) or in the time to first recurrence. The authors reported, however, that there was a statistically significantly longer time between subsequent recurrences among treated patients in comparison with those given the placebo. They also noted that more patients on placebo were withdrawn from the study because of apparent treatment failure, and that this may have biased the results against treatment with etretinate. [The Working Group noted that the statistical approach described in this report was unconventional and did not include a 'time-to-failure' component.]

Yoshida *et al.* (1986) studied 174 patients with superficial bladder tumours that had been treated by trans-urethral resection. Ninety-four subjects were randomized to receive etretinate at 10 mg/day and 80 to receive no treatment. Patients were examined for recurrence every three months. Nine of the patients in the group receiving etretinate and eight controls dropped out of the study. The recurrence rate over the two-year observation period was 18% in the group given etretinate and 38% in the controls ($p < 0.1$; Kaplan-Meier). Etretinate was reported to have reduced the rate of recurrence of multiple tumours and tumours smaller than 1 cm. [The Working Group noted that patients were randomized in this trial by the envelope method, which allows breaking of randomization and that the control group did not receive a placebo.]

Hirao *et al.* (1987) included 130 patients with superficial bladder cancer treated by trans-urethral electroresection in a randomized study in which a number of agents administered intravesically or orally were evaluated. Twenty patients who received the agents orally were allocated to receive etretinate at 10 mg/day for two years. The tumours of five patients given etretinate and eight of 27 controls recurred. The actuarial non-recurrence rate at 48 months was 69% in the group given etretinate and 58% in controls (not significant).

4.1.2.2 Head-and-neck cancers
Bolla *et al.* (1994) studied the effect of etretinate on the development of second primary tumours in 316 patients who had been treated for squamous-cell carcinoma of the head and neck. Therapy with etretinate consisted of a loading dose of 50 mg/day for the first month, followed by 25 mg/day for up to 24 months. Randomly allocated controls received a placebo by the same schedule. Treatment began no later than 15 days after surgery or the initiation of radiotherapy. Over a median 41-month follow-up period, there were no differences between the groups in overall survival or disease-free survival. Second primary tumours occurred in 28 patients given etretinate and 29 given placebo.

In a subsequent report (Bolla *et al.*, 1996), based on a mean follow-up of 65 months, 42 new primary tumours were found in the etretinate-treated group and 40 in the placebo group (not significant).

4.1.3 Intermediary end-points
4.1.3.1 Lung
Gouveia *et al.* (1982) determined by means of bronchoscopy and bronchial biopsy the degree of metaplasia in 70 volunteers who had smoked at least 15 pack-years. The 34 who had an index of metaplasia > 15% were given a six-month course of etretinate at 25 mg/day. No control group was included. At six months, a second bronchoscopy with repeat bronchial biopsies was performed. Of 11 subjects who had completed the therapy at the time of this preliminary communication and who had continued to smoke, two showed a reduction in the index of metaplasia from that before treatment.

As an extension of this study, Misset *et al.* (1986) reported on 40 heavy smokers who had received six months' treatment with etretinate at 25 mg/day. The majority of patients who had continued to smoke had a reduced index of metaplasia, but eight appeared to have increased scores.

Arnold *et al.* (1992) evaluated the effect of etretinate on the presence of bronchial atypia in the sputum of 150 current smokers with at least a

15-pack-year history of smoking, mild bronchial atypia in at least two samples of sputum or moderate or severe atypia in one sample. The subjects were selected from a pool of 2223 potential participants attending one of two clinics in Ontario, Canada. Eligible subjects were randomized to receive 25 mg/day etretinate orally or an identical placebo, for six months. The pre-treatment distributions of the characteristics of the 75 subjects allocated to etretinate and the 75 allocated to placebo were almost identical, although the only two subjects with severe dysplasia were allocated to receive etretinate. Compliance with the intervention was good in both groups. In a comparison of the pre- and post-treatment distribution of atypia, an overall reduction was seen in each group; the final distributions were virtually identical, approximately 20 subjects in each group having no atypia.

4.1.3.2 Oral cavity

Koch (1981) studied the effects of two dose regimens of etretinate in 48 patients with leukoplakia, 12 of whom were heavy smokers. There was no control group. One group of 21 patients received etretinate at 75 mg/day orally for six weeks, and a second group of 24 patients received 50 mg/day orally plus a 0.1% paste locally. After termination of therapy, five patients in the first group and seven in the second showed complete remission, while 10 and 13 in the two groups, respectively, showed partial regression of their lesions. There were no cases of progression. Relapses occurred after completion of therapy. [The Working Group noted that the long-term results tabulated 24 months after completion of therapy were difficult to interpret.]

4.1.3.3 Skin

The most frequently studied intermediary end-point for skin neoplasia is actinic keratosis, which is difficult to follow-up longitudinally and may regress spontaneously. Retinoid therapy produces mucocutaneous changes, which may make it easier for patients and investigators to identify the treated or control status of subjects and may also complicate recognition of neoplastic skin lesions.

Moriarty et al. (1982) included 50 patients with actinic keratosis in a double-blind cross-over trial to compare the effects of etretinate at 75 mg/day

with a placebo. After the first phase of two months, five of 22 evaluable patients who had received etretinate showed complete remission and 14 partial remission of their lesions, whereas the corresponding numbers in the 23 patients given placebo were none and one, respectively. In the second phase, after cross-over, five of 22 evaluable patients who had received etretinate showed complete remission and 13 had partial remission of their lesions. The placebo group consisted of 22 patients, of whom 3 dropped out. Of the remaining 19, one had complete remission and none had partial remission. The authors stated that the results were so conclusive that statistical analysis was not required. [The Working Group noted that the findings in the placebo group during the second phase of the study, after cross-over, are difficult to interpret but suggest that there was very rapid recurrence of lesions after cessation of treatment with etretinate.]

Grupper and Berretti (1983) treated 80 patients with premalignant or malignant skin conditions with etretinate at 1 mg/kg bw per day initially, followed by a progressive reduction to 0.75 mg/kg bw and then 0.5 mg/kg bw per day or less for up to five months. There was no control group. Twenty-two of 26 patients given etretinate who initially had multiple actinic keratoses and all six patients who had keratoacanthomas showed complete clearance. The remaining patients, who had squamous- or basal-cell carcinomas, had poorer responses. After cessation of therapy, 16 of those who initially had actinic keratoses and one of those who had keratoacanthomas showed relapse of their lesions.

Watson (1986) included 15 patients with severe multiple actinic keratoses in an eight-month double-blind cross-over trial. Etretinate was given at a dose of 1 mg/kg bw per day for two weeks for a maximum dose of 75 mg, and slightly lower doses were given subsequently, depending on the side-effects. The end-points evaluated were the numbers of lesions on representative involved areas and the size of the largest lesions. During the first four months, improvement was seen in eight of nine patients who received etretinate and one of six on placebo, while none of the patients on etretinate and five on placebo showed worsening of their lesions. During the second four-month cross-over phase, the lesions of all six patients given etretinate and one on placebo improved; only one patient given placebo showed worsening. The apparent protective effect in the second four-month period may have been due to prolonged retention of etretinate in the tissues. [The Working Group noted that no formal statistical analysis of the results was reported.]

4.2 Experimental models
4.2.1 Cancer and preneoplastic lesions
These studies are summarized in Table 1.

4.2.1.1 Skin
Mouse: Three groups of 15–20 inbred, albino, hair-less (Skh-hr1) female mice, 10–12 weeks of age, were exposed to ultraviolet radiation (UVR) on five consecutive days each week for 12 weeks. The UVR fluence used was initially 0.53 J/cm² but was raised to 1.6 J/cm² after 12 weeks, when it was maintained at that rate for a maximum of 25 weeks but the frequency reduced to twice weekly. The three groups received 0, 120 or 600 µg of etretinate by gavage in 0.1 ml of peanut oil three times weekly beginning two weeks before the start of UVR and continuing until death. Etretinate did not statistically significantly modulate skin tumour development in terms of time to onset of tumours, total tumour yield or the type of tumours produced (Kelly *et al.*, 1989).

Female Swiss albino mice weighing 20–22 g were shaved and received two applications of 150 µg of 7,12-dimethylbenz[*a*]anthracene (DMBA) in 0.2 ml acetone onto the skin with an interval of 14 days between applications. Three weeks after DMBA treatment, 0.5 mg of croton oil was applied twice weekly for three to eight months. Treatment with etretinate was begun when the average diameter of the papillomas was 3 mm. At that time, groups of four mice were treated either intraperitoneally or intragastrically with etretinate dissolved in arachis oil and administered once weekly (12.5–400 mg/kg bw) or daily (5–40 mg/kg bw) for two weeks. Control mice received the vehicle alone. The sum of the diameters of the papillomas per animal was reduced from 26 mm in controls to 17 mm at the dose of 12.5 mg/kg bw given intraperitoneally and to 6.6 mm at the dose of 200 mg/kg bw dose given intraperitoneally ($p < 0.05$, Student's *t* test). Intragastric treatment with 25–400 mg/kg bw etretinate produced similar

results. The intermediate doses resulted in papillomas of intermediate size. Intraperitoneal injection of etretinate thus appeared to be more effective than oral administration and daily treatment more effective than weekly administration in regressing established papillomas (Bollag, 1974).

Groups of 30 female Charles River CD-1 mice, seven to nine weeks of age, were treated once with 0.2 µmol of DMBA in acetone for tumour initiation and with 8 nmol of 12-*O*-tetradecanoylphorbol 13-acetate (TPA) two times per week for tumour promotion for 20 weeks. Etretinate was applied topically at a dose of 140 nmol 1 h before each application of TPA. The development of papillomas was checked weekly by visual observation. The incidence of papillomas at 20 weeks was about 90% in acetone-treated controls and about 40% in those treated with etretinate, and the tumour multiplicity was about 10 papillomas per mouse in controls and about 1.5 papillomas per mouse in those given etretinate. [The numbers were estimated from graphs; no statistics were given.] (Verma *et al.*, 1979).

Rabbit: Both auricles of 21 domestic rabbits [strain and sex not specified] were painted with 1% DMBA in petrolatum on five days per week, and 11 of the animals were also treated with 30 mg (later reduced to 20 mg) etretinate (8–10 mg/kg bw) by gavage on five days per week. Two animals served as untreated controls. After eight or nine weeks of treatment, six of the seven surviving controls developed a total of 25 keratoacanthoma-like tumours, while no tumours developed in the seven surviving treated animals [no statistics given] (Mahrle & Berger, 1982).

4.2.1.2 Oesophagus
Rat: A total of 38 male and 38 female Sprague-Dawley rats, 100 days of age, were divided in three experimental groups (eight controls of each sex and two groups of 15 male and 15 female treated animals), and all were given weekly subcutaneous injections of *N*-nitrosomethylbenzylamine at a dose of 2.5 mg/kg bw as a 0.1% aqueous solution for 15 weeks. The treated groups received etretinate in the diet throughout the study at concentrations of 0, 30 or 100 mg/kg of diet, the last dose being reduced to 60 mg/kg of diet after six weeks. The animals were maintained on their respective diets for life and were killed when moribund.

Table 1. Effects of etretinate on carcinogenesis in experimental animals

Cancer site	Species, sex, age at carcinogen treatment	No. of animals per group	Carcinogen dose, route	Etretinate dose, route	Treatment relative to carcinogen	Incidence Control	Incidence Treated	Multiplicity Control	Multiplicity Treated	Efficacy	Reference
Skin	Mouse, SKh-hr 1, female	20	UVR, 0.53–1.6 J/cm² in 12 wks, 5 d/wk followed by 1.6 J/cm² for maximum 13 wks, twice per wk	120 and 600 µg 3 times per wk by gavage	– 2 wk to end	70/25[a] 70/25[a]	59/32[a] 56/41[a]	5.7 5.7	5.8 7.6	Not effective	Kelly et al. (1989)
Skin	Mouse, Swiss female	4	DMBA, 150 µg twice and croton oil two wks after DMBA twice per wk	Once per wk by gavage or i.p. at 12.5–400 mg/kg bw or daily at 5–40 mg/kg bw for 2 wks	After papilloma developed	NR	NR	NR	NR	Effective in reducing papilloma size	Bollag (1974)
Skin	Mouse, CD-1, female	30	DMBA, 0.2 µmole once and TPA, 8 nmole twice per wk for 20 wks	140 nmole twice per wk for 20 wks	+ 2 wk – 20 wk	90	40	10	1.5	Effective	Verma et al. (1979)
Skin	Rabbit, domestic [strain and sex not specified]	7 (survivors)	DMBA (1% in petrolatum), 5 d per wk	30–20 mg (8–10 mg/kg bw), gavage, 5 d per wk	d 0 – wk 9	86	0	3.6[b]	0	Effective	Mahrle & Berger (1982)
Oeso-phagus	Rat, Sprague-Dawley, males and females	8/sex (controls) 15/sex (treated)	NMBA, 2.5 mg/kg bw per wk for 15 wks	30 mg/kg diet, for life 60 mg/kg diet, for life	d 0 to end d 0 to end	69 69	67 57*	NR NR	NR NR	Ineffective Effective	Schmähl & Habs (1981)

Table 1 (contd)

Cancer site	Species sex, age at carcinogen treatment	No. of animals per group	Carcinogen dose, route	Etretinate dose, route	Treatment relative to carcinogen	Incidence Control	Incidence Treated	Multiplicity Control	Multiplicity Treated	Efficacy	Reference
Forestomach	Mouse, C57BL, female	56–68	DMBA, 25 mg/kg bw by gavage; TPA, 10 mg/kg bw by gavage every wk until day 253	0.17 0.51 1.53 mg/kg bw	d 7 to end	62 62 62	56 48 35*	NR NR NR	NR NR NR	Not effective Not effectve Effective	Wagner et al. (1983)
Colon	Rat, BD-6, male	25–30	DMH, 20 mg/kg bw s.c. for 20 wks	50 mg/kg bw	d 0 to end	92	71*	1.8	1.65	Effective	Hadjiolov & Grueva (1986)
Lung	Rat, Wistar, male	48 (control) 46 (treated)	Plutonium dioxide (nose-only inhalation) d −15, 5 mg benzo[a]pyrene, haematite, intratracheal, d 0	25 mg/kg bw by gavage per wk	d 0 to end	72	63	NR	NR	No effect	Nolibe et al. (1983)
Lung	Mouse, CD-1, female	137 (control) 44 treated	SQ 18506, 1 mg/kg bw by gavage	75 mg/kg bw by gavage	− 18 h	1	11*	NR	NR	Tumour enhancing effect	Dunsford et al. (1984)
Urinary bladder	Rat, Fischer 344, male	15 (control) 18–29 treated	NBHBA, 0.025% in drinking-water for 8 wks	50 mg/kg diet	− 8 wk to d 0 d 0 to wk 8 + 8 wk to +16 wk − 8 wk to end	100 100 100 100	17* 56* 55* 77*	NR NR NR NR	NR NR NR NR	Effective Effective Effective Effective	Murasaki et al. (1980)
				100 mg/kg diet	− 8 wk to d 0 d 0 to wk 8 +8 wk to +16 wk	100 100 100	41* 31* 40*	NR NR NR	NR NR NR	Effective Effective Effective	Murasaki et al. (1980)

Table 1 (contd)

Cancer site	Species, sex, age at carcinogen treatment	No. of animals per group	Carcinogen dose, route	Etretinate dose, route	Treatment relative to carcinogen	Incidence Control	Incidence Treated	Multiplicity Control	Multiplicity Treated	Efficacy	Reference
Haemato-poetic system (leukaemia)	Rat, Long-Evans, males and females	29–48 males and females/group	DMBA, i.v. 10–30 mg/kg bw, 4 pulse doses to offspring	20 mg/kg bw by gavage, daily, for life	d 0 to end	90	85	NR	NR	Ineffective	Berger & Schmähl (1986)
Skin	Rabbits, domestic Japanese white [sex not specified]	6	0.1 ml Shope papilloma-virus (SPV) 10^{-1} (1000 ID_{50}) or SPV 10^{-2} (100 ID_{50}) per site (2–4 sites)	200 mg/kg im twice per wk [total no. not specified]	After	NR	NR	NR	NR	Effective[a]	Ito (1981)
Connective tissue	Hamster, Syrian golden [sex not specified]	32–56 controls 32–76 treated	Rous sarcoma virus (Schmidt-Ruppin), s.c., inoculation at 1 day of age	100 mg/kg, bw i.p. 3 wks of age and wkly thereafter	+3 wks to end	56 75	5 0	NR NR	NR	Effective	Frankel et al. (1980)
	Chicken [not further specified]	20	Rous sarcoma virus (Bryan), inoculation via wing web at 5 d of age	50 mg/kg bw 25 mg/kg bw 25 mg/kg bw	d 0 d +5 d +18	100	5	NR	NR	Effective	Frankel et al. (1980)

UVR, ultraviolet radiation; NR, not reported; DMBA, 7,12-dimethylbenz[a]anthracene; i.p., intraperitoneal; TPA, 12-O-tetradecanoylphorbol 13-acetate NMBA, N-nitrosomethybenzylamine; DMH, dimethylhydrazine; s.c., subcutaneous; NBHBA, N-butyl-N-(4-hydroxybutyl)nitrosamine; SQ 18506, 5-amino-3-[2-(5-nitro-2-furyl)vinyl]-1,2,4-oxadiazole; i.m., intramuscular; wk, week

[a] % animals with papillomas/% animals with carcinomas

[b] 1.8 tumours per auricle

[c] inhibition of tumour growth rate

* Statistically significant (see text)

Squamous-cell carcinomas of the oesophagus developed in 11/16 controls, 20/30 animals in the group receiving etretinate at 30 mg/kg and 17/30 in the group receiving 60 mg/kg. The tumour incidence in the group given the low dose of etretinate was not significantly different from the age-standardized expected frequency in controls, but the tumour incidence in the group given the high dose was significantly reduced ($p < 0.025$, χ^2 test (Schmähl & Habs, 1981).

4.2.1.3 Forestomach

Mouse: A total of 277 female C57BL mice, about 12 weeks of age, were divided into five groups and treated by gavage with a single dose of 25 mg/kg bw DMBA. On day 7, 10 mg/kg bw TPA were given orally and repeated every week until termination of the study on day 253, and etretinate was administered in the diet at doses of 0.17, 0.51 or 1.53 mg/kg bw. A fourth group given 4.59 mg/kg bw was excluded from evaluation because of severe toxic effects. The incidence of tumours (papilloma or carcinoma of the forestomach) was 62% in controls, whereas only 35% of animals given the high dose of etretinate developed forestomach tumours ($p < 0.001$; Peto's trend test involving all groups) (Wagner *et al.*, 1983). [The Working Group noted marked weight loss and reduced survival in the group given 1.53 mg/kg bw etretinate and that papillomas and carcinomas were counted together.]

4.2.1.4 Colon

Rat: Groups of 25 (controls) and 30 (treated) male BD-6 rats weighing 160 g [age not specified] were treated subcutaneously with dimethylhydrazine at a dose of 20 mg/kg bw weekly for 20 weeks. The treated group was simultaneously injected intramuscularly with 50 mg/kg bw etretinate weekly for 20 weeks. The animals were killed after 48 weeks. Adenocarcinomas of the colon were found in 20/28 rats treated with etretinate and 23/25 controls ($p < 0.05$, Student's *t* test), although the average number of tumours per rat was similar (Hadjiolov & Grueva, 1986).

4.2.1.5 Lung

Mouse: Groups of 137 controls and 44 treated female CD-1 mice, six weeks of age, received the antiparasitic nitrovinylfuran SQ 18506 (*trans*-5-amino-3-[2-(5-nitro-2-furyl)vinyl]-1,2,4-oxadiazole), which has been shown to be carcinogenic in rodents, at a dose of 1 mg/kg bw by gastric intubation. The compound was homogenized in 25% glycerol and administered twice daily for five days. Three such treatments were given at intervals of four weeks. Etretinate at 75 mg/kg bw was given by gavage 18 h before the first dose of SQ 18506 in each course of treatment. The cancers observed most commonly were squamous-cell carcinomas of the forestomach, lymphomas, myeloid leukaemias and sarcomas. Etretinate had no effect on the incidence of these tumours, but lung adenocarcinomas occurred in 5/44 animals given etretinate and 1/137 controls ($p < 0.05$, Fisher-Irwin exact test) (Dunsford *et al.*, 1984).

Rat: Two groups of 48 (controls) and 46 (treated) male Wistar rats, eight weeks of age, were submitted to nose-only inhalation of plutonium dioxide 15 days before intratracheal instillations of benzo[*a*]pyrene and haematite (5 mg each) in 0.2 ml saline. Etretinate was given to the rats by gavage at a dose of 25 mg/kg bw weekly from day 0 for life. The incidence of squamous-cell carcinomas of the lung in the carcinogen-exposed rats (72%) was not significantly modified by long-term administration of etretinate (63%) [No statistical methods were described.] (Nolibe *et al.*, 1983).

4.2.1.6 Urinary bladder

Rat: Five groups of 15–29 male Fischer 344 rats [age not specified] were given 0.025% N-nitrosobutyl-N-(4-hydroxylbutyl)amine (NBHBA) in the drinking-water for eight weeks, and etretinate was administered in the diet at a concentration of 50 mg/kg. The effects of etretinate on NBHBA-induced bladder carcinogenesis were evaluated when given eight weeks before, for eight weeks during or for eight weeks after carcinogen administration and when given continuously throughout the experiment. Treatment with NBHBA alone resulted in the induction of bladder papillomas in all rats (15/15), whereas the incidence of papillomas was decreased in animals given etretinate before (5/29), during (10/18) or after (12/22) NBHBA ($p < 0.01$; statistical test not given) and in those given etretinate continuously (77%; $p < 0.05$). The group given etretinate before NBHBA also had a significantly decreased incidence of bladder carcinomas, from 8/15 in controls to 6/29 in etretinate-treated animals ($p < 0.05$ [test not given], while the other groups given etretinate showed no significantly lower incidence of carcinomas (Murasaki et al., 1980).

In a second, similar study, four groups of 15–26 male Fischer 344 rats were given etretinate at 100 mg/kg diet for eight weeks before, during or after treatment with NBHBA. Treatment with NBHBA alone induced papillomas in all rats, while the incidence was significantly lower in groups given etretinate before (9/22; $p < 0.001$), during (8/26; $p < 0.001$) or after (10/25; $p < 0.001$) NBHBA [statistical methods not given in detail]. Carcinomas developed in 8/15 rats in the group treated with NBHBA alone and in 2/22 ($p < 0.01$) given etretinate before NBHBA, 0/26 ($p < 0.001$) given etretinate with NBHBA and 2/25 ($p < 0.01$) given etretinate after NBHBA (Murasaki et al., 1980).

4.2.1.7 Leukaemia

Rat: Five groups of 29–48 male and female Long-Evans rat pups received DMBA intravenously at doses of 30, 10, 20 and 10 mg/kg bw on days 27, 42, 57 and 70 of life, respectively, and etretinate daily by gavage at a dose of 5 or 20 mg/kg bw for life on the day after the first, second, third or fourth DMBA injection. Etretinate did not reduce the incidence of leukaemia or mammary tumours (Berger & Schmähl, 1986).

4.2.1.8 Virus-induced tumours

(a)   Shope papilloma virus

A group of 12 domestic Japanese white rabbits [sex not specified] developed 23 papillomas 12–14 days after inoculation with Shope papilloma virus onto the clipped and shaved skin. Six rabbits bearing 12 papillomas were selected and injected intramuscularly with 200 mg/kg bw etretinate twice weekly [total numbers of treatments not specified]. The remaining six rabbits, bearing 11 papillomas, served as controls. After two weeks, the tumours in the controls continued to grow, whereas those in treated animals showed marked growth retardation, and about 60% of all the tumours regressed completely during the 4–10 weeks after cessation of treatment. Once regression had occurred, there was no regrowth [no statistics given] (Ito, 1981).

(b)   Rous sarcoma virus

Golden Syrian hamsters [sex unspecified] were inoculated subcutaneously with Rous sarcoma virus (Schmidt-Ruppin) at one day of age. Three weeks later, 56 control hamsters received peanut oil alone and 32 animals received etretinate at 100 mg/kg bw suspended in peanut oil intraperitoneally each week. After 130 days, no tumours were observed in the etretinate-treated hamsters, whereas large sarcomas occurred at the injection site in 42/56 control animals. In a second experiment, 4/76 etretinate-treated hamsters and 18/32 controls developed tumours [no statistics given] (Frankel et al., 1980).

Forty chickens [not further specified] were inoculated in the wing web with Rous sarcoma virus (Bryan) at five days of age; 20 of these were simultaneously treated intramuscularly with etretinate at 50 mg/kg bw in peanut oil and 20 with peanut oil alone, followed by 25 mg/kg bw etretinate or peanut oil 5 and 18 days later. After 41 days of observation, 1/20 chickens given etretinate developed palpable tumours at the injection site, whereas large invasive sarcomas developed in all control chickens [no statistics given] (Frankel et al., 1980).

4.2.2   Intermediate biomarkers

No data were available to the Working Group.

4.2.3   Cellular studies

4.2.3.1   In vitro

Etretinate is highly lipophilic and is insoluble in water. In most of the tests described below it was supplied to the cells dissolved in dimethylsulfoxide (DMSO) or ethanol, and the final concentration of the solvent was usually added to control samples. When the cells were exposed for more than two days, the medium was changed every two or three days.

(a)   Effect on cell proliferation (see Table 2)

The antiproliferative effects of etretinate have been investigated in vitro in cancer cells and in normal epidermal cells. Although etretinate is de-esterified to acitretin, the presence of acitretin in the culture medium or in the cells was not assessed in any of the studies. In studies of antiproliferative effects, etretinate was generally less effective than acitretin, all-trans-retinoic acid and 13-cis-retinoic acid.

Table 2. Effects of etretinate on cell proliferation, differentiation and tumour promotion *in vitro*

Cell line; end-point	Vehicle	Concentration (mol/L) and exposure	Response	Comments	Reference
Cell proliferation					
Human melanoma; colony-forming ability	DMSO	10^{-9} to 10^{-5} for 1 h	Decreased AIG in 4/6	No dose–response relationship	Meyskens & Salmon (1979)
Murine and human melanoma cell lines; proliferation	Methanol	10^{-11} to 10^{-5} for 7 days	Decreased proliferation in the murine cell line, no effect in the two human cell lines		Gaukroger et al. (1985)
Murine melanoma cell line; proliferation and melanogenesis	Ethanol	10^{-5} for 6 days	Decreased proliferation, 2–3-fold increase in melanogenesis	Too high single concentration, less active than all-*trans*-retinoic acid	Lauharanta et al. (1985)
Epstein-Barr virus-transformed lymphoblastoid cell lines; proliferation and differentiation	DMSO	3×10^{-7} to 10^{-5} for 3, 5, 7, 10 days	Decreased proliferation	Less active than all-*trans*-retinoic acid	Pomponi et al. (1996)
Normal human epidermal cells; proliferation	Ethanol	10^{-7} to 10^{-4} for 1–2 weeks	25–30% decrease in proliferation	No dose–response relationship, less active than all-*trans*-retinoic acid and 13-*cis*-retinoic acid	Hashimoto et al. (1985)
Normal pig epidermal cells; TdR incorporation	DMSO	10^{-7} to 10^{-4} for 24 h	No effect on proliferation	Less active than acitretin	Hashimoto et al. (1990)
Normal neonatal murine epidermal cells; DNA synthesis	DMSO	10^{-8} to 10^{-4} for 4 days	Decreased proliferation in fast-growing (high Ca^{++}) cells, increased proliferation in slow-growing (low Ca^{++}) cells	Less active than acitretin	Tong et al. (1988)
Normal human keratinocytes; proliferation	DMSO	10^{-12} to 10^{-6} for 48 h	10–15% increase in proliferation. No effect on proliferation in cells grown in growth factor-deficient medium	Effect depended on culture conditions	Zhang et al. (1994)
Normal human endothelial cells from skin vessels; proliferation and differentiation (immunocytochemical differentiation)	DMSO	10^{-8} to 10^{-5} for 6 days	No effect on proliferation or differentiation	Less active than acitretin	Imcke et al. (1991)
Normal chick vascular smooth-muscle cells: cell proliferation and differentiation (elastin synthesis)	Not reported	10^{-9} to 10^{-5} for 48 h	Slightly decreased proliferation Increased differentiation	Less active than all-*trans*-retinoic acid	Hayashi et al. (1995a)

			Table 2. (contd)		
Cell line; end-point	Vehicle	Concentration (mol/L) and exposure	Response	Comments	Reference

Cell differentiation

Hamster trachea; reversal of metaplasia	DMSO	10^{-11} to 10^{-6} for 10 days	Reversal of metaplasia	Less active than all-*trans*-retinoic acid	Newton *et al.* (1980)
Human myelomono-cytic cell lines (HL60, U937); cell viability and differentiation (NBT reduction)	DMSO	10^{-6} for 4 or 6 days	No effect on viability or differentiation	all-*trans*-Retinoic acid was active	Chomienne *et al.* (1986)
HL-60; differentiation (morphology, NBT reduction)	DMSO	10^{-6} for 5 days	No effect on differentiation	all-*trans*-Retinoic acid induced differentiation	Ladoux *et al.* (1987)
Bone-marrow mono-nuclear cells from myelodysplastic patients; differentiation (morphology and immunophenotyping)	Ethanol	10^{-6} for 6 days	No effect on differentiation	13-*cis*-Retinoic acid induced differentiation	Hast *et al.* (1986)
Human teratocarcinoma (PA-1)	Not reported	10^{-8} to 10^{-6} for 4 days	Contact inhibition of growth, changes in cell morphology, altered composition of intra-cellular and membrane proteins, increased inter-cellular communication, reduced activity of alkaline phosphatase	As active as all-*trans*-retinoic acid	Taylor *et al.* (1990)
Normal human epi-dermal cells; keratin expression and envelope formation	Not reported	10^{-8} to 10^{-5} for 9 days	Increased keratin K14: K16 ratio expression, decreased envelope formation	Less active than acitretin	West *et al.* (1992)
Normal human dermal and epidermal cells; surface area, differentiation (involucrin and CRABP II mRNA levels)	DMSO	10^{-6} for 2 weeks	Decreased epidermal surface area, decreased CRABP II and mRNA levels		Sanquer *et al.* (1993)
Normal pig skin explant cultures; growth and keratin formation	DMSO	10^{-7} to 10^{-5} for 4 days	Slightly increased epidermal outgrowth, no effect on keratin formation	Less active than acitretin	Aoyagi *et al.* (1981a,b)

Table 2. (contd)					
Cell line; end-point	Vehicle	Concentration (mol/L) and exposure	Response	Comments	Reference
Fetal mouse lung and neonatal rat tracheas exposed to 3,4-benzo-pyrene and cigarette smoke condensate; mitotic activity, differentiation	Not reported	5.6×10^{-6} for 12–14 days with the carcinogen or for 4 days after the carcinogen	Decreased hyperpro-liferation, restoration of secretory and ciliary function		Lasnitzki & Bollag (1982)
Human keratino-cytes exposed to TCDD; differentiation (CLE)	DMSO	10^{-11} to 10^{-6} separately and simul-taneously with\	Increased CLE formation at low concentrations followed by decreased CLE formation at 10^{-6} acid and retinol	Dose–response related decrease in differentiation by all-*trans*-retinoic	Berkers *et al.* (1995)

TdR, ^{13}H-thymidine; DMSO, dimethylsulfoxide; AIG, anchorage-independent growth; CRABP, cellular retinoic acid binding protein; TCDD, 2,3,7,8-tetrachlorodibenzo-*para*-dioxin; CLE, cross-linked envelope; NBT, nitroblue tetrazolium test

Etretinate reduced the colony-forming ability in soft agar of four out of six samples of fresh human melanoma cells obtained at biopsy from patients. The inhibitory effect was seen at a low concentration of the drug (10^{-9} mol/L) and did not increase at higher concentrations. The cells were exposed for only 1 h (Meyskens & Salmon, 1979). [The Working Group noted that the assay is for toxicity and that the short exposure excluded the detection of cytostatic effects.]

Etretinate inhibited the growth of a murine melanoma (PG19) cell line but affected the growth of two human melanoma cell lines only minimally when tested at concentrations of 10^{-11}–10^{-5} mol/L for seven days (Gaukroger *et al.*, 1985). Another murine melanoma (S91) cell line was sensitive to the antiproliferative effect of etretinate at a concentration of 10^{-5} mol/L for six days. Etretinate-treated cells were conspicuously flatter and more spread out than untreated cells. The effect on proliferation was reversible, as usually occurs with retinoids, and was associated with a two- to three-fold increase in melanogenesis. Etretinate was less active than all-*trans*-retinoic acid in inhibiting proliferation and in inducing melanogenesis (Lauharanta *et al.*, 1985). The proliferation of rat

bladder carcinoma cells was not affected by etretinate even at a concentration of 10^{-4} mol/L for 1 h (Fujita & Yoshida, 1984). [The Working Group noted the very high concentration used.] In Epstein-Barr virus-transformed lymphoblastoid cell lines, etretinate inhibited cell proliferation in a dose-dependent manner without inducing differentiation. It was markedly less efficacious than all-*trans*-retinoic acid (Pomponi *et al.*, 1996).

The antiproliferative activity of etretinate has also been investigated in untransformed cells, which were mostly epithelial. When human epidermal cells obtained from foreskins and grown as primary cultures were treated with etretinate for one week, a slight reduction in proliferation was seen which was not dose-dependent. A reduction in cell area, perhaps due to interference with cell-to-cell or cell-to-substrate attachment, was also observed. In this system, etretinate was less potent than all-*trans*-retinoic acid and 13-*cis*-retinoic acid (Hashimoto *et al.*, 1985). In pig epidermal cells, etretinate, in contrast to acitretin, had no effect on cell proliferation when tested for 24 h (Hashimoto *et al.*, 1990).

The state of proliferation of keratinocytes can influence the action of etretinate. Different rates of proliferation of neonatal murine epidermal ker-atinocytes were obtained by growing cells in media with high or low concentrations of Ca++. Etretinate caused dose-dependent inhibition of DNA synthe-sis in rapidly growing cells cultured in a medium with a high concentration of Ca++ but stimulated DNA synthesis in slowly growing cells in a medium with a low concentration of Ca++ (Tong et al., 1988). Acitretin had effects similar to those of etretinate but was more effective. Etretinate tested for 48 h in normal human keratinocytes caused growth promotion when the cells were grown in keratinocyte-complete growth medium but had no effect when the cells were grown in growth factor-deficient medium (Zhang et al., 1994).

Unlike acitretin, etretinate did not inhibit the proliferation or the differentiation of primary cultures of endothelial cells obtained from small vessels and capillaries of human skin (Imcke et al., 1991). In contrast, treatment with etretinate for 48 h inhibited the proliferation of vascular smooth-muscle cells from chick embryos by 30–40%, and the inhibition was associated with stimulation of elastin synthesis. Etretinate was less effective than all-trans-retinoic acid (Hayashi et al., 1995a).

(b)   Effects on cell differentiation (see Table 2)
Explants of trachea from vitamin A-deficient ham-sters have been used to measure the effects of retinoids on the squamous metaplasia that usually results when this tissue is cultured in the absence of vitamin A. Etretinate dissolved in DMSO reversed the metaplasia, with a median effective dose of 2×10^{-8} mol/L when applied over 10 days. The median effective dose of all-trans-retinoic acid under these conditions was 3×10^{-11} mol/L, indicating that etretinate was significantly less potent. Over 90% of the control cultures showed metaplasia (Newton et al., 1980).

Etretinate did not affect differentiation of lymphoid cells. In the human myelomonocytic cell lines HL-60 and U937, often used to test the efficacy of differentiating agents, all-trans-retinoic acid and 13-cis-retinoic acid induced differentiation but etretinate at 10^{-6} mol/L for four or six days was completely inactive in both these cells and in fresh human leukaemic blasts (Chomienne et al., 1986; Ladoux et al., 1987). Similarly, etretinate was inactive in bone-marrow mononuclear cells from patients with myelodys-

plastic syndrome (Hast et al., 1986). In contrast, in a teratocarcinoma-derived cell line (PA-1), etreti-nate induced differentiation in terms of mor-phology, cytoskeletal organization, intercellular communication and cell surface glycoprotein expression, at concentrations that had no antiproliferative effect. In this system, etretinate was as active as all-trans-retinoic acid (Taylor et al., 1990).

Etretinate can modify the differentiation profile of keratinocytes. In epidermal cells isolated from skin biopsies, etretinate decreased the relative amount of keratin 16, with a consequent marked increase in the ratio of keratin 14 to keratin 16. It was less active than acitretin in altering this ratio but was more potent than acitretin in inhibiting envelope formation (West et al., 1992). Differentiation of human epidermal cells can be accomplished by growing them on a collagen gel at the air–liquid interphase. Etretinate decreased the epidermal surface area of cultures exposed to air to a similar degree as all-trans-retinoic acid, whereas it had no effect in submerged cultures. The effect was associated with down-regulation of the mRNA of cellular retinoic acid-binding protein (CRABP) II and of involucrin, a precursor of the cross-linked envelope (Sanquer et al., 1993). In explant cultures obtained from pig dorsal skin, etretinate slightly stimulated epidermal outgrowth without affecting keratin formation. In the same system, acitretin significantly stimulated epider-mal outgrowth (Aoyagi et al., 1981a,b).

(c)   Effects on carcinogen-induced neoplastic
        transformation and on abnormal differentia-
        tion (see Table 2)
Exposure of rodent bronchial and tracheal epithe-lium grown in organ culture to 3,4-benzopyrene or to cigarette smoke condensate leads to hyperplasia. Moreover, the secretory epithelium in the bronchial epithelium is inhibited, and the number of goblet cells in the trachea is reduced and the cilia become clumped. Addition of etretinate for 12–14 days with the carcinogen or for four days after the carcinogen inhibited or reversed these effects (Lasnitzki & Bollag, 1982).

Altered keratinocyte differentiation is induced in humans by dioxins. In primary human ker-atinocyte cultures from neonatal or adult foreskin, differentiation measured as incorporation of

[35]S-methionine-labelled proteins into the cross-linked envelopes, was increased by 2,3,7,8-tetra-chlorodibenzo-*para*-dioxin (TCDD). Etretinate added simultaneously with TCDD at a low concentration (10^{-10} mol/L) induced a significant increase in the formation of cross-linked envelopes but a decrease at a higher concentration (10^{-6} mol/L). In the same system, all-*trans*-retinoic acid antagonized the induction of differentiation by TCDD in a dose-dependent manner (Berkers *et al.*, 1995).

(d) Effects on immune function (see Table 3)
Etretinate, unlike 13-*cis*-retinoic acid, had no effect on DNA synthesis or on cell morphology when added for a short time (5 h) to guinea-pig and human lymphoid cell cultures (Nordlind & Thyberg, 1983). In experiments in which human lymphocyte proliferation was induced by various mitogens, etretinate inhibited only phytohaemag-glutinin-induced proliferation (Dupuy *et al.*, 1989). Etretinate at an extremely high concentration (10^{-4} mol/L) for three days inhibited the proliferation of human peripheral blood mononuclear cells and their mitogen response to phytohaemagglu-tinin (Chaidaroglou *et al.*, 1998). [The Working Group noted the extremely high concentration used.] Incubation of lectin-induced rat thymocytes with etretinate for three days caused a dose-dependent inhibition of proliferation even at a concentrations as low as 1×10^{-7} mol/L. In the same experiments, etretinate did not inhibit production of interleukin (IL)-1 by rat peritoneal macrophages or IL-1-dependent events in T-cell activation, whereas it suppressed IL-2-stimulated T-cell proliferation (Stosic-Grujicic & Simic, 1992). Etretinate did not inhibit the generation of O_2 or production of H_2O_2 in zymosan-stimulated polymorphonuclear leuko-cytes, although, unlike acitretin and all-*trans*-retinoic acid, it slightly stimulated generation of hydroxy radicals (OH$^{\bullet}$) (Yoshioka *et al.*, 1986). The effects of etretinate on the production of cytokines *in vitro* appear to depend on the cell type and culture conditions. Etretinate caused a dose-dependent increase in the production of IL-1 in murine ker-atinocytes (Tokura *et al.*, 1992), but it did not affect unstimulated or tumour necrotizing factor-α-stimu-lated IL-1α or IL-8 secretion in normal human ker-atinocytes. Nevertheless, it inhibited the secretion of these two cytokines when it was induced by phyto-haemagglutinin (Zhang *et al.*, 1994). Etretinate had no

effect on IL-1α-induced IL-6 production by human lung fibroblasts (Zitnik *et al.*, 1994).

4.2.3.2 Antimutagenicity in short-term tests
In Chinese hamster V79 cells exposed to mitomycin-C at 0.03 μg/ml for 3 h, exposure for 24 h to etretinate at doses of 1–4 μg/ml did not alter the induction of sister chromatid exchange by mitomycin-C (Siranni *et al.*, 1981).

4.3   Mechanisms of cancer prevention
As etretinate is converted to acitretin, the mechanisms of action described in the Handbook on that compound apply.

4.3.1   *Effects on cell differentiation*
Most studies of the mechanisms of action of etretinate have addressed the mechanisms that might account for its effects on differentiation in epidermal cells. Etretinate can alter the course of epidermal differentiation and the concomitant expression of differentiation-specific epidermal proteins. After topical treatment of hairless rhino mice, etretinate induced the synthesis of keratins K6, K16 and K17 and suppressed filaggrin in the epidermis, whereas it reduced proteolysis of keratins in the stratum corneum (Eichner *et al.*, 1992). In epidermal cells isolated from skin biopsy samples and cultured *in vitro*, the decrease in the relative amount of K16 induced by etretinate markedly increased the ratio of K14 to K16. A similar increase in the ratio of K14 to K16 was found in epidermal lesions of etretinate-treated patients (West *et al.*, 1992). In skin biopsy samples from patients with psoriasis vulgaris, etretinate reduced keratinocyte hyperplasia and, unexpectedly, enhanced keratinocyte differentiation, as evidenced by increased filaggrin production, increased numbers and size of keratohyalin granules, greater abundance of keratin filaments and increased secretion of intercellular lipids (Gottlieb *et al.*, 1996). In human dermis and epidermis grown in culture and induced to undergo differentiation by being lifted into the air, etretinate down-regulated the expression of involucrin mRNA (Sanquer *et al.*, 1993). In one patient with keratoderma striatum, the filagrin pattern returned to normal during etretinate therapy, whereas the altered involucrin pattern was not affected. The tonofibrils and kera-tohyalin granules were reduced in number and size

Table 3. Effects of etretinate on immune function *in vitro*

Test system; end-point	Vehicle	Concentration (mol/L) and exposure	Response	Comments	Reference
Guinea-pig and human lymphoid cells; DNA synthesis, cell morphology	Acetone	1.4×10^{-6}, 1.4×10^{-5} for 5 h	No effect		Nordlind & Thyberg (1983)
Human lymphocyte mitogenic response to PHA, MLR and MECLR; cell viability	DMSO	10^{-8} to 10^{-5} for 4–6 days	Inhibition of mitogenic response to PHA; no consistent response	Less active than acitretin	Dupuy *et al.* (1989)
Human peripheral blood mononuclear cells; mitogenic response to PHA and TPA, TdR incorporation	DMSO	10^{-6} to 10^{-4} for 3 days	No effect on mitogenic response to PHA; inhibition of mitogenic response to TPA at high concentration and stimulation at lower concentration		Chaidaroglou *et al.* (1998)
PHA- and ConA-activated rat thymocytes, and macrophages; TdR incorporation, cytokine production	DMSO	2×10^{-8} to 2×10^{-4} for 3 days	Inhibition of proliferation No effect on IL-1 production		Stosic-Grujicic & Simic (1992)
Zymosan-stimulated polymorphonuclear leukocytes; generation of reactive oxygen species	50% DMSO, 50% ethanol	2×10^{-6} to 2×10^{-4} during stimulation	No effect on O_2 or H_2O_2 production; slight stimulation of generation of OH[*]	Acitretin and all-*trans*-retinoic acid reduced generation of OH[*]	Yoshioka *et al.* (1986)
Murine epidermal keratinocytes; IL-1 production	DMSO	8×10^{-9} to 8×10^{-6} for 1–3 days	Stimulation (2.5-fold) of IL-1 activity, no effect on cell proliferation	Less active than all-*trans*-retinoic acid	Tokura *et al.* (1992)
Normal human keratinocytes: IL-1α-induced IL-8 production	DMSO	10^{-12} to 10^{-6} for 48 h	No effect on unstimulated or TNFα-stimulated secretion; inhibition of PHA-induced secretion		Zhang *et al.* (1994)
Normal human lung fibroblasts; IL-6 production	Not reported	10^{-6} for 48 h	No effect on IL-1α-induced IL-6 production		Zitnik *et al.* (1994)

PHA, phytohaemagglutinin; MLR, mixed lymphocyte reaction; MECLR, mixed epidermal cell lymphocyte reaction; DMSO, dimethylsulfoxide; TPA, 12-*O*-tetradecanoylphorbol 13-acetate; ConA, concanavalin A; TdR, [13]H-thymidine; IL, interleukin; TNFα, tumour necrotizing factor α

(Fartasch *et al.,* 1990). Etretinate may also cause changes in keratinocyte membranes, since the lectin binding of keratinocytes from1 the skin of guinea-pigs treated with etretinate changed after treatment (Nomura *et al.,* 1994). Galactose incorporation into epidermal glycoproteins was increased in explant cultures from pig ear skin treated with etretinate (King & Pope, 1984). Slight effects of etretinate on extracellular collagen and collagenase synthesis or activity have been reported. In cultured human skin fibroblasts, etretinate only slightly inhibited collagenase expression (Bauer *et al.,* 1983), and it did not affect type IV collagenolytic activity in human melanoma cells (Oikarinen & Salo, 1986). In one patient with lichen sclerosis and atro-phisms, clinical improvement seen after treament with etretinate was not accompanied by enhanced collagen synthesis (Niinimaki *et al.,* 1989). In contrast, etretinate inhibited TGFβ1-stimulated type-1 collagen production by normal human lung fibroblasts in culture (Redlich *et al.,* 1995).

The content of steroid receptors may positively correlate with the degree of mammary tumour differentiation. Mammary tumours from dogs treated with etretinate showed an increased cytoplasmic oestrogen receptor content, which may suggest that etretinate induced differentiating effects in the mammary gland cells (Cappelletti *et al.,* 1988).

4.3.2 Inhibition of cell proliferation and oncogene expression

The enzyme ornithine decarboxylase is induced during proliferation. Etretinate completely inhibited induction by TPA of ornithine decarboxylase mRNA in a simian virus 40-transformed human keratinocyte cell line (Xue *et al.,* 1996). It also markedly inhibited Epstein-Barr virus induction by croton oil and *n*-butyrate in Raji infected cells (Zeng *et al.,* 1981). The immunoreactivity of p53 in premalignant and malignant lesions indicates that expression of this oncogene plays a role in skin cancer; however, etretinate did not affect the expression of *p53* in premalignant and malignant cutaneous lesions of kidney transplant recipients (Gibson *et al.,* 1997).

4.3.3 Effects on immune function and cytokine production

Although etretinate, unlike retinyl palmitate and 13-*cis*-retinoic acid, did not enhance the cell-mediated immune response of mice to sheep red blood cells (Athanassiades, 1981), clinical studies indicate that it can activate T cells. In patients with psoriasis or other dermatoses, etretinate treatment at 1 mg/kg bw per day for 28 days significantly increased the reactions to recall antigens (Fulton *et al.,* 1982). In another study in patients with psoriasis, etretinate at 1 mg/kg bw per day for two months stimulated the number of peripheral T lymphocytes, which was lower than that of control subjects (David *et al.,* 1990). The cytotoxic activity of neutrophils, which before therapy was greater in patients with psoriasis than in control subjects, was decreased by etretinate treatment at 1 mg/kg bw for 28 days (Ellis *et al.,* 1985a). Etretinate also decreased the migration of neutrophils from the bloodstream to human skin (Dubertret *et al.,* 1982). It did not affect generation of the leukocyte chemotactic factor leukotriene B_4 from rat polymorphonuclear leukocytes stimulated by calcium ionophores (Bray, 1984), but an inverse relationship was found between the dose of etretinate and the number of intraepidermal infiltrating polymorphonuclear leukocytes after epicutaneous application of leukotriene B_4 (Lammers & van de Kerkhof, 1987). Natural killer cell activity has been found to be decreased in most patients with psoriasis, and etretinate increased the number and activity of these cells in several studies (Jansén *et al.,* 1985; McKerrow *et al.,* 1988; Majewski *et al.,* 1989). In one case the increase was transient, in that the natural killer cell activity rose during the first two months of treatment but returned thereafter to the starting value (Jansén *et al.,* 1985). Etretinate abolished the manifestation of chronic graft-versus-host disease in semi-allogenic recipient rats (Stosic-Grujicic *et al.,* 1996). In patients with psoriasis, etretinate had no effect on the elevated serum IL-1 concentrations, but it caused a substantial decrease in serum tumour necrotizing factor-α and interferon concentrations (Shiohara *et al.,* 1992).

4.3.4 Effects on angiogenesis

Etretinate inhibited angiogenesis induced by a human epidermoid cancer cell line, although it was less effective than acitretin. When the same effect was tested in a non-tumorigenic cell line, etretinate had a stimulatory effect (Rudnicka *et al.,* 1991).

5. Other Beneficial Effects

Etretinate has been shown to be of benefit to patients with psoriasis and cutaneous disorders of keratinization. Infants treated with etretinate at doses of up to 1.3 mg per day for up to six weeks have had no clear adverse reactions. The drug is efficacious in the treatment of congenital lamellar ichthyosis (Collin *et al.*, 1989; Rogers & Scarf, 1989; Lawlor & Peiris, 1985a,b; Ward & Jones, 1989; Nayar & Chin, 1992).

Harlequin fetus is the most severe manifestation of autosomal recessive nonbullous congenital icthyosis erythroderma, which is a distinct autosomal recessive ichthyosis or the phenotypic expression of several genotypes. Left untreated, infants with this syndrome almost always die shortly after birth, following sepsis and excessive loss of fluid, electrolyte and protein through the thick, inelastic, water-permeable skin. With constant nursing care, maintenance of body temperature, control of infection and initial treatment with etretinate at 2.5 mg/day from birth through to the age of six weeks and then 1.5 mg/day to the age of 10 months, these infants can survive, and development of motor and vocabulary skills can be consistent with the norm by 6–24 months of age (Collin *et al.*, 1989; Lawlor & Peiris, 1985b). These infants may also have renal, thymic, thyroid and pulmonary malformations and develop pulmonary infection, respiratory difficulty and feeding problems and die despite administration of etretinate (Waisman *et al.*, 1989). While long-term follow-up of these children has not been reported, they appear to tolerate this protocol without the typical signs of retinoid intoxication.

6. Carcinogenicity

6.1 Humans

No epidemiological studies were available to the Working Group.

Isolated case reports of neoplasms occurring after treatment with etretinate have been published. One report described a case of malignant B-cell lymphoma and one of Hodgkin disease (Woll *et al.*, 1987); a second reported one case of Hodgkin disease, one malignant teratoma of the testis and a squamous-cell carcinoma of

the anus (Harrison, 1987), and a third was of a case of Hodgkin disease (Desablens *et al.*, 1989).

6.2 Experimental models

No studies were available to the Working Group in which the effects of etretinate on cancer development in the absence of carcinogen treatment were evaluated; however, etretinate enhanced lung carcinogenesis (see section 4.2.1).

7. Other Toxic Effects

7.1 Adverse effects

7.1.1 Humans

Several authoritative reviews have appeared on the clinical toxicology of etretinate (Orfanos, 1980; Peck, 1981; Lauharanta, 1982; Ward *et al.*, 1983; Lippman *et al.*, 1987; Orfanos *et al.*, 1987). The longest experience with the toxicity of synthetic retinoids is associated with their therapeutic use in dermatological practice, as many patients have been treated continuously with etretinate for 15–20 years (Kamm, 1982). The usual initial dose is 0.5–1 mg/kg bw per day for two to four weeks. After 8–16 weeks, the maintenance dose is 0.25–0.75 mg/kg per day. The maximum daily dose is 75–100 mg/day, and the lowest effective dose is 10 mg/day.

The toxic effects observed are summarized in Table 4 (Halioua & Saurat, 1990).

(a)   Dermatological toxicity

The standard mucocutaneous symptoms associated with treatment with etretinate at 0.25–1 mg/kg bw per day orally are dose-dependent and vary widely in frequency and severity. Cheilitis is seen in the majority of patients but this symptom rapidly resolves upon discontinuation of the drug. Epistaxis can result from drying of nasal membranes. An erythematous rash may develop in up to 50% of patients treated for psoriasis. An exaggerated healing response typical of the effects of retinoids on granulation tissue may result at the sites of wounds or healing lesions (Lauharanta, 1980; Ward *et al.*, 1983; Ellis & Voorhees, 1987). There was an isolated report of fatal epidermal necrolysis associated with treatment with this drug (McIvor, 1992).

Alopecia occurred in nine of 56 patients given 40–75 mg/day (0.7–0.9 mg/kg bw per day) for more

Table 4. Toxic effects reported with standard long-term use of etretinate

Body system	Adverse effect
Mucocutaneous	Xerosis, skin fragility, mucous membrane dryness, dermatitis, exuberant granulation tissue, photosensitivity, changes in hair and nails
Skeletal	Vertebral abnormalities, diffuse idiopathic hyperostosis, osteophytes on vertebral bodies, calcification of anterior spinal ligament and other tendons, extraspinal involvement, osseous hyperostosis
Hepatic	Elevated liver enzyme activity, severe hepatotoxic damage
Biochemical and haematological	Hypertriglyceridaemia, hypercholesterolaemia, elevated creatinine kinase activity, anaemia, monocytosis, lymphoma
Ocular	Blepharitis, conjunctivitis, night blindness
Neurological	Headache, intracranial hypertension, depression, otitis externa, earache
Muscular	Myalgia, muscle weakness, myopathy
Other	Sexual dysfunction (male and female), menstrual changes, gynaecomastia, fatigue, nausea, renal oedema

From Halioua & Saurat (1990)

than four weeks (Lauharanta, 1982). When the dose was increased to 0.9–1.5 mg/kg bw per day (Hönigsmann et al., 1978; Orfanos et al., 1978; Binazzi & Cicilioni, 1979), alopecia affected 21–29% of patients (Goerz & Orfanos, 1978; Lassus, 1980). Women seem to be preferentially affected (Foged & Jacobsen, 1982). Alopecia becomes evident within five to six weeks of continuous dosing (Mahrle et al., 1979), and it is the principal reason given for discontinuation of treatment (Goerz & Orfanos, 1978; Lassus, 1980; Lauharanta, 1982). The condition resolves within one to two months after drug withdrawal (Mahrle et al., 1979; Lauharanta, 1982). Some patients given the drug at 25–50 mg/day have reversible, dose-dependent hair kinking, which generally begins 3–12 months after initiation of oral therapy (Graham et al., 1985). A case of increased curliness of scalp hair (pili torti) was reported in a 15-year-old girl given 0.3 mg/kg bw day (Hays & Camisa, 1985); similar reports of patients with previously straight hair are anecdotal (Ellis & Voorhees, 1987).

Fingernail growth increased and the nails became dystrophic, thin and clear and were shed in 2/10 patients given etretinate for 12 weeks (Galosi et al., 1985). The nails returned to normal after cessation of treatment (Ferguson et al., 1983). In about 10% of patients given a therapeutic course at 0.25–1 mg/kg bw per day, a mucin-like material (thought to be synthesized by keratinocytes undergoing mucous metaplasia) accumulates in the skin, leading to a shiny, smooth texture (Ellis & Voorhees, 1987).

Palmoplantar desquamation, scaling and alopecia were observed more commonly among patients given etretinate at 0.25–1 mg/kg per day than in those receiving 13-cis-retinoic acid at 0.5–1 mg/kg bw per day (Cunningham & Ehmann, 1983). Granulation about the toes, groin and nails can affect about 15% of etretinate-treated patients (Campbell et al., 1983; Hodak et al., 1984; Wolska et al., 1985). In up to 50% of patients, a reversible 'retinoid dermatitis' can develop (Crivellato, 1982; Molin et al., 1985; Ellis & Voorhees, 1987). Bone and joint pain occurs in 25–50% of treated patients, and older patients appear to be more severely affected. Fewer than 10% of patients experience myalgia, but affected individuals voluntarily restrict regular exercise or strenuous physical activity while taking the drug (Orfanos et al., 1987).

Cheilitis is the most frequent side-effect in etretinate-treated patients (Table 5). In 10% of patients so affected, this progresses to rhagades (Lauharanta, 1982). Etretinate less frequently induces skin fragility (Neild et al., 1985), dry

Table 5. Incidences of mucocutaneous side effects with standard oral etretinate therapy

Condition	Incidence (%)
Cheilitis	42–100
Dry mouth	21–95
Dry nasal mucosa	21–87.5
Epistaxis, petechiae	5
Facial dermatitis	5–7
Palmoplantar desquamation	17–40
Desquamation	23–94
Skin thinning	6–93
Skin fragility	25
Xerosis	20–30
Dermatitis	5
Alopecia	3–69
Conjunctivitis or ocular irritation	5–50
Pruritus	15–25

Summarized from Windhorst & Nigra (1982); Cunningham & Ehmann (1983); Ward et al. (1983); Orfanos et al. (1987)

nose and mouth, paronychia, bruise, dermatitis, epistaxis, xerosis, pruritus and conjunctivitis (see Table 5 and references cited therein).

(b)   Skeletal toxicity
Long-term treatment with etretinate was often associated with skeletal changes, including demineralization of bones and extraosseous calcification (Kaplan & Haettich, 1991). These changes often occurred in the vertebrae, more often in the cervical rather than the thoracic or lumbar spine. Extraspinal tendon and ligament calcification most often affected the ankle, pelvis, knee, shoulder and then elbow joints. In one clinical trial, 38 of 45 patients with psoriasis or other disorders of keratinization treated with an average dose of 0.8 mg/kg for a mean of 60 months had radiographic evidence of extraspinal tendon and ligament calcification. Of 38 patients given etretinate for an average of five years, 32 had radiographic evidence of extraspinal ligament and tendon calcification (DiGiovanna et al., 1986). Vertebral disk degeneration, osteoporosis, spinal hyperostosis with calcification of the spinal ligaments and periosteal thickening occurred in a substantial fraction of adults receiving oral etretinate at doses as low as 25–50 mg/day for years (Burge & Ryan, 1985; Ellis et al., 1985b; Logan, 1987; Halkier-Sorensen & Andresen, 1989).

While brief therapy with etretinate in children usually results in no clinically discernible skeletal toxicity, prolonged treatment at > 1 mg/kg bw per day has resulted in thinning of the long bones, focal osteoporosis, fracture after minor trauma and premature epiphyseal closure (Rosinska et al., 1988; Lowe & David, 1998). Children given etretinate at doses up to 2.5 mg/kg bw per day for five or six years experienced premature closure of the epiphyseal plate (Prendiville et al., 1986). While some cases of etretinate-induced skeletal toxicity progress with prolonged therapy (Sillevis-Smitt & de Mari, 1984), others fail to show clinically detectable evidence of such changes (Brun & Baran, 1986), particularly when the dose is reduced (< 1 mg/kg bw per day) promptly when the patient's condition improves (Tamayo & Ruiz-Maldonado, 1981; Traupe & Happle, 1985; Paige et al., 1992). When the dose is maintained at 0.2–0.5 mg/kg bw per day or at no more than 1 mg/kg bw per day, the margin of safety is increased. No skeletal toxicity was seen in infants started on treatment as young as two weeks, in children as old as 11 years and in young adults given the drug continuously for one month to 11 years (Glover et al., 1987; Rosinska et al., 1988; Paige et al., 1992).

The highest dose reported to have no skeletal toxicity was 25–50 mg/day in an eight-year-old child who had been treated for six years (Presbury, 1984), and a dose of 2 mg/kg bw per day for 36–42 months was tolerated without clinically evident detrimental effects (Tamayo & Ruiz-Maldonado, 1981). No significant bone abnormalities were found on physical examination, technetium bone scans and X-rays of cervical, thoracic and lumbar vertebrae of patients as young as six years who were maintained on standard long-term (6–100 months) therapy with etretinate (Mills & Marks, 1993). Genetic profile, physical activity and level of psychological stimulation confound direct evaluation of delayed or deficient development in affected individuals given higher doses for 16–42 months from as early as seven months of age (Tamayo & Ruiz-Maldonado, 1980, 1981). Since etretinate can have developmental toxicity in children, it has been proposed that its prescription be limited to those with severe recalcitrant disease that seriously impairs their quality of life (Shelnitz *et al.*, 1987).

(c)   Hepatotoxicity

The principal danger associated with standard therapy with etretinate is the onset of chronic, aggressive hepatitis (Fredriksson & Pettersson, 1978; Glazer *et al.*, 1982; van Voorst Vader *et al.*, 1984), which can progress to toxic centrilobular necrosis (Thune & Mork, 1980). In general, the clinical signs of liver involvement begin within the first four weeks of treatment (Roenigk *et al.*, 1985; Roenigk, 1989). While 90% of patients treated with etretinate do not develop histologically or clinically significant hepatotoxicity (Foged *et al.*, 1984; Glazer *et al.*, 1984), about 1% develop frank hepatitis. Elevated activities of serum aspartate and alanine aminotransferases occur in 18 and 23%, respectively, of patients receiving etretinate orally (Fontan *et al.*, 1983; Kaplan *et al.*, 1983). Hyperbilirubinaemia was reported in patients on etretinate, but only after more than four years of therapy (Ott, 1981). The increased activities of liver enzymes returned to pretreatment values upon cessation of treatment (Mahrle *et al.*, 1979; Lauharanta, 1982).

Prior exposure to methotrexate for psoriasis at a total administered dose of 480–11 860 mg increased the risk for hepatotoxicity; in about 10% of these patients, the disease progressed from fibrosis to cirrhosis. No significant dmage to the liver was found during etretinate therapy (Roenigk *et al.*, 1985).

Approximately 20–30% of all patients receiving standard therapy with etretinate develop temporary abnormalities in liver function that are reversible when the dose is reduced or the drug is withdrawn. Etretinate may be more hepatotoxic than other synthetic retinoids because of its higher concentration in the liver. Of 652 patients treated in clinical trials, 10 had clinical or histological hepatitis that was considered to be possibly or probably related to treatment. The liver function in eight of these patients returned to normal after discontinuation of etretinate (Gollnick, 1981). Rare cases of severe hepatotoxic damage have been reported, which appear to result from hypersensitivity to the drug (Sanchez *et al.*, 1993).

(d)   Metabolic and biochemical effects

The induction of hyperlipidaemia is one of the most common side-effects of retinoid therapy in general, and the increased risk for atherosclerosis associated with long-term treatment is of considerable concern. Administration of etretinate results in elevated serum concentrations of cholesterol (> 300 mg/dl) and triglycerides (> 250 mg/dl) in 25–50% of all patients (Michaëlsson *et al.*, 1981; Ellis *et al.*, 1982; Gollnick & Orfanos, 1985). Of 652 patients on etretinate, 16% developed hypercholesterolaemia and 45% developed hypertriglyceridaemia (Gollnick, 1981). The hyperlipidaemia is attributable to increased production of very-low-density lipoprotein. Large increases in triglyceride concentrations are reported to occur only in individuals with pre-existing hypertriglyceridaemia, but smaller increases in the concentrations of triglycerides, cholesterol and apoprotein B and decreases in those of high-density lipoprotein and cholesterol are very common (Marsden, 1989).

Patients with predisposing factors such as obesity, alcohol abuse, diabetes and smoking habits appear to have a higher incidence of hyperlipidaemia when treated with etretinate. Although the exact mechanism of retinoid-induced hyperlipidaemia is unknown, it may increase the absorption of dietary lipids, increase chylomicron production or reduce its clearance, increase the synthesis of triglycerides and cholesterol in the liver and increase the synthesis or decrease the catabolism of low-density lipoproteins (Ellis *et al.*, 1982; Marsden, 1989). Other less frequent biochemical effects seen with etretinate therapy include the development of pseudoporphyria (McDonagh & Harrington, 1989) and elevated creatinine kinase activity. Some studies have also shown an effect of etretinate on the therapeutic efficacy of concomitant medications, such as warfarin (Ostlere *et al.*, 1991) and oral contraceptives (Berbis *et al.*, 1987).

(e)   Ocular, central nervous system and other toxicity

The ocular manifestations seen with etretinate therapy include both conjunctival symptoms and rare retinal dysfunction associated with depletion of retinol (Weber *et al.*, 1988). Effects on the central nervous system such as headache and impaired vision may be associated with benign intracranial hypertension induced by etretinate (Peck, 1982; Bonnetblanc *et al.*, 1983; Viraben *et al.*, 1985). Depression has been associated with use of etretinate at 75–100 mg/day, particularly among people who consume copious quantities of ethanol, but is less frequent when the dose of etretinate is reduced to < 50 mg/day (Logan, 1987; Henderson & Highet, 1989). Muscle damage (Hodak *et al.*, 1987) and renal impairment (Cribier *et al.*, 1992) have also been described.

Photosensitivity is usually not a result of exposure to etretinate, and the threshold for erythema can actually be increased (Ippen *et al.*, 1978; Mahrle *et al.*, 1982). Sensitivity to light can be increased in a minority of patients (Collins *et al.*, 1986), and photophobia developed in two of 23 patients given etretinate at 75–100 mg/day for three weeks (Ippen *et al.*, 1978). Cases of night blindness, iritis, subcapsular cataract, corneal erosion, reductions in visual activity with blurring and retinal haemorrhage have been recorded among patients receiving etretinate orally (Viraben *et al.*, 1985).

Cases of gynaecomastia have also been reported (Carmichael & Paul, 1989). Inflammation of the external ear canal due to accumulation of excess cerumen and associated pain can occur but are seldom reported in the literature (Kramer, 1982; Juhlin, 1983).

7.1.2 Experimental studies

The toxicity of etretinate was studied in rats at doses up to 20 mg/kg bw per day and in dogs at doses up to 30 mg/kg bw per day during the initial development of this drug as an anti-psoriatic agent. The most striking manifestation of toxicity in rodents was bone fractures, but this osteolytic response was not seen in dogs. Other dose-related changes in animals treated with etretinate included alopecia, erythema, reductions in body weight and food consumption, stiffness and alterations in gait, haematological changes and changes in serum chemistry and testicular atrophy with evidence of reduced spermatogenesis (reviewed by Kamm, 1982).

The ocular toxicity of etretinate was examined in rabbits, which showed degenerative changes in the meibomian gland (Kremer *et al.*, 1994).

7.2 Reproductive and developmental effects

7.2.1 Humans

7.2.1.1 Reproductive effects

While cases of dysmenorrhoea (Halkier-Sorensen, 1987), male impotence (Halkier-Sorensen, 1988; Krause, 1988; Reynolds, 1991) and loss of libido (Halkier-Sorensen, 1987) in patients treated with etretinate have been reported, these are isolated, and the extent to which etretinate contributed to these observations is not clear (Krause, 1988). The changes resolved without sequelae after withdrawal of the drug. There is no evidence that etretinate interferes with the actions of oral contraceptives or progesterone in women given etretinate orally at 0.7–1 mg/kg bw per day (Berbis *et al.*, 1987).

In 23 men given etretinate at 25–75 mg/day for three months, there was no effect on sperm count, total sperm output or morphology or on spermatogenesis (Schill *et al.*, 1981; Török, 1984; Török *et al.*, 1987). Morphological examination of semen from 11 men showed no change in absolute or progressive motility, and the wife of one patient conceived during treatment and gave birth to a healthy baby (Török, 1984).

7.2.1.2 Developmental effects

The first cases of teratogenicity associated with exposure to etretinate before or during pregnancy were recognized in 1983 (Happle *et al.*, 1984), and seven infants with congenital defects and one fetal death had been recorded by 1985 (reviewed by Rosa, 1992). By 1986, eight infants afflicted by etretinate embryopathy had been identified (Kietzmann *et al.*, 1986; Orfanos *et al.*, 1987), and by 1988, 22 cases occurring after continuous exposure during pregnancy had been reported (Rosa, 1992). Between 1976 (when etretinate was first introduced in the United Kingdom) and December 1990, 83 pregnancies, including 12 in the USA, in which the women reported having been exposed to etretinate had been reported; in 16 of these, the infant was normal at birth, and in 47 the pregnancy was terminated. Malformations occurred after daily exposure to 0.4–1.5 mg/kg bw (Rosa *et al.*, 1986). Far fewer pregnancies and elected abortions (Chan *et al.*, 1995) have been reported in association with use of etretinate than with 13-*cis*-retinoic acid, probably because it is indicated for an older population than that in which 13-*cis*-retinoic acid is used (Lehucher Ceyrac *et al.*, 1992).

The terata arising after exposure to etretinate include meningomyelocoele, malformation of the chondrocranium and viscerocranium, the tetralogy of Fallot, ventricular septal defect, anophthalmia, malformations of the hip, ankle and forearm, syndactyly, short digits, imperforate anus and genitourinary disorders such as absent penis or meatus urinarius (Happle *et al.*, 1984; Lambert *et al.*, 1988; Martinez-Tallo *et al.*, 1989; Geiger *et al.*, 1994). Only one of 23 newborns with a history of exposure to etretinate *in utero* showed even borderline microtia (Rosa, 1992), whereas this occurs in 70% of infants with 13-*cis*-retinoic acid-associated embryopathy (Lynberg *et al.*, 1990). Digit and limb malformations (unilateral hypoplasia; Grote *et al.*, 1985) occurred in 31% of these infants and in 2% of those with equivalent exposure to 13-*cis*-retinoic acid. Cardiac terata were far less prevalent in infants exposed to etretinate (16%) than in those exposed to 13-*cis*-retinoic acid (42%).

While fetuses conceived shortly after cessation of therapy with 13-*cis*-retinoic acid are not at increased risk for developmental toxicity (Dai *et al.*, 1992), congenital malformations have been recorded among aborted fetuses (Happle *et al.*, 1984; Lambert *et al.*, 1988; Verloes *et al.*, 1990) and among infants born to mothers who had discontinued therapy with etretinate 4–12 months before conception (Grote *et al.*, 1985; Lammer, 1988; Geiger *et al.*, 1994). By 1988, 11 such cases had been reported (Rosa, 1992). Cardiovascular (abnormal vena cava, atrial septal defect) and renal (horseshoe kidney) terata were reported in a 23-week-old fetus aborted by a mother who had discontinued use of etretinate at 0.5 mg/kg bw per day seven to eight months before conception (Verloes *et al.*, 1990).

Between 1976 and 1991, 123 women reported pregnancies within two years of cessation of etretinate use. Of these, 34% (42) either aborted spontaneously or elected termination; malformations were seen in 10. The true extent of the problem is unknown, however, and calculation of risk is compromised by failure to report spontaneous abortions accurately, failure to examine and report abortuses that have been exposed to etretinate before or during pregnancy and failure to delineate

and to separate those infants with terata that may be due to factors other than etretinate. For example, one infant with malformations not typical of retinoid embryopathy (premature with inguinal hernia) was included in one summary (Mitchell, 1992); another case (Lammer, 1988) has been questioned in that the defects resembled those of the CHARGE syndrome (coloboma, heart defects, choanal atresia, retardation, genital and ear anomalies), which is of genetic origin (Blake & Wyse, 1988).

Not all mothers who conceive after discontinuing use of etretinate gave birth to infants with congenital malformations, even when exposure continued into the first trimester (Cordero *et al.*, 1981; Ruther & Kietzmann, 1984; Jäger *et al.*, 1985; Vahlquist & Rollman, 1990). By 1988, six normal pregnancies had been reported after use of etretinate had been stopped one to nine months before conception (Rosa, 1992). Given the delay between direct exposure to etretinate and abnormal pregnancy outcome and identification of inherited syndromes of terata with features in common with etretinate embryopathy, debate on the case reports has been vigorous (Blake & Wyse, 1988; Greaves, 1988).

In view of the elimination half-time of about 100 days (DiGiovanna *et al.*, 1989) and the fact that 99% of the body burden of etretinate is removed within seven elimination half-times, the calculated period of theoretical excess risk is less than 700 days before conception (Geiger *et al.*, 1994). The precise duration of the increased teratogenic risk after cessation of use of etretinate is unknown, but it is generally recommended that post-therapy contraception be continued for at least two years after treatment (Rinck *et al.*, 1989). Clinical experience has demonstrated that the risk for embryonic death associated with exposure to etretinate is greatest during the first three weeks of pregnancy, and the risk for teratogenic effects is highest when exposure occurs during weeks 4–8 of pregnancy. When exposure occurs after that time or ceases two years before conception, the risk for major malformations is close to that expected for the general population (Geiger *et al.*, 1994).

7.2.2 Experimental models

In animals, etretinate is converted to its acid metabolites, acitretin and 13-*cis*-acitretin (Löfberg *et al.*, 1990; Bouvy *et al.*, 1992), which are assumed to be the proximate teratogens since etretinate has no activity in various assays *in vitro* (see below).

7.2.2.1 Reproductive effects

Male rats became infertile after receiving daily doses of etretinate at 5 or 25 mg/kg bw for four weeks. Animals at the low dose were normal, but many effects were seen at the high dose: some of the rats died, and the rest had bone fractures in the paws, smudges around the eyes, decreased spontaneous activity and decreased body weight and they were infertile, as seen by a decrease in serum testosterone concentration, a decrease in sperm motility and number, abnormal sperm shape, atrophy of the seminiferous tubules and Leydig cells, necrosis of spermatocytes and atrophy of the seminal vesicle and prostatic epithelium. They also showed atrophy of acidophils but an increased number of gonadotrophs in the pituitary gland (Hayashi *et al.*, 1995b). Guinea-pigs exposed to 25 mg/kg bw for six weeks showed similar effects on the testes: decreased spermatogenic activity, lack of mature sperm and reduced diameters of the seminiferous tubules (Tsambaos *et al.*, 1980).

7.2.2.2 Developmental effects

Administration of etretinate to hamsters on day 8 of gestation at a dose of 44 mg/kg bw resulted in 100% abnormal fetuses, while administration of 22 mg/kg bw resulted in 88% abnormal fetuses. The median effective dose for abnormalities was 5.7 mg/kg bw, indicating that it is nearly twice as potent as all-*trans*-retinoic acid. The defects observed included shortening and oligodactyly of the limbs, exencephaly, encephalocoele, spina bifida, exophthalmos, clefting and agnathia, fused and hooked ribs and aplastic or hypoplastic tail (Williams *et al.*, 1984).

In mice, administration of etretinate on day 11 of gestation produced cleft palate and shortening of the long bones of the limb. The number of abnormal fetuses increased with increasing dose: 25 mg/kg bw resulted in 52% abnormal embryos, while 100 mg/kg bw resulted in 98% abnormal embryos. The median effective dose for abnormalities was 26 mg/kg bw, which was similar to that of all-*trans*-retinoic acid. Earlier administration resulted in much more severe abnormalities (Reiners *et al.*, 1988; Kochhar *et al.*, 1989). In mice given a dose of 50 mg/kg bw on day 8.25 of

gestation, microcephaly, exophthalmos, smaller zygomatic arches leading to a narrower and shorter facial skeleton, persistence of Meckel's cartilage, absent pinna and spina bifida were observed. The offspring had smaller brains with a hypoplastic cerebellum. Examination of embryos after 24 h revealed extensive cell death in the rhombomeres and rhombic lip (which makes the cerebellum) and in the neural crest (which makes the cranial skeleton). As the branchial arches were also smaller, many of the abnormalities can be attributed to the induction of cell death in specific embryonic populations (Alles & Sulik, 1992).

Administration of etretinate on day 9 of gestation at a dose of 60 mg/kg bw resulted in 100% abnormal embryos, but the abnormalities were concentrated at the caudal end of the embryo rather than in the head (Mesrobian *et al.*, 1994). No spina bifida or limb abnormalities were seen; rather, 100% had imperforate anus and tail abnormalities and a high rate of urethral atresia. Surprisingly, excessive cell death was not observed, in contrast to that seen after administration on day 8.25 (Alles & Sulik, 1992). In a study of the development of anorectal malformations after the same administration regimen (60 mg/kg bw on day 9), there was decreased cell proliferation in the cloacal membrane and either excessive apoptosis or lack of apoptosis, depending on the region of study. Thus, the cellular dynamics of this region of the embryo were severely altered (Kubota *et al.*, 1998).

Etretinate was given to mice at 10 or 25 mg/kg bw on day 6, 7 or 8 of gestation. It was not teratogenic when given on day 6 or 7, and day 8 was considered to be the earliest susceptible time for the embryos (Agnish *et al.*, 1990).

In a more refined method, to avoid giving single large doses of etretinate on particular days of gestation, a low dose is infused continually into the stomach of pregnant mice. Infusion of a dose of 2.5 mg/kg bw on days 8–15 of development resulted in a very high frequency of limb defects, cleft palate, micrognathia, phalangeal defects and tail defects (Löfberg *et al.*, 1990). Similar results were obtained after daily administration of etretinate to mouse embryos over the period of gestation of 7–17 days; the lowest teratogenic dose was 4 mg/kg bw (Kistler, 1987).

Visceral and cardiac heterotaxy were induced by administration of a dose of 15 mg/kg bw on day

7. The heart defects were severe and included transposition of the great arteries, aortic arch abnormalities and complete atrial defect (Kim *et al.*, 1995).

A similar pattern of abnormalities is seen in rats. At doses of 5–10 mg/kg bw, exencephaly and spina bifida were seen after administration on days 7–8 of gestation, craniofacial malformations in 100% of embryos when given on days 8.5–9, and digital and tail malformations when given on days 9.5–11 (Granström & Kullaa-Mikkonen, 1990a; Granström *et al.*, 1990, 1991). The lowest teratogenic dose for rat embryos was reported to be 8 mg/kg bw (Kistler, 1987); no teratogenesis was seen with doses of 1, 3 or 6 mg/kg bw, but typical teratogenic effects occurred at 10, 15 and 25 mg/kg bw (Agnish *et al.*, 1990). The craniofacial malformations induced by etretinate included micrognathia, displaced and smaller Meckel's cartilage, facial and palatal clefts, reduced nasal width, flattened face and reduced number of cranial neural crest cells. Other abnormalities that have been reported include an abnormal hypophysis, hypoplasia of the submandibular salivary glands and tooth aplasia. In similar studies of craniofacial malformations induced by a dose of 10 mg/kg bw on day 8.5 of gestation, microtia and meningocoele were observed with cranial displacement of the otocyst, which is a classical sign of retinoid teratogenicity. The non-cranial malformations reported include omphalocoele and cardiac and renal malformations (Granström *et al.*, 1991; Jacobsson & Granström, 1997). The craniofacial malformations could be prevented by prior administration of vitamin B_6 (Jacobsson & Granström 1996). At the same dose (10 mg/kg bw) on days 8.5–10.5 of gestation, the characteristic craniofacial defects noted above were accompanied by auricular displacement or absent outer ears, skin tags between the auricle and the mouth, ossicles of the inner ear that were small, altered in position or fused, shorter cochlea with fewer turns and hypoplastic stapedial artery and facial nerve (Granström, 1990; Granstrom *et al.*, 1991; Jacobsson & Granström, 1997). Defective fusion of the nasal processes, resulting in fistulas and clefts and missing or reduced nasal cartilages, has also been reported (Granström & Kullaa-Mikkonen, 1990b).

In these studies of craniofacial defects in rats, etretinate was found to be four times as teratogenic as all-*trans*-retinoic acid. In a comparative study of several retinoids, however, the opposite was found to be the case: all-*trans*-retinoic acid was more teratogenic than etretinate. In this study, the craniofacial defects were accompanied by thymus abnormalities, urogenital defects including hydronephrosis, dilated ureter, genital agenesis, undescended testis and cardiac vessel defects. As in mice, imperforate anus and caudal agenesis were also reported in the rat embryos (Turton *et al.*, 1992).

7.2.2.3 In vitro

In striking contrast to the results described above, etretinate is virtually inactive *in vitro*. It did not inhibit chondrogenesis in mouse limb bud cultures, whereas the activity of acitretin was similar to that of all-*trans*-retinoic acid (Kistler, 1987; Reiners *et al.*, 1988; Kochhar *et al.*, 1989). Indeed, when esterases were added to the culture medium, etretinate was activated (Kochhar *et al.*, 1989). Etretinate also had no effect in whole-embryo cultures of rats at the maximum soluble concentration (Steele *et al.*, 1987). [The Working Group concluded that since etretinate is metabolized to acitretin, which itself is active *in vivo*, acitretin is the proximate teratogen.]

7.3   Genetic and related effects

Etretinate at a concentration of 1–50 mg/ml had no effect on sister chromatid exchange frequency in exponentially growing Chinese hamster V79 cells (Sirianni *et al.*, 1981).

8.   Summary of Data

8.1   Chemistry, occurrence and human exposure

Etretinate [ethyl all-*trans*-3,7-dimethyl-9-(4-methoxy-2,3,6-trimetriphenyl)nona-2,4,6,8-tetraenoate) is a synthetic retinoid of the aromatic class which is structurally related to all-*trans*-retinoic acid. Because of its conjugated tetraene structure, etretinate has characteristic absorption in the ultraviolet and visible spectra and readily undergoes photoisomerization in solution to multiple geometric isomers. Etretinate is a highly lipophilic molecule which is readily partitioned into hydrophobic compartments, including human adipose tissue.

Etretinate is a purely synthetic compound which can readily be prepared by various routes. Human exposure occurs entirely during treatment with formulations for oral administration, primarily for dermatological indications. Etretinate has been replaced by acitretin in most countries. The recommended doses were 0.25–1.5 mg/kg bw per day.

A variety of normal-phase and reversed-phase high-performance liquid chromatographic methods is available for the detection and quantification of etretinate and its geometric isomers.

8.2 Metabolism and kinetics

Etretinate must be metabolized to its free acid form in order to exert biological activity. The pharmacokinetics of etretinate has been studied extensively, particularly in patients with psoriasis. In both humans and experimental animals, the tissue distribution of etretinate is influenced primarily by its lipophilicity.

8.3 Cancer-preventive effects

8.3.1 Humans

Etretinate was evaluated in six randomized trials for its efficacy in preventing the recurrence of superficial tumours of the urinary bladder. None showed unequivocal evidence of an effect of treatment; efficacy was suggested in analyses of some end-points. Controls receiving placebo were used in three of these trials, whereas the controls in the largest study were untreated.

Etretinate was not effective in preventing second primary tumours in subjects with head-and-neck tumours when compared with those given placebo.

In two reports of the same study without a separate control group, etretinate was reported to reduce an index of metaplasia in bronchial biopsy samples from heavy smokers. In a randomized trial involving 150 subjects, however, etretinate showed no efficacy in reducing atypia in sputum samples when compared with placebo.

In one study with no controls in which etretinate was given orally at a high dose or orally at a moderate dose plus topical application as a paste, regression of leukoplakia of the mouth was reported, more notably when topical application was added.

In one study with no controls, oral treatment with etretinate appeared to reduce the severity of actinic keratotic and keratocanthoma lesions of the skin. In two double-blind cross-over trials involving patients with actinic keratosis, improvement in terms of the number and size of lesions was reported in patients treated orally with etretinate, although no statistical analysis was reported for either trial.

8.3.2 Experimental models

The cancer-preventive efficacy of etretinate has been assessed in mouse, rat and rabbit models and in virus-induced tumours. It was ineffective in a skin tumorigenesis model in mice but effective in a similar model in rabbits. In one study in mice, etretinate reduced the size of skin papillomas. It was effective in various models of digestive tract carcinogenesis in mice and rats.

In single studies, etretinate was ineffective in preventing either leukaemia or lung tumours but was effective in preventing urinary bladder carcinogenesis in rats. It was effective in three studies in models of benign tumours induced in mice by Shope papilloma virus and malignant tumours induced by Rous sarcoma virus.

In some experimental models, etretinate enhanced the tumorigenic effects of carcinogens.

Etretinate has been shown to modify differentiation in several models *in vitro*: in hamsters, squamous metaplasia induced by vitamin A deficiency was reversed. Since metaplasia is considered to be a potential precursor of neoplasia, this activity of etretinate is considered to be significant. In respiratory tracts exposed to carcinogens, it inhibited loss of mucus secretion and ciliary action. In many studies with human and animal keratinocytes, etretinate causes changes in differentiation similar to those seen after treatment with all-*trans*-retinoic acid, and in one study it modified the toxic effects of 2,3,7,8-tetrachlorodibenzo-*para*-dioxin. In contrast to all-*trans*-retinoic acid, it did not induce differentiation in promyelocytic leukaemic cell lines. It inhibited proliferation in murine and human melanoma cell lines, in lymphoblastoid lines and in normal keratinocytes. Because of differences in the experimental protocols, it is not clear whether etretinate is selectively active against tumour cells. In all cases, it was less active than all-*trans*-retinoic acid. Etretinate has been studied in many models of immune function *in vitro*, but no consistent responses were reported.

8.3.3 Mechanisms of cancer prevention

The active form of etretinate is acitretin. There have been no detailed studies of the mechanism of action of etretinate. Its ability to inhibit the induction of ornithine decarboxylase in keratinocytes after treatment with phytohaemag-glutinin suggests that, like all-*trans*-retinoic acid, it acts in the promotional phase of carcinogenesis.

8.4 Other beneficial effects

Etretinate was demonstrated to be of benefit to patients with psoriasis or congenital lamellar ichthyosis.

8.5 Carcinogenic effects
8.5.1 Human studies

Only case reports were available to the Working Group.

8.5.2 Experimental models

No data were available to the Working Group; however, in one study of prevention, etretinate enhanced lung carcinogenesis in rats.

8.6 Other toxic effects
8.6.1 Humans

Long-term treatment with etretinate for dermato-logical disorders may result in several toxic effects, including mucocutaneous, skeletal, hepatic, ocular, neurological (headache) and neuromuscular complications, and abnormal concentrations of serum lipids. Children given etretinate can experience progressive skeletal toxicity.

Etretinate is a confirmed human teratogen. In view of its long elimination half-life of 100 days, pregnancy should be avoided for at least two years after exposure. Terata arising from exposure include meningomyelocoele, malformations of the chrondrocranium and viscerocranium, the tetralogy of Fallot, ventricular septal defect, anophthalmia, malformations of the hip, ankle and forearm, syndactyly, short digits, imperforate anus and genitourinary disorders. Malformations occur after daily exposure to 0.4–1.5 mg/kg bw. Clinical experience shows that the risk of death of embryos exposed to etretinate is greatest when exposure occurs during the first three weeks of pregnancy. The teratogenic risk is highest when exposure occurs during weeks 4–8 of pregnancy.

8.6.2 Experimental models

Studies of toxicity in experimental animals reflect the spectrum of effects observed in human beings. It causes sterility in males after long-term administration at high doses. It was not active in two tests for teratogenicity *in vitro*, but it is metabolized *in vivo* to acitretin, which is a potent teratogen, and therefore produced the typical retinoid embryopathy of the central nervous system, craniofacial region, limbs, heart, genitourinary tract and tail. In general, etretinate appears to be more teratogenic than all-*trans*-retinoic acid in experimental animals.

Etretinate did not induce sister chromatid exchange in hamster cells in a single study.

9. Recommendations for Research

9.1 General recommendations for etretinate and other retinoids

See section 9 of the Handbook on all-*trans*-retinoic acid.

9.2 Recommendations specific to etretinate

None.

10. Evaluation

10.1 Cancer-preventive activity
10.1.1 Humans

There is *inadequate evidence* that etretinate has cancer-preventive activity in humans.

10.1.2 Experimental animals

There is *limited evidence* that etretinate has cancer-preventive activity in experimental animals. This evaluation is based on the observation of inhibitory effects in single studies with models of skin, digestive tract and urinary bladder carcinogenesis and in three models of virus-induced tumours.

10.2 Overall evaluation

There is *inadequate evidence* for the cancer-preventive activity of etretinate in humans and *limited evidence* in experimental animals. Etretinate is toxic and a confirmed human teratogen, and is no longer available for use in most countries.

11.   References

Agnish, N.D., Vane, F.M., Rusin, G., DiNardo, B. & Dashman, T. (1990) Teratogenicity of etretinate during early pregnancy in the rat and its correlation with maternal plasma concentrations of the drug. *Teratology,* **42**, 25–33

Alfthan, O., Tarkkanen, J., Gröhn, P., Heinonen, E., Pyrhönen, S. & Säilä, K. (1983) Tigason® (etretinate) in prevention of recurrence of superficial bladder tumors. A double-blind clinical trial. *Eur. Urol.,* **9**, 6–9

Alles, A.J. & Sulik, K.K. (1992) Pathogenesis of retinoid-induced hindbrain malformations in an experimental model. *Clin. Dysmorphol.,* **1**, 187–200

Annesley, T., Giacherio, D., Wilkerson, K., Grekin, R. & Ellis, C. (1984) Analysis of retinoids by high-performance liquid chromatography using programmed gradient separation. *J. Chromatogr.,* **305**, 199–203

Aoyagi, T., Kamigaki, K., Saruta, M., Iizuka, H. & Miura, Y. (1981a) Retinoid inhibits keratin formation of pig skin explants. *J. Dermatol.,* **8**, 207–213

Aoyagi, T., Kamigaki, K., Kato, N., Fukaya, T., Iizuka, H. & Miura, Y. (1981b) Retinoid stimulates epidermal outgrowth of pig skin explants. *J. Dermatol.,* **8**, 197–205

Arnold, A.M., Browman, G.P., Levine, M.N., D'Souza, T., Johnstone, B., Skingley, P., Turner-Smith, L., Cayco, R., Booker, L., Newhouse, M. & Hryniuk, W.M. (1992) The effect of the synthetic retinoid etretinate on sputum cytology: Results from a randomised trial. *Br. J. Cancer,* **65**, 737–743

Athanassiades, T.J. (1981) Adjuvant effect of vitamin A palmitate and analogs on cell-mediated immunity. *J. Natl Cancer Inst.,* **67**, 1153–1156

Aurell, M.J., Ceita, L., Mestres, R., Parra, M. & Tortajada, A. (1995) Trienediolates of hexadienoic acids in synthesis. Addition to unsaturated ketones. A convergent approach to the synthesis of retinoic acids. *Tetrahedron,* **51**, 3915–3928

Bauer, E.A., Seltzer, J.L. & Eisen, A.Z. (1983) Retinoic acid inhibition of collagenase and gelatinase expression in human skin fibroblast cultures. Evidence for a dual mechanism. *J. Invest. Dermatol.,* **81**, 162–169

Berbis, P., Bounameaux, Y., Rognin, C., Hartmann, D. & Privat, Y. (1987) Study on the influence of etretinate on biologic activity of oral contraceptives. *J. Am. Acad. Dermatol.,* **17**, 302–303

Berger, M.R. & Schmähl, D. (1986) Protection by the alkyllysophospholipid, 1-octadecyl-2-methoxy-*rac*-glycero-3-phosphocholine, but not by the retinoid etretinate against leukemia development in DMBA-treated Long-Evans rats. *Cancer Lett.,* **30**, 73–78

Berkers, J.A., Hassing, I., Spenkelink, B., Brouwer, A. & Blaauboer, B.J. (1995) Interactive effects of 2,3,7,8-tetrachlorodibenzo-p-dioxin and retinoids on proliferation and differentiation in cultured human keratinocytes: Quantification of cross-linked envelope formation. *Arch. Toxicol.,* **69**, 368–378

Bestmann, H.J. & Ermann, P. (1984) Retinoids and carotenoids. Synthesis of (13*Z*)-retinoic acids. *Liebigs Ann. Chem.,* 1740–1745

Binazzi, M. & Cicilioni, E.G. (1979) Systemic treatment of Darier's disease with a new retinoid (RO 10-9359). *Arch. Dermatol. Res.,* **264**, 365–367

Blake, K.D. & Wyse, R.K.H. (1988) Embryopathy in infant conceived one year after termination of maternal etretinate: A reappraisal. *Lancet,* **ii**, 1254

Bolla, M., Lefur, R., Ton Van, J., Domenge, C., Badet, J.M., Koskas, Y. & Laplanche, A. (1994) Prevention of second primary tumours with etretinate in squamous cell carcinoma of the oral cavity and oropharynx. Results of a multicentric double-blind randomised study. *Eur. J. Cancer,* **30A**, 767–772

Bolla, M., Laplanche, A., Lefur, R., Ton Van, J., Domenge, C., Lefebvre, J.L. & Luboinski, B. (1996) Prevention of second primary tumours with a second generation retinoid in squamous cell carcinoma of oral cavity and oropharynx: Long term follow-up. *Eur. J. Cancer,* **32A**, 375–376

Bollag, W. (1974) Therapeutic effects of an aromatic retinoic acid analog on chemically induced skin papillomas and carcinomas of mice. *Eur. J. Cancer,* **10**, 731–737

Bollag, W., Ruegg, R. & Ryser, G. (1978) 9-Phenyl 5,6-dimethyl-nona-2,4,6,8-tetraeonic acid compounds. United States Patent, No. 4 105 681 (8 August 1978)

Bonnetblanc, J.M., Hugon, J., Dumas, M. & Rupin, D. (1983) Intracranial hypertension with etretinate. *Lancet,* **ii**, 974

Bouvy, M.L., Sturkenboom, M.C., Cornel, M.C., de Jong-van den Berg, L.T., Stricker, B.H. & Wesseling, H. (1992) Acitretin (Neotigason®). A review of pharmacokinetics and teratogenicity and hypothesis on metabolic pathways. *Pharm. Weekbl. Sci.,* **14**, 33–37

Bray, M.A. (1984) Retinoids are potent inhibitors of the generation of rat leukocyte leukotriene B4-like activity in vitro. *Eur. J. Pharmacol.,* **98**, 61–67

Brun, P. & Baran, R. (1986) Neonatal ichthyosis treated for seven years with etretinate without side-effects on growth or ossification: A case report. *Curr. Ther. Res.,* **40**, 657–663

Budavari, S., O'Neil, M.J., Smith, A. & Heckelman, P.E. (1989) *The Merck Index. An Encyclopedia of Chemicals, Drugs, and Biologicals.* 11th Ed. Rahway, NJ, Merck & Co.

Burge, S. & Ryan, T. (1985) Diffuse hyperostosis associated with etretinate. *Lancet*, **ii**, 397–398

Campbell, J.P., Grekin, R.C., Ellis, C.N., Matsuda John, S.S., Swanson, N.A. & Voorhees, J.J. (1983) Retinoid therapy is associated with excess granulation tissue responses. *J. Am. Acad. Dermatol.*, **9**, 708–713

Cappelletti, V., Granata, G., Miodini, P., Coradini, D., Di Fronzo, G., Cairoli, F., Colombo, G., Nava, A. & Scanziani, E. (1988) Modulation of receptor levels in canine breast tumors by administration of tamoxifen and etretinate either alone or in combination. *Anticancer Res.*, **8**, 1297–1301

Carillet, V., Morliere, P., Maziere, J.C., Huppe, G., Santus, R. & Dubertret, L. (1990) In vitro interactions of the aromatic retinoids Ro 10-9359 (etretinate) and Ro 10-1670 (acitretin), its main metabolite, with human serum lipoproteins and albumin. *Biochim. Biophys. Acta*, **1055**, 98–101

Carmichael, A.J. & Paul, C.J. (1989) Reversible gynaecomastia associated with etretinate. *Br. J. Dermatol.*, **120**, 317–325

Chaidaroglou, A., Degiannis, D., Koniavitou, K., Georgiou, S. & Tsambaos, D. (1998) In vitro effects of retinoids on mitogen-induced peripheral blood leucocyte responses. *Arch. Dermatol. Res.*, **290**, 205–210

Chan, A., Keane, R.J., Hanna, M. & Abbott, M. (1995) Terminations of pregnancy for exposure to oral retinoids in South Australia, 1985–1993. *Aust. N. Z. J. Obstet. Gynaecol.*, **35**, 422–426

Charbit, L., Mangin, P., Rognin, C. & Cukier, J. (1983) Etretinate in the prevention of recurrences of superficial bladder tumors. Clinical trial using the double-blind method. *J. Urol. Paris*, **89**, 247–249

Chien, D.S., Sandri, R.B. & Tang-Liu, D.S. (1992) Systemic pharmacokinetics of acitretin, etretinate, isotretinoin, and acetylenic retinoids in guinea pigs and obese rats. *Drug Metab. Dispos.*, **20**, 211–217

Chomienne, C., Balitrand, N. & Abita, J.P. (1986) Inefficacy of the synthetic aromatic retinoid etretinate and of its free acid on the in-vitro differentiation of leukemic cells. *Leuk. Res.*, **10**, 1079–1081

Collin, S., Copsey, A. & Ferguson, S. (1989) A harlequin baby survives. *Nurs. Times*, **85**, 28–31

Collins, M.R., James, W.D. & Rodman, O.G. (1986) Etretinate photosensitivity. *J. Am. Acad. Dermatol.*, **14**, 274–274

Cordero, A.A., Allevato, M.A. & Donatti, L. (1981) Ro 10-9359 and pregnancy. In: Orfanos, C.E., Braun-Falco, O., Farber, E.M., Grupper, C., Polano, M.K. & Schuppli, R., eds, *Retinoids. Advances in Basic Research and Therapy.* Berlin, Springer Verlag, p. 501

Cribier, B., Welsch, M. & Heid, E. (1992) Renal impairment probably induced by etretinate. *Dermatology*, **185**, 266–268

Crivellato, E. (1982) A rosacea-like eruption induced by Tigason (Ro 10-9359) treatment. *Acta Derm. Venereol.*, **62**, 450–452

Cunningham, W.J. & Ehmann, C.W. (1983) Clinical aspects of the retinoids. *Semin. Dermatol.*, **2**, 145–160

Dai, W.S., LaBraico, J.M. & Stern, R.S. (1992) Epidemiology of isotretinoin exposure during pregnancy. *J. Am. Acad. Dermatol.*, **26**, 599–606

David, M., Shohat, B., Hodak, E. & Sandbank, M. (1990) Effect of etretinate on peripheral T lymphocytes in psoriatic patients before, during and after 6 months of therapy. *Dermatologica*, **180**, 86–89

De Leenheer, A.P., Lambert, W.E., De Bersaques, J.P. & Kint, A.H. (1990) High-performance liquid chromatographic determination of etretinate and all-*trans*- and 13-*cis*-acitretin in human plasma. *J. Chromatogr.*, **500**, 637–642

Decker, M.A. & Zimmerman, C.L. (1995) Simultaneous determination of etretinate, acitretin and their metabolites in perfusate, perfusate plasma, bile or hepatic tissue with reversed-phase high-performance liquid chromatography. *J. Chromatogr. B. Biomed. Appl.*, **667**, 105–113

Desablens, B., Muir, J.F. & Andrejak, M. (1989) Manifestations of Hodgkin's disease caused by retinoids? *Therapie*, **44**, 301–302

DiGiovanna, J.J., Gross, E.G., McClean, S.W., Ruddel, M.E., Gantt, G. & Peck, G.L. (1984) Etretinate: Effect of milk intake on absorption. *J. Invest. Dermatol.*, **82**, 636–640

DiGiovanna, J.J., Helfgott, R.K., Gerber, L.H. & Peck, G.L. (1986) Extraspinal tendon and ligament calcification associated with long-term therapy with etretinate. *N. Engl. J. Med.*, **315**, 1177–1182

DiGiovanna, J.J., Zech, L.A., Ruddel, M.E., Gantt, G. & Peck, G.L. (1989) Etretinate. Persistent serum levels after long-term therapy. *Arch. Dermatol.*, **125**, 246–251

Dubertret, L., Lebreton, C. & Touraine, R. (1982) Inhibition of neutrophil migration by etretinate and its main metabolite. *Br. J. Dermatol.*, **107**, 681–685

Dunsford, H.A., Dolan, P.M., Seed, J.L. & Bueding, E. (1984) Effects of multiple putative anticarcinogens on the carcinogenicity of *trans*-5-amino-3-[2-(5-nitro-2-furyl)vinyl]-1,2,4-oxadiazole. *J. Natl Cancer Inst.*, **73**, 161–168

Dupuy, P., Bagot, M., Heslan, M. & Dubertret, L. (1989) Synthetic retinoids inhibit the antigen presenting properties of epidermal cells in vitro. *J. Invest. Dermatol.*, **93**, 455–459

Eichner, R., Kahn, M., Capetola, R.J., Gendimenico, G.J. & Mezick, J.A. (1992) Effects of topical retinoids on cytoskeletal proteins: Implications for retinoid effects on epidermal differentiation. *J. Invest. Dermatol.*, **98**, 154–161

Eisenhardt, E.U. & Bickel, M.H. (1994) Kinetics of tissue distribution and elimination of retinoid drugs in the rat. II. Etretinate. *Drug Metab. Dispos.*, **22**, 31–35

Ellis, C.N. & Voorhees, J.J. (1987) Etretinate therapy. *J. Am. Acad. Dermatol.*, **16**, 267–291

Ellis, C.N., Swanson, N.A., Grekin, R.C., Goldstein, N.G., Bassett, D.R., Anderson, T.F. & Voorhees, J.J. (1982) Etretinate therapy causes increases in lipid levels in patients with psoriasis. *Arch. Dermatol.*, **118**, 559–562

Ellis, C.N., Kang, S., Grekin, R.C., LoBuglio, A.F. & Voorhees, J.J. (1985a) Etretinate therapy for psoriasis. Reduction of antibody-dependent cell-mediated cytotoxicity of polymorphonuclear leukocytes. *Arch. Dermatol.*, **121**, 877–880

Ellis, C.N., Pennes, D.R., Madison, K.C., Gilbert, M., Martel, W., Voorhees, J.J. & Cunningham, W.J. (1985b) Skeletal radiographic changes during retinoid therapy. In: Saurat, J.H., ed., *Retinoids. New Trends of Research and Therapy*. Basel, Karger, pp. 440–444

Englert, G., Weber, S. & Klaus, M. (1978) Isolation by HPLC and identification by NMR spectroscopy of 11 mono-, di- and tri-*cis* isomers of an aromatic analogue of retinoic acid, ethyl all-*trans*-9-(4-methoxy-2,3,6-trimethylphenyl)-3,7-dimethyl-nona-2,4,6,8-tetraenoate. *Helv. Chim. Acta*, **61**, 2697–2708

Evans, R.M. (1988) The steroid and thyroid hormone receptor superfamily. *Science*, **240**, 889–895

Fartasch, M., Vigneswaran, N., Diepgen, T.L. & Hornstein, O.P. (1990) Abnormalities of keratinocyte maturation and differentiation in keratosis palmoplantaris striata. Immunohistochemical and ultrastructural study before and during etretinate therapy. *Am. J. Dermatopathol.*, **12**, 275–282

Ferguson, M.M., Simpson, N.B. & Hammersley, N. (1983) Severe nail dystrophy associated with retinoid therapy. *Lancet*, **ii**, 974–974

Foged, E.K. & Jacobsen, F.K. (1982) Side effects due to RO 10-9359 (Tigason). A retrospective study. *Dermatologica*, **164**, 395–403

Foged, E., Bjerring, P., Kragballe, K., Sogaard, H. & Zachariae, H. (1984) Histologic changes in the liver during etretinate treatment. *J. Am. Acad. Dermatol.*, **11**, 580–583

Fontan, B., Bonafe, J.L. & Moatti, J.P. (1983) Toxic effects of the aromatic retinoid etretinate. *Arch. Dermatol.*, **119**, 187–188

Frankel, J.W., Horton, E.J., Winters, A.L., Samis, H.V. & Ito, Y. (1980) Inhibitory effects of an aromatic retinoid (Ro 10-9359) on viral tumorigenesis. *Intervirology*, **14**, 321–325

Fredriksson, T. & Pettersson, U. (1978) Severe psoriasis—Oral therapy with a new retinoid. *Dermatologica*, **157**, 238–244

Fujita, J. & Yoshida, O. (1984) Inhibitory effects of aromatic retinoic acid analog, administered alone or in combination with mitomycin C, on the *in vitro* growth of rat bladder carcinoma cells. *Hinyokika Kiyo*, **30**, 1627–1631

Fulton, R.A., Souteyrand, P. & Thivolet, J. (1982) Influence of retinoid Ro 10-9359 on cell-mediated immunity in vivo. *Dermatologica*, **165**, 568–572

Gale, J.B. (1993) Recent advances in the chemistry and biology of retinoids. In: Ellis, G.P. & Luscombe, D.K., eds, *Progress in Medicinal Chemistry*. Amsterdam, Elsevier Science, pp. 1–55

Galosi, A., Plewig, G. & Braun-Falco, O. (1985) The effect of aromatic retinoid Ro 10-9359 (etretinate) on fingernail growth. *Arch. Dermatol. Res.*, **277**, 138–140

Gaukroger, J.M., Wilson, L. & MacKie, R. (1985) Cytotoxicity of etretinate and vindesine. *Br. J. Cancer*, **52**, 369–375

Geiger, J.M., Baudin, M. & Saurat, J.H. (1994) Teratogenic risk with etretinate and acitretin treatment. *Dermatology*, **189**, 109–116

Gibson, G.E., O'Grady, A., Kay, E.W., Leader, M. & Murphy, G.M. (1997) p53 tumor suppressor gene protein expression in premalignant and malignant skin lesions of kidney transplant recipients. *J. Am. Acad. Dermatol.*, **36**, 924–931

Giguère, V., Ong, E.S., Segui, P. & Evans, R.M. (1987) Identification of a receptor for the morphogen retinoic acid. *Nature*, **330**, 624–629

Glazer, S.D., Roenigk, H.H., Jr, Yokoo, H. & Sparberg, M. (1982) A study of potential hepatotoxicity of etretinate used in the treatment of psoriasis. *J. Am. Acad. Dermatol.*, **6**, 683–687

Glazer, S.D., Roenigk, H.H.J., Yokoo, H., Sparberg, M. & Paravicini, U. (1984) Ultrastructural survey and tissue analysis of human livers after a 6-month course of etretinate. *J. Am. Acad. Dermatol.*, **10**, 632–638

Glover, M.T., Peters, A.M. & Atherton, D.J. (1987) Surveillance for skeletal toxicity of children treated with etretinate. *Br. J. Dermatol.*, **116**, 609–614

Goerz, G. & Orfanos, C.E. (1978) Systemic treatment of psoriasis with a new aromatic retinoid. Preliminary evaluation of a multicenter controlled study in the Federal Republic of Germany. *Dermatologica*, **157** (Suppl. 1), 38–44

Goldfarb, M.T. & Ellis, C.N. (1998) Clinical use of etretinate and acitretin. In: Roenigk, H.H. & Maibach, H.I., eds, *Psoriasis*, 3rd Ed. New York, Marcel Dekker, pp. 663–670

Gollnick, H. (1981) Elevated levels of triglycerides in patients with skin disease treated with oral aromatic retinoid. In: Orfanos, C.E., Braun-Falco, O., Farber, E.M., Grupper, C., Polano, M.K. & Schuppli, R., eds, *Retinoids. Advances in Basic Research and Therapy.* Berlin, Springer-Verlag, pp. 503–505

Gollnick, H. & Orfanos, C.E. (1985) Etretinate: Pro and con. Risk–benefit analysis of systemic retinoid therapy in psoriasis and recent developments: Free aromatic acid, arotinoids. *Hautarzt.*, **36**, 2–9

Gollnick, H., Ehlert, R., Rinck, G. & Orfanos, C.E. (1990) Retinoids: An overview of pharmacokinetics and therapeutic value. *Meth. Enzymol.*, **190**, 291–304

Gottlieb, S., Hayes, E., Gilleaudeau, P., Cardinale, I., Gottlieb, A.B. & Krueger, J.G. (1996) Cellular actions of etretinate in psoriasis: Enhanced epidermal differentiation and reduced cell-mediated inflammation are unexpected outcomes. *J. Cutan. Pathol.*, **23**, 404–418

Gouveia, J., Mathé, G., Hercend, T., Gros, F., Lemaigre, G., Santelli, G., Homasson, J.P., Gaillard, J.P., Angebault, M., Bonniot, J.P., Lededente, A., Marsac, J., Parrot, R. & Pretet, S. (1982) Degree of bronchial metaplasia in heavy smokers and its regression after treatment with a retinoid. *Lancet*, **i**, 710–712

Graham, R.M., James, M.P., Ferguson, D.J. & Guerrier, C.W. (1985) Acquired kinking of the hair associated with etretinate therapy. *Clin. Exp. Dermatol.*, **10**, 426–431

Granström, G. (1990) Retinoid-induced ear malformations. *Otolaryngol. Head Neck Surg.*, **103**, 702–709

Granström, G. & Kullaa-Mikkonen, A. (1990a) Experimental craniofacial malformations induced by retinoids and resembling branchial arch syndromes. *Scand. J. Plast. Reconstr. Surg. Hand Surg.*, **24**, 3–12

Granström, G. & Kullaa-Mikkonen, A. (1990b) Retinoid-induced nasal malformations. *ORL J. Otorhinolaryngol. Relat. Spec.*, **52**, 239–248

Granström, G., Kullaa-Mikkonen, A. & Zellin, G. (1990) Malformations of the maxillofacial region induced by retinoids in an experimental system. *Int. J. Oral Maxillofac. Surg.*, **19**, 167–171

Granström, G., Jacobsson, C. & Magnusson, B.C. (1991) Enzyme histochemical analysis of craniofacial malformations induced by retinoids. *Scand. J. Plast. Reconstr. Surg. Hand Surg.*, **25**, 133–141

Greaves, M.W. (1988) Embryopathy in infant conceived one year after termination of maternal etretinate: A reappraisal. *Lancet*, **ii**, 1254

Grote, W., Harms, D., Janig, U., Kietzmann, H., Ravens, U. & Schwarze, I. (1985) Malformation of fetus conceived 4 months after termination of maternal etretinate treatment. *Lancet*, **i**, 1276

Grupper, C. & Berretti, B. (1983) Cutaneous neoplasia and etretinate. In: Spitzy, K. H. & Karrer, K., eds, *Proceedings of the 13th International Congress of Chemo-therapy*, Vienna, Austria, Vienna, B.H. Egermann, pp. 24–27

Hadjiolov, D. & Grueva, D. (1986) Effect of combined Tigason and selenium treatment on colon carcinogenesis. *J. Cancer Res. Clin. Oncol.*, **112**, 285–286

Halioua, B. & Saurat, J.H. (1990) Risk:benefit ratio in the treatment of psoriasis with systemic retinoids. *Br. J. Dermatol.*, **122** (Suppl. 36), 135–150

Halkier-Sorensen, L. (1987) Menstrual changes in a patient treated with etretinate. *Lancet*, **ii**, 636

Halkier-Sorensen, L. (1988) Sexual dysfunction in a patient treated with etretinate. *Acta Derm. Venereol.*, **68**, 90–91

Halkier-Sorensen, L. & Andresen, J. (1989) A retrospective study of bone changes in adults treated with etretinate. *J. Am. Acad. Dermatol.*, **20**, 83–87

Hänni, R., Bigler, F., Vetter, W., Englert, G. & Loeliger, P. (1977) The metabolism of the retinoid Ro 10-9359. Isolation and identification of the major metabolites in human plasma, urine and feces. Synthesis of three urinary metabolites. *Helv. Chim. Acta*, **60**, 2309–2325

Happle, R., Traupe, H., Bounameaux, Y. & Fisch, T. (1984) Teratogenic effects of etretinate in humans. *Dtsch. Med. Wochenschr.*, **109**, 1476–1480

Harrison, P.V. (1987) Retinoids and malignancy. *Lancet*, **ii**, 801

Hashimoto, T., Dykes, P.J. & Marks, R. (1985) Retinoid-induced inhibition of growth and reduction of spreading of human epidermal cells in culture. *Br. J. Dermatol.*, **112**, 637–646

Hashimoto, Y., Ohkuma, N. & Iizuka, H. (1990) Effects of retinoids on DNA synthesis of pig epidermis: Its relation to epidermal beta-adrenergic adenylate cyclase response and to epidermal superoxide dismutase activity. *J. Dermatol. Sci.*, **1**, 303–309

Hast, R., Beksac, M., Axdorph, S., Sjogren, A.M., Ost, A. & Reizenstein, P. (1986) Effects of retinoids on in vitro differentiation of bone marrow cells in the myelodysplastic syndrome. *Med. Oncol. Tumor Pharmacother.*, **3**, 35–38

Hayashi, A., Suzuki, T. & Tajima, S. (1995a) Modulations of elastin expression and cell proliferation by retinoids in cultured vascular smooth muscle cells. *J. Biochem. Tokyo*, **117**, 132–136

Hayashi, M., Takizawa, S., Fukatsu, N., Imamura, I., Shimura, K. & Horii, I. (1995b) Male fertility in rats treated with etretinate for 4 weeks. *J. Toxicol. Sci.*, **20**, 281–296

Hays, S.B. & Camisa, C. (1985) Acquired pili torti in two patients treated with synthetic retinoids. *Cutis*, **35**, 466–468

Henderson, C.A. & Highet, A.S. (1989) Depression induced by etretinate. *Br. Med. J.*, **298**, 964

Heyman, R.A., Mangelsdorf, D.J., Dyck, J.A., Stein, R.B., Eichele, G., Evans, R.M. & Thaller, C. (1992) 9-*cis* Retinoic acid is a high affinity ligand for the retinoid X receptor. *Cell*, **68**, 397–406

Hill, D.L. & Sani, B.P. (1991) Metabolic disposition and development of new chemopreventive retinoids. *Drug Metab. Rev.*, **23**, 413–438

Hirao, Y., Okajima, E., Ohara, S., Ozono, S., Hiramatsu, T., Yoshida, K., Yamada, K., Aoyama, H., Hashimoto, M. & Watanabe, S. (1987) Prophylactic treatment for superficial bladder cancer following transurethral resection. *Cancer Chemother. Pharmacol.*, **20** (Suppl.), S85–S90

Hodak, E., David, M. & Feuerman, E.J. (1984) Excess granulation tissue during etretinate therapy. *J. Am. Acad. Dermatol.*, **11**, 1166–1167

Hodak, E., David, M., Gadoth, N. & Sandbank, M. (1987) Etretinate-induced skeletal muscle damage. *Br. J. Dermatol.*, **116**, 623–626

Hönigsmann, H., Fritsch, P. & Jaschke, E. (1978) Hyperkeratotic variant of Darier's disease. Successful oral treatment using an aromatic retinoid (Ro 10-9395). *Hautarzt*, **29**, 601–603

Imcke, E., Ruszczak, Z., Mayer-da Silva, A., Detmar, M. & Orfanos, C.E. (1991) Cultivation of human dermal microvascular endothelial cells in vitro: Immunocytochemical and ultrastructural characterization and effect of treatment with three synthetic retinoids. *Arch. Dermatol. Res.*, **283**, 149–157

Ippen, H., Hofbauer, M. & Schauder, S. (1978) Influence of a systemically administered aromatic retinoid (Ro 10-9359) on the light sensitivity. *Derm. Beruf. Umwelt.*, **26**, 88–90

Ito, Y. (1981) Effect of an aromatic retinoic acid analog (Ro 10-9359) on growth of virus-induced papilloma (Shope) and related neoplasia of rabbits. *Eur. J. Cancer*, **17**, 35–42

Jacobsson, C. & Granström, G. (1996) Prevention of etretinate-induced craniofacial malformations by vitamin B_6 in the rat. *Eur. J. Oral Sci.*, **104**, 583–588

Jacobsson, C. & Granström, G. (1997) Etretinate-induced malformation of the first two branchial arches: Differential staining and microdissection study of embryonic cartilage. *ORL J. Otorhinolaryngol. Relat. Spec.*, **59**, 147–154

Jäger, K., Schiller, F. & Stech, P. (1985) Congenital ichthyosiforme erythroderma, pregnancy under aromatic retinoid treatment. *Hautarzt*, **36**, 150–153

Jakobsen, P., Larsen, F.G. & Larsen, C.G. (1987) Simultaneous determination of the aromatic retinoids etretin and etretinate and their main metabolites by reversed-phase liquid chromatography. *J. Chromatogr.*, **415**, 413–418

Jansén, C.T., Viander, M. & Koulu, L. (1985) Effect of oral retinoid treatment on human natural killer cell activity. *Dermatologica*, **171**, 220–225

Juhlin, L. (1983) Ear ache during etretinate treatment. *Acta Derm. Venereol.*, **63**, 181–182

Kamm, J.J. (1982) Toxicology, carcinogenicity, and teratogenicity of some orally administered retinoids. *J. Am. Acad. Dermatol.*, **6**, 652–659

Kaplan, G. & Haettich, B. (1991) Rheumatological symptoms due to retinoids. *Baillieres Clin. Rheumatol.*, **5**, 77–97

Kaplan, R.P., Russell, D.H. & Lowe, N.J. (1983) Etretinate therapy for psoriasis: Clinical responses, remission times, epidermal DNA and polyamine responses. *J. Am. Acad. Dermatol.*, **8**, 95–102

Kelly, G.E., Meikle, W.D. & Sheil, A.G. (1989) Effects of oral retinoid (vitamin A and etretinate) therapy on photocarcinogenesis in hairless mice. *Photochem. Photobiol.*, **50**, 213–215

Kietzmann, H., Schwarze, I., Grote, W., Ravens, U., Jänig, U. & Harms, D. (1986) Embryonal malformation following etretinate therapy of Darier's disease in the mother. *Dtsch. Med. Wochenschr.*, **111**, 60–62

Kim, S.H., Son, C.S., Lee, J.W., Tockgo, Y.C. & Chun, Y.H. (1995) Visceral heterotaxy syndrome induced by reti-noids in mouse embryo. *J. Korean Med. Sci.*, **10**, 250–257

King, I.A. & Pope, F.M. (1984) Retinoids increase the incorporation of D-[³H]galactose into epidermal glycoproteins. *Biochem. Biophys. Res. Commun.*, **121**, 364–371

Kistler, A. (1987) Limb bud cell cultures for estimating the teratogenic potential of compounds. Validation of the test system with retinoids. *Arch. Toxicol.*, **60**, 403–414

Koch, H.F. (1981) Effect of retinoids on precancerous lesions of oral mucosa. In: Orfanos, C.E., ed., *Retinoids. Advances in Basic Research and Therapy.* Berlin, Springer Verlag, pp. 307–312

Kochhar, D.M., Penner, J.D. & Minutella, L.M. (1989) Biotransformation of etretinate and developmental toxicity of etretin and other aromatic retinoids in teratogenesis bioassays. *Drug Metab. Dispos.*, **17**, 618–624

Kramer, M. (1982) Excessive cerumen production due to the aromatic retinoid Tigason in a patient with Darier's disease. *Acta Derm. Venereol.*, **62**, 267–268

Krari, N., Mauras, Y. & Allain, P. (1989) Effects of etretinate on the distribution of elements in rats. *Biol. Trace Elem. Res.*, **22**, 113–118

Krause, W. (1988) Diagnosis of erectile dysfunction in etretinate treatment. *Acta Derm. Venereol.*, **68**, 458–458

Kremer, I., Gaton, D.D., David, M., Gaton, E. & Shapiro, A. (1994) Toxic effects of systemic retinoids on meibomian glands. *Ophthalmic Res.*, **26**, 124–128

Kubota, Y., Shimotake, T., Yanagihara, J. & Iwai, N. (1998) Development of anorectal malformations using etretinate. *J. Pediatr. Surg.*, **33**, 127–129

Ladoux, A., Cragoe, E.J.J., Geny, B., Abita, J.P. & Frelin, C. (1987) Differentiation of human promyelocytic HL 60 cells by retinoic acid is accompanied by an increase in the intracellular pH. The role of the Na$^+$/H$^+$ exchange system. *J. Biol. Chem.*, **262**, 811–816

Lambert, D., Dalac, S., Escallier, F., Foucher, J.L. & Mounicq, F. (1988) Malformation of fetus after maternal etretinate treatment. *Nouv. Dermatol.*, **7**, 448–451

Lammer, E.J. (1988) Embryopathy in infant conceived one year after termination of maternal etretinate. *Lancet*, **ii**, 1080–1081

Lammers, A.M. & van de Kerkhof, P.C. (1987) Etretinate modulates the leukotriene B$_4$ induced intra-epidermal accumulation of polymorphonuclear leukocytes. *Br. J. Dermatol.*, **117**, 297–300

Larsen, F.G. (1994) Pharmacokinetics of etretinate and acitretin with special reference to treatment of psoriasis. *Acta Derm. Venereol. Suppl. Stockh.*, **190**, 1–33

Lasnitzki, I. & Bollag, W. (1982) Prevention and reversal by a retinoid of 3,4-benzpyrene- and cigarette smoke condensate-induced hyperplasia and metaplasia of rodent respiratory epithelia in organ culture. *Cancer Treat. Rep.*, **66**, 1375–1380

Lassus, A. (1980) Systemic treatment of psoriasis with an oral retinoic acid derivative (Ro 10-9359). *Br. J. Dermatol.*, **102**, 195–202

Lauharanta, J. (1980) Retinoids in the treatment and prevention of dermatoses and epithelial neoplasias. *Ann. Clin. Res.*, **12**, 123–130

Lauharanta, J. (1982) Clinical, ultrastructural and biochemical effects of an aromatic retinoid (etretinate) on psoriasis and Darier's disease. *Acta Derm. Venereol. Suppl. Stockh.*, **101**, 1–29

Lauharanta, J., Käpyaho, K. & Kanerva, L. (1985) Changes in three-dimensional structure of cultured S91 mouse melanoma cells associated with growth inhibition and induction of melanogenesis by retinoids. *Arch. Dermatol. Res.*, **277**, 147–150

Lawlor, F. & Peiris, S. (1985a) Harlequin fetus successfully treated with etretinate. *Br. J. Dermatol.*, **112**, 585–590

Lawlor, F. & Peiris, S. (1985b) Progress of a harlequin fetus treated with etretinate. *J. R. Soc. Med.*, **78** (Suppl. 11), 19–20

Lehucher Ceyrac, D., Serfaty, D. & Lefrancq, H. (1992) Retinoids and contraception. *Dermatology*, **184**, 161–170

Lippman, S.M., Kessler, J.F. & Meyskens, F.L.., Jr (1987) Retinoids as preventive and therapeutic anticancer agents (Part II). *Cancer Treat. Rep.*, **71**, 493–515

Logan, R.A. (1987) Efficacy of etretinate for the PUVA-dependent psoriatic. *Clin. Exp. Dermatol.*, **12**, 98–102

Löfberg, B., Reiners, J., Spielmann, H. & Nau, H. (1990) Teratogenicity of steady-state concentrations of etretinate and metabolite acitretin maintained in maternal plasma and embryo by intragastric infusion during organogenesis in the mouse: A possible model for the extended elimination phase in human therapy. *Dev. Pharmacol. Ther.*, **15**, 45–51

Lowe, N.J. & David, M. (1998) Toxicity. In: Lowe, N. & Marks, R., eds, *Retinoids. A Clinicians' Guide*. St Louis, MO, Mosby, pp. 149–165

Lucek, R.W. & Colburn, W.A. (1985) Clinical pharmacokinetics of the retinoids. *Clin. Pharmacokinet.*, **10**, 38–62

Lucek, R.W., Dickerson, J., Carter, D.E., Bugge, C.J., Crews, T., Vane, F.M., Cunningham, W. & Colburn, W.A. (1988) Pharmacokinetics of ^{14}C-etretinate in healthy volunteers and two patients with biliary T-tube drainage. *Biopharm. Drug Dispos.*, **9**, 487–499

Lynberg, M.C., Khoury, M.J., Lammer, E.J., Waller, K.O., Cordero, J.F. & Erickson, J.D. (1990) Sensitivity, specificity, and positive predictive value of multiple malformations in isotretinoin embryopathy surveillance. *Teratology*, **42**, 513–519

Mahrle, G. & Berger, H. (1982) DMBA-induced tumors and their prevention by aromatic retinoid (Ro 10-9359). *Arch. Dermatol. Res.*, **272**, 37–47

Mahrle, G., Orfanos, C.E., Ippen, H. & Hofbauer, M. (1979) Hair growth, liver function and light sensitivity during oral retinoid therapy for psoriasis. *Dtsch. Med. Wochenschr.*, **104**, 473–477

Mahrle, G., Meyer-Hamme, S. & Ippen, H. (1982) Oral treatment of keratinizing disorders of skin and mucous membranes with etretinate. Comparative study of 113 patients. *Arch. Dermatol.*, **118**, 97–100

Majewski, S., Wolska, H., Jablonska, S. & Wasik, M. (1989) Effects of systemic etretinate treatment on natural cytotoxicity, immune angiogenesis and neutrophil adherence in patients with various forms of psoriasis. *Arch. Immunol. Ther. Exp. Warsz*, **37**, 459–464

Makin, S.M., Mikerin, I.E., Shavrygina, O.A. & Lanina, T.I. (1989) Stereoselective synthesis of the aromatic analogs of retinal and retinoic acid. *Zh. Org. Khim.*, **25**, 792–797

Marsden, J. (1986) Hyperlipidaemia due to isotretinoin and etretinate: Possible mechanisms and consequences. *Br. J. Dermatol.*, **114**, 401–407

Marsden, J.R. (1989) Lipid metabolism and retinoid therapy. *Pharmacol. Ther.*, **40**, 55–65

Martinez-Tallo, M.E., Galan-Gomez, E., Cordero-Carrasco, J.L., Hidalgo-Barquero, E.H., Campo-Sampedro, F.M. & Cardesa-Garcia, J.J. (1989) Penile agenesis and syndrome of multiple abnormalities associated with the ingestion of retinoic acid by the mother. *An. Esp. Pediatr.*, **31**, 399–400

McDonagh, A.J. & Harrington, C.I. (1989) Pseudo-porphyria complicating etretinate therapy. *Clin. Exp. Dermatol.*, **14**, 437–438

McIvor, A. (1992) Fatal toxic epidermal necrolysis associated with etretinate. *Br. Med. J.*, **304**, 548

McKerrow, K.J., Mackie, R.M., Lesko, M.J. & Pearson, C. (1988) The effect of oral retinoid therapy on the normal human immune system. *Br. J. Dermatol.*, **119**, 313–320

Mesrobian, H.G., Sessions, R.P., Lloyd, R.A. & Sulik, K.K. (1994) Cloacal and urogenital abnormalities induced by etretinate in mice. *J. Urol.*, **152**, 675–678

Meyskens, F.L., Jr & Salmon, S.E. (1979) Inhibition of human melanoma colony formation by retinoids. *Cancer Res.*, **39**, 4055–4057

Michaëlsson, G., Bergqvist, A., Vahlquist, A. & Vessby, B. (1981) The influence of 'Tigason' (Ro 10-9359) on the serum lipoproteins in man. *Br. J. Dermatol.*, **105**, 201–205

Mills, C.M. & Marks, R. (1993) Adverse reactions to oral retinoids. An update. *Drug Saf.*, **9**, 280–290

Misset, J.L., Mathe, G., Santelli, G., Gouveia, J., Homasson, J.P., Sudre, M.C. & Gaget, H. (1986) Regression of bronchial epidermoid metaplasia in heavy smokers with etretinate treatment. *Cancer Detect. Prev.*, **9**, 167–170

Mitchell, A.A. (1992) Oral retinoids. What should the prescriber known about their teratogenic hazards among women of child-bearing potential? *Drug Saf.*, **7**, 79–85

Molin, L., Thomsen, K., Volden, G. & Lange Wantzin, G. (1985) Retinoid dermatitis mimicking progression in mycosis fungoides: A report from the Scandinavian Mycosis Fungoides Group. *Acta Derm. Venereol.*, **65**, 69–71

Moriarty, M., Dunn, J., Darragh, A., Lambe, R. & Brick, I. (1982) Etretinate in treatment of actinic keratosis. A double-blind crossover study. *Lancet*, **i**, 364–365

Murasaki, G., Miyata, Y., Babaya, K., Arai, M., Fukushima, S. & Ito, N. (1980) Inhibitory effect of an aromatic retinoic acid analog on urinary bladder carcinogenesis in rats treated with N-butyl-N-(4-hydroxybutyl)nitrosamine. *Gann*, **71**, 333–340

Nayar, M. & Chin, G.Y. (1992) Harlequin fetus treated with etretinate. *Pediatr. Dermatol.*, **9**, 311–314

Neild, V.S., Moss, R.F., Marsden, R.A., Sanderson, K.V. & Fawcett, H.A. (1985) Retinoid-induced skin fragility in a patient with hepatic disease. *Clin. Exp. Dermatol.*, **10**, 459–465

Newton, D.L., Henderson, W.R. & Sporn, M.B. (1980) Structure–activity relationships of retinoids in hamster tracheal organ culture. *Cancer Res.*, **40**, 3413–3425

Niinimäki, A., Kallioinen, M. & Oikarinen, A. (1989) Etretinate reduces connective tissue degeneration in lichen sclerosus et atrophicus. *Acta Derm. Venereol.*, **69**, 439–442

Nolibe, D., Masse, R., Lafuma, J. & Florentin, I. (1983) Effect of chronic administration of a synthetic aromatic retinoid (Ro 10-9359) on the development of lung squamous metaplasia and epidermoid cancer in rats. *Adv. Exp. Med. Biol.*, **166**, 269–277

Nomura, H., Maeyama, Y., Matsuzaki, M. & Sasai, Y. (1994) The effect of orally-administered retinoid on lectin binding in guinea pig keratinocytes. *Kurume Med. J.*, **41**, 143–148

Nordlind, K. & Thyberg, J. (1983) In vitro effects of 13-cis-retinoic acid (Ro 4-3780) and etretinate (Ro 10-9359) on DNA synthesis and fine structure of guinea pig and human lymphoid cells. *Int. Arch. Allergy Appl. Immunol.*, **71**, 363–367

Oikarinen, A. & Salo, T. (1986) Effects of retinoids on type IV collagenolytic activity in melanoma cells. *Acta Derm. Venereol.*, 66, 346-348

Orfanos, C.E. (1980) Oral retinoids—Present status. *Br. J. Dermatol.*, 103, 473–481

Orfanos, C.E., Kurka, M. & Strunk, V. (1978) Oral treatment of keratosis follicularis with a new aromatic retinoid. *Arch. Dermatol.*, 114, 1211–1214

Orfanos, C.E., Ehlert, R. & Gollnick, H. (1987) The retinoids. A review of their clinical pharmacology and therapeutic use. *Drugs*, 34, 459–503

Orfanos, C.E., Zouboulis, C.C., Almond-Roesler, B. & Geilen, C.C. (1997) Current use and future potential role of retinoids in dermatology. *Drugs*, 53, 358–388

Ostlere, L.S., Langtry, J.A., Jones, S. & Staughton, R.C. (1991) Reduced therapeutic effect of warfarin caused by etretinate. *Br. J. Dermatol.*, 124, 505

Ott, F. (1981) Long-term biological tolerance of Ro 10-9359. In: Orfanos, C.E., ed., *Retinoids. Advances in Basic Research and Therapy*. Berlin, Springer Verlag, pp. 355–357

Paige, D.G., Judge, M.R., Shaw, D.G., Atherton, D.J. & Harper, J.I. (1992) Long-term etretinate therapy in childhood. *Br. J. Dermatol.*, 127, 23–24

Palmskog, G. (1980) Determination of plasma levels of two aromatic retinoic acid analogues with antipsoriatic activity by high-performance liquid chromatography. *J. Chromatogr.*, 221, 345–351

Paravicini, U. & Busslinger, A. (1983) Determination of etretinate and its main metabolite in human plasma using normal-phase high-performance liquid chromatography. *J. Chromatogr.*, 276, 359–366

Paravicini, U., Stockel, K., MacNamara, P.J., Hänni, R. & Busslinger, A. (1981) On metabolism and pharmacokinetics of an aromatic retinoid. *Ann. N. Y. Acad. Sci.*, 359, 54–67

Paul, C. & Dubertret, L. (1998) Acitretin and etretinate: Strategy for use and long-term side effects. In: Roenigk, H.H. & Maibach, H.I., eds, *Psoriasis*, 3rd Ed. New York, Marcel Dekker, pp. 671–683

Peck, G.L. (1981) Retinoids in clinical dermatology. In: Fleischmajer, R., ed., *Progress in Diseases of the Skin*. New York, Grune & Stratton, pp. 227–269

Peck, G.L. (1982) Retinoids. Therapeutic use in dermatology. *Drugs*, 24, 341–351

Peck, G.L. (1984) Synthetic retinoids in dermatology. In: Sporn, M.B., Roberts, A.B. & Goodman, D.S., eds, *The Retinoids*. Orlando, FL, Academic Press, pp. 391–411

Pedersen, H., Wolf, H., Jensen, S.K., Lund, F., Hansen, E., Olsen, P.R. & Sorensen, B.L. (1984) Administration of a retinoid as prophylaxis of recurrent non-invasive bladder tumors. *Scand. J. Urol. Nephrol.*, 18, 121–123

Petkovich, M., Brand, N.J., Krust, A. & Chambon, P. (1987) A human retinoic acid receptor which belongs to the family of nuclear receptors. *Nature*, 330, 444–450

Pomponi, F., Cariati, R., Zancai, P., De Paoli, P., Rizzo, S., Tedeschi, R.M., Pivetta, B., De Vita, S., Boiocchi, M. & Dolcetti, R. (1996) Retinoids irreversibly inhibit in vitro growth of Epstein-Barr virus-immortalized B lymphocytes. *Blood*, 88, 3147–3159

Prendiville, J., Bingham, E.A. & Burrows, D. (1986) Premature epiphyseal closure—A complication of etretinate therapy in children. *J. Am. Acad. Dermatol.*, 15, 1259–1262

Presbury, D.G. (1984) Intractable skin disorders treated with the aromatic retinoid etretinate. *S. Afr. Med. J.*, 65, 501–502

Redlich, C.A., Delisser, H.M. & Elias, J.A. (1995) Retinoic acid inhibition of transforming growth factor-β-induced collagen production by human lung fibroblasts. *Am. J. Respir. Cell. Mol. Biol.*, 12, 287–295

Reiners, J., Löfberg, B., Kraft, J.C., Kochhar, D.M. & Nau, H. (1988) Transplacental pharmacokinetics of teratogenic doses of etretinate and other aromatic retinoids in mice. *Reprod. Toxicol.*, 2, 19–29

Reynolds, O.D. (1991) Erectile dysfunction in etretinate treatment. *Arch. Dermatol.*, 127, 425–426

Rinck, G., Gollnick, H. & Orfanos, C.E. (1989) Duration of contraception after etretinate. *Lancet*, i, 845–846

Roenigk, H.H., Jr (1989) Liver toxicity of retinoid therapy. *Pharmacol. Ther.*, 40, 145–155

Roenigk, H.H., Jr, Gibstine, C., Glazer, S., Sparberg, M. & Yokoo, H. (1985) Serial liver biopsies in psoriatic patients receiving long-term etretinate. *Br. J. Dermatol.*, 112, 77–81

Rogers, M. & Scarf, C. (1989) Harlequin baby treated with etretinate. *Pediatr. Dermatol.*, 6, 216–221

Rollman, O., Berne, C. & Vahlquist, A. (1989) Etretinate and human adrenal function. *J. Am. Acad. Dermatol.*, 20, 133–134

Rosa, F.W. (1992) Retinoid embryopathy in humans. In: Koren, G., ed., *Retinoids in Clinical Practice. The Risk–Benefit Ratio*. New York, Marcel Dekker, pp. 77–109

Rosa, F.W., Wilk, A.L. & Kelsey, F.O. (1986) Teratogen update: Vitamin A congeners. *Teratology*, 33, 355–364

Rosinska, D., Wolska, H., Jablonska, S. & Konca, I. (1988) Etretinate in severe psoriasis of children. *Pediatr. Dermatol.*, 5, 266–272

Rudnicka, L., Marczak, M., Szmurlo, A., Makiela, B., Skiendzielewska, A., Skopinska, M., Majewski, S. & Jablonska, S. (1991) Acitretin decreases tumor cell-induced angiogenesis. *Skin Pharmacol.*, **4**, 150–153

Ruther, T.H. & Kietzmann, H. (1984) Pegnancy after therapy with etretinate. *Akt. Derm.*, **10**, 62–63

Sanchez, M.R., Ross, B., Rotterdam, H., Salik, J., Brodie, R. & Freedberg, I.M. (1993) Retinoid hepatitis. *J. Am. Acad. Dermatol.*, **28**, 853–858

Sanquer, S., Eller, M.S. & Gilchrest, B.A. (1993) Retinoids and state of differentiation modulate CRABP II gene expression in a skin equivalent. *J. Invest. Dermatol.*, **100**, 148–153

Schill, W.B., Wagner, A., Nikolowski, J. & Plewig, G. (1981) Aromatic retinoid and 13-*cis*-retinoic acid: Spermatological investigations. In: Orfanos, C.E., Braun-Falco, O., Farber, E.M., Grupper, C., Polano, M.K. & Schuppli, R., eds, *Retinoids. Advances in Basic Research and Therapy*. Berlin, Springer Verlag, pp. 389–395

Schmähl, D. & Habs, M. (1981) Experiments on the influence of an aromatic retinoid on the chemical carcinogenesis induced by N-nitroso-methylbenzyl-amine in rats. *Drug Res.*, **31**, 677–679

Shelnitz, L.S., Esterly, N.B. & Honig, P.J. (1987) Etretinate therapy for generalized pustular psoriasis in children. *Arch. Dermatol.*, **123**, 230–233

Shiohara, T., Imanishi, K., Sagawa, Y. & Nagashima, M. (1992) Differential effects of cyclosporine and etretinate on serum cytokine levels in patients with psoriasis. *J. Am. Acad. Dermatol.*, **27**, 568–574

Sillevis Smitt, J.H. & de Mari, F. (1984) A serious side-effect of etretinate (Tigason®). *Clin. Exp. Dermatol.*, **9**, 554–556

Sirianni, S.R., Chen, H.H. & Huang, C.C. (1981) Effects of retinoids on plating efficiency, sister-chromatid exchange (SCE) and mitomycin-C-induced SCE in cultured Chinese hamster cells. *Mutat. Res.*, **90**, 175–182

Soukup, M., Broger, E. & Widmer, E. (1989) New approaches to some aromatic retinoids. *Helv. Chim. Acta*, **72**, 370–376

Steele, C.E., Marlow, R., Turton, J. & Hicks, R.M. (1987) In-vitro teratogenicity of retinoids. *Br. J. Exp. Pathol.*, **68**, 215–223

Stosic-Grujicic, S. & Simic, M.M. (1992) *In vitro* effects of retinoid RO 10-9359 on lectin-induced activation and proliferation of T-lymphocytes. *Int. J. Immunopharmacol.*, **14**, 903–914

Stosic-Grujicic, S., Ejdus, L., Mijatovic, S., Jovanovic, S. & Ostojic, N. (1996) Etretinate (Ro 10-9359) prevents autoimmune syndrome associated with chronic graft-versus-host disease in rats. *Transplant Proc.*, **28**, 3258–3258

Studer, U.E., Biedermann, C., Chollet, D., Karrer, P., Kraft, R., Toggenburg, H. & Vonbank, F. (1984) Prevention of recurrent superficial bladder tumors by oral etretinate: Preliminary results of a randomized, double blind multicenter trial in Switzerland. *J. Urol.*, **131**, 47–49

Studer, U.E., Jenzer, S., Biedermann, C., Chollet, D., Kraft, R., von Toggenburg, H. & Vonbank, F. (1995) Adjuvant treatment with a vitamin A analogue (etretinate) after transurethral resection of superficial bladder tumors. Final analysis of a prospective, randomized multicenter trial in Switzerland. *Eur. Urol.*, **28**, 284–290

Tamayo, L. & Ruiz-Maldonado, R. (1980) Oral retinoid (Ro 10-9359) in children with lamellar ichthyosis, epidermolytic hyperkeratosis and symmetrical progressive erythrokeratoderma. *Dermatologica*, **161**, 305–314

Tamayo, L. & Ruiz-Maldonado, R. (1981) Long-term follow-up of 30 children under oral retinoid Ro 10-9359. In: Orfanos, C.E., Braun-Falco, O., Farber, E.M., Grupper, C., Polano, M.K. & Schuppli, R., eds, *Retinoids. Advances in Basic Research and Therapy*. Berlin, Springer Verlag, pp. 287–294

Taylor, D.D., Taylor, C.G., Black, P.H., Jiang, C.G. & Chou, I.N. (1990) Alterations of cellular characteristics of a human ovarian teratocarcinoma cell line after in vitro treatment with retinoids. *Differentiation*, **43**, 123–130

Thongnopnua, P. & Zimmerman, C.L. (1988) Simultaneous microassay for etretinate and its active metabolite, etretin, by reversed-phase high-performance liquid chromatography. *J. Chromatogr.*, **433**, 345–351

Thune, P. & Mork, N.J. (1980) A case of centrolobular toxic necrosis of the liver due to aromatic retinoid—Tigason (Ro 10-9359). *Dermatologica*, **160**, 405–408

Tokura, Y., Edelson, R.L. & Gasparro, F.P. (1992) Retinoid augmentation of bioactive interleukin-1 production by murine keratinocytes. *Br. J. Dermatol.*, **126**, 485–495

Tong, P.S., Mayes, D.M. & Wheeler, L.A. (1988) Differential effects of retinoids on DNA synthesis in calcium-regulated murine epidermal keratinocyte cultures. *J. Invest. Dermatol.*, **90**, 861–868

Török, L. (1984) Spermatological examinations in males treated with etretinate. In: Cunliffe, W.J. & Miller, A.J., eds, *Retinoid Therapy. A Review of Clinical and Laboratory Research*. Lancaster, MTP Press, pp. 161–164

Török, L., Kadar, L. & Kasa, M. (1987) Spermatological investigations in patients treated with etretinate and isotretinoin. *Andrologia*, **19**, 629–633

Traupe, H. & Happle, R. (1985) Etretinate therapy in children with severe keratinization defects. *Eur. J. Pediatr.*, **143**, 166–169

Tsambaos, D., Hundeiker, M., Mahrle, G. & Orfanos, C.E. (1980) Reversible impairment of spermatogenesis induced by aromatic retinoid in guinea pigs. *Arch. Dermatol. Res.*, **267**, 153–159

Turton, J.A., Willars, G.B., Haselden, J.N., Ward, S.J., Steele, C.E. & Hicks, R.M. (1992) Comparative teratogenicity of nine retinoids in the rat. *Int. J. Exp. Pathol.*, **73**, 551–563

Vahlquist, A. & Rollman, O. (1990) Etretinate and the risk for teratogenicity: Drug monitoring in a pregnant woman for 9 months after stopping treatment. *Br. J. Dermatol.*, **123**, 131

Vane, F.M., Buggé, C.J. & Rodriguez, L.C. (1989a) Identification of etretinate metabolites in human bile. *Drug Metab. Dispos.*, **17**, 275–279

Vane, F.M., Buggé, J.L. & Rodriguez, L.C. (1989b) Identification of etretinate metabolites in human blood. *Drug Metab. Dispos.*, **17**, 280–285

Verloes, A., Dodinval, P., Koulischer, L., Lambotte, R. & Bonnivert, J. (1990) Etretinate embryotoxicity 7 months after discontinuation of treatment. *Am. J. Med. Genet.*, **37**, 437–438

Verma, A.K., Shapas, B.G., Rice, H.M. & Boutwell, R.K. (1979) Correlation of the inhibition by retinoids of tumor promoter-induced mouse epidermal ornithine decarboxylase activity and of skin tumor promotion. *Cancer Res.*, **39**, 419–425

Viraben, R., Mathieu, C. & Fontan, B. (1985) Benign intracranial hypertension during etretinate therapy for mycosis fungoides. *J. Am. Acad. Dermatol.*, **13**, 515–517

van Voorst Vader, P.C., Houthoff, H.J., Eggink, H.F. & Gips, C.H. (1984) Etretinate (Tigason) hepatitis in 2 patients. *Dermatologica*, **168**, 41–46

Wagner, G., Habs, M. & Schmähl, D. (1983) Inhibition of the promotion phase in two-step carcinogenesis in forestomach epithelium of mice by the aromatic retinoid etretinate. *Drug Res.*, **33**, 851–852

Waisman, Y., Rachmel, A., Metzker, A., Wielunsky, E., Nitzan, M., Rotem, A. & Steinherz, R. (1989) Failure of etretinate therapy in twins with severe congenital lamellar ichthyosis. *Pediatr. Dermatol.*, **6**, 226–228

Ward, P.S. & Jones, R.D. (1989) Successful treatment of a harlequin fetus. *Arch. Dis. Child.*, **64**, 1309–1311

Ward, A., Brogden, R.N., Heel, R.C., Speight, T.M. & Avery, G.S. (1983) Etretinate. A review of its pharmacological properties and therapeutic efficacy in psoriasis and other skin disorders. *Drugs*, **26**, 9–43

Watson, A.B. (1986) Preventative effect of etretinate therapy on multiple actinic keratoses. *Cancer Detect. Prev.*, **9**, 161–165

Weber, U., Melnik, B., Goerz, G. & Michaelis, L. (1988) Abnormal retinal function associated with long-term etretinate? *Lancet*, **i**, 235–236

West, M.R., Page, J.M., Turner, D.M., Wood, E.J., Holland, D.B., Cunliffe, W.J. & Rupniak, H.T. (1992) Simple assays of retinoid activity as potential screens for compounds that may be useful in treatment of psoriasis. *J. Invest. Dermatol.*, **99**, 95–100

Williams, K.J., Ferm, V.H. & Willhite, C.C. (1984) Teratogenic dose–response relationships of etretinate in the golden hamster. *Fundam. Appl. Toxicol.*, **4**, 977–982

Windhorst, D.B. & Nigra, T. (1982) General clinical toxicology of oral retinoids. *J. Am. Acad. Dermatol.*, **6**, 675–682

Woll, P.J., Kostrzewski, A. & Glen-Bott, A.M. (1987) Lymphoma in patients taking etretinate. *Lancet*, **ii**, 563–564

Wolska, H., Jablonska, S., Langner, A. & Fraczykowska, M. (1985) Etretinate therapy in generalized pustular psoriasis (Zumbusch type). Immediate and long-term results. *Dermatologica*, **171**, 297–304

Wyss, R. (1990) Determination of retinoids in plasma by high-performance liquid chromatography and automated column switching. *Meth. Enzymol.*, **189**, 146–155

Wyss, R. & Bucheli, F. (1988) Determination of highly protein bound drugs in plasma using high-performance liquid chromatography and column switching, exemplified by the retinoids. *J. Chromatogr.*, **456**, 33–43

Xue, G.Z., Zheng, Z.S., Chen, R.Z., Lloyd, M.B. & Prystowsky, J.H. (1996) Phorbol 12-myristate 13-acetate inhibits epidermal growth factor signalling in human keratinocytes, leading to decreased orni-thine decarboxylase activity. *Biochem. J.*, **319**, 641–648

Yoshida, O., Miyakawa, M., Watanabe, H., Mishina, T., Okajima, E., Hirao, Y., Matushima, M., Nihira, H. & Nakatsu, H. (1986) Prophylactic effect of etretinate on the recurrence of superficial bladder tumors—Results of a randomized control study. *Hinyokika Kiyo*, **32**, 1349–1358

Yoshioka, A., Miyachi, Y., Imamura, S. & Niwa, Y. (1986)
Anti-oxidant effects of retinoids on inflammatory
skin diseases. *Arch. Dermatol. Res.*, **278**, 177–183

Zeng, Y., Zhou, H.M. & Xu, S.P. (1981) Inhibitory effect of
retinoids on Epstein-Barr virus induction in Raji cells.
Intervirology, **16**, 29–32

Zhang, J.Z., Maruyama, K., Ono, I., Nihei, Y., Iwatsuki, K.
& Kaneko, F. (1994) Effects of etretinate on keratinocyte proliferation and secretion of interleukin-
1α (IL-1α) and IL-8. *J. Dermatol.*, **21**, 633–638

Zitnik, R.J., Kotloff, R.M., Latifpour, J., Zheng, T.,
Whiting, N.L., Schwalb, J. & Elias, J.A. (1994) Retinoic
acid inhibition of IL-1-induced IL-6 production by
human lung fibroblasts. *J. Immunol.*, **152**, 1419–1427

Handbook 6

Acitretin

1. Chemical and Physical Characteristics

1.1 Nomenclature

Acitretin is the free acid form of etretinate and belongs to the class of aromatic synthetic retinoids in which the lipophilic trimethylcyclohexenyl group of retinoic acid has been replaced by an aromatic ring (Figure 1). In the case of acitretin, the cyclohexenyl group has been replaced by a 4-methoxy-2,3,6-trimethylphenyl group, while the all-*trans*-tetraene structure of the retinoic acid side-chain has been retained. Acitretin, like retinoic acid, is a carboxylic acid and hence has direct biological activity and, unlike etretinate, does not require metabolic conversion for activity.

In this nomenclature, the side-chain of acitretin is numbered starting from the carboxylic acid (Figure 1). Since acitretin is a synthetic derivative of retinoic acid, however, the retinoid numbering system is often used for acitretin and its derivatives. The common numbering system for retinoic acid and its application to the basic skeleton of acitretin are shown in Figure 2. Derivatives of acitretin are often given this common numbering system. For example, (2Z,4E, 6E,8E)-3,7-dimethyl-9-(4-methoxy-2,3,6-trimethylphenyl)nona-2,4,6,8-tetraenoic acid, a geometric isomer of acitretin, is commonly referred to as 13-*cis*-acitretin (Figure 2), and the methyl groups attached to the tetraene side-chain are often referred to as the C-9 and C-13 methyls, in keeping with the retinoid nomenclature.

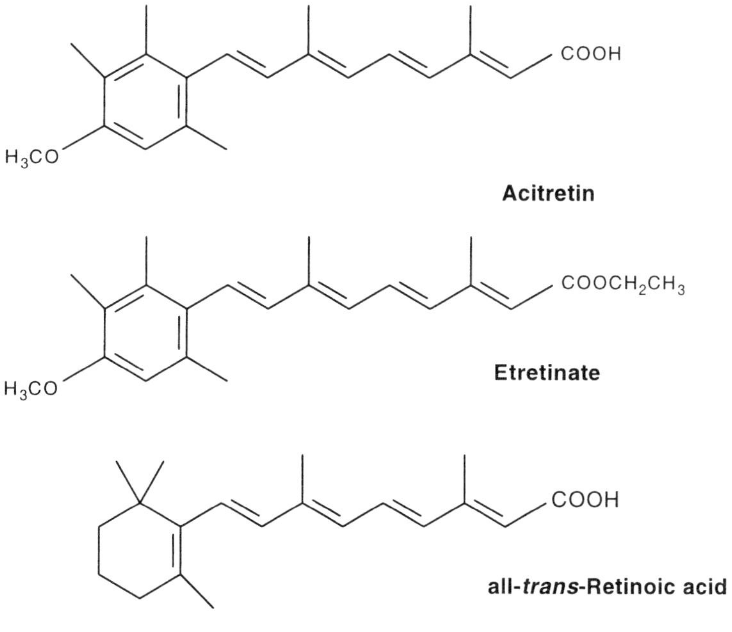

Figure 1. Structures of acitretin, etretinate and all-*trans*-retinoic acid

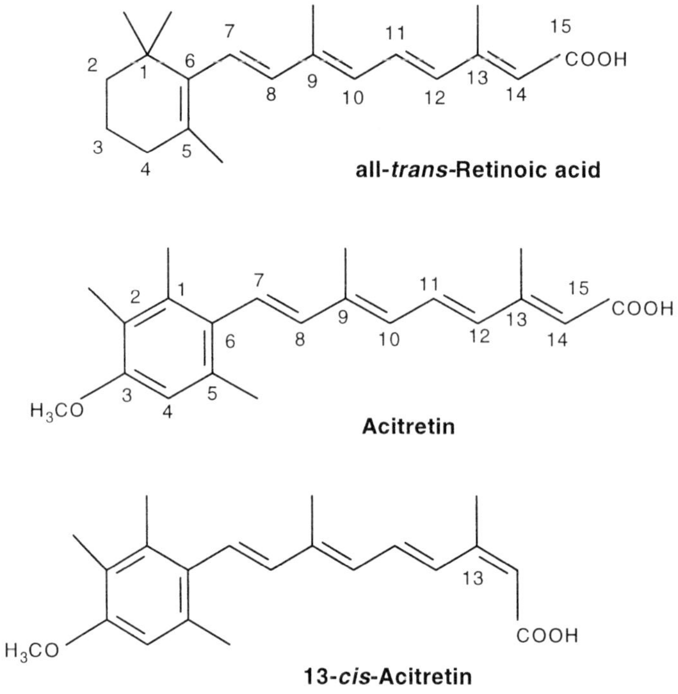

all-*trans*-Retinoic acid

Acitretin

13-*cis*-Acitretin

Figure 2. Common numbering scheme for retinoids

1.2   Name
Chemical Abstract Services Registry Number
160024-33-9

IUPAC Systematic name
all-*trans*-3,7-Dimethyl-9-(4-methoxy-2,3,6-tri-methylphenyl)nona-2,4,6,8-tetraenoic acid

Synonyms
Acitretin, Etretin, Soriaten®, RO 10-9359

1.3   Structural formula

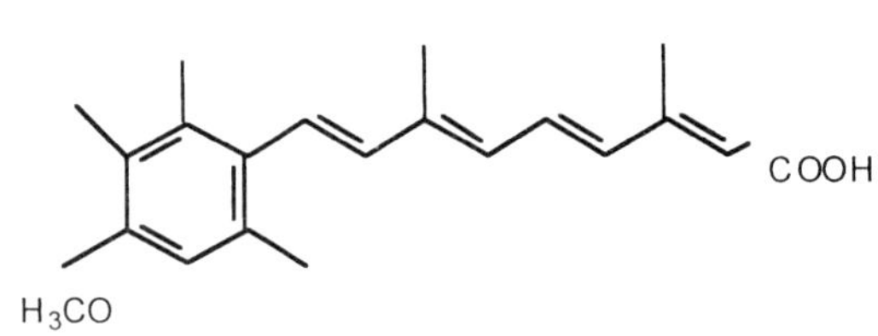

H_3CO
Composition: $C_{21}H_{26}O_3$

Relative molecular mass: 326

1.4   Physical and chemical properties

Melting-point
228–230 °C (Budavari *et al.*, 1989)

Spectroscopy
UV and visible spectrum: λ_{max} = 352 nm in methanol (Makin *et al.*, 1989)

^{1}H-NMR (CDCl$_3$, 270 MHz): δ 2.10 (3H, s), 2.28, 2.24 and 2.14 (9H, 3s), 2.37 (3H, s), 3.80 (3H, s), 5.80 (1H, s), 6.20 (1H, d, *J* = 11.4 Hz), 6.24 (1H, d, *J* = 16.3 Hz), 6.40 (1H, d, *J* = 15.04 Hz), 6.60 (1H, s), 6.70 (1H, d, *J* = 16.3 Hz), 7.09 (1H, dd, *J* = 15.02, 11.4 Hz) (Aurell *et al.*, 1995).

^{13}C-NMR (CDCl$_3$): δ 11.80, 12.85, 13.85, 17.35, 21.36, 55.40, 110.25, 119.10, 122.85, 128.65, 130.00, 130.40,130.55, 133.55, 133.85, 135.80, 135.85, 138.20, 138.95, 152.30, 156.25, 166.85 (Aurell *et al.*, 1995)

Infrared spectrum
v_{max} 3600–3300 (O-H), 1700 (C=O), 1600 (C=C) cm^{-1} (Aurell *et al.*, 1995)

Geometrical isomers
Sixteen possible isomers

Photochemical properties
Acitretin is a yellow to greenish-yellow powder with an absorption maximum (λ_{max}) at 352 nm (methanol) in the UV–visible spectrum (Makin *et al.*, 1989). Because of its conjugated tetraene structure, acitretin can readily undergo photo-isomerization reactions when exposed to light, particularly in solution.

Solubility
Soluble in most organic solvents, fats and oils; low solubility in water probably similar to that of all-*trans*-retinoic acid, i.e. 0.21 µmol/L (Szuts & Harosi, 1991)

Relationships between chemical structure and biological activity
The pharmacological activity of acitretin is likely to be due primarily to activation of the retinoic acid receptors (RARs). The physiological ligand for the RARs is all-*trans*-retinoic acid (Giguère *et al.*, 1987; Petkovich *et al.*, 1987), and extensive studies of structure–activity relationships with retinoid analogues have established that a terminal carboxylic acid group and a lipophilic head group are required for interaction with the RARs (Gale, 1993). The lipophilic head group required for RAR activity is provided by the 4-methoxy-2,3,6-trimethylphenyl group of acitretin. The planar all-*trans* configuration and the terminal carboxylic acid group of the acitretin side-chain appear to be optimal for RAR activity, but 9-*cis*-retinoic acid, the putative physiological ligand for the retinoid X receptors, also activates RARs (Heyman *et al.*, 1992), and it is possible that the 9-*cis* isomer of acitretin can also activate RARs.

2. Occurrence, Production, Use, Human Exposure and Analysis

2.1 Occurrence
Acitretin is not a naturally occurring compound but can readily be synthesized by a variety of routes.

2.2 Production
In the synthesis of acitretin, outlined in Scheme 1, the aryl-substituted pentadienal, **1**, is used as the starting material (Makin *et al.*, 1989). Reaction of **1** with the diester **2** in the presence of ethanolic sodium hydroxide gave the dicarboxylic acid, **3**.

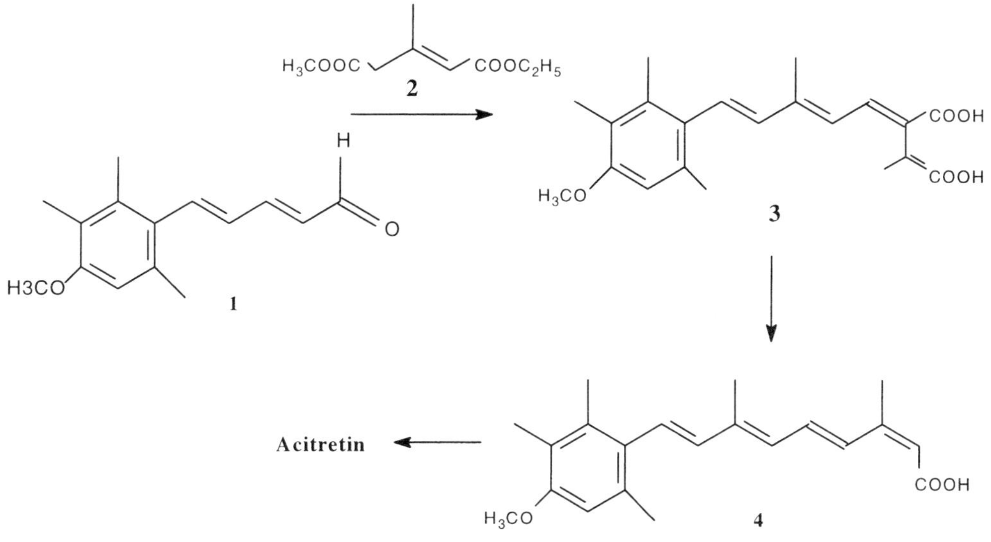

Scheme 1

Decarboxylation of **3** gave primarily the 13-*cis* isomer of acitretin, compound **4**. Isomerization of a benzene and ether solution of **4** in the presence of catalytic amounts of iodine followed by recrystallation afforded acitretin.

An alternative synthesis of acitretin is described in section 2.2 of Handbook 5 (scheme 3). Several other syntheses described for etretinate can be used for acitretin, since etretinate is readily hydrolysed to acitretin. Two of these syntheses are described in section 2.2 of Handbook 5 (schemes 1 and 2). Syntheses of etretinate, derivatives of etretinate and geometric isomers of these compounds have also been described by Bestmann and Ermann (1984). The large-scale synthesis of acitretin and various derivatives, including etretinate, has been described by Bollag *et al.* (1978).

2.3   Use

Acitretin has been approved by the appropriate regulatory authorities in many countries for the oral treatment of severe psoriasis, including erythrodermic and generalized pustular psoriasis (Goldfarb & Ellis, 1998; Paul & Dubertret, 1998). Several double-blind comparative clinical trials with acitretin and etretinate showed that the efficacy of the two drugs in psoriasis is essentially identical. Thus, acitretin is being used in the treatment of a variety of other skin diseases, cancers and premalignant conditions which respond to etretinate, including mycosis fungoides, basal-cell carcinoma, actinic keratoses, keratoacanthoma and epidermodysplasia verruciformis (Paul & Dubertret, 1998) and has largely replaced etretinate on the market. It is recommended that acitretin be administered with a meal.

2.4   Human exposure

Acitretin is marketed in 10-mg and 25-mg gelatin capsules for oral administration. The manufacturer recommends individualization of dosage in order to achieve an optimal therapeutic index. In general, it is recommended that acitretin therapy be initiated at an initial dose of 25 or 50 mg/day given as a single dose with the main meal. After an initial response to therapy, maintenance doses of 25–50 mg/day may be used. Goldfarb and Ellis (1998) recommended slightly lower doses of acitretin than of etretinate and that two-thirds of the dose of etretinate be used when switching from etretinate to acitretin. A starting dose of 0.5 mg/kg bw per day is recommended for plaque psoriasis. Slightly higher initial doses are recommended for pustular psoriasis and slightly lower doses for erythrodermic psoriasis. Acitretin is contraindicated in women of childbearing potential, and negative results in a pregnancy test in serum prior to initiation of therapy and strict contraception during treatment and for at least two years after drug withdrawal are required (Bouvy *et al.*, 1992; Stricker *et al.*, 1992; for more details, see section 7.2.1).

2.5   Analysis

Numerous methods based on high-performance liquid chromatography (HPLC) have been described for the quantitative analysis in plasma of acitretin, etretinate and their geometric isomers. The limit of detection of a reversed-phase HPLC method for analysis of etretinate and acitretin in plasma was 10 ng/ml (Palmskog, 1980), while that of a normal-phase HPLC method for the same two compounds was 4 ng/ml (Paravicini & Busslinger, 1983). An alternative reversed-phase HPLC method for the simultaneous determination of etretinate and acitretin in rat blood required much smaller sample volumes and allowed for serial sampling (Thongnopnua & Zimmerman, 1988). Another normal-phase HPLC method which allowed for the determination of etretinate, acitretin and the 13-*cis* isomer of acitretin, with a detection limit of 3 ng/ml, was used to study the long-term pharmacokinetics of etretinate in patients with psoriasis who had been changed from etretinate to acitretin therapy (De Leenheer *et al.*, 1990). A reversed-phase HPLC method with shorter retention times was also used to detect these three compounds in human plasma (Jakobsen *et al.*, 1987). A programmed-gradient HPLC system for the analysis of etretinate, its metabolites and other retinoids in plasma allowed shortened analysis and better peak shapes (Annesley *et al.*, 1984). Problems of recovery arising from strong binding of retinoids to plasma proteins were addressed by column-switching techniques (Wyss & Bucheli, 1988; Wyss, 1990).

HPLC methods were used to isolate metabolites from the faeces and urine of persons treated with tritium-labelled acitretin. The structures of the metabolites were elucidated by mass spectrometry and ^{1}H-NMR spectroscopy (Hänni *et al.*, 1977). Bile samples collected from patients treated with ^{14}C-labelled etretinate were analysed by HPLC after β-glucuronidase treatment, and the structures of the metabolites were determined by mass spectrometry and ^{1}H-NMR spectroscopy (Vane *et al.*, 1989a). Similarly, HPLC methods were used to isolate metabolites from the blood of persons with psoriasis treated with etretinate, and spectroscopic techniques were used to elucidate their structures (Vane *et al.*, 1989b). Another reversed-phase HPLC method has been developed for the simultaneous assay of etretinate, acitretin and their metabolites in whole perfusate, perfusate plasma, bile and hepatic tissue obtained in a perfused rat liver model, and was used to study the first-pass hepatic metabolism of etretinate and acitretin (Decker & Zimmerman, 1995). A reliable method has been reported involving normal-phase HPLC and ultraviolet detection which allows improved quantification of acitretin and 13-*cis*-acitretin in human plasma (Meyer *et al.*, 1991). A rapid HPLC method for the simultaneous, specific analysis of acitretin and its 13-*cis* isomer in blood, plasma and urine has been used to measure the concentrations of the compounds in patients receiving acitretin therapy (Al-Mallah *et al.*, 1987). A very sensitive method involving microbore liquidchromatography–negative chemical ionization mass spectrometry has been used to measure acitretin and its 13-*cis* metabolite in human plasma at a detection limit of 1 ng/ml (Fayer *et al.*, 1991). A highly sensitive HPLC method has been used to quantify acitretin and 13-*cis*-acitretin in the plasma and skin of patients being treated for psoriasis with acitretin (Laugier *et al.*, 1989).

3. Metabolism, Kinetics and Genetic Variation

Acitretin was developed clinically because the extreme lipophilicity of etretinate led to its storage in adipose tissue and hence to an extended half-life of elimination (Paravicini *et al.*, 1981). Acitretin, because of its free carboxyl group, is much less lipophilic than etretinate and as a consequence has a much shorter half-life: 50 h compared with approximately four months for etretinate (Brindley, 1989; Goldfarb & Ellis, 1998). In the circulation, more than 99.9% of acitretin is bound to plasma proteins, primarily albumin.

3.1 Humans

About 60% of an oral dose of acitretin is bioavailable, with a wide range of 36–95%. The pharmokinetics of acitretin has been studied extensively, and the results have been summarized (Pilkington & Brogden, 1992; Larsen, 1994). Typically, the maximum plasma concentrations detected in healthy volunteers about 2–3.3 h after ingestion of a single oral dose of 50 mg of acitretin were 200–400 ng/ml, and the mean terminal elimination half-life was 2.5–6.7 h. In these studies, the maximum concentration of the metabolite 13-*cis*-acitretin was reached 4–22 h after administration, and its mean terminal elimination half-life was 50–60 h.

Most studies of the pharmacokinetics of multiple oral doses of acitretin have involved patients with psoriasis receiving 30–50 mg/day for up to six months (Larsen, 1994). [The Working Group noted that the half-life depends markedly on the dosing schedule, the tissue considered and when the measurements are made after dosing.] Under the conditions used by Larsen (1994), the maximum plasma concentrations of the drug were 230–400 ng/ml and were recorded 1–4 h after administration. In 11 patients with psoriasis, the time to the mean peak concentration was 3.5 h after 50 mg/day for two months (Larsen *et al.*, 1991; Koo *et al.*, 1997). The elimination half-life was 2 h after single oral doses and about 50 h after multiple dosing (Gollnick *et al.*, 1990). Within one month of treatment with an oral dose of acitretin at 30 mg/day, the steady-state concentration of acitretin in the epidermis of 12 patients with psoriasis was 17 ng/g, with a significant correlation to plasma levels. Acitretin is fairly well absorbed from the gastrointestinal tract, the average concentrations in the dermis being 177 ng/g after one month of treatment and 227 ng/g after six months. The concentration in adipose tissue (98 ng/g) exceeded that in skin (28 ng/g) within 5 h of consumption of a dose of 25 mg (Koo *et al.*, 1997).

The concentrations of acitretin in blood and epidermis after a therapeutic dose are generally one-fourth those of etretinate. Since acitretin contains a comparatively polar carboxylic acid (pK$_a$ 3.7), it is less likely to be sequestered in adipose tissue (Larsen *et al.*, 1992). It is eliminated by excretion of its metabolites in the liver and kidney. After a single 50-mg oral dose of ^{14}C-acitretin, 21% of the radiolabel in six healthy volunteers was found in urine and 63% in faeces. The immediate major metabolite of acitretin is its 13-*cis* isomer, isoacitretin (Koo *et al.*, 1997). After administration of acitretin to animals or humans, both acitretin and its 13-*cis* isomer are observed in plasma. Glutathione catalyses the interconversion of acitretin and its 13-*cis* isomer (Jewell & McNamara, 1990). all-*trans*-Acitretin and 13-*cis*-acitretin are demethylated and are subsequently eliminated in the bile as the acyl-β-glucuronide derivatives or through the kidney as soluble metabolites with shorter side-chains (Koo *et al.*, 1997). Acitretin and 13-*cis*-acitretin are transferred into breast milk, acitretin being distributed almost exclusively in the lipid fractions of the milk. The estimated amount of the drug consumed by suckling infants corresponded to about 1.5% of a single maternal dose of 40 mg (Rollman & Pihl-Lundin, 1990).

When 12 patients with psoriasis ceased taking acitretin, the terminal elimination half-life of the drug was 16–110 h, whereas that of the 13-*cis* metabolite was 36–250 h (Larsen *et al.*, 1991).

Etretinate is detectable in the plasma of patients taking acitretin, and the concentration is affected by alcohol consumption (Larsen *et al.*, 1993a; Maier & Hönigsmann, 1996). In human liver preparations, acitretin may be esterified to etretinate in a reaction requiring ethanol and coenzyme A (Schmitt-Hoffmann *et al.*, 1995). The recommended two-year period of contraception after etretinate therapy has been considered to be applicable to acitretin (Lambert *et al.*, 1994). The elimination half-life of acitretin is much shorter than that of etretinate in most patients.

3.2 Experimental models

Radiolabelled acitretin administered intravenously was ultimately distributed in the skin and in adipose tissue where its storage was moderate and short-lived. The metabolite 13-*cis*-acitretin was detected in all tissues but not in plasma. After 6 h, < 1% of the intravenously injected dose remained in rat plasma as acitretin (Eisenhardt & Bickel, 1994). In isolated perfused rat liver, acitretin undergoes α-oxidation, chain shortening, *O*-demethylation and glucuronidation; isoacitretin undergoes glucuronidation as the major route of metabolism (Cotler *et al.*, 1992).

The percutaneous absorption of [^{14}C]acitretin from an isopropyl myristate formulation (160 μg acitretin per 2.5 cm^2) was approximately twice as high in hairless guinea-pigs as in rhesus monkeys after a 24-h exposure. Administration of up to 10 mg/kg bw per day to rats for six weeks altered the composition of liver microsomal phospholipid and induced cytochrome P450 enzyme activities (Tsambaos *et al.*, 1994). Pretreatment with acitretin orally at a dose of 10 mg/kg bw per day did not significantly alter the systemic clearance, volume of distribution or mean residence time of acitretin in male or female rats (Small & McNamara, 1994). The complex of microsomal UDP-glucuronosyl transferases in rat liver catalyses the formation of β-glucuronides from all-*trans*-retinoic acid and other retinoids, including acitretin (Genchi *et al.*, 1996).

4. Cancer-preventive Effects

4.1 Humans
4.1.1 Epidemiological studies
No data were available to the Working Group.

4.1.2 Intervention trials
Bavinck *et al.* (1995) evaluated the effect of acitretin on the development of squamous- and basal-cell carcinomas in a group of 44 renal transplant recipients with more than 10 keratotic skin lesions on the hands and forearms. Twenty-one patients were allocated to receive acitretin at 30 mg daily and 23 to placebo, for six months. Two patients allocated to acitretin and four to placebo withdrew before the first follow-up visit and were not included in the analysis. The pre-treatment characteristics of the remainder were similar. There was a significantly lower incidence of new skin tumours in the treated group ($p < 0.01$). During the six-month treatment period, two of the 19 patients given acitretin developed squamous-cell carcinomas, whereas nine of the 19 given placebo developed a total of 18 new skin cancers, of which 15 were squamous-cell carcinomas, two were basal-cell carcinomas and one was a case of Bowen disease. After cessation of treatment, the number of skin cancers appeared to increase.

4.1.3 Intermediate end-points

Bavinck *et al.* (1995; see above) also evaluated the effect of acitretin on the prevalence of keratotic skin lesions. A reduction was noted in the group receiving acitretin when compared with those given placebo during the six-month period of treatment. The treated patients showed a 13% reduction from baseline in the number of keratotic lesions, whereas the number of lesions in the placebo group increased by 28% ($p = 0.008$). The treated group had an increased incidence of lesions after cessation of treatment.

4.2 Experimental models

4.2.1 Cancer and preneoplastic lesions

These studies are summarized in Table 1.

Mouse: In a study of the effects of acitretin in C3H/HeNCrj mice, which are susceptible to spontaneous development of hepatomas, the control group was fed basal diet whereas the treatment group received 0.01% acitretin for 60 weeks, which was reduced from 0.01% to 0.005% at week 4 because of toxicity manifested as a reduction in body weight. Hepatomas [identified only macroscopically] developed in 12/13 control mice and 8/14 of those treated with acitretin ($p < 0.05$, Student's *t* test) (Muto & Moriwaki, 1984). [The Working Group noted the marked decrease in body weight in acitretin-treated mice.]

Rat: Groups of 40 male Fischer 344 rats were fed a diet containing 0.06% 3′-methyldimethylazobenzene for 20 weeks to induce hepatocellular carcinomas and were given acitretin at 10 mg/kg bw by gavage on five days per week for the entire period of 20 weeks. Acitretin reduced the incidence of hyperplastic nodules and hepatocellular carcinoma from 22/40 in controls to 13/40 in the treated group ($p < 0.01$, Student's *t* test) (Muto & Moriwaki, 1984). [The Working Group noted the marked decrease in body weight in acitretin-treated rats.]

4.2.2 Intermediate biomarkers

No data were available to the Working Group.

4.2.3 In-vitro models

4.2.3.1 Cellular studies

These studies are summarized in Table 2.

Acitretin, like its parent drug etretinate, is highly lipophilic and insoluble in water. In tests *in vitro* it has therefore been dissolved in dimethylsulfoxide (DMSO) or ethanol. The cells were usually exposed to the drug for at least two days; when the exposure was for longer than four days, the medium was changed every two or three days.

(a) Effects on cell proliferation

The antiproliferative effects of acitretin have been assessed in transformed cells of various histotypes and in normal epidermal cells. In studies of the growth inhibitory activity of acitretin, it was always more effective than its parent drug etretinate, and it is considered to be the active metabolite. Acitretin reduces the proliferation of various tumour cell lines, including human breast cancer cells (T47D and MCF-7) (Wetherhall & Taylor, 1986; Frey *et al.*, 1991), acute myelocytic leukaemia (HL-60), squamous carcinoma (SCC4, SCC15 and A431) (Frey *et al.*, 1991) and 1/4 Kaposi sarcoma cells (Corbeil *et al.*, 1994). The combination of acitretin with tamoxifen and interferon-α enhanced the antiproliferative effect (Fontana, 1987; Frey *et al.*, 1991). In all these cells, acitretin was less active than all-*trans*-retinoic acid. Acitretin had no effect on cell proliferation in rat bladder carcinoma cells exposed for only 1 h, even at a concentration of 10^{-4} mol/L (Fujita & Yoshida, 1984). [The Working Group noted the very high concentration used.]

No correlation was found between the sensitivity of four murine sarcomas and four murine carcinomas to etretinate *in vivo* and their sensitivity to acitretin *in vitro*; acitretin inhibited the growth of two carcinomas. The antiproliferative effect of acitretin in transformed and nontransformed epidermal cells has been shown to depend on the culture conditions and cell proliferation (Eccles *et al.*, 1985). Acitretin inhibited the proliferation of normal human vaginal keratinocytes and of early-passage dysplastic epithelial cell lines derived from vaginal lesions. At late passages, the premalignant cell lines showed a more transformed phenotype and became less sensitive to acitretin. Like all-*trans*-retinoic acid and 13-*cis*-retinoic acid, acitretin was less effective in cells grown in a medium with a low concentration of Ca^{++} (Hietanen *et al.*, 1998). In neonatal murine epidermal keratinocytes with different rates of proliferation obtained by growing cells in media with high or low concentrations of Ca^{++}, etretinate caused

Table 1. Prevention or regression of liver tumours by acitretin

Species, sex, age at carcinogen treatment	No. of animals per group	Carcinogen, dose, route	Acitretin (dose, route)	Duration in relation to carcinogen	Hepatoma bearing animals (%)		Multiplicity		Efficacy
					Control	Treated	Control	Treated	
Mice C3H/HeNCrj [sex not specified]	13–14		0.01% in diet, 4 wks, 0.005%, 56 wks	Throughout life	92	57	1.9	0.7*	Effective**
Rats, Fischer 344, male	40	3'-MeDAB, 0.06% in diet for 20 wks	10 mg/kg bw by gavage 5 d/week	day 0 to end	55	33	0.9	0.4*	Effective**

From Muto & Moriwaki (1984). 3'-MeDAB, 3'-methyldimethylazobenzene; wk, week; d, day

*Statistically significant (see text)

** Associated with reductions in body weight

dose-dependent inhibition of DNA synthesis in rapidly growing cells cultured in a medium with a high concentration of Ca^{++} but stimulated DNA synthesis in slowly growing cells in a medium with a low concentration of Ca^{++} (Tong *et al.*, 1988).

In a model of a skin equivalent, acitretin inhibited the growth of epidermal cells, but when dermal fibroblasts were present in the culture, reflecting the situation *in vivo*, acitretin had no effect on cell proliferation (Sanquer *et al.*, 1993). The effects of acitretin contrasted with those of all-*trans*-retinoic acid and 13-*cis*-retinoic acid, which stimulated the epidermis alone but inhibited epidermal growth in the presence of viable dermal fibroblasts. In pig epidermis, acitretin significantly decreased thymidine incorporation even after a short (24-h) exposure (Hashimoto *et al.*, 1990). In fibroblast lines from normal and psoriatic skin, acetretin was cytostatic in psoriatic cells but had no effect on normal skin fibroblasts (Priestley, 1987). In primary cultures of human sebocytes, acitretin at a high concentration (10^{-5} mol/L) had minimal effects on cell proliferation and decreased lipogenesis. Acitretin markedly decreased the synthesis of triglycerides, wax or stearyl esters and free fatty acids, whereas all-*trans*-retinoic acid and 13-*cis*-retinoic acid were potent inhibitors of both cell proliferation and lipid synthesis (Zouboulis *et al.*, 1991). Acitretin inhibited endothelial cell proliferation in a dose- and time-dependent manner in endothelial cells obtained from small vessels and capillaries of human skin (Imcke *et al.*, 1991).

(b)   Effects on cell differentiation
Explants of trachea from vitamin A-deficient hamsters have been used to measure the effects of retinoids on the squamous metaplasia that usually results when this tissue is cultured in the absence of vitamin A. Acitretin dissolved in DMSO reversed the metaplasia, with a median effective dose of 5 x 10^{-9} mol/L when applied over 10 days. The median effective dose of all-*trans*-retinoic acid under these conditions was 3 x 10^{-11} mol/L, indicating that acitretin was significantly less potent. Over 90% of the control cultures showed metaplasia (Newton *et al.*, 1980).

In the human myelomonocytic cell lines HL-60 and U937, often used to test the efficacy of differentiating agents, all-*trans*-retinoic acid and 13-*cis*-

retinoic acid induced differentiation but acitretin was completely inactive (Chomienne *et al.*, 1986). Acitretin at a higher dose induced a moderate increase in the differentiation of HL-60 cells but not U937 cells, but it was much less effective than all-*trans*-retinoic acid and 13-*cis*-retinoic acid. Differentiation induced by acitretin, but not by these two retinoids, was potentiated by interferon-β but not by interleukin-4 (Peck & Bollag, 1991). The addition of acitretin at a high concentration (10^{-5} mol/L) for five days strongly reduced keratin formation in cultured explants of pig skin (Aoyagi *et al.*, 1981a). In the same experimental system, acitretin was much more effective than etretinate in stimulating epidermal outgrowth, and this stimulation resulted in reduced keratin formation (Aoyagi *et al.*, 1981b). In human epidermal cells isolated from skin biopsy samples and cultured on a 3T3 cell feeder layer, addition of acitretin decreased the relative amount of keratin 16, thus markedly increasing the ratio of keratin 14 to keratin 16 (West *et al.*, 1992).

(c)   Effects on immune function
The ability of acitretin to interfere with lymphocyte proliferation has been examined in few studies. Exposure for three days to acitretin at a concentration much higher than those achievable *in vivo* (7 x 10^{-5} mol/L) inhibited the stimulation of human lymphocytes induced by various lectins (Bauer & Orfanos, 1981). It reduced proliferation induced by the mixed epidermal cell–lymphocyte reaction by 20–30% but only when the epidermal cells had been exposed to acitretin. In the mixed lymphocyte reaction, a decrease of 10–15% was found only at a concentration of 10^{-5} mol/L (Dupuy *et al.*, 1989). At an extremely high concentration (10^{-4} mol/L), acitretin inhibited human peripheral blood mononuclear cells and phytohaemagglutinin-stimulated proliferation (Chaidaroglou *et al.*, 1998). [The Working Group noted the very high concentration used.] In stimulated polymorphonuclear leukocytes, acitretin, unlike etretinate, suppressed generation of hydroxy radicals (Yoshioka *et al.*, 1986).

4.2.3.2   Antimutagenicity in short-term tests
No data were available to the Working Group.

Table 2. Effect of acitretin on cell proliferation, differentiation, tumour promotion and immune function

Cell line; end-point	Vehicle	Concentration (mol/L)	Response	Comments	Reference
Cell proliferation					
Human breast cancer cell line (T47D); proliferation	DMSO	10^{-9} to 10^{-5} for 7 days	Decreased proliferation	Less potent than ATRA	Wetherall & Taylor (1986)
Human breast cancer cell line (MCF7); proliferation	Ethanol	10^{-8} for 6 days	Decreased proliferation	Additive interaction with tamoxifen	Fontana (1987)
Human cancer cell lines (MFC-7, HL-60, SCC_4, SCC_{15}, A431); proliferation	DMSO	3×10^{-8} to 3×10^{-5} for 7 days	Decreased proliferation at the highest dose in all 5 cell lines	Less potent than ATRA; enhanced effect with IFNα	Frey et al. (1991)
Human Kaposi sarcoma cell lines; TdR incorporation	DMSO	10^{-9} to 10^{-5} for 2 days	Decreased TdR incorporation in 1/4 lines	Less potent than ATRA	Corbeil et al. (1994)
Murine sarcomas (4) and carcinomas (4); proliferation	Ethanol	10^{-8} to 10^{-6} for 7, 9 days	Decreased proliferation in 2 carcinomas		Eccles et al. (1985)
Human keratinocyte cell lines derived from vaginal intraepithelial neoplasia, normal vaginal keratinocytes and fibroblasts; proliferation	DMSO	10^{-9} to 10^{-5} for 4 days	Decreased proliferation of early-passage cell lines and of normal keratinocytes; reduced inhibition in late-passages and in low Ca^{++} medium	IFNα-2A potentiates the antiproliferative effect	Hietanen et al. (1998)
Normal murine epidermal cells; DNA synthesis	DMSO	10^{-8} to 10^{-4} for 4 days	Decreased proliferation in fast-growing (high Ca^{++}) cells; increased proliferation in slow-growing (low Ca^{++}) cells	More potent than etretinate	Tong et al. (1988)
Normal human epidermal cells; TdR incorporation,	DMSO	10^{-7} to 10^{-6} for 2 weeks	Decreased proliferation in epidermal cells. No effect in epidermis when grown with dermis fibroblasts	Effects opposite to those of ATRA and 13-cis-RA	Sanquer et al. (1993)
Normal pig epidermis	DMSO	10^{-7} to 10^{-4} for 24 h	Decreased TdR incorporation	More potent than etretinate	Hashimoto et al. (1990)
Normal and psoriatic skin fibroblasts; proliferation	DMSO	10^{-7} to 10^{-4} for 3 days	Cytostatic in psoriatic cells; no effect in normal skin		Priestley (1987)
Normal human sebocytes; TdR incorporation, lipid lipogenesis	DMSO	10^{-8} to 10^{-5} for 7–14 days	No effect on proliferation; decreased lipid synthesis	Less potent than ATRA and 13-cis-RA	Zouboulis et al. (1991)

Table 2 (contd)					
Cell-line; end-point	Vehicle	Concentration (mol/L)	Response	Comments	Reference
Normal human endothelial cells from skin vessels; proliferation and differentiation	DMSO	10^{-8} to 10^{-5} for 6 days	Decreased proliferation; no effect on HLA-DR or ICAM-1	More potent than etretinate	Imcke et al. (1991)
Cell differentiation					
Human myelomono-cytic cell lines (HL-60, U937) and fresh human leukaemic blast cells; cell viability and differ-entiation (NBT reduction)	DMSO	10^{-7} to 10^{-6} for 4 or 6 days	No effect on viability; No effect on differentiation	ATRA is active	Chomienne et al. (1986)
Human myelomono-cytic cell lines (HL-60, U937); differentiation (NBT reduction)	DMSO	10^{-5} for 2 days	Moderate increase in differentiation of HL-69 cells; potentiation of differentiation by IFNβ and not by IL-4	Less potent than ATRA and 13-cis-RA	Peck & Bollag (1991)
Normal pig skin explant cultures; keratin formation	Not reported	10^{-5} for 5 days	Modified keratin formation	High concentration	Aoyagi et al. (1981a)
Normal pig skin explant cultures; growth and keratin formation	DMSO	10^{-7} to 10^{-5} for 4 days	Stimulated growth and reduced keratin formation		Aoyagi et al. (1981b)
Normal human epidermal cells; keratin expression and envelope formation	Not reported	10^{-8} to 10^{-5} for 9 days	Increased keratin 14:16 ratio; decreased envelope formation	More potent than etretinate but less potent than ATRA	West et al. (1992)
Immune function					
Human lymphocytes; response to lectins	DMSO	7×10^{-8} to 7×10^{-5} for 3 days	Inhibition of PHA- and Con A-induced stimulation	Effective	Bauer & Orfanos (1981)
Human lymphocytes; mitogenic response to PHA, MLR and MECLR; cell viability	DMSO	10^{-8} to 10^{-5} for 4–6 days	Inhibition (20–30%) of MECLR-induced proliferation; no consistent inhibition of PHA mitogenic response		Dupuy et al. (1989)
Zymosan-stimulated polymorphonuclear lymphocytes; reactive oxygen species generation	50% DMSO 50% ethanol	2×10^{-6} to 2×10^{-4} during stimulation	Inhibition of OH$^{\bullet}$ generation		Yoshioka et al. (1986)

DMSO, dimethylsulfoxide; ATRA, all-trans-retinoic acid; IFN, interferon; TdR, ^{3}H-thymidine; 13-cis-RA, 13-cis-retinoic acid; NBT, nitroblue tetrazolium test; IL, interleukin, PHA, phytohaemagglutinin; MLR, mixed lymphocyte reaction; MECLR, mixed epidermal cell–lymphocyte reaction; ConA, concanavalin A

4.3 Mechanisms of cancer prevention

Information on the biological action of acitretin was obtained from studies of patients with skin disease.

4.3.1 Effects on cell differentiation

Acitretin modifies cell membrane glycosylation. In primary cultures of epidermal and dermal cells, acitretin stimulated the biosynthesis of cell and matrix glycosaminglycans (Shapiro & Mott, 1981), and this occurred at a low concentration (10^{-7} mol/L) and declined as the concentration increased (Priestley, 1987). Acitretin, like etretinate, inhibited tumour necrosis factor $(TGF)\beta 1$-stimulated type 1 collagen production by normal human lung fibroblasts. The pattern of keratinocyte proteins in cells removed from the dermal layer and grown in culture was modified by acitretin (Redlich et al., 1995). Acitretin, like etretinate, inhibited non-disulfide, disulfide and envelope proteins, whereas it stimulated kerato-hyaline-associated proteins (Stadler et al., 1987). Acitretin was twice as active as etretinate in decreasing the relative amount of keratin 16 and consequently in causing a marked increase in the ratio of keratin 14:16 (West et al., 1992). In primary human sebocyte cultures, acitretin decreased lipogenesis at concentrations that did not affect cell proliferation (Zouboulis et al., 1991).

4.3.2 Inhibition of cell proliferation

The only suggestion for a mechanism by which acitretin inhibits cell proliferation is that it inhibits the activity of ornithine decarboxylase (Xue et al., 1996).

4.3.3 Effects on immune function and cytokine production

Few studies have addressed the effects of acitretin on immune function. It was more active than etretinate in decreasing the migration of neutrophils from the bloodstream to human skin when applied locally (Dubertret et al., 1982). A two- to threefold increase in epidermal interleukin-1 was found in acitretin-treated hairless rats when compared with control rats (Schmitt et al., 1987). Acitretin also increased interleukin-1 production in keratinocytes grown in vitro (Tokura et al., 1992).

4.3.4 Effects on angiogenesis

Acitretin inhibited angiogenesis evoked by intra-dermal injection of human epidermoid cancer cell lines in mice and was more effective than etretinate at an equivalent dose (Rudnicka et al., 1991).

5. Other Beneficial Effects

Acitretin has been shown in clinical trials to be of benefit in the treatment of severe psoriasis, including erythrodermic and generalized pustular psoriasis. Relevant references are given in the General Remarks.

6. Carcinogenicity

6.1 Humans

No data were available to the Working Group.

6.2 Experimental models

No data were available to the Working Group.

7. Other Toxic Effects

7.1 Adverse effects
7.1.1 Humans

Pilkington and Brogden (1992) and Gollnick (1996) summarized the multicentre clinical trials in which acitretin was compared with etretinate. Acitretin has a lower therapeutic index than etretinate, and while the total incidence of adverse effects is higher with etretinate, the symptoms were more severe with acitretin. Clinical experience with these drugs has demonstrated that the hazards posed are very similar. Because acitretin is less lipophilic and has a much shorter elimination half-life than etretinate, it has replaced etretinate in 34 countries (Lacour et al., 1996). The doses used in the treatment of moderate-to-severe psoriasis are 10–75 mg/day (Pilkington & Brogden, 1992).

Most of the information about the toxicity of acetretin is derived from dermatological studies, which indicate that the incidence of idiosyncratic hepatitis, musculoskeletal problems and hyper-lipidaemia is comparable to that seen with etretinate (Halioua & Saurat, 1990). Rare effects that may be associated with acitretin treatment include pancreatitis, pseudotumour cerebri, keratoconus (Larsen *et al.*, 1993b), myopathy (Lister *et al.*, 1996) and vulvo-vaginal candidiasis (Sturkenboom *et al.*, 1995). A unique contraindication to the use of acitretin is the ingestion of alcohol (see section 3.1).

7.1.1.1 Skeletal toxicity

Like other retinoids, acitretin can be toxic to the bone in children (reviewed by Orfanos *et al.*, 1997). When the dose of acitretin given to 29 paediatric patients was limited to < 0.4 mg/kg bw per day, only one child experienced osteo-articular symptoms (transient knee pain), and no remarkable effects were found on physical examination or X-ray of this patient (Lacour *et al.*, 1996). Nevertheless, maintenance doses of 0.5–0.75 mg/kg bw per day have been used successfully (Salleras *et al.*, 1995). Although skeletal changes are seen in adults given 0.5 mg/kg bw per day for two years (Mork *et al.*, 1992), acitretin can be given to children over long periods with no such complications if all four limbs and the lateral spine are screened radiologically before treatment, the dose is maintained at 0.49 ± 0.12 mg/kg bw per day and the patients are observed carefully for musculoskeletal complaints (Lacour *et al.*, 1996).

7.1.1.2 Effects during chemotherapy

Acitretin has been evaluated in combination with interferon α-2a for the treatment of cutaneous T-cell lymphomas. The combination increased the number of flu-like symptoms, skin dryness, hair loss, increased triglyceride concentrations and neurological or psychiatric symptoms when compared with interferon α-2a plus psoralen–ultraviolet A therapy. The rate of complete response in 98 patients was no greater with acitretin plus interferon α-2a at 25–50 mg/week for 48 weeks than with the interferon α-2a plus phototherapy (38% vs 70%; $p \leq 0.008$; χ^2 test) (Stadler *et al.*, 1998).

7.1.2 *Experimental models*

Short- and long-term studies in rats and dogs showed dose-related, reversible toxic effects typical of the retinoids. In rats, these included decreased body-weight gain and increased serum cholesterol, triglyceride and lipoprotein concentrations and alkaline phosphatase activity. Fractures and evidence of healed fractures were observed. The doses

that produced these effects were one to two times the recommended human therapeutic dose. In dogs at doses up to 10 times the human dose, the signs of intolerance included erythema, skin hypertrophy and hyperplasia. Most of these side-effects were readily reversed upon cessation of treatment (Arky, 1998).

7.2 Reproductive and developmental effects
7.2.1 *Humans*
7.2.1.1 *Reproductive effects*

Sperm concentration, sperm morphology, total sperm motility and ejaculate volume were unchanged in four patients with psoriasis and six healthy volunteers aged 21–61 years who were given acitretin at 50 mg/day for six weeks, with individual dose adjustment to 25–50 mg/day for the next six weeks (Sigg *et al.*, 1987; Parsch *et al.*, 1990). No significant alterations from pretreatment values occurred during or after treatment in follicle-stimulating hormone, luteinizing hormone or testosterone, and there was no evidence of alterations in male reproductive function up to three months after discontinuation of treatment (Parsch *et al.*, 1990).

In nine fertile women aged 17–40 who were given acitretin at 25–40 mg/day (0.2–0.8 mg/kg bw per day) and maintained on laevonorgestrel or ethinyloestradiol, acitretin did not interfere with the antiovulatory actions of these combined oral contraceptives (Berbis *et al.*, 1988).

7.2.1.2 *Developmental effects*

Acitretin is contraindicated in women of child-bearing potential, and negative results in pregnancy test before initiation of therapy and strict contraception during treatment and for at least two years after drug withdrawal are required (Bouvy *et al.*, 1992; Stricker *et al.*, 1992). The prolonged elimination half-time of its ethyl ester metabolite—more than one year in some patients (Lambert *et al.*, 1990, 1992)—indicates the need for prolonged contraception in potentially fertile women.

Of 75 women whose exposure during pregnancy had been reported before December 1993, 67 had been exposed for a median of 15 months before the pregnancy. Thirty-seven of these women had normal infants (Table 3). The remaining pregnancies were terminated after elective abortion or by spontaneous embryonic or fetal death *in utero* or ended with the birth of a malformed infant (Geiger *et al.*, 1994).

Exposure to acitretin at 1 mg/kg bw per day from 10 days after conception through week 10 was embryolethal. Autopsy revealed symmetrical short limbs, oligodactyly, absence of nails, microstomia, micrognathia, bilateral low-set microtia with preauricular skin tags, imperforate auditory meatus and atrioventricular septal defect (de Die-Smulders *et al.*, 1995). In another case, in which the mother received 50 mg/day during the first 19 weeks of pregnancy, autopsy of the fetus showed microtia and malformations of the face and limbs. In a third example, the infant of a mother who received 20 mg/day during the first eight months of her pregnancy was born with impaired hearing (Geiger *et al.*, 1994).

Because of the initial reports that the efficacy of acitretin, the main pharmacologically active metabolite of etretinate, was equivalent to that of etretinate in the therapy of psoriasis (Bjerke & Geiger, 1989) and because of its shorter terminal elimination half-time (2.4 vs 120 days) (Paravicini *et al.*, 1985; Larsen *et al.*, 1988), acitretin was thought to be more suitable than etretinate for use in women of child-bearing potential (O'Brien, 1990). Identification of the acitretin esterification pathway in humans (Chou *et al.*, 1992; Larsen, 1994; Laugier *et al.*, 1994; Maier & Hönigsmann, 1996), however, has reduced the potential value of acitretin as a substitute for etretinate. Although etretinate and acitretin are comparable in terms of efficacy, etretinate tends to be better tolerated (reviewed by Gollnick, 1996). Etretinate given at a dose of 25–50 mg/day for 5–24 months was still present in the circulation 500 days later (Lambert *et al.*, 1990).

7.2.2 *Experimental models*

7.2.2.1 *Reproductive effects*

No data were available to the Working Group.

7.2.2.2 *Developmental effects*

In mice given acitretin at 200 mg/kg bw on day 11 of gestation, typical retinoid-related effects were induced, including cleft palate and shortening of the long bones of the limbs (Kochhar *et al.*, 1988; Reiners *et al.*, 1988). In mice given 100 mg/kg bw

on day 11, cleft palate and limb bone shortening were also seen, but the 13-*cis* isomer was not teratogenic at this dose (Löfberg *et al.*, 1990). Acitretin was considerably less potent than etretinate in these studies, but when tested *in vitro* for inhibition of chondrogenesis, acitretin was as potent as all-*trans*-retinoic acid (Kistler, 1987; Kochhar *et al.*, 1988; Reiners *et al.*, 1988). The lowest teratogenic dose for mice was found to be 3 mg/kg bw given not as a single large dose on one day but as daily doses on days 7–17 of gestation. In these experiments, the 13-*cis* metabolite of acitretin was also considerably less active than the parent all-*trans* isomer (Kistler & Hummler, 1985; Kistler, 1987).

In rats, acitretin at 25 or 50 mg/kg bw increased the rate of embryo resorption; at the higher dose, almost all of the surviving embryos were abnormal. The malformations of the central nervous system included exencephaly, hydrocephaly and spina bifida; those in the craniofacial region were micrognathia, agnathia, clefting, ear deformities, anophthalmia and exophthalmia; those of the urogenital system were genital agenesis, undescended testes, hydronephrosis and dilated ureter; and those at the caudal end were imperforate anus and hindlimb and tail defects. No cardiac abnormalities were observed (Turton *et al.*, 1992). The lowest teratogenic dose for rat embryos was 15 mg/kg bw, and, in contrast to the effect in mice embryos, 13-*cis*-acitretin was slightly more teratogenic than the all-*trans* isomer (Kistler & Hummler, 1985; Kistler, 1987). When mid-gestation rat embryos were cultured for 48 h in the presence of acitretin, a concentration of 1 µg/ml caused embryonic abnormalities, measured as retarded growth and differentiation, a reduction in the number of pharyngeal arches and delayed closure of the anterior neuropore. At this concentration, acitretin was as potent as 13-*cis*-retinoic acid but only half as potent as all-*trans*-retinoic acid (Steele *et al.*, 1987).

Rabbit embryos were more sensitive to acitretin than mice or rats, the lowest teratogenic dose being 0.6 mg/kg bw (Kistler & Hummler, 1985; Kistler, 1987).

7.3 Genetic and related effects

No data were available to the Working Group.

Table 3. Exposure to acitretin and pregnancy outcome			
Outcome	Exposed during pregnancy	Exposed before pregnancy[a]	Total
Newborns			
• normal	1	36	37
• with typical jaw, ear and cardiac malformations	–	–	0
• with other malformations	1	4	5
Spontaneous abortion	4	9	13
Late fetal death	–	–	0
Induced abortion			
• no information	1	15	16
• normal fetus	–	3	3
• with typical jaw, ear and cardiac malformations	1	–	1
• with other malformations	–	–	0
Total	8	67	75

Modified from Geiger *et al.* (1994)

[a] Range: 6 weeks to 23 months, median: 5 months

8. Summary of Data

8.1 Chemistry, occurrence and human exposure

Acitretin [all-*trans*-3,7-dimethyl-9-(4-methoxy-2,3,6-trimethylphenyl)nona-2,4,6,8-tetraenoic acid] is a synthetic retinoid of the aromatic class which is structurally related to all-*trans*-retinoic acid. Because of its conjugated tetraene structure, acitretin has a characteristic absorption in the ultraviolet and visible spectrum and is readily photoisomerized in solution to multiple geometric isomers. Acitretin has a free carboxylic acid and as a consequence is much less lipophilic than its ethyl ester derivative, etretinate; however, like other acidic retinoids, it is lipophilic and is partitioned into hydrophobic compartments.

Acitretin can be prepared by various routes from readily available starting materials. Human exposure is due entirely to treatment with oral formulations, primarily for dermatological indications.

The recommended doses of acitretin are 25–50 mg/day.

Various normal-phase and reversed-phase high-performance liquid chromatographic methods are available for the detection and quantification of acitretin and its geometric isomers.

8.2 Metabolism and kinetics

The pharmacokinetics of acitretin has been extensively studied, particularly in patients with psoriasis. Acitretin is eliminated from the body more rapidly than etretinate, and less is sequestered in adipose tissue. Its metabolites are eliminated via the hepatic and renal routes, but acitretin can be esterified to etretinate *in vivo*.

8.3 Cancer-preventive effects
8.3.1 Humans

In one trial with 44 renal transplant patients, acitretin reduced the frequency of occurrence of squamous-cell cancers of the skin when compared with placebo. In the same trial, the prevalence of keratotic skin lesions was also reduced by acitretin. When treatment was stopped, the numbers of cancers and keratotic skin lesions increased.

8.3.2 Experimental models

In single studies, acitretin reduced the incidence of spontaneous and chemically induced liver tumours in mice and rats in conjunction with reductions in body weight.

Acitretin was evaluated for its ability to inhibit proliferation or to induce differentiation of tumour and normal cells *in vitro*. Acitretin was more active than etretinate, and both were less active than all-*trans*-retinoic acid and 13-*cis*-retinoic acid. Acitretin reversed squamous metaplasia in hamster trachea resulting from vitamin A deficiency. It had an anti-proliferative effect on some but not all tumour cell lines that were tested. Several studies with epidermal cells showed that the effects of acitretin depended on the culture conditions and/or the proliferation rate. It did not induce differentiation of leukaemic cells *in vitro*. In normal epidermal cells, it decreased envelope formation and modified the pattern of keratin. In studies of lymphocyte proliferation *in vitro*, the effects depended on the concentration of acitretin and on the mitogen used to induce proliferation.

8.3.3 Mechanisms of cancer prevention

The differentiating effect of acitretin on epidermal cells may be associated with modifications in the pattern of keratin expression and membrane glycosylation; however, the effect seems to depend on the concentration of the drug. The only mechanism that can be associated with the anti-proliferative activity of acitretin is inhibition of ornithine decarboxylase activity, which is increased in hyperproliferative states. The effects of acitretin on immune function have not been studied extensively. It stimulated the production of interleukin-1 both *in vitro* and *in vivo*, which might result in activation of lymphoid cells. In one study, acitretin inhibited angiogenesis, an effect that might contribute to its cancer-preventive activity.

8.4 Other beneficial effects

Acitretin is of benefit to patients suffering from psoriasis, including erythrodermic and generalized pustular forms.

8.5 Carcinogenic effects

No data were available to the Working Group.

8.6 Other toxic effects
8.6.1 Humans

At therapeutic doses, acitretin may produce hepatotoxicity, pancreatitis and pseudotumour cerebri. Ophthalmic toxicity, hyperostosis and lipid abnormalities have also been reported. These side-effects are readily reversible upon cessation of treatment in all but a small proportion of patients. Since acitretin is the active metabolite of etretinate and in view of case reports of malformations, acitretin is considered to be a human teratogen and is contraindicated in women of child-bearing potential. The recommended post-medication period during which pregnancy should be avoided is two years. No effects of acitretin were observed on spermatogenesis in humans in two studies. The efficacy of the oral contraceptives laevonorgestrel and ethinyloestradiol was not affected by treatment with acitretin in one study.

8.6.2 Experimental models

No published studies on the toxic effects of acitretin were available to the Working Group. In studies of cancer-preventive effects in experimental animals (see section 8.3.2), weight loss was associated with administration of acitretin.

Reproductive toxicity has not been reported in male animals. Acitretin is a potent teratogen in experimental animals, inducing the classical embryopathy seen with retinoids, with effects on the central nervous system, craniofacial region, urogenital system, limbs and tail in a range of animal models. Acitretin is slightly less potent as a teratogen than all-*trans*-retinoic acid.

9. Recommendations for Research

9.1 General recommendations for acitretin and other retinoids

See section 9 of the Handbook on all-*trans*-retinoic acid.

9.2 Recommendations specific to acitretin

None.

10. Evaluation

10.1 Cancer-preventive activity
10.1.1 Humans
There is *inadequate evidence* that acitretin has cancer-preventive activity in humans.

10.1.2. Experimental animals
There is *inadequate evidence* that acitretin has cancer-preventive activity in experimental animals.

10.2 Overall evaluation
There is inadequate evidence in humans and in experimental animals for the cancer-preventive activity of acitretin. Since acitretin is a derivative of etretinate, however, it probably has cancer-preventive efficacy similar to that of etretinate. Furthermore, it is less toxic than etretinate, although it is a potent teratogen in experimental animals and is considered to be a teratogen in humans.

11. References

Al-Mallah, N.R., Bun, H., Coassolo, P., Aubert, C. & Cano, J.P. (1987) Determination of the aromatic retinoids (etretin and isoetretin) in biological fluids by high-performance liquid chromatography. *J. Chromatogr.*, **421**, 177–186

Annesley, T., Giacherio, D., Wilkerson, K., Grekin, R. & Ellis, C. (1984) Analysis of retinoids by high-performance liquid chromatography using programmed gradient separation. *J. Chromatogr.*, **305**, 199–203

Aoyagi, T., Kamigaki, K., Kato, N., Fukaya, T., Iizuka, H. & Miura, Y. (1981a) Retinoid stimulates epidermal outgrowth of pig skin explants. *J. Dermatol.*, **8**, 197–205

Aoyagi, T., Kamigaki, K., Saruta, M., Iizuka, H. & Miura, Y. (1981b) Retinoid inhibits keratin formation of pig skin explants. *J. Dermatol.*, **8**, 207–213

Arky, R. (1998) *Physicians' Desk Reference*, 52nd Ed. Montvale, NJ, Medical Economics Company, p. 2498

Aurell, M.J., Ceita, L., Mestres, R., Parra, M. & Tortajada, A. (1995) Trienediolates of hexadienoic acids in synthesis. Addition to unsaturated ketones. A convergent approach to the synthesis of retinoic acids. *Tetrahedron*, **51**, 3915–3928

Bauer, R. & Orfanos, C.E. (1981) Trimethyl-methoxyphenyl-retinoic acid (Ro 10-1670) inhibits mitogen-induced DNA-synthesis in peripheral blood lymphocytes *in vitro*. *Br. J. Dermatol.*, **105**, 19–24

Bavinck, J.N., Tieben, L.M., van der Woude, F.J., Tegzess, A.M., Hermans, J., ter Schegget, J. & Vermeer, B.J. (1995) Prevention of skin cancer and reduction of keratotic skin lesions during acitretin therapy in renal transplant recipients: A double-blind, placebo-controlled study. *J. Clin. Oncol.*, **13**, 1933–1938

Berbis, P., Bun, H., Geiger, J.M., Rognin, C., Durand, Serradimigni, A., Hartmann, D. & Privat, Y. (1988) Acitretin (RO10-1670) and oral contraceptives: Interaction study. *Arch. Dermatol. Res.*, **280**, 388–389

Bestmann, H.J. & Ermann, P. (1984) Retinoids and carotenoids. Synthesis of (13Z)-retinoic acids. *Liebigs Ann. Chem.*, 1740–1745

Bjerke, J.R. & Geiger, J.M. (1989) Acitretin versus etretinate in severe psoriasis. A double-blind randomized Nordic multicenter study in 168 patients. *Acta Derm. Venereol. Suppl. Stockh.*, **146**, 206–207

Bollag, W., Ruegg, R. & Ryser, G. (1978) 9-Phenyl 5,6-dimethyl-nona-2,4,6,8-tetraeonic acid compounds. United States Patent 41 05 681 (8 August 1978)

Bouvy, M.L., Sturkenboom, M.C., Cornel, M.C., de Jong-van den Berg, L.T., Stricker, B.H. & Wesseling, H. (1992) Acitretin (Neotigason®). A review of pharmacokinetics and teratogenicity and hypothesis on metabolic pathways. *Pharm. Weekbl. Sci.*, **14**, 33–37

Brindley, C.J. (1989) Overview of recent clinical pharmacokinetic studies with acitretin (Ro 10-1670, etretin). *Dermatologica*, **178**, 79–87

Budavari, S., O'Neil, M.J., Smith, A. & Heckelman, P.E. (1989) *The Merck Index. An Encyclopedia of Chemicals, Drugs, and Biologicals*, 11th Ed. Rahway, NJ, Merck & Co.

Chaidaroglou, A., Degiannis, D., Koniavitou, K., Georgiou, S. & Tsambaos, D. (1998) In vitro effects of retinoids on mitogen-induced peripheral blood leucocyte responses. *Arch. Dermatol. Res.*, **290**, 205–210

Chomienne, C., Balitrand, N. & Abita, J.P. (1986) Inefficacy of the synthetic aromatic retinoid etretinate and of its free acid on the in-vitro differentiation of leukemic cells. *Leuk. Res.*, **10**, 1079–1081

Chou, R.C., Wyss, R., Huselton, C.A. & Wiegand, U.W. (1992) A potentially new metabolic pathway: Ethyl esterification of acitretin. *Xenobiotica*, **22**, 993–1002

Corbeil, J., Rapaport, E., Richman, D.D. & Looney, D.J. (1994) Antiproliferative effect of retinoid compounds on Kaposi's sarcoma cells. *J. Clin. Invest.*, **93**, 1981–1986

Cotler, S., Chang, D., Henderson, L., Garland, W. & Town, C. (1992) The metabolism of acitretin and isoacitretin in the in situ isolated perfused rat liver. *Xenobiotica*, **22**, 1229–1237

Decker, M.A. & Zimmerman, C.L. (1995) Simultaneous determination of etretinate, acitretin and their metabolites in perfusate, perfusate plasma, bile or hepatic tissue with reversed-phase high-performance liquid chromatography. *J. Chromatogr. B. Biomed. Appl.*, **667**, 105–113

De Leenheer, A.P., Lambert, W.E., De Bersaques, J.P. & Kint, A.H. (1990) High-performance liquid chromatographic determination of etretinate and all-*trans*- and 13-*cis*-acitretin in human plasma. *J. Chromatogr.*, **500**, 637–642

de Die-Smulders, C.E., Sturkenboom, M.C., Veraart, J., van Katwijk, C., Sastrowijoto, P. & van der Linden, E. (1995) Severe limb defects and craniofacial anomalies in a fetus conceived during acitretin therapy. *Teratology*, **52**, 215–219

Dubertret, L., Lebreton, C. & Touraine, R. (1982) Inhibition of neutrophil migration by etretinate and its main metabolite. *Br. J. Dermatol.*, **107**, 681–685

Dupuy, P., Bagot, M., Heslan, M. & Dubertret, L. (1989) Synthetic retinoids inhibit the antigen presenting properties of epidermal cells in vitro. *J. Invest. Dermatol.*, **93**, 455–459

Eccles, S.A., Barnett, S.C. & Alexander, P. (1985) Inhibition of growth and spontaneous metastasis of syngeneic transplantable tumors by an aromatic retinoic acid analogue. 1. Relationship between tumour immunogenicity and responsiveness. *Cancer Immunol. Immunother.*, **19**, 109–114

Eisenhardt, E.U. & Bickel, M.H. (1994) Kinetics of tissue distribution and elimination of retinoid drugs in the rat. I. Acitretin. *Drug Metab. Dispos.*, **22**, 26–30

Englert, G., Weber, S. & Klaus, M. (1978) Isolation by HPLC and identification by NMR spectroscopy of 11 mono-, di- and tri-*cis* isomers of an aromatic analogue of retinoic acid, ethyl all- *trans*-9-(4-methoxy-2,3,6-trimethylphenyl)-3,7-dimethyl-nona-2,4,6,8-tetraenoate. *Helv. Chim. Acta*, **61**, 2697–2708

Evans, R.M. (1988) The steroid and thyroid hormone receptor superfamily. *Science*, **240**, 889–895

Fayer, B.E., Huselton, C.A., Garland, W.A. & Liberato, D.J. (1991) Quantification of acitretin in human plasma by microbore liquid chromatography–negative chemical ionization mass spectrometry. *J. Chromatogr.*, **568**, 135–144

Fontana, J.A. (1987) Interaction of retinoids and tamoxifen on the inhibition of human mammary carcinoma cell proliferation. *Exp. Cell Biol.*, **55**, 136–144

Frey, J.R., Peck, R. & Bollag, W. (1991) Antiproliferative activity of retinoids, interferon alpha and their combination in five human transformed cell lines. *Cancer Lett.*, **57**, 223–227

Fujita, J. & Yoshida, O. (1984) Inhibitory effects of aromatic retinoic acid analog, administered alone or in combination with mitomycin C, on the *in vitro* growth of rat bladder carcinoma cells. *Hinyokika Kiyo*, **30**, 1627–1631

Gale, J.B. (1993) Recent advances in the chemistry and biology of retinoids. In: Ellis, G.P. & Luscombe, D.K., eds, *Progress in Medicinal Chemistry.* Amsterdam, Elsevier Science, pp. 1–55

Geiger, J.M., Baudin, M. & Saurat, J.H. (1994) Teratogenic risk with etretinate and acitretin treatment. *Dermatology*, **189**, 109–116

Genchi, G., Wang, W., Barua, A., Bidlack, W.R. & Olson, J.A. (1996) Formation of β-glucuronides and of β-galacturonides of various retinoids catalyzed by induced and noninduced microsomal UDP-glucuronosyltransferases of rat liver. *Biochim. Biophys. Acta*, **1289**, 284–290

Giguère, V., Ong, E.S., Segui, P. & Evans, R.M. (1987) Identification of a receptor for the morphogen retinoic acid. *Nature*, **330**, 624–629

Goldfarb, M.T. & Ellis, C.N. (1998) Clinical use of etretinate and acitretin. In: Roenigk, H.H. & Maibach, H.I., eds, *Psoriasis*, 3rd Ed. New York, Marcel Dekker, pp. 663–670

Gollnick, H.P. (1996) Oral retinoids—Efficacy and toxicity in psoriasis. *Br. J. Dermatol.*, **135** (Suppl. 49), 6–17

Gollnick, H., Ehlert, R., Rinck, G. & Orfanos, C.E. (1990) Retinoids: An overview of pharmacokinetics and therapeutic value. *Methods Enzymol.*, **190**, 291–304

Halioua, B. & Saurat, J.H. (1990) Risk:benefit ratio in the treatment of psoriasis with systemic retinoids. *Br. J. Dermatol.*, **122** (Suppl. 36), 135–150

Hänni, R., Bigler, F., Vetter, W., Englert, G. & Loeliger, P. (1977) The metabolism of the retinoid Ro 10-9359. Isolation and identification of the major metabolites in human plasma, urine and feces. Synthesis of three urinary metabolites. *Helv. Chim. Acta*, **60**, 2309–2325

Hashimoto, Y., Ohkuma, N. & Iizuka, H. (1990) Effects of retinoids on DNA synthesis of pig epidermis: Its relation to epidermal beta-adrenergic adenylate cyclase response and to epidermal superoxide dismutase activity. *J. Dermatol. Sci.*, **1**, 303–309

Heyman, R.A., Mangelsdorf, D.J., Dyck, J.A., Stein, R.B., Eichele, G., Evans, R.M. & Thaller, C. (1992) 9-*cis* Retinoic acid is a high affinity ligand for the retinoid X receptor. *Cell*, **68**, 397–406

Hietanen, S., Auvinen, E., Syrjänen, K. & Syrjänen, S. (1998) Anti-proliferative effect of retinoids and interferon-α-2a on vaginal cell lines derived from squamous intra-epithelial lesions. *Int. J. Cancer*, **78**, 338–345

Imcke, E., Ruszczak, Z., Mayer-da Silva, A., Detmar, M. & Orfanos, C.E. (1991) Cultivation of human dermal microvascular endothelial cells in vitro: Immunocytochemical and ultrastructural characterization and effect of treatment with three synthetic retinoids. *Arch. Dermatol. Res.*, **283**, 149–157

Jakobsen, P., Larsen, F.G. & Larsen, C.G. (1987) Simultaneous determination of the aromatic retinoids etretin and etretinate and their main metabolites by reversed-phase liquid chromatography. *J. Chromatogr.*, **415**, 413–418

Jewell, R.C. & McNamara, P.J. (1990) Glutathione catalysis of interconversion of acitretin and its 13-*cis* isomer isoacitretin. *J. Pharm. Sci.*, **79**, 444–446

Kistler, A. (1987) Limb bud cell cultures for estimating the teratogenic potential of compounds. Validation of the test system with retinoids. *Arch. Toxicol.*, **60**, 403–414

Kistler, A. & Hummler, H. (1985) Teratogenesis and reproductive safety evaluation of the retinoid etretin (Ro 10-1670). *Arch. Toxicol.*, **58**, 50–56

Kochhar, D.M., Penner, J.D. & Satre, M.A. (1988) Derivation of retinoic acid and metabolites from a teratogenic dose of retinol (vitamin A) in mice. *Toxicol. Appl. Pharmacol.*, **96**, 429–441

Koo, J., Nguyen, Q. & Gambla, C. (1997) Advances in psoriasis therapy. *Adv. Dermatol.*, **12**, 47–73

Lacour, M., Mehta, N.B., Atherton, D.J. & Harper, J.I. (1996) An appraisal of acitretin therapy in children with inherited disorders of keratinization. *Br. J. Dermatol.*, **134**, 1023–1029

Lambert, W.E., De Leenheer, A.P., De Bersaques, J.P. & Kint, A. (1990) Persistent etretinate levels in plasma after changing the therapy to acitretin. *Arch. Dermatol. Res.*, **282**, 343–344

Lambert, W.E., Meyer, E., De Leenheer, A.P., De Bersaques, J. & Kint, A.H. (1992) Pharmacokinetics and drug interactions of etretinate and acitretin. *J. Am. Acad. Dermatol.*, **27**, S19–S22

Lambert, W.E., Meyer, E., De Leenheer, A.P., De Bersaques, J. & Kint, A.H. (1994) Pharmacokinetics of acitretin. *Acta Derm. Venereol. Suppl. Stockh.*, **186**, 122–123

Larsen, F.G. (1994) Pharmacokinetics of etretinate and acitretin with special reference to treatment of psoriasis. *Acta Derm. Venereol. Suppl. Stockh.*, **190**, 1–33

Larsen, F.G., Jakobsen, P., Larsen, C.G., Kragballe, K. & Nielsen-Kudsk, F. (1988) Pharmacokinetics of etretin and etretinate during long-term treatment of psoriasis patients. *Pharmacol. Toxicol.*, **62**, 159–165

Larsen, F.G., Jakobsen, P., Eriksen, H., Gronhoj, J., Kragballe, K. & Nielsen Kudsk, F. (1991) The pharmacokinetics of acitretin and its 13-*cis*-metabolite in psoriatic patients. *J. Clin. Pharmacol.*, **31**, 477–483

Larsen, F.G., Vahlquist, C., Andersson, E., Törma, H., Kragballe, K. & Vahlquist, A. (1992) Oral acitretin in psoriasis: Drug and vitamin A concentrations in plasma, skin and adipose tissue. *Acta Derm. Venereol.*, **72**, 84–88

Larsen, F.G., Jakobsen, P., Knudsen, J., Weismann, K., Kragballe, K. & Nielsen Kudsk, F. (1993a) Conversion of acitretin to etretinate in psoriatic patients is influenced by ethanol. *J. Invest. Dermatol.*, **100**, 623–627

Larsen, F.G., Andersen, S.R., Weismann, K., Julian, K. & Tfelt Hansen, P. (1993b) Keratoconus as a possible side-effect of acitretin (neotigason) therapy. *Acta Derm. Venereol.*, **73**, 156–156

Laugier, J.P., Berbis, P., Brindley, C., Bun, H., Geiger, J.M., Privat, Y. & Durand, A. (1989) Determination of acitretin and 13-*cis*-acitretin in skin. *Skin Pharmacol.*, **2**, 181–186

Laugier, J.P., de Sousa, G., Bun, H., Geiger, J.M., Surber, C. & Rahmani, R. (1994) Acitretin biotransformation into etretinate: Role of ethanol on in vitro hepatic metabolism. *Dermatology*, **188**, 122–125

Lister, R.K., Lecky, B.R., Lewis, J.M. & Young, C.A. (1996) Acitretin-induced myopathy. *Br. J. Dermatol.*, **134**, 989–990

Löfberg, B., Chahoud, I., Bochert, G. & Nau, H. (1990) Teratogenicity of the 13-*cis* and all-*trans*-isomers of the aromatic retinoid etretin: Correlation to transplacental pharmacokinetics in mice during organogenesis after a single oral dose. *Teratology*, **41**, 707–716

Maier, H. & Hönigsmann, H. (1996) Concentration of etretinate in plasma and subcutaneous fat after long-term acitretin. *Lancet*, **348**, 1107–1107

Makin, S.M., Mikerin, I.E., Shavrygina, O.A. & Lanina, T.I. (1989) Stereoselective synthesis of the aromatic analogs of retinal and retinoic acid. *Zh. Org. Khim.*, **25**, 792–797

Meyer, E., Lambert, W.E., De Leenheer, A.P., Bersaques, J.P. & Kint, A.H. (1991) Improved quantitation of 13-*cis*- and all-*trans*-acitretin in human plasma by normal-phase high-performance liquid chromatography. *J. Chromatogr.*, **570**, 149–156

Mork, N.J., Kolbenstvedt, A. & Austad, J. (1992) Efficacy and skeletal side effects of two years' acitretin treatment. *Acta Derm. Venereol.*, **72**, 445–448

Muto, Y. & Moriwaki, H. (1984) Antitumor activity of vitamin A and its derivatives. *J. Natl Cancer Inst.*, **73**, 1389–1393

Newton, D.L., Henderson, W.R. & Sporn, M.B. (1980) Structure–activity relationships of retinoids in hamster tracheal organ culture. *Cancer Res.*, **40**, 3413–3425

O'Brien, T.J. (1990) Etretin. A replacement for etretinate. *Int. J. Dermatol.*, **29**, 270–271

Orfanos, C.E., Zouboulis, C.C., Almond-Roesler, B. & Geilen, C.C. (1997) Current use and future potential role of retinoids in dermatology. *Drugs*, **53**, 358–388

Palmskog, G. (1980) Determination of plasma levels of two aromatic retinoic acid analogues with antipsoriatic activity by high-performance liquid chromatography. *J. Chromatogr.*, **221**, 345–351

Paravicini, U. & Busslinger, A. (1983) Determination of etretinate and its main metabolite in human plasma using normal-phase high-performance liquid chromatography. *J. Chromatogr.*, **276**, 359–366

Paravicini, U., Stockel, K., MacNamara, P.J., Hänni, R. & Busslinger, A. (1981) On metabolism and pharmacokinetics of an aromatic retinoid. *Ann. N.Y. Acad. Sci.*, **359**, 54–67

Paravicini, U., Camenzind, M., Gower, M., Geiger, J.M. & Saurat, J.H. (1985) Multiple dose pharmacokinetics of Ro 10-1670, the main metabolite of etretinate (Tigason®). In: Saurat, J.H., ed., *Retinoids. New Trends in Research and Therapy*. Basel, Krager, pp. 289–292

Parsch, E.M., Ruzicka, T., Przybilla, B. & Schill, W.B. (1990) Andrological investigations in men treated with acitretin (Ro 10-1670). *Andrologia*, **22**, 479–482

Paul, C. & Dubertret, L. (1998) Acitretin and etretinate: Strategy for use and long-term side effects. In: Roenigk, H.H. & Maibach, H.I., eds, *Psoriasis*, 3rd Ed. New York, Marcel Dekker, pp. 671–683

Peck, R. & Bollag, W. (1991) Potentiation of retinoid-induced differentiation of HL-60 and U937 cell lines by cytokines. *Eur. J. Cancer*, **27**, 53–57

Petkovich, M., Brand, N.J., Krust, A. & Chambon, P. (1987) A human retinoic acid receptor which belongs to the family of nuclear receptors. *Nature*, **330**, 444–450

Pilkington, T. & Brogden, R.N. (1992) Acitretin. A review of its pharmacology and therapeutic use. *Drugs*, **43**, 597–627

Priestley, G.C. (1987) Proliferation and glycosaminoglycans secretion in fibroblasts from psoriatic skin: Differential responses to retinoids. *Br. J. Dermatol.*, **117**, 575–583

Redlich, C.A., Delisser, H.M. & Elias, J.A. (1995) Retinoic acid inhibition of transforming growth factor-β-induced collagen production by human lung fibroblasts. *Am. J. Respir. Cell. Mol. Biol.*, **12**, 287–295

Reiners, J., Löfberg, B., Kraft, J.C., Kochhar, D.M. & Nau, H. (1988) Transplacental pharmacokinetics of teratogenic doses of etretinate and other aromatic retinoids in mice. *Reprod. Toxicol.*, **2**, 19–29

Rollman, O. & Pihl-Lundin, I. (1990) Acitretin excretion into human breast milk. *Acta Derm. Venereol.*, **70**, 487–490

Rudnicka, L., Marczak, M., Szmurlo, A., Makiela, B., Skiendzielewska, A., Skopinska, M., Majewski, S. & Jablonska, S. (1991) Acitretin decreases tumor cell-induced angiogenesis. *Skin Pharmacol.*, **4**, 150–153

Salleras, M., Sanchez-Regana, M. & Umbert, P. (1995) Congenital erythrodermic psoriasis: Case report and literature review. *Pediatr. Dermatol.*, **12**, 231–234

Sanquer, S., Eller, M.S. & Gilchrest, B.A. (1993) Retinoids and state of differentiation modulate CRABP II gene expression in a skin equivalent. *J. Invest. Dermatol.*, **100**, 148–153

Schmitt, A., Hauser, C., Didierjean, L., Merot, Y., Dayer, J.M. & Saurat, J.H. (1987) Systemic administration of etretin increases epidermal interleukin I in the rat. *Br. J. Dermatol.*, **116**, 615–622

Schmitt Hoffmann, A.H., Dittrich, S., Saulnier, E., Schenk, P. & Chou, R.C. (1995) Mechanistic studies on the ethyl-esterification of acitretin by human liver preparations in vitro. *Life Sci.*, **57**, L407–L412

Shapiro, S.S. & Mott, D.J. (1981) Modulation of glycosaminoglycan biosynthesis by retinoids. *Ann. N.Y. Acad. Sci.*, **359**, 306–321

Sigg, C., Bruckner-Tuderman, L. & Gilardi, S. (1987) Andrological investigations in patients treated with etretin. *Dermatologica*, **175**, 48–49

Small, D.S. & McNamara, P.J. (1994) Hepatic enzyme induction potential of acitretin in male and female Sprague-Dawley rats. *J. Pharm. Sci.*, **83**, 662–667

Stadler, R., Müller, R., Detmar, M. & Orfanos, C.E. (1987) Retinoids and keratinocyte differentiation in vitro. *Dermatologica*, **175** (Suppl. 1), 45–55

Stadler, R., Otte, H.G., Luger, T., Henz, B.M., Kühl, P., Zwingers, T. & Sterry, W. (1998) Prospective randomized multicenter clinical trial on the use of interferon α-2a plus acitretin versus interferon α-2a plus PUVA in patients with cutaneous T-cell lymphoma stages I and II. *Blood*, **92**, 3578–3581

Steele, C.E., Marlow, R., Turton, J. & Hicks, R.M. (1987) In-vitro teratogenicity of retinoids. *Br. J. Exp. Pathol.*, **68**, 215–223

Stricker, B.H., Barendregt, M., Herings, R.M., de Jong-van den Berg, L.T., Cornel, M.C. & de Smet, P.A. (1992) Ad-hoc tracing of a cohort of patients exposed to acitretine (Neotigason®) on a nation-wide scale. *Eur. J. Clin. Pharmacol.*, **42**, 555–557

Sturkenboom, M.C., Middelbeek, A., de Jong-van den Berg, L.T., van den Berg, P.B., Stricker, B.H. & Wesseling, H. (1995) Vulvo–vaginal candidiasis associated with acitretin. *J. Clin. Epidemiol.*, **48**, 991–997

Szuts, E.Z. & Harosi, F.I. (1991) Solubility of retinoids in water. *Arch. Biochem. Biophys.*, **287**, 297–304

Thongnopnua, P. & Zimmerman, C.L. (1988) Simultaneous microassay for etretinate and its active metabolite, etretin, by reversed-phase high-performance liquid chromatography. *J. Chromatogr.*, **433**, 345–351

Tokura, Y., Edelson, R.L. & Gasparro, F.P. (1992) Retinoid augmentation of bioactive interleukin-1 production by murine keratinocytes. *Br. J. Dermatol.*, **126**, 485–495

Tong, P.S., Mayes, D.M. & Wheeler, L.A. (1988) Differential effects of retinoids on DNA synthesis in calcium-regulated murine epidermal keratinocyte cultures. *J. Invest. Dermatol.*, **90**, 861–868

Tsambaos, D., Bolsen, K., Georgiou, S., Kalofoutis, A. & Goerz, G. (1994) Effects of oral administration of acitretin on rat liver microsomal phospholipids, P-450 content and monooxygenase activities. *Skin Pharmacol.*, **7**, 320–323

Turton, J.A., Willars, G.B., Haselden, J.N., Ward, S.J., Steele, C.E. & Hicks, R.M. (1992) Comparative teratogenicity of nine retinoids in the rat. *Int. J. Exp. Pathol.*, **73**, 551–563

Vane, F.M., Buggé, C.J. & Rodriguez, L.C. (1989a) Identification of etretinate metabolites in human bile. *Drug Metab. Dispos.*, **17**, 275–279

Vane, F.M., Buggé, J.L. & Rodriguez, L.C. (1989b) Identification of etretinate metabolites in human blood. *Drug Metab. Dispos.*, **17**, 280–285

West, M.R., Page, J.M., Turner, D.M., Wood, E.J., Holland, D.B., Cunliffe, W.J. & Rupniak, H.T. (1992) Simple assays of retinoid activity as potential screens for compounds that may be useful in treatment of psoriasis. *J. Invest. Dermatol.*, **99**, 95–100

Wetherall, N.T. & Taylor, C.M. (1986) The effects of retinoid treatment and antiestrogens on the growth of T47D human breast cancer cells. *Eur. J. Cancer Clin. Oncol.*, **22**, 53–59

Wyss, R. (1990) Determination of retinoids in plasma by high-performance liquid chromatography and automated column switching. *Methods Enzymol.*, **189**, 146–155

Wyss, R. & Bucheli, F. (1988) Determination of highly protein bound drugs in plasma using high-performance liquid chromatography and column switching, exemplified by the retinoids. *J. Chromatogr.*, **456**, 33–43

Xue, G.Z., Zheng, Z.S., Chen, R.Z., Lloyd, M.B. & Prystowsky, J.H. (1996) Phorbol 12-myristate 13-acetate inhibits epidermal growth factor signalling in human keratinocytes, leading to decreased ornithine decarboxylase activity. *Biochem. J.*, **319**, 641–648

Yoshioka, A., Miyachi, Y., Imamura, S. & Niwa, Y. (1986) Anti-oxidant effects of retinoids on inflammatory skin diseases. *Arch. Dermatol. Res.*, **278**, 177–183

Zouboulis, C.C., Korge, B., Akamatsu, H., Xia, L.Q., Schiller, S., Gollnick, H. & Orfanos, C.E. (1991) Effects of 13-*cis*-retinoic acid, all-*trans*-retinoic acid, and acitretin on the proliferation, lipid synthesis and keratin expression of cultured human sebocytes in vitro. *J. Invest. Dermatol.*, **96**, 792–797

N-Ethylretinamide

1. Chemical and Physical Characteristics

1.1 Nomenclature
See General Remarks, Section 1.4

1.2 Name
Chemical Abstracts Services Registry Number
33631-41-3

IUPAC Systematic name
N-Ethyl (2E,4E,6E,8E)-3,7-dimethyl-9-(2,2,6-tri-methylcyclohexenyl)-2,4,6,8-nonatetraenamide

Synonyms
all-*trans*-N-Ethylretinamide, NER, N-ethyl all-*trans*-retinamide, N-ethyl (E)-3,7-dimethyl-9-(2,2,6-trimethylcyclohexenyl)-2,4,6,8-nonate-traenamide, N-ethyl retinamide, Ro 8-4968.

1.3 Structural formula

CONHEt

Composition: $C_{22}H_{33}NO$
Relative molecular mass: 326.3

1.4 Physical and chemical properties
Description
Pale-yellow crystals

Melting-point
137–138 °C

Spectroscopy
UV and visible: λ_{max} 347 nm; $E_{1\,cm}^{1\%}$ 1540 (Bollag *et al.*, 1976); λ_{max} (ethanol) 347 nm (ε = 50 300 M^{-1} cm^{-1}) (Zanotti *et al.*, 1993).

Solubility
Soluble in organic solvents

Stability
Unstable to light, oxygen and heat

2. Occurrence, Production, Use, Human Exposure and Analysis

2.1 Occurrence
N-Ethylretinamide, a synthetic compound, is not present in food, and human exposure is limited to medical treatment.

2.2 Production
N-Ethylretinamide is prepared by treatment of an etheral solution of all-*trans*-retinoyl chloride with ethylamine at 0 °C, followed by room temperature for 4 h and reflux temperature for 2 h (Bollag *et al.*, 1976). The acid chloride is prepared by treatment of all-*trans*-retinoic acid with thionyl chloride. The compound became available from the United States National Cancer Institute Chemical Repository in 1998.

2.3 Use
N-Ethylretinamide has not been used extensively in humans.

2.4 Human exposure
N-Ethylretinamide has been used in some trials for psoriasis (Runne *et al.*, 1973).

2.5 Analysis
N-Ethylretinamide can be separated by reversed-phase high-performance liquid chromatography and quantified by its ultraviolet absorption at 347 nm (Shih *et al.*, 1988).

3. Metabolism, Kinetics and Genetic Variation

3.1 Humans
No data were available to the Working Group.

3.2   Experimental models

Enzymatic activity present in rat liver microsomes hydrolysed N-ethylretinamide to all-*trans*-retinoic acid. The reaction was more rapid than that for 4-hydroxyphenylretinamide (Shih *et al.*, 1988).

4.   Cancer-preventive Effects

4.1   Humans

No data were available to the Working Group.

4.2   Experimental models

4.2.1   Cancer and preneoplastic lesions

These studies are summarized in Table 1.

4.2.1.1   Trachea

Hamster: Groups of 63 male Syrian hamsters were given intratracheal instillations of N-methyl-N-nitrosourea (MNU), [amount not stated] once a week for 12 weeks and one week after the last exposure were placed on diets containing N-ethylretinamide at 1 mmol/kg of diet (327 mg/kg of diet) for six months, at which time they were killed and examined for tracheal neoplasms. None of 12 hamsters given only N-ethylretinamide developed an epithelial neoplasm, but of the animals dosed with MNU and fed a control diet, 16% developed epithelial neoplasms and 6% had carcinomas. Of hamsters dosed with MNU and fed the diet containing N-ethylretinamide, 38% developed epithelial neoplasms and 19% had carcinomas. The incidence of epithelial neoplasms and carcinomas in N-ethylretinamide-treated hamsters was significantly greater than that in controls ($p < 0.01$ and < 0.05, respectively; χ^2 test; Stinson *et al.*, 1981).

4.2.1.2   Liver

Mouse: Groups of 25–29 B6D2F1 mice were given a single intraperitoneal injection of N-nitrosodiethylamine (NDEA) at 50 or 100 mg/kg bw and one week later were fed a diet containing N-ethylretinamide at 0.5 or 1 mmol/kg of diet for 12 months. In mice given the low dose of NDEA, the incidence of liver carcinomas increased from 0% in controls to 62% and 72% in the groups fed diets containing the low and high doses of N-ethylretinamide, respectively. In mice given the high dose of NDEA, the incidence of liver carcinomas increased from 15% in controls to 64% and 100%, respectively

($p < 0.01$, χ^2 test). In groups of mice fed diets containing N-ethylretinamide and killed at 9 or 12 months, hepatocellular carcinomas were found in 2 of 30 animals, and benign tumours were found in 6 additional mice (see section 6.2; McCormick *et al.*, 1990).

4.2.1.3   Pancreas

Hamster: Groups of 10–12 controls and 23–26 treated male and female Syrian hamsters, eight weeks of age, were given a single subcutaneous dose of N-nitrosobis(2-oxopropyl)amine (NBOPA) at 40 mg/kg bw. One week later, they were placed on diets containing N-ethylretinamide at concentrations of 0.05, 0.1 or 0.2 mmol/kg of diet. The animals were killed 33 weeks after administration of the carcinogen and examined for pancreatic cancers. The tumour incidence in animals of each sex was not significantly different from that in controls. In females, the number of pancreatic carcinomas per animal at all three doses increased from 1.2 to 2.6 ($p < 0.01$, χ^2 test). In males, the carcinoma multiplicity was 1.5 in controls and 2.3 in treated animals (not significant; Birt *et al.*, 1981).

Groups of 20–24 control and 25–40 treated male and female hamsters were given a single subcutaneous dose of 10 or 40 mg/kg bw NBOPA and one week later were placed on diets containing N-ethylretinamide at 0.5 or 1 mmol/kg of diet. The hamsters were killed 40 weeks after administration of the high dose of the carcinogen or 50 weeks after the low dose and examined for pancreatic cancers. The number of ductular carcinomas per animal was significantly increased in both male and female hamsters given the high dose of NBOPA and either concentration of N-ethylretinamide, from 0.3 to 1 for females and from 0.3 to 1.1 for males ($p < 0.05$, χ^2 test). No significant difference in tumour incidence or multiplicity was seen in animals given the low dose of NBOPA (Birt *et al.*, 1983).

4.2.1.4   Urinary bladder

Mouse: Groups of 97 control and 75 treated male B6D2F$_1$ mice were given N-nitrosobutyl-N-(4-hydroxybutyl)amine (NBHBA) at 5 or 10 mg/animal by gastric intubation twice a week for nine weeks with diets containing N-ethylretinamide at 0.5 or 1 mmol/kg of diet. The animals

Table 1. Effects of N-ethylretinamide on carcinogenesis in animals

Cancer site	Species sex, age at carcinogen treatment	No. of animals per group	Carcinogen dose, route	N-Ethyl-retinamide dose and route (mmol/kg diet)	Duration in relation to carcinogen	Incidence Control	Treated	Multiplicity Control	Treated	Efficacy	Reference
Trachea	Male Syrian hamsters, 20 wks	63	MNU (0.5%, intra-tracheally [total amount not stated] once a wk, 12 wks)	None 1	−1 wk to end (6 months)	6	19*	NR	NR	Tumour enhancing	Stinson et al. (1981)
Liver	Female B6D2F₁ mice, 4–5 wks	25–29	NDEA (50 mg/kg bw, i.p.)	1 0.5	−1 wk to end	0	72* 62*	NR	NR	Tumour enhancing	McCormick et al. (1990)
		27–29	NDEA (100 mg/kg bw, i.p.)	None 1 0.5	−1 wk to end	15	100* 64*	NR	NR	Tumour enhancing	
Pancreas	Female Syrian hamsters	10 23	NBOPA (40 mg/kg bw, s.c.)	0.05–0.2ᵃ	−1 wk to end (33 wks)	40	43	1.2	2.6*	Tumour enhancing	Birt et al. (1981)
	Male Syrian hamsters	12 26	NBOPA (40 mg/kg bw, s.c.)	0.005–0.2ᵃ	−1 wk to end (33 wks)	50	50	1.5	2.3	Ineffective	Birt et al. (1983)
	Female Syrian hamsters	20 (control) 37 (treated)	NBOPA (40 mg/kg bw, s.c.)	0.5–1ᵇ	+ 1 wk to wk 40	30	43	0.3	1.0*	Tumour enhancing	Birt et al. (1983)
	Male Syrian hamsters	24 (control) 40 (treated)	NBPOA (40 mg/kg bw, s.c.)	0.5–1ᵇ	+ 1 wk to wk 40	21	50	0.3	1.1*	Tumour enhancing	Birt et al. (1983)
	Female Syrian hamsters	23 (control) 25 (treated)	NBOPA (10 mg/kg bw, s.c.)	0.5–1ᵇ	+ 1 wk to wk 50	27	24	0.3	0.4	Ineffective	Birt et al. (1983)
	Male Syrian hamsters	22 (control) 30 (treated)	NBOPA (10 mg/kg bw, s.c.)	0.5–1ᵇ	+ 1 wk to wk 50	18	33	0.2	0.4	Ineffective	Birt et al. (1983)

Table 1. (contd)

Cancer site	Species sex, age at carcinogen treatment	No. of animals per group	Carcinogen dose, route	N-Ethyl-retinamide dose and route (mmol/kg diet)	Duration in relation to carcincgen	Incidence Control	Treated	Multiplicity Control	Treated	Efficacy	Reference
Bladder	Male B6D2F1 mice	(75–97)	NBHBA (5 or 10 mg/animal by gavage twice/wk for 9 wks)[c]	0.5 1.0	– 1 wk to end	37	33	NR	NR	Ineffective	Thompson et al. (1981)
	Male Fischer 344 rats, 6–7 wks	60 (control) 30 (treated)	NBHBA (200 mg, p.o. twice a wk. 8 wks)	2	–1 wk to 6 month	92	83	2.25	1.76	Ineffective	Thompson et al. (1981)
	Female Fischer 344 rats, 6–7 wks	80 (control) 40 (treated)	NBHBA (150 mg, p.o. twice a wk, 6 wks)	2	–1 wk to 6 month	35	12*	0.49	0.13*	Effective	Thompson et al. (1981)
	Male B6D2F$_1$ mice, 6–7 wks	99	NBHBA (7.5 mg, by gavage once a wk, 8 wks	1.5	– 1 wk to 7 month	35	21*	NR	NR	Effective	Moon et al. (1982)
	Female Fischer 344 rats, 50–60 g bw	200 (control) 100 (treated)	FANFT (0.2% in the diet, 10 wks)	1 2	– 1 wk to 50 wks	53	63 78*	NR	NR	Tumour enhancing	Croft et al. (1981)
Colon	Male Fischer 344 rats, 9 wks	40	MNU (0.5 mg, twice per wk, 8 wks, intrarectal)	2	– 5 d to 32 wks	60	65	1.71	1.65	Ineffective	Wenk et al. (1981)
		50	MNU (0.5 mg, twice per wk, 6 wks, intrarectal)	2	– 5 d to + 44 wks	62	63	1.55	1.58	Ineffective	Wenk et al. (1981)
		50	MNU (0.5 mg, twice per wk, 4 wks, intrarectal)	2	– 5 d + 52 wks	31	30	1.40	1.20	Ineffective	Wenk et al. (1981)

MNU, N-methyl-N-nitrosourea; i.v., intravenous; NDEA, N-nitrosodiethylamine; i.p., intraperitoneal; NBOPA, N-nitrosobis(2-oxopropyl)amine; s.c., subcutaneous; NBHBA, N-nitrosobutyl-N-(4-hydroxybutyl)amine; p.o., oral; FANFT, N-[4-(5-nitrofuryl)-2-thiazolyl]formamide; NR, not reported

*Significantly different from controls

[a] Data combined for three N-ethylretinamide doses

[b] Data combined for two N-ethylretinamide doses

[c] Data combined for two carcinogen doses

were killed six months after the first dose of carcinogen and examined for bladder carcinomas. Since the incidence of bladder cancer was similar at the two doses of carcinogen, the values were combined. *N*-Ethylretinamide at a dose of 0.5 mmol/kg of diet did not significantly affect the incidence of carcinomas, but at 1 mmol/kg of diet, the incidence was 21%, which was significantly lower ($p < 0.025$, χ^2 test) than that in controls (37%; Thompson *et al.*, 1981).

Groups of 99 control and 99 treated male B6D2F$_1$ mice were given NBHBA at 7.5 mg/animal once a week for eight weeks. One week after the final dose, the mice were placed on a diet containing *N*-ethylretinamide at 1.5 mmol/kg of diet. The animals were killed 210 days after the first dose of carcinogen and were examined for bladder carcinomas. *N*-Ethylretinamide reduced the incidence of carcinomas from 35 to 21% ($p < 0.05$, χ^2 test) (Moon *et al.*, 1982).

Rat: Groups of 60–80 control and 30–40 treated male and female Fischer 344 rats were given NBHBA by gastric intubation. Males were given 200 mg/animal twice a week for eight weeks, and females received 150 mg/animal for six weeks. One week after the final dose, the rats were placed on diets containing *N*-ethylretinamide at 2 mmol/kg diet. In females, the incidence of bladder carcinomas was 35% in controls and 12% in *N*-ethylretinamide-treated animals ($p < 0.01$, χ^2 test), and the multiplicity was reduced from 0.49 to 0.13 ($p < 0.01$, χ^2 test). In male rats, the incidence of bladder carcinomas was 92% in controls and 83% in treated animals (not significant), and the multiplicity was 2.2 in controls and 1.8 in treated animals (not significant) (Thompson *et al.*, 1981).

Groups of 200 control and 100 treated female Fischer 344 rats weighing 50–60 g were given a diet containing 0.2% *N*-[4-(5-nitro-2-furyl)-2-thiazolyl]-formamide (FANFT) for 10 weeks and one week later were given diets containing *N*-ethylretinamide at 1 or 2 mmol/kg diet. The rats were killed 50 weeks after the first exposure to the carcinogen. The incidence of bladder carcinomas was 53% in controls, 63% at the low dose and 78% at the high dose ($p < 0.001$ [test not specified]) (Croft *et al.*, 1981).

4.2.1.5 Colon
Rat: Groups of 40–50 male Fischer 344 rats, nine weeks of age, were given MNU intrarectally at a dose of 0.5 mg per animal twice a week for four, six or eight weeks. Five days after the last dose, they were placed on diets containing *N*-ethylretinamide at 2 mmol/kg diet. The animals were killed at 52, 44 or 32 weeks after the initial dose of carcinogen. There were no appreciable differences in the incidences or multiplicity of colon carcinomas between control and treated animals (Wenk *et al.*, 1981).

4.2.2 Intermediate biomarkers
No data were available to the Working Group.

4.2.3 In-vitro models
4.2.3.1 Cellular studies

(a) Inhibition of neoplastic transformation
Neoplastically transformed foci can be produced in cultured C3H/10T/1/2 cells by application of 3-methylcholanthrene or by exposure to ionizing radiation, and various retinoids reduce the incidence of such foci. Complete inhibition of transformation was achieved when *N*-ethylretinamide was applied seven days after removal of the carcinogen and continued throughout the four-week assay. The activity was therefore not a result of changes in the metabolic activation of the carcinogen or repair of pre-carcinogenic lesions. Activity was observed at concentrations that were marginally toxic, and the inhibition was reversible upon withdrawal of the retinoids, although this was not tested with *N*-ethylretinamide. The activity of the retinoids was thus not due to cytotoxicity. A dose–response relationship was seen for reductions in focus formation with doses of 10^{-5} to 3×10^{-7} mol/L, the median effective dose being about 10^{-6} mol/L (Bertram, 1980; see Table 2). *N*-Ethylretinamide was marginally more potent than all-*trans*-retinoic acid, but the relatively low activity of all-*trans*-retinoic acid in these cells has been shown to be due to its rapid catabolism. Its activity can be increased by a factor of 1000 by simultaneous treatment with liarozole (Acevedo & Bertram, 1995), an inhibitor of an inducible cytochrome P450 4-hydroxylase enzyme which inactivates all-*trans*-retinoic acid. [The Working Group noted that it is not known if *N*-ethylretinamide is subject to similar inactivation.]

Table 2. Inhibition of cell transformation and differentiation by *N*-ethylretinamide *in vitro*

End-point	Treatment	Concentration (mol/L)	No. of foci/no. dishes	Preventive efficacy (% vehicle control)	Comments	Reference
Cell transformation	MCA 2.5 µg/ml 7 days after, then weekly	10^{-5} 3×10^{-6} 10^{-6} 3×10^{-7} Acetone Control	0/12 5/12 13/12 23.12 80/36	0 18.8 48.8 86.2 100	2–3 times more potent than all-*trans*-retinoic acid	Bertram (1980)
Differentiation	Hamster trachea; vitamin A deficiency		+	IC_{50} 1 nmol/L	30 times less potent than all-*trans*-retinoic acid	Newton *et al.* (1980)
Differentiation	Chick skin; vitamin A deficiency		+	IC_{80}, 2.2 µmol/L	Similar to all *trans*-retinoic acid	Wilkoff *et al.* (1976)

MCA, 3-methylcholanthrene; IC, inhibitory concentration

(b)   Inhibition of cell differentiation.
Explants of trachea from vitamin A-deficient hamster have been used to measure the efficacy of retinoids in preventing the squamous metaplasia that usually results when this tissue is cultured in the absence of vitamin A. *N*-Ethylretinamide dissolved in dimethylsulfoxide reversed the metaplasia, at a median effective dose of about 10^{-9} mol/L when applied over 10 days. The activity of all-*trans*-retinoic acid when tested under the same conditions was 3×10^{-11} mol/L. Thus, *N*-ethylretinamide was significantly less active than the parent retinoid. More than 90% of the control cultures that had received no retinoid for the entire 10-day culture period showed metaplasia with keratin and keratohyalin granules (Newton *et al.*, 1980).

N-Ethylretinamide was also evaluated for its capacity to inhibit squamous keratinization in chick embryo metatarsal skin, which occurs in culture in the absence of adequate vitamin A. When *N*-ethylretinamide dissolved in ethanol or dimethylsulfoxide was administered for 6–8 days at a concentration of 2.2×10^{-6} mol/L, keratinization was inhibited in about 80% of exposed chick

skin. all-*trans*-Retinoic acid had equivalent activity in this assay system. In the absence of exogenously added vitamin A, all the skin explants underwent squamous differentiation (Wilkoff *et al.*, 1976).

4.2.3.2   Antimutagenicity in short-term tests
No data were available to the Working Group.

4.3   Mechanisms of cancer prevention
N-Ethylretinamide inhibited transformation induced in C3H10T1/2 cells by the carcinogen, 3-methylcholanthrene (Bertram, 1980). Since the retinoid was added to the cultures seven days after removal of the carcinogen, it is not likely to have had an effect on carcinogen uptake or metabolic activation. The capacity of *N*-ethylretinamide to modulate epithelial differentiation in chick embryo skin is equivalent to that of all-*trans*-retinoic acid (Wilkoff *et al.*, 1976). This activity is evidently mediated through effects on gene activation, although *N*-ethylretinamide has no measurable affinity for the retinoid receptors (Kim *et al.*, 1994). It is not clear if *N*-ethylretinamide acts without hydrolytic cleavage to all-*trans*-retinoic acid, which occurs in a slow

enzymatic reaction catalysed by an enzyme present in liver microsomes (Shih *et al.*, 1988).

The mechanism by which *N*-ethylretinamide prevents cancer in the models of carcinogenesis in which it is effective is unknown.

5.   Other Beneficial Effects

No data were available to the Working Group.

6.   Carcinogenicity

6.1   Humans

No data were available to the Working Group.

6.2   Experimental models

Thirty female B6D2F$_1$ mice, 4–5 weeks of age, were fed a diet containing *N*-ethylretinamide at 1 mmol/kg of diet for 9 or 12 months. Eight animals developed hepatocellular tumours, two of which were carcinomas. No such tumours developed in control mice or in mice fed *N*-ethylretinamide at a lower dose (0.5 nmol/kg of diet; McCormick *et al.*, 1990).

N-Ethylretinamide enhanced the incidences of tracheal tumours in hamsters receiving intratracheal instillations of MNU (Stinson *et al.*, 1981), of pancreatic tumours in hamsters treated with NBOPA (Birt *et al.*, 1981, 1983), of liver tumours in mice treated with NDEA (McCormick et al., 1990) and of bladder tumours in rats given FANFT (Croft *et al.*, 1981; see section 4.2.1).

7.   Other Toxic Effects

7.1   Adverse effects
7.1.1   Humans

Increased concentrations of serum lipids and increased erythrocyte sedimentation rates were seen after oral administration of a total dose of 8400 mg of *N*-ethylretinamide over three weeks to 26 patients with psoriasis. A few of the patients complained of headache, diarrhoea and vomiting (Runne *et al.*, 1973).

7.1.2   Experimental models
7.1.2.1   Acute and short-term toxicity
The toxicity of both the all-*trans* and the 13-*cis* isomers of *N*-ethylretinamide have been investigated in

rats and mice after peroral and intraperitoneal administration (Sani & Meeks, 1983). The estimated LD$_{50}$ in mice was 33 mg/kg bw for all-*trans*-retinoic acid and 1801 mg/kg bw for *N*-ethylretinamide. In 21-day studies in mice given *N*-ethylretinamide at doses of 100–1800 mg/kg bw, the haemoglobin, haematocrit, erythrocyte, leukocyte and reticulocyte counts were decreased at doses as low as 400 mg/kg bw. The anaemia-generating effect of the 13-*cis* derivative was milder than that of the all-*trans* isomer. Treatment with the *N*-ethylretinamides also increased plasma alkaline phosphatase activity and decreased serum albumin concentrations. No bone fractures were seen. Higher doses of *N*-ethylretinamide were associated with histopathological evidence of degenerative liver lesions.

7.1.2.2   Long-term toxicity
The anaemia seen after treatment with *N*-ethylretinamide was confirmed in a one-year study in rats and was related in part to retinoid-induced bone remodelling. Groups of rats given *N*-ethylretinamide at a dose of 321 or 654 mg/kg bw were compared with groups on normal diets and diets containing placebo and also with groups treated with *N*-(2-hydroxyethyl)-, *N*-butyl-, *N*-(4-hydroxyphenyl)-, *N*-tetrazol-5-yl- or 13-*cis*-*N*-ethyl-retinamides or with etretinate. The retinoids caused a narrowing of the medullary cavity and a subsequent reduction in haematopoietic capacity. The osteopathy induced by *N*-ethylretinamide was dose-dependent. At several of the doses tested, *N*-ethylretinamide and some of the other retinamides also caused significant increases in lymphoid tissue weight and peripheral blood lymphocytosis (Turton *et al.*, 1985).

7.2   Reproductive and developmental effects
7.2.1   Humans
No data were available to the Working Group.

7.2.2   Experimental models
7.2.2.1   Reproductive effects
N-Ethylretinamide induced sterility in male hamsters fed diets containing 327 mg/kg for six months. Atrophy of the terminal epithelium was observed, and the testicular weights had decreased by 75% (Stinson *et al.*, 1980).

7.2.2.2   Developmental effects

Treatment of mice with N-ethylretinamide at doses of 100–400 mg/kg bw on day 11 of gestation did not cause terata but mildly increased the rate of embryo resorption, indicating that the compound is minimally embryotoxic (Kochhar *et al.*, 1992). The embryo resorption rates were not increased in rats given a dose of 300 or 600 mg/kg bw, and at 600 mg/kg only 20% of the embryos were abnormal. The abnormalities were mild: only optic abnormalities were seen in the craniofacial region, and occasional incidences of dilated ureter were found in the caudal region (Turton *et al.*, 1992). In mice and rats, a dose of at least 300 mg/kg bw was required to induce teratogenic effects (Kistler, 1987). In rat whole-embryo cultures, the concentration of N-ethylretinamide required to produce teratogenic effects (failure of yolk sac circulation, delayed closure of the anterior neuropore, reduced number of somites) was 50–100 times that of all-*trans*-retinoic acid (Steele *et al.*, 1987).

A single oral dose of 75 mg/kg bw of all-*trans*- or 13-*cis*-retinoic acid given to pregnant hamsters increased the incidence of malformations in the offspring, but equimolar doses of N-ethylretinamide or 13-*cis*-N-ethylretinamide were not embryotoxic (Willhite & Shealy, 1984).

In an assay based on the inhibition of chondrogenesis of limb bud cells *in vitro*, N-ethylretinamide was active only at very high doses, 1–50 mmol/L (Kistler, 1987).

7.3   Genetic and related effects

No data were available to the Working Group.

8.   Summary of Data

8.1   Chemistry, occurrence and human exposure

N-Ethylretinamide is a synthetic derivative of all-*trans*-retinoic acid. It has not been approved for use in humans.

8.2   Metabolism and kinetics

N-Ethylretinamide is slowly hydrolysed, albeit more rapidly than 4-hydroxyphenylretinamide, to all-*trans*-retinoic acid by rat liver microsomes *in vitro*. No information was available about its metabolism in humans.

8.3   Cancer-preventive effects
8.3.1   Humans

No data were available to the Working Group.

8.3.2   Experimental models

The cancer-preventive efficacy of N-ethylretinamide has been evaluated in models of respiratory tract and pancreas carcinogenesis in hamsters, of liver carcinogenesis in mice, of urinary bladder carcinogenesis in mice and rats and of colon carcinogenesis in rats. The tumour incidence was enhanced in the trachea and pancreas of hamsters, in the liver in mice and, in one study, in the urinary bladder in rats. N-Ethylretinamide had cancer-preventive effects in some studies of urinary bladder carcinogenesis in mice and rats but was ineffective in models of colon carcinogenesis.

N-Ethylretinamide inhibited carcinogen-induced neoplastic transformation at concentrations similar to those at which all-*trans*-retinoic acid had this effect. In the hamster trachea it was less potent than all-*trans*-retinoic acid in reversing squamous metaplasia; when tested in chick skin for an equivalent end-point, its activity was similar to that of all-*trans*-retinoic acid.

8.3.3   Mechanisms of cancer prevention

No relevant data were available to the Working Group.

8.4   Other beneficial effects

No data were available to the Working Group.

8.5   Carcinogenicity
8.5.1   Humans

No data were available to the Working Group.

8.5.2   Experimental models

N-Ethylretinamide was tested for carcinogenicity in one study in mice by oral administration. An increased incidence of benign and malignant liver tumours was observed. It also had tumour-enhancing effects at several sites in several species.

8.6   Other toxic effects
8.6.1   Humans

N-Ethylretinamide has been evaluated for toxic effects in human beings in only one study, which showed increased concentrations of serum lipids after oral administration. The toxic effects seen in preclinical studies include anaemia, osteopathy and liver abnormalities.

8.6.2 Experimental models

The spectrum of effects in short-term studies of the toxicity of *N*-ethylretinamide in animals is more limited than that of other synthetic retinamide analogues, such as 4-hydroxyphenylretinamide. In a long-term study in rats, *N*-ethylretinamide induced osteopathy and haematopoietic toxicity. Like other retinoids, *N*-ethylretinamide is toxic to the male reproductive tract after long-term exposure. Its teratological effects are mild and seen only at very high doses.

9. Recommendations for Research

9.1 General recommendations for *N*-ethyl-retinamide and other retinoids

See section 9 of the Handbook on all-*trans*-retinoic acid.

9.2 Recommendations specific to *N*-ethyl-retinamide

None.

10. Evaluation

10.1 Cancer-preventive activity
10.1.1 Humans

There is *inadequate evidence* that *N*-ethylretinamide has cancer-preventive activity in humans.

10.1.2 Experimental animals

There is *evidence suggesting lack of* cancer-preventive activity of *N*-ethylretinamide in experimental animals.

10.2 Overall evaluation

There are no data on the cancer-preventive activity of *N*-ethylretinamide in humans, but there is evidence that it enhances carcinogenicity in some experimental models.

N-Ethylretinamide has not been approved for human use and is no longer produced.

11. References

Acevedo, P. & Bertram, J.S. (1995) Liarozole potentiates the cancer chemopreventive activity of and the up-regulation of gap junctional communication and connexin43 expression by retinoic acid and beta-carotene in 10T1/2 cells. *Carcinogenesis*, **16**, 2215–2222

Bertram, J.S. (1980) Structure–activity relationships among various retinoids and their ability to inhibit neoplastic transformation and to increase cell adhesion in the C3H/10T1/2 CL8 cell line. *Cancer Res.*, **40**, 3141–3146

Birt, D.F., Sayed, S., Davies, M.H. & Pour, P. (1981) Sex differences in the effects of retinoids on carcinogenesis by N-nitrosobis(2-oxopropyl)amine in Syrian hamsters. *Cancer Lett.*, **14**, 13–21

Birt, D.F., Davies, M.H., Pour, P.M. & Salmasi, S. (1983) Lack of inhibition by retinoids of bis(2-oxopropyl)-nitrosamine-induced carcinogenesis in Syrian hamsters. *Carcinogenesis*, **4**, 1215–1220

Bollag, W., Ruegg, R. & Gottlieb, R. (1976) Vitamin A acid amides. Hoffmann–La Roche Inc., *United States Patent* 3 950 418

Croft, W.A., Croft, M.A., Paulus, K.P., Williams, J.H., Wang, C.Y. & Lower, G.M., Jr (1981) Synthetic retinamides: Effect on urinary bladder carcinogenesis by FANFT in Fischer rats. *Carcinogenesis*, **2**, 515–517

Kim, Y.W., Sharma, R.P. & Li, J.K. (1994) Characterization of heterologously expressed recombinant retinoic acid receptors with natural or synthetic retinoids. *J. Biochem. Toxicol.*, **9**, 225–234

Kistler, A. (1987) Limb bud cell cultures for estimating the teratogenic potential of compounds. Validation of the test system with retinoids. *Arch. Toxicol.*, **60**, 403–414

Kochhar, D.M., Shealy, Y.F., Penner, J.D. & Jiang, H. (1992) Retinamides: Hydrolytic conversion of retinoylglycine to retinoic acid in pregnant mice contributes to teratogenicity. *Teratology*, **45**, 175–185

McCormick, D.L., Hollister, J.L., Bagg, B.J. & Long, R.E. (1990) Enhancement of murine hepatocarcinogenesis by all-*trans*-retinoic acid and two synthetic retinamides. *Carcinogenesis*, **11**, 1605–1609

Moon, R.C., McCormick, D.L., Becci, P.J., Shealy, Y.F., Frickel, F., Paust, J. & Sporn, M.B. (1982) Influence of 15 retinoic acid amides on urinary bladder carcinogenesis in the mouse. *Carcinogenesis*, **3**, 1469–1472

Newton, D.L., Henderson, W.R. & Sporn, M.B. (1980) Structure–activity relationships of retinoids in hamster tracheal organ culture. *Cancer Res.*, **40**, 3413–3425

Runne, U., Orfanos, C.E. & Gartmann, H. (1973) Oral therapy of psoriasis using two vitamin A acid-derivatives. *Arch. Dermatol. Forsch.*, **247**, 171–180

Sani, B.P. & Meeks, R.G. (1983) Subacute toxicity of all-*trans*- and 13-*cis*-isomers of *N*-ethyl retinamide, *N*-2-hydroxyethyl retinamide, and *N*-4-hydroxyphenyl retinamide. *Toxicol. Appl. Pharmacol.*, **70**, 228–235

Shih, T.W., Shealy, Y.F. & Hill, D.L. (1988) Enzymatic hydrolysis of retinamides. *Drug Metab. Dispos.*, **16**, 337–340

Steele, C.E., Marlow, R., Turton, J. & Hicks, R.M. (1987) In-vitro teratogenicity of retinoids. *Br. J. Exp. Pathol.*, **68**, 215–223

Stinson, S.F., Reznik–Schüller, H., Reznik, G. & Donahoe, R. (1980) Atrophy induced in the tubules of the testes of Syrian hamsters by two retinoids. *Toxicology*, **17**, 343–353

Stinson, S.F., Reznik, G. & Donahoe, R. (1981) Effect of three retinoids on tracheal carcinogenesis with *N*-methyl-*N*-nitrosourea in hamsters. *J. Natl Cancer Inst.*, **66**, 947–951

Thompson, H.J., Becci, P.J., Grubbs, C.J., Shealy, Y.F., Stanek, E.J., Brown, C.C., Sporn, M.B. & Moon, R.C. (1981) Inhibition of urinary bladder cancer by *N*-(ethyl)-all-*trans*-retinamide and *N*-(2-hydroxyethyl)-all-*trans*-retinamide in rats and mice. *Cancer Res.*, **41**, 933–936

Turton, J.A., Hicks, R.M., Gwynne, J., Hunt, R. & Hawkey, C.M. (1985) Retinoid toxicity. *Ciba Found. Symp.*, **113**, 220–251

Turton, J.A., Willars, G.B., Haselden, J.N., Ward, S.J., Steele, C.E. & Hicks, R.M. (1992) Comparative teratogenicity of nine retinoids in the rat. *Int. J. Exp. Pathol.*, **73**, 551–563

Wenk, M.L., Ward, J.M., Reznik, G. & Dean, J. (1981) Effects of three retinoids on colon adenocarcinomas, sarcomas and hyperplastic polyps induced by intrarectal *N*-methyl-*N*-nitrosourea administration in male F344 rats. *Carcinogenesis*, **2**, 1161–1166

Wilkoff, L.J., Peckham, J.C., Dulmadge, E.A., Mowry, R.W. & Chopra, D.P. (1976) Evaluation of vitamin A analogs in modulating epithelial differentiation of 13-day chick embryo metatarsal skin explants. *Cancer Res.*, **36**, 964–972

Willhite, C.C. & Shealy, Y.F. (1984) Amelioration of embryotoxicity by structural modification of the terminal group of cancer chemopreventive retinoids. *J. Natl Cancer Inst.*, **72**, 689–695

Zanotti, G., Malpeli, G. & Berni, R. (1993) The interaction of *N*-ethyl retinamide with plasma retinol-binding protein (RBP) and the crystal structure of the retinoid-RBP complex at 1.9-Å resolution. *J. Biol. Chem.*, **268**, 24873–24879

Targretin

1. Chemical and Physical Characteristics

1.1 Nomenclature

See General Remarks, section 1.4,

1.2 Name

Chemical Abstracts Services Registry number
153559-49-0

IUPAC Systematic name
4-[1-(5,6,7,8-Tetrahydro-3,5,5,8,8-pentamethyl-2-naphthalenyl)ethenyl]benzoic acid

Synonyms
Bexarotene, LG1069, LGD1069, LGD1001069, SR11247

1.3 Structural formula

Composition: $C_{24}H_{28}O_2$
Relative molecular mass: 348.2

1.4 Physical and chemical properties

Description
Fine white crystals (ethyl acetate or hexane)

Melting-point
234 °C

Spectroscopy
UV spectrum: λ_{max} 264 nm (ε 16 400 in methane)

^{1}H-NMR spectrum (CDCl$_3$): δ 1.28 (s, 6H, CH$_3$), 1.31 (s, 6H, CH$_3$), 1.70 (s, 4H, CH$_2$), 1.95 (s, 3H, CH$_3$), 5.35 and 5.83 (s, 2H, C=CH$_2$), 7.08 (s, 1H, ArH), 7.13 (s, 1H, ArH), 7.28 (d, J = 8.1 Hz, 2H, ArH), 8.03 (d, J = 8.1 Hz, 2H, ArH)

High-resolution mass spectrum: (FAB-MS): (M + H) calculated for $C1_4H_{29}O_2$ 349.2168, found 349.2178

Infrared spectrum:
(KBr) 2959, 1677, 1278 cm^{-1}

Solubility
Soluble in organic solvents (see section 1.4 on all-*trans*-retinoic acid)

Stability
More stable than all-*trans*-retinoic acid

2. Occurrence, Production, Use, Human Exposure and Analysis

2.1 Occurrence

Human exposure to this synthetic retinoid is limited to patients receiving it as a drug. It does not occur in the diet.

2.2 Production

Targretin was prepared in four steps from toluene by the general route outlined in Figure 1 (Boehm *et al.*, 1994).

The procedure of Dawson *et al.* (1995) has only minor differences, including conversion of **2** to **3** with ClCH$_2$CH$_2$Cl as the solvent, addition at 0 °C, reaction at room temperature and conversion of **3** to **4** with KN(SiMe$_3$)$_2$ as the base and reaction at room temperature.

2.3 Use

Several clinical trials have been conducted to assess the efficacy of targretin in the treatment of cancers, including advanced breast cancer (capsules in a phase-II trial); cutaneous T-cell lymphoma (gel in a phase-I and capsules in a phase-II/III trial); advanced lung cancer (capsules in a phase-II/III trial); Kaposi sarcoma (capsules in a phase-II/III trial); prostate cancer (phase-II trial);

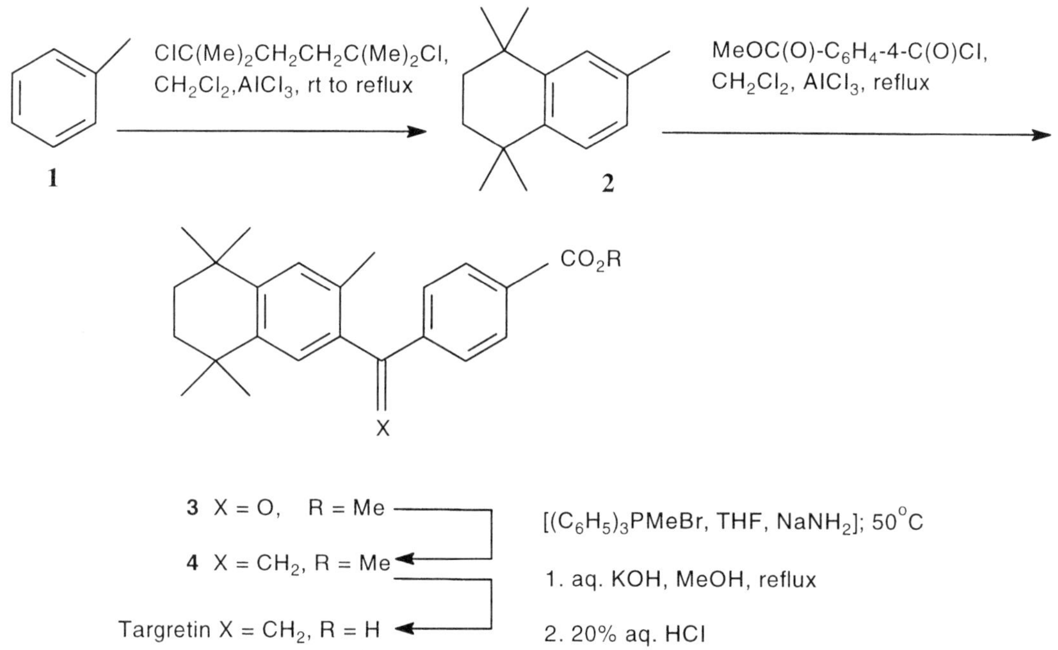

ClC(Me)$_2$CH$_2$CH$_2$C(Me)$_2$Cl,
CH$_2$Cl$_2$,AlCl$_3$, rt to reflux

1 ⟶ **2**

MeOC(O)-C$_6$H$_4$-4-C(O)Cl,
CH$_2$Cl$_2$, AlCl$_3$, reflux

CO$_2$R

X

3 X = O,   R = Me

4 X = CH$_2$, R = Me

Targretin X = CH$_2$, R = H

[(C$_6$H$_5$)$_3$PMeBr, THF, NaNH$_2$]; 50°C

1. aq. KOH, MeOH, reflux

2. 20% aq. HCl

Figure 1. Synthesis of Targretin

renal cancer (phase-II trial); ovarian cancer (phase-I trial) and head-and-neck cancer (phase-I trial) (Rizvi *et al.*, 1996; Rigas *et al.*, 1997). Patients with cutaneous T-cell lymphoma responded well, whereas patients with advanced cancers showed mild retinoid toxicity (Miller *et al.*, 1997).

2.4   Human exposure
The maximum tolerated dose was considered to be 300 mg/m² (Miller *et al.*, 1997).

2.5   Analysis
Targretin can be separated by thin-layer chromatography (10% methane and 90% chloroform; R$_f$ 0.5) (Boehm *et al.*, 1994). Gas chromatography–mass spectrometry has been used to determine targretin and its metabolites in studies of human pharmacokinetics (Miller *et al.*, 1997). High-performance liquid chromatography is also appropriate for the analysis of targretin (Howell *et al.*, 1998).

3.   Metabolism, Kinetics and Genetic Variation

3.1   Humans
Studies of pharmocokinetics provide no evidence of auto-induction of metabolism. At a dose of 400 mg/m², the concentration of targretin in blood was about 300 ng/ml. The elimination half-life was 1–2 h (Miller *et al.*, 1997).

3.2   Experimental models
Although targretin increases the activity of hepatic cytochrome P450 enzymes in rats, little is known about its metabolism. It is converted to the 6- or 7-monohydroxy and glucuronide derivatives by rat liver microsomes (Howell *et al.*, 1998).

4.   Cancer-preventive Effects

4.1   Humans
No data were available to the Working Group.

4.2 Experimental models

4.2.1 Cancer and preneoplastic lesions

Groups of 17–18 female rats, 50 days of age, received intravenous injections of N-methyl-N-nitrosourea (MNU) at a dose of 50 mg/kg bw, and, one week later, the vehicle or targretin was administered five times per week at a dose of 30 or 100 mg/kg bw by oral gavage. After 12 weeks, rats in the control group had a 100% incidence of mammary carcinomas and an average of three carcinomas per rat, whereas rats given the low and high doses of targretin had incidences of 22% and 12% and tumour multiplicities of 0.33 and 0.18, respectively (Table 1; $p < 0.001$, ANOVA) (Gottardis et al., 1996). [The Working Group noted the short duration of the experiment.]

4.2.2 Intermediate biomarkers

No data were available to the Working Group.

4.2.3 In-vitro models

4.2.3.1 Cellular studies

(a) Inhibition of cell proliferation

In HL-60 myelocytic leukaemia cells, targretin had low antiproliferative activity at doses between 10^{-8} and 10^{-6} mol/L. At the highest concentration tested, it reduced proliferation by about 20%, an effect that requires only about 10^{-9} mol/L of all-$trans$-retinoic acid (Kizaki et al., 1996).

(b) Inhibition of cell differentiation

Targretin has been evaluated in two human myelocytic leukaemia cell lines used as models of differentiation: the HL-60 and the U937 lines. It was active at high concentrations in both. In HL-60 cells, expression of a differentiation marker CD11b was increased after six days of culture. Activity was seen at doses between 10^{-9} and 10^{-7} mol/L, the highest concentration tested. Simultaneous treatment with all-$trans$-retinoic acid caused marked synergy of response (Kizaki et al., 1996). When targretin was tested in U937 cells, it was marginally active, inducing differentiation (measured as an oxidative burst) at concentrations of 10^{-8} to 10^{-6} mol/L. This action was strongly enhanced by the retinoic acid receptor (RAR)-specific retinoid Ro 13-7410 at 10^{-7} mol/L (Defacque et al., 1997).

4.2.3.2 Antimutagenicity in short-term tests

No data were available to the Working Group.

4.3 Mechanisms of cancer prevention

4.3.1 Receptor selectivity

Targretin was initially reported to bind selectively to retinoid X receptors (RXRs). It was most active in the presence of RXRs α, β and γ and was inactive in the presence of the RARs α, β and γ (Boehm et al., 1994, 1995). Targretin was subsequently reported to show RAR cross-reactivity (Dawson et al., 1995; Umemiya et al., 1997). Targretin has a 12–100 times higher relative binding affinity for RXRs than for RARs ($K_d = 16$–31 nmol/L) (Table 2). Table 2 also shows the results of co-transfection assays, which measure the capacity of compounds to activate gene expression through each of the six known retinoid receptors. In these assays, targretin (median effective concentration, 20–28 nmol/L) was > 600 times more active with RXRs than with RARs (Gottardis et al., 1996; Umemiya et al., 1997).

4.3.2 Studies in animals

The study of MNU-induced breast carcinogenesis in rats (see section 4.2.1) provides some information about the mechanism whereby targretin can reduce tumour incidence. Since treatment began after administration of the carcinogen, effects on initiation can be excluded. Although the plasma concentrations of oestradiol, progesterone and prolactin were unchanged, targretin reduced the uterine weight and partially inhibited the increases in uterine weight resulting from treatment with oestrogen or tamoxifen (Gottardis et al., 1996). [The Working Group noted that targretin appears to have anti-oestrogenic activity in the uterus and may have similar effects in the breast.]

4.3.3 Cell cultures

Targretin was only moderately active in cell culture models of differentiation, but its activity was greatly increased by addition of RAR or vitamin D receptor agonists (Kizaki et al., 1996; Defacque et al., 1997), which suggests that differentiation in these cells is driven by RAR–RXR or vitamin D receptor–RXR heterodimers.

5. Other Beneficial Effects

No data were available to the Working Group.

Table 1. Effects of targretin on mammary gland carcinogenesis in animals

Species sex, age at carcinogen treatment	No. of animals per group	Carcinogen dose/route	Targretin dose and route	Duration in relation to carcinogen	Incidence		Multiplicity		Efficacy	Reference
					Control	Treated	Control	Treated		
Female Sprague-Dawley rat	18	MNU (50 mg/kg bw, i.v.)	30 mg/kg b.w. (5 per wk p.o. for 12 wks)	– 1 wk – 12 wks	100	22*	3.0	0.33*	Effective	Gottardis *et al.* (1996)
			100 mg/kg bw (5 per wk p.o. for 12 wks)	– 1 wk – 12 wks		12*		0.18*	Effective	

MNU, *N*-methyl-*N*-nitrosourea; i.v., intravenous; p.o., oral
* Significantly different from controls (see text)

Receptor	Relative binding activity (nmol/L)		Median effective concentration (nmol/L)[a]
	Gottardis *et al.* (1996)	Umemiya *et al.* (1997)	Gottardis *et al.* (1996)
RARα	5950	180	> 10 000
RARβ	7624	50	> 10 000
RARγ	4221	130	> 10 000
RXRα	31	16	30–46
RXRβ	16	6	30–46
RXRγ	20	8	30–46

Table 2. Relative binding affinity of targretin to retinoic acid receptors (RARs) and retinoid X receptors (RXRs)

[a]At 10 µmol/L in transient transfections, targretin gives a response equal to 20% of the maximal response to all-*trans*-retinoic acid.

6. Carcinogenicity

No data were available to the Working Group.

7. Other Toxic Effects

7.1 Adverse effects
7.1.1 Humans

A study was performed in 52 patients with advanced cancer to determine the safety, clinical tolerance and pharmacokinetics of targretin at doses of 5–500 mg/m² for 1–41 weeks. Reversible, asymptomatic increases in the activity of liver enzymes were the most common dose-limiting adverse effect. The cumulative incidence of increased alkaline phosphatase activity and hypercalcaemia also increased with dose. Overall, 17% of the study group was so affected. Dry mucous membranes and dry skin occurred in 41% of the patients, and two developed a diffuse maculopapular skin rash. Other reactions included leukopenia and hyperlipidaemia. Reduction of the dose by 25–50% resolved the more severe neutropenia and the increases in aspartate aminotransferase activity. Toxic effects characteristic of the retinoids, such as cheilitis, headache, myalgia and arthralgia were mild or absent. Most of the headaches required no or occasional analgesia. The maximum tolerated dose was considered to be 300 mg/m² on the basis of the haematological and hepatic biochemical abnormalities at higher doses. The mucocutaneous toxicity of targretin was less frequent and milder than that seen in most patients treated with all-*trans*- or 13-*cis*-retinoic acid (Miller *et al.*, 1997).

In a preliminary report of a phase-I/II study of targretin in 26 patients with recurrent squamous-cell carcinoma of the head and neck, the dose was escalated from 10 mg/m² to 300 mg/m² twice daily. Two cases of pancreatitis were seen at the highest dose, including one episode of fatal haemorrhagic pancreatitis in a patient who continued to drink alcohol during the study. Hypertriglyceridaemia of grade 2 or higher was also seen in six patients (Papadimitrakopoulou *et al.*, 1998).

As reported in an abstract, treatment with targretin produced alterations primarily in cholesterol metabolism, with effects on plasma cholesterol and low-density lipoprotein cholesterol (Nervi *et al.*, 1997).

7.1.2 Experimental models

In a model of mammary carcinoma in which Sprague-Dawley rats received targretin at 30 or 100 mg/kg bw per day on five days per week for 13 weeks, one week after a single dose of MNU, none of the classical signs of retinoid-associated toxicity was seen, except for mild alopecia. In particular, targretin did not induce osteopathy at doses similar to those of all-*trans*-retinoic acid needed to achieve the same degree of chemoprevention in this model within the same time (Gottardis *et al.*, 1996).

7.2 Reproductive and developmental effects
7.2.1 Humans
No data were available to the Working.

7.2.2 Experimental models
Targretin was not teratogenic in mice given single doses of 5–20 mg/kg bw on day 8 or 11 of gestation. When it was administered with a below-threshold dose of Am580, a ligand with relative selectivity for the RARα, or CD437, with relative selectivity for the RARγ, synergistic effects on a number of structural defects were observed. Spina bifida and ear and mandible defects, but not exencephaly, were induced when this regimen was given on day 8 and cleft palate and limb defects when it was given on day 11 of gestation. The synergistic response increased with increasing doses of targretin (Elmazar *et al.*, 1996). [The Working Group noted that these results were confirmed with additional RXR ligands and indicate that RXR ligands of low teratogenic potency can induce a strong teratogenic response when combined with low doses of RAR ligands which do not induce structural defects.]

7.3 Genetic and related effects
No data were available to the Working Group.

8. Summary of Data

8.1 Chemistry, occurrence and human exposure
Targretin {4-[1-(5,6,7,8-tetrahydro-3,5,5,8,8-penta-methyl-2-naphthalenyl)ethenyl]benzoic acid} is a synthetic aromatic retinoid. It is a lipophilic molecule that is more stable than all-*trans*-retinoic acid. Human exposure to targretin is limited to patients participating in clinical trials.

8.2 Metabolism and kinetics
Few data are available. Certain metabolites have been implicated *in vitro*.

8.3 Cancer-preventive effects
8.3.1 Humans
No data were available to the Working Group.

8.3.2 Experimental models
In a single study of three months' duration, targretin was effective in preventing mammary cancer induced by N-methyl-N-nitrosourea in rats.

In two models of differentiation in human cells *in vitro*, targretin was less active than retinoic acid receptor-selective agonists; however, in both models supra-additive activity was seen when the cells were treated simultaneously with targretin and the retinoic acid receptor-selective agonists.

8.3.3 Mechanisms of cancer prevention
There are insufficient data to establish the mechanism of action of targretin.

8.4 Other beneficial effects
No data were available to the Working Group.

8.5 Carcinogenicity
No data were available to the Working Group.

8.6 Other toxic effects
8.6.1 Humans
Reversible, asymptomatic increases in the activity of hepatic enzymes were the dose-limiting adverse side-effects observed most commonly in phase I studies of targretin. Other reactions included leukopenia, hyperlipidaemia and hypercalcaemia. Mild mucocutaneous lesions and headache were seen infrequently after exposure to targretin.

8.6.2 Experimental models
In one short-term study in rats, targretin caused mild alopecia. In a single study, it was not teratogenic in mice when administered alone, but synergistic effects were seen when it was given in conjunction with agonists of retinoic acid receptors.

9. Recommendations for Research

9.1 General recommendations for targretin and other retinoids
See section 9 of the Handbook on all-*trans*-retinoic acid.

9.2 Recommendations specific to targretin

1. Evaluate the role of retinoid X receptors in the inhibition of experimental carcinogens using targretin (and other synthetic ligands) selective for retinoid X receptors.
2. Elucidate the mechanisms by which retinoic acid receptors and selective agonists enhance the effect of targretin.

10. Evaluation

10.1 Cancer-preventive activity
10.1.1 Humans
There is *inadequate evidence* that targretin has cancer-preventive activity in humans.

10.1.2 Experimental animals
There is *inadequate evidence* that targretin has cancer-preventive activity in experimental animals.

10.2 Overall evaluation
There are no data on the cancer-preventive activity of targretin in humans.

11. References

Boehm, M.F., Zhang, L., Badea, B.A., White, S.K., Mais, D.E., Berger, E., Suto, C.M., Goldman, M.E. & Heyman, R.A. (1994) Synthesis and structure–activity relationships of novel retinoid X receptor-selective retinoids. *J. Med. Chem., 37,* 2930–2941

Boehm, M.F., Zhang, L., Zhi, L., McClurg, M.R., Berger, E., Wagoner, M., Mais, D.E., Suto, C.M., Davies, J.A., Heyman, R.A. & Nadzan, A.M. (1995) Design and synthesis of potent retinoid X receptor selective ligands that induce apoptosis in leukemia cells. *J. Med. Chem., 38,* 3146–3155

Dawson, M.I., Jong, L., Hobbs, P.D., Cameron, J.F., Chao, W.R., Pfahl, M., Lee, M.O. & Shroot, B. (1995) Conformational effects on retinoid receptor selectivity. 2. Effects of retinoid bridging group on retinoid X receptor activity and selectivity. *J. Med. Chem., 38,* 3368–3383

Defacque, H., Sévilla, C., Piquemal, D., Rochette–Egly, C., Marti, J. & Commes, T. (1997) Potentiation of VD-induced monocytic leukemia cell differentiation by retinoids involves both RAR and RXR signaling pathways. *Leukemia, 11,* 221–227

Elmazar, M.M., Reichert, U., Shroot, B. & Nau, H. (1996) Pattern of retinoid-induced teratogenic effects: Possible relationship with relative selectivity for nuclear retinoid receptors RARα, RAR β, and RARγ. *Teratology, 53,* 158–167

Gottardis, M.M., Bischoff, E.D., Shirley, M.A., Wagoner, M.A., Lamph, W.W. & Heyman, R.A. (1996) Chemoprevention of mammary carcinoma by LGD1069 (targretin): An RXR-selective ligand. *Cancer Res., 56,* 5566–5570

Howell, S.R., Shirley, M.A. & Ulm, E.H. (1998) Effects of retinoid treatment of rats on hepatic microsomal metabolism and cytochromes P450. Correlation between retinoic acid receptor/retinoid X receptor selectivity and effects on metabolic enzymes. *Drug Metab. Dispos., 26,* 234–239

Kizaki, M., Dawson, M.I., Heyman, R., Elster, E., Morosetti, R., Pakkala, S., Chen, D.L., Ueno, H., Chao, W., Morikawa, M., Ikeda, Y., Heber, D., Pfahl, M. & Koeffler, H.P. (1996) Effects of novel retinoid X receptor-selective ligands on myeloid leukemia differentiation and proliferation in vitro. *Blood, 87,* 1977–1984

Miller, V.A., Benedetti, F.M., Rigas, J.R., Verret, A.L., Pfister, D.G., Straus, D., Kris, M.G., Crisp, M., Heyman, R., Loewen, G.R., Truglia, J.A. & Warrell, R.P.J. (1997) Initial clinical trial of a selective retinoid X receptor ligand, LGD1069. *J. Clin. Oncol., 15,* 790–795

Nervi, A.M., Rigas, J.R., Miller, V.A., Levine, D.M., Dain, B.J. & Warrell, R.P.J. (1997) Plasma lipoproteins associated with three novel retinoids: all-*trans* Retinoic acid, 9-*cis* retinoic acid, and oral targretin™. *J. Invest. Med., 45,* 260A–260A

Papadimitrakopoulou, V., Khuri, F.R., Lippman, S.M., Shin, D.M., Ginsberg, L., Glisson, B.S., Martinez, L., Loewen, G., Truglia, J. & Hong, W.K. (1998) Phase I/II evaluation of targretin (LGD1069), a novel, RXR-specific retinoid, in patients with recurrent squamous cell carcinoma of the head and neck. *Proc. Am. Soc. Clin. Oncol., 17,* 1512–1512

Rigas, J.R., Maurer, L.H., Meyer, L.P., Hammond, S.M., Crisp, M.R., Parker, B.A. & Truglia, J.A. (1997) Targretin, a selective retinoid X receptor ligand (LGD1069), vinorelbine and cisplatin for the treatment of non-small cell lung cancer (NSCLC): A phase I/II trial. *Proc. Am. Soc. Clin. Oncol., 16,* A1724–A1724

Rizvi, N.A., Marshall, J.L., Loewen, G.R., Ulm, E.H., Gill, G.M., Truglia, J.A., Ness, E., Clarke, R. & Hawkins, M.J. (1996) A phase I study of targretin™, an RXR-selective retinoid agonist. *Proc. Am. Assoc. Cancer Res.*, **37**, 165–165

Umemiya, H., Kagechika, H., Fukasawa, H., Kawachi, E., Ebisawa, M., Hashimoto, Y., Eisenmann, G., Erb, C., Pornon, A., Chambon, P., Gronemeyer, H. & Shudo, K. (1997) Action mechanism of retinoid-synergistic dibenzodiazepines. *Biochem. Biophys. Res. Commun.*, **233**, 121–125

Handbook 9

LGD 1550

1. Chemical and Physical Characteristics

1.1 Nomenclature
See note on nomenclature of retinoids in the General Remarks, section 1.4.

1.2 Name
Chemical Abstracts Services Registry Number 178600-20-9

IUPAC systematic name
(all-*E*)-7-[3,5-Bis(1,1-dimethylethyl)phenyl]-3-methyl-2,4,6-octatrienoic acid

Synonyms
AGN 193101; ALRT 1550; ALRT1550; all-*trans*-7-[3,5-bis-1,1-dimethylethyl)phenyl]-3-methyl-2,4,6-octatrienoic acid; (2*E*,4*E*,6*E*)-7-(3,5-di-*tert*-butylphenyl)-3-methyl-2,4,6-octatrienoic acid; (2*E*,4*E*,6*E*)-7-(3,5-di-*tert*-butylphenyl)-3-methylocta-2,4,6-trienoic acid, (*E*)-7-(3,5-di-*tert*-butylphenyl)-3-methyl-2,4,6-octatrienoic acid; LG1550; LGD100550

1.3 Structural formula

Composition: $C_{23}H_{32}O_2$
Relative molecular mass: 340.24

1.4 Physical and chemical properties
Appearance
Pale-yellow needles

Melting point
196–198 °C

Spectroscopy
^{1}H-NMR (CDCl$_3$): δ 1.35 (s, 18H, 6 CH$_3$), 222.29 (s, 3H, CH$_3$), 2.41 (s, 3H, CH$_3$), 5.84 (s, 1H, C=CH), 6.41 (d, *J* = 15 Hz, 1H, C=CH), 6.54 (d, *J* = 11 Hz, 1H, C=CHO, 7.08 (m, 1H, C=CH), 7.32 (d, *J* = 1 Hz, 2H, ArH), 7.39 (t, *J* = 1 Hz, 1H, ArH)

High-resolution mass spectrum
Calculated for $C_{23}H_{32}O_2$, 340.2402, found 340.2394 (see Zhang *et al.*, 1996)

Solubility
Soluble in organic solvents (see all-*trans*-Retinoic acid, section 1.4)

Stability
Unstable to light, oxygen and heat (see all-*trans*-Retinoic acid, section 1.4)

2. Occurrence, Production, Use, Human Exposure and Analysis

2.1 Occurrence
LGD 1550 is a synthetic drug, and human exposure is limited to patients receiving it.

2.2 Production
LGD 1550 was prepared in five steps from 3,5-di-*tert*-benzoic acid, as shown in Figure 1 (Zhang *et al.*, 1996).

2.3 Use
Phase-I/II trials of the use of LGD 1550 in combination with cisplatin and radiation for head-and-neck cancer, in combination with chemotherapy for ovarian cancer and in combination with interferon for advanced cervical cancer are under way.

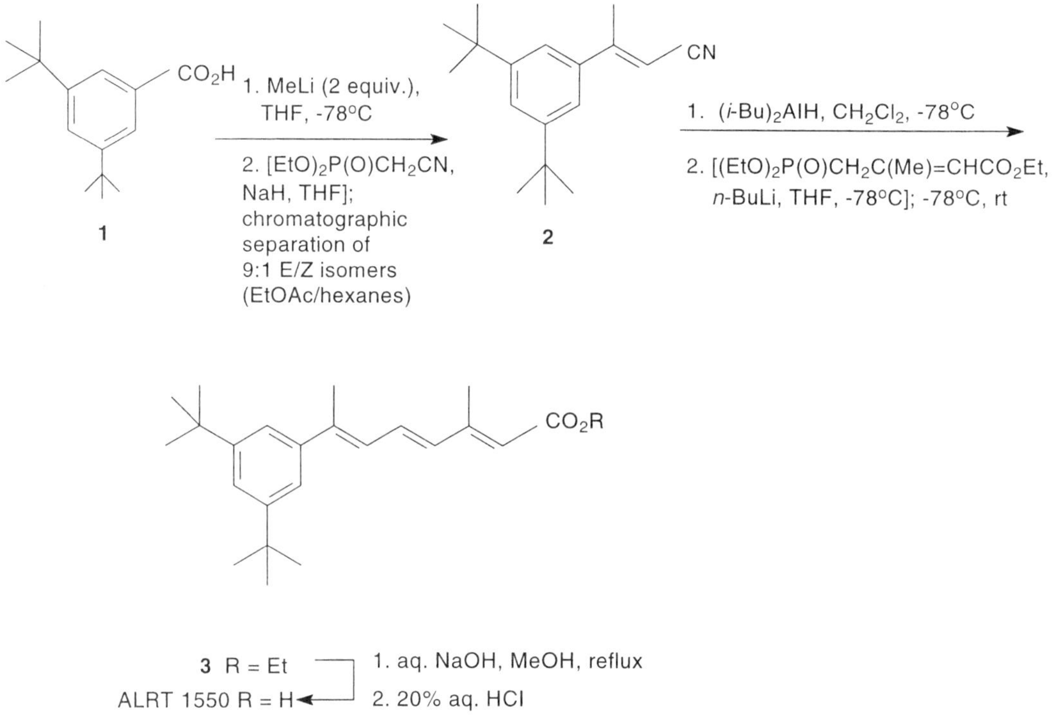

Figure 1. Synthesis of LGD 1550

2.4   Human exposure

LGD 1550 is being tested in phase-I/II trials for cancer therapy.

2.5   Analysis

LGD 1550 can be separated by thin-layer chromatography (10% methanol and 90% chloroform): R_f 0.6 (Zhang *et al.*, 1996). High-performance liquid chromatography has also been used for analysis of this retinoid (Howell *et al.*, 1998).

3.   Metabolism, Kinetics and Genetic Variation

3.1   Humans

A phase-I/II study indicated a plasma half-life for LGD 1550 of 5 h. The concentrations in plasma were similar on days 1, 15 and 29, as determined from the integrated areas under the curves of con-

centration–time, indicating that the clearance of LGD 1550 is not self-induced (Soignet *et al.*, 1998).

3.2   Experimental models

The metabolites of LGD 1550 formed by rat liver microsomes, although not identified, are presumed to be mono-hydroxylated or acyl-glucuronidated structures (Howell *et al.*, 1998).

4.   Cancer-preventive Effects

4.1   Humans

No data were available to the Working Group.

4.2   Experimental models
4.2.1   *Cancer and preneoplastic lesions*

No data were available to the Working Group.

4.2.2   *Intermediate biomarkers*

No data were available to the Working Group.

4.2.3 In-vitro models

4.2.3.1 Cellular studies

These studies are summarized in Table 1.

LGD 1550 dissolved in 10% dimethylsulfoxide and 90% ethanol was studied for antiproliferative activity by addition for four days to a culture of the human cervical carcinoma cell line ME180. Incorporation of radioactive thymidine was then measured over a concentration of $10^{-12}–10^{-6}$ mol/L. LGD 1550 was active, with a median inhibitory concentration of 1 nmol/L, whereas all-*trans*-retinoic acid was active under the same assay conditions only at 300 nmol/L. The activity of LGD 1550 correlated with its increased ability to activate retinoic acid receptors (Zhang *et al.*, 1996).

LGD 1550 potently inhibited proliferation of human breast cancer cell lines, irrespective of their oestrogen-receptor status. The activity correlated with expression of RARα. In responsive cells such as T-47 D, SK-BR-3 and HS 578T, LGD 1550 was sig-nificantly more active than 9-*cis*-retinoic acid, LGD 1550 having a median effective concentration of 1–4 nmol/L (Fitzgerald *et al.*, 1997).

In a study reported only in an abstract, the antiproliferative effect of LGD 1550 was examined in UMCSS-22B cells from a human head-and-neck carcinoma. The median inhibitory concentration with continuous exposure was stated to be 0.22 nmol/L [method for determining proliferation not stated]. LGD 1550 acted synergistically with interferon and cisplatin in this assay (Shalinsky *et al.*, 1996).

4.2.3.2 Antimutagenicity in short-term tests

No data were available to the Working Group.

4.3 Mechanisms of cancer prevention

Some of the biological effects of LGD 1550 may be mediated by its selective binding to retinoic acid receptors (RARs). Table 2 shows the relative binding affinity of LGD 1550 to the RARs and retinoid X

Table 1. Antiproliferative activity of LGD 1550

End-point	Assay	Result	Potency (IC_{50}; nmol/L)	Comments	Reference
Proliferation (^{3}H-thymidine incorporation)	ME180 cervical carcinoma cells	Active	1	300 times more potent than all-*trans*-retinoic acid	Zhang *et al.* (1996)
Proliferation	Head-and-neck squamous carcinoma cells	Active	0.22	370 times more potent than 9-*cis*-retinoic acid Potentiates activity of interferon	Shalinsky *et al.* (1996)

IC_{50}, concentration that inhibits proliferation by 50%

Table 2. Relative binding affinity of LGD 1550 to retinoic acid receptors (RARs) and retinoid X receptors (RXRs)

Receptor	Relative binding affinity	EC_{50} (nmol/L)
RARα	1.1	4.0
RARβ	0.7	2.2
RARγ	1.9	0.3
RXRα	224	> 1000
RXRβ	560	> 1000
RXRγ	320	> 1000

From Shalinsky *et al.* (1996) and Zhang *et al.* (1996). EC_{50}, median effective concentration. The results are an average of four or five experiments with triplicate determinations.

receptors (RXRs). LGD 1550 binds to the RARs 100–800 times more potently than to RXRs (Zhang *et al.*, 1996; Shalinsky *et al.*, 1997). Table 2 also shows the results of co-transfection assays (Shalinsky *et al.*, 1997), which measure the capacity of compounds to activate gene expression through each of the six known retinoid receptors. LGD 1550, with a median effective concentration of 0.3–4 nmol/L, was > 250 times more active with the RARs than with the RXRs. In both the binding and the co-transfection assays, LGD 1550 was > 10 times more potent than all-*trans*-retinoic acid.

5. Other Beneficial Effects

No data were available to the Working Group.

6. Carcinogenicity

No data were available to the Working Group.

7. Other Toxic Effects

7.1 Adverse effects
7.1.1 Humans
No data were available to the Working Group.

7.1.2 Experimental models
Athymic nude mice, six to seven weeks of age, received LGD 1550 in sesame oil by oral intubation at daily doses of 0, 3, 10, 30, 50 or 100 µg/kg bw, five days per week for up to eight weeks. The compound was well tolerated at doses up to 10 µg/kg bw per day, but there was a dose-dependent reduction in body-weight gain with increasing dose. Mice at 100 µg/kg bw per day lost about 25% of their body weight and were killed on day 11. Mild, moderate and severe mucocutaneous irritation occurred at 30, 50 and 75 µg/kg bw per day, respectively. The maximum tolerated oral dose was 50 µg/kg bw per day (Shalinsky *et al* 1997).

7.2 Reproductive and developmental effects
No data were available to the Working Group.

7.3 Genetic and related effects
No data were available to the Working Group.

8. Summary of Data

8.1 Chemistry, occurrence and human exposure
LGD 1550 (all-*trans*-7-[3,5-bis(1,1-dimethylethyl)-phenyl]-3-methyl-2,4,6-octatrienoic acid) is a synthetic aromatic retinoid that is structurally related to all-*trans*-retinoic acid. Because of its conjugated triene structure, LGD 1550 has a characteristic absorption in the ultraviolet and visible spectrum and can readily photoisomerize in solution to multiple geometric isomers. Human exposure is limited to patients undergoing clinical trials.

8.2 Metabolism and kinetics
Few data are available.

8.3 Cancer-preventive effects
8.3.1 Humans
No data were available to the Working Group.

8.3.2 Experimental models
No data were available to the Working Group. LGD 1550 inhibited proliferation of human breast cancer cells that express retinoic acid receptor-α, but not in cells that did not express this receptor.

8.3.3 Mechanisms of cancer prevention
There were insufficient data to determine the mechanism of action of LGD 1550.

8.4 Other beneficial effects
No data were available to the Working Group.

8.5 Carcinogenicity
No data were available to the Working Group.

8.6 Other toxic effects
8.6.1 Humans
No data were available to the Working Group.

8.6.2 Experimental models
In one study, short-term administration of LGD 1550 to athymic nude mice induced mucocutaneous irritation. No data were available on the reproductive or developmental effects of LGD 1550 in experimental animals, or on its genetic effects in short-term assays.

9.   Recommendations for research

9.1   General recommendations for LGD 1550 and other retinoids

See section 9 of the Handbook on all-*trans*-retinoic acid.

9.2   Recommendations specific to LGD 1550
None.

10.   Evaluation

10.1   Cancer-preventive activity
10.1.1   Humans
There is *inadequate evidence* that LGD 1550 has cancer-preventive activity in humans.

10.1.2   Experimental animals
There is *inadequate evidence* that LGD 1550 has cancer-preventive activity in experimental animals.

10.2   Overall evaluation
There are no data on the cancer-preventive activity of LGD 1550 in humans.

11.   References

Fitzgerald, P., Teng, M., Chandraratna, R.A., Heyman, R.A. & Allegretto, E.A. (1997) Retinoic acid receptor α expression correlates with retinoid-induced growth inhibition of human breast cancer cells regardless of estrogen receptor status. *Cancer Res.*, **57**, 2642–2650

Howell, S.R., Shirley, M.A. & Ulm, E.H. (1998) Effects of retinoid treatment of rats on hepatic microsomal metabolism and cytochromes P450. Correlation between retinoic acid receptor/retinoid X receptor selectivity and effects on metabolic enzymes. *Drug Metab. Dispos.*, **26**, 234–239

Shalinsky, D.R., Sheeter, L.M., Bischoff, E.D., Boehm, M., Nadzan, A.M. & Heyman, R.A. (1996) ALRT1550, a potent RAR-selective retinoid, synergistically inhibits growth of UMSCC-22B cells in combination with interferon-α2β or cisplatin *in vitro*. *Proc. Am. Assoc. Cancer Res.*, **37**, 293–293

Shalinsky, D.R., Bischoff, E.D., Lamph, W.W., Zhang, L., Boehm, M.F., Davies, P.J., Nadzan, A.M. & Heyman, R.A. (1997) A novel retinoic acid receptor-selective retinoid, ALRT1550, has potent antitumor activity against human oral squamous carcinoma xenografts in nude mice. *Cancer Res.*, **57**, 162–168

Soignet, S.L., Miller, V.A., Chen, Y.W., Parker, B.A., Amyotte, S.A., Cato, A., Matsumoto, R.M. & Warrell, R.P.J. (1998) Phase 1–2 study of a retinoic acid receptor-selective high-affinity ligand (LGD1550). *Proc. Am. Soc. Clin. Oncol.*, **17**, 826–826

Zhang, L., Nadzan, A.M., Heyman, R.A., Love, D.L., Mais, D.E., Croston, G., Lamph, W.W. & Boehm, M.F. (1996) Discovery of novel retinoic acid receptor agonists having potent antiproliferative activity in cervical cancer cells. *J. Med. Chem.*, **39**, 2659–2663

CORRIGENDUM

Volume 2. Carotenoids

Would the reader please note the following corrigendum:

Page 41, 4th line of the left-hand column should read μmol/L in both places.

Achevé d'imprimer sur rotative
par l'Imprimerie Darantiere à Dijon-Quetigny
en décembre 1999

Dépôt légal : décembre 1999
N° d'impression : 99-1379

Imprimé en France